To Tony Putra —

a great Physician

With Best wishes

John Hill

THE
ESOPHAGUS
MEDICAL & SURGICAL MANAGEMENT

Lucius Hill, M.D., F.A.C.S.

Clinical Professor of Surgery,
University of Washington,
Surgeon, Virginia Mason and Swedish Medical Center,
Seattle, Washington

Richard Kozarek, M.D.

Section of Therapeutic Endoscopy, The Mason Clinic,
Associate Clinical Professor, University of Washington,
Seattle, Washington

Richard McCallum, M.D.

Head, Division of Gastroenterology,
University of Virginia School of Medicine,
Charlottesville, Virginia

C. Dale Mercer, M.D., F.R.C.S.(C)

Assistant Professor of Surgery, Queen's University,
Director of Surgical Esophageal Research,
Queen's University, Kingston, Ontario

1988
W. B. SAUNDERS COMPANY
Harcourt Brace Jovanovich, Inc.
Philadelphia □ London □ Toronto □ Montreal □ Sydney □ Tokyo

W. B. SAUNDERS COMPANY
Harcourt Brace Jovanovich, Inc.

The Curtis Center
Independence Square West
Philadelphia, PA 19106

Library of Congress Cataloging-in-Publication Data

The Esophagus.

1. Esophagus—Diseases—Treatment. 2. Esophagus—
Surgery. I. Hill, Lucius D. [DNLM: 1. Esophageal
Diseases. 2. Esophagus. WI 250 E793]
RC815.7.E77 1988   616.3′2   87-16642
ISBN 0-7216-2348-4

Editor: Lisa McAllister
Designer: Karen O'Keefe
Production Manager: Bill Preston
Manuscript Editor: Lee Walters
Illustration Coordinator: Peg Shaw
Indexer: Helene Taylor
Cover illustration rendered by Jo Ann Clifford.

The Esophagus: Medical and Surgical Management   ISBN   0-7216-2348-4

Last digit is the print number: 9   8   7   6   5   4   3   2   1

Contributors

Italo Braghetto, M.D. ■ Assistant Professor of Surgery, Faculty of Medicine, University of Chile, Santiago, Chile; Assistant Professor of Surgery, Department of Surgery, Hospital J.J. Aguirre, University of Chile, Santiago ■ *Highly Selective Vagotomy, Posterior Gastropexy, and Calibration of the Cardia for Reflux Esophagitis*

Lyman A. Brewer III, M.D., Ph.D., Sc.D. (Hon.) ■ Distinguished Professor of Surgery, Loma Linda School of Medicine, Loma Linda, California; Honorary Clinical Professor of Surgery, University of California, Irvine, California; Emeritus Clinical Professor of Surgery, University of Southern California, Los Angeles, California; Distinguished Physician, Pettis Memorial Veterans Administration Hospital, Loma Linda, California; Senior Attending Surgeon, Los Angeles County/University of Southern California Hospital, Los Angeles, California; Affiliate Surgeon, Hospital of the Good Samaritan, Los Angeles, California ■ *Historical Notes on Surgery of the Esophagus*

Donald O. Castell, M.D. ■ Professor of Medicine, Chief, Gastroenterology Section, Bowman Gray School of Medicine, Winston-Salem, North Carolina; Chief of Gastroenterology, North Carolina Baptist Hospital, Winston-Salem, North Carolina ■ *Physiology*

Dennis L. Christie ■ Chief of Pediatric Gastroenterology, Virginia Mason and Children's Medical Center, Seattle, Washington ■ *Gastroesophageal Reflux in the Pediatric Patient*

C. Cordiano, M.D. ■ Professor of Emergency Surgery and Chief of Postgraduate School of Emergency Surgery, University of Verona, Italy; Chief, III Divisione Clinicizzata Di Chirurgia Generale, Centro Ospedaliero Di Borgo, Trento-Verona, Italy ■ *The "Nill" Procedure*

Attila Csendes, M.D. ■ Professor of Surgery, Faculty of Medicine, University of Chile, Santiago, Chile; Professor of Surgery, Department of Surgery, Hospital J.J. Aguirre, University of Chile, Santiago, Chile ■ *Highly Selective Vagotomy, Posterior Gastropexy, and Calibration of the Cardia for Reflux Esophagitis*

Howard C. Filston, M.D. ■ Professor of Pediatric Surgery and Pediatrics, Duke University Medical School, Durham, North Carolina; Chief, Pediatric Surgery, Duke Hospital, Durham, North Carolina ■ *Surgical Aspects of Congenital Anomalies of the Esophagus*

Martin D. Gelfand, M.D. ■ Clinical Associate Professor of Medicine, University of Washington, Seattle, Washington; Head, Section of Gastroenterology, Virginia Mason Medical Center, Seattle, Washington ■ *Motility Disorders*

Rodger C. Haggitt, M.D. ■ Professor of Pathology and Adjunct Professor of Medicine, University of Washington, Seattle, Washington; Director, Hospital Pathology, University Hospital, Seattle, Washington ■ *Barrett's Esophagus and Esophageal Adenocarcinoma*

Lucius D. Hill, M.D. ■ Clinical Professor of Surgery, University of Washington, Seattle, Washington; Surgeon, Swedish and Virginia Mason Medical Center, Seattle, Washington ■ *Anatomy of the Esophagus; Surgery for Hiatal Hernia and Esophagitis; Nissen Fundoplication; Surgery for Peptic Esophageal Stricture; Paraesophageal Hernia; Failed Antireflux Procedures; Surgery for Motility Disorders of the Esophagus; Rings, Webs, and Diverticula; Perforation, Rupture, and Injury of the Esophagus; Benign Tumors and Cysts of the Esophagus*

Riivo Ilves, B.A.Sc., M.A.Sc., M.D., F.R.C.S.(C), F.A.C.S. ■ Lecturer, Department of Surgery, University of Toronto, Toronto, Ontario; Thoracic Surgeon, St. Joseph's Health Centre, Northwestern General Hospital, Toronto, Ontario ■ *Carcinoma of the Esophagus*

G. Inaspettato, M.D. ■ Professor of Surgical Endoscopy, University of Verona, Verona, Italy; Assistant Professor of Surgery, IIIa Divisione Clinicizzata Di Chirurgia Generale, Centro Ospedaliero Di Borgo, Trento-Verona, Italy ■ *The "Nill" Procedure*

Richard A. Kozarek, M.D. ▪ Associate Clinical Professor of Medicine, University of Washington, Seattle, Washington; Section of Therapeutic Endoscopy, Virginia Mason Medical Center, Seattle, Washington ▪ *Esophageal Endoscopy, Dilation, and Intraesophageal Prosthetic Devices; Caustic and Medication-Induced Esophagitis; Endoscopic Variceal Sclerotherapy; Neodymium-YAG Laser Applications in the Esophagus; Esophageal Foreign Bodies and Food Impaction*

Augusto Larrain, M.D. ▪ Associate Professor of Surgery, Faculty of Medicine, University of Chile, Santiago, Chile; Department of Surgery, Instituto Nacional de Enfermedades Respiratorias y Cirugía Torácica, Santiago, Chile; Staff Member, Department of Surgery, Clinica Las Condes, Santiago, Chile ▪ *Respiratory Complications of Gastroesophageal Reflux*

Donald E. Low, M.D., F.R.C.S.(C) ▪ Howard Wright Fellow in Surgical Research, Virginia Mason Medical Center, Seattle, Washington; Department of Surgery, Swedish Hospital Medical Center, Seattle, Washington ▪ *Esophageal Endoscopy, Dilation, and Intraesophageal Prosthetic Devices*

Steven D. MacFarlane, M.D. ▪ General and Vascular Surgeon, Stevens Memorial Hospital, Edmonds, Washington ▪ *Carcinoma of the Esophagus*

Richard W. McCallum, M.D., F.A.C.P., F.A.C.G., F.R.A.C.P. ▪ The Paul Janssen Professor of Medicine, University of Virginia School of Medicine, Charlottesville, Virginia; Chief, Division of Gastroenterology, University of Virginia Medical Center, Charlottesville, Virginia; Staff Member, University of Virginia Hospital and Medical Center, Charlottesville, Virginia; Staff Member and Director of Gastroenterology Training at Salem Veterans Administration Hospital, Salem, Virginia ▪ *The Medical Approach to the Treatment of Gastroesophageal Reflux*

C. Dale Mercer, M.D., F.R.C.S.C. ▪ Assistant Professor and Director, Surgical Esophageal Research Group, Queen's University, Kingston, Ontario; Attending Staff, Kingston General Hospital and Hôtel Dieu Hospital, Kingston, Ontario ▪ *Anatomy of the Esophagus; Surgery for Hiatal Hernia and Esophagitis; Paraesophageal Hernia; Surgery for Motility Disorders of the Esophagus; Rings, Webs, and Diverticula; Perforation, Rupture, and Injury of the Esophagus; Benign Tumors and Cysts of the Esophagus*

G. Alec Patterson, F.R.C.S., F.A.C.S. ▪ Assistant Professor, University of Toronto, Toronto, Ontario ▪ *Esophageal Replacement, Bypass, and Intubation*

John M. Petersen, D.O. ■ Former Fellow, Medical Division of Gastroenterology, Yale University, New Haven, Connecticut ■ *The Medical Approach to the Treatment of Gastroesophageal Reflux*

Charles E. Pope II ■ Professor, Medicine, University of Washington, Seattle, Washington; Chief, Gastroenterology, Seattle Veterans Administration Medical Center, Seattle, Washington ■ *Complications of Gastroesophageal Reflux; Respiratory Complications of Gastroesophageal Reflux*

R. W. Postlethwait, M.D. ■ Professor of Surgery Emeritus, Duke University, Durham, North Carolina ■ *Surgical Aspects of Congenital Anomalies of the Esophagus*

Brian J. Reid, M.D., Ph.D. ■ Acting Assistant Professor of Medicine, University of Washington, Seattle, Washington; Attending Gastroenterologist, University of Washington, University Hospital, Harborview Hospital, Providence Medical Center, Seattle, Washington ■ *Barrett's Esophagus and Esophageal Adenocarcinoma*

L. Rodella, M.D. ■ Assistant, Postgraduate School of Emergency Surgery, University of Verona, Italy; Assistant, III Divisione Clinicizzata Di Chirurgia Generale, Centro Ospedaliero Di Borgo, Trento-Verona, Italy ■ *The "Nill" Procedure*

Cyrus E. Rubin, M.D. ■ Professor of Medicine and Pathology, University of Washington, Seattle, Washington; Attending Gastroenterologist, University Hospital, University of Washington, Seattle, Washington; Consultant, Veterans Administration Hospital, Harborview Hospital, Providence, Washington; Attending, Medical Center, Group Health Cooperative, and Children's Orthopaedic, Seattle, Washington ■ *Barrett's Esophagus and Esophageal Adenocarcinoma*

Colin O. H. Russell, M.B.Ch.B., M.S., F.R.A.C.S. ■ Senior Lecturer, Monash University, Melbourne, Australia; Consultant Surgeon, Monash Medical Centre, Melbourne, Australia; Visiting Surgeon, Prince Henry's Hospital, Melbourne, Australia ■ *Symptoms of Esophageal Disease; Functional Evaluation of the Esophagus*

Kjell Thor, M.D., Ph.D. ■ Associate Professor of Surgery, Karolinska Institute, Stockholm, Sweden; Assistant Chief Surgeon, Department of Surgery, Ersta Hospital, Stockholm, Sweden ■ *Surgery for Hiatal Hernia and Esophagitis; The Modified Toupet Procedure; Mark IV Anti-Reflux Procedure; Surgery for Motility Disorders of the Esophagus*

N. Velasco, M.D. ■ Former Howard Wright Research Fellow and Surgeon, Santiago, Chile ■ *Paraesophageal Hernia*

Foreword

"Why, in God's name, in our days, is there such a difference between the physician and the surgeon? It ought to be understood that no one can be a good physician who has no idea of surgical operations, and that a surgeon is nothing if ignorant of medicine. In a word one must be familiar with both departments of medicine." These words could serve as the text of this book. As a matter of fact, they were spoken by LanFranc, a founder of French surgery, who died nearly seven centuries ago.

Despite similar admonitions, until recently medical gastroenterologists and digestive tract disease surgeons essentially have been competitors. Rivalry has been keen; mutual trust and understanding have been absent. Even today, the domain of endoscopy continues to be disputed by both disciplines.

The editors of this book are certain it is time that hatchets should be buried and that the wisdom of both physicians and surgeons be available to all who are concerned with diseases of the esophagus. Such cooperation has already become essential in such specialties as cardiovascular disease and has redounded to the benefit of physicians' and surgeons' mutual patients.

However, to produce a book that appeals to all doctors of medicine is another matter. Physicians have been annoyed by the emphasis placed on details of operative techniques, and surgeons have drowned in the sea of words in some medical texts. Nevertheless, all doctors of medicine recognize that the boundaries between medicine and surgery continue to be eroded by many factors. Endoscopists have developed an essentially independent specialty. Physiologists have begun to unravel the mysteries of esophageal motility. Cancer of the esophagus now is a matter not only for surgeons but also for radiotherapists and chemotherapists, and, most recently, for those interested in the laser vaporization of tumors. No one can or should remain ignorant of such contributions.

The result of such investigations is the production of a large amount of relatively new knowledge that merits compilation. The attempt of the editors is not to turn out superspecialists who are equally able in both medicine and surgery but to make the information gathered from each quarter available to everyone else.

Thus physicians treating what has been identified by one of the authors as a particularly common complaint—reflux esophagitis—can find clinical and laboratory criteria that will help them to decide which medicines to use or when to refer the patient to a surgeon. Endoscopists can learn the limits of sclerotherapy and when shunts should be employed.

It cannot be expected that this volume, complete as it is, will quiet all controversies; however, data are presented that should aid any practitioner in making decisions. The competing operations for reflux esophagitis are all given a fair hearing. Other problems are addressed, such as the management of Barrett's esophagus and the optimum treatment of cancer, but they are left as unsolved problems for the future.

All who read this volume will gain a clear grasp of what actually is known today about diseases of the esophagus and acquire some definition of what needs to be done in the future. In this venture, it may be that the editors will succeeed even more fully than they expect. They may generate a trend that will meld the combined knowledge about other specific viscera of all disciplines in a similar manner, in a form that is digestible and informative for all doctors of medicine, regardless of their specialties.

CLAUDE E. WELCH, M.D., F.A.C.S.

Senior Surgeon
Massachusetts General Hospital
Clinical Professor of Surgery (Emeritus)
Harvard Medical School

Preface

Gastroesophageal reflux disease is recognized as the most common upper gastrointestinal tract abnormality in humans. The overall incidence of esophageal disease is increasing dramatically. It is timely, therefore, that our experience should be combined with that of experts from around the world in a volume dealing with these common disorders. There have been several volumes devoted to the surgery of eosphageal disease and several volumes devoted to medical management, but few, if any, have tried to strike a balance between presenting both the medical and surgical aspects of esophageal disorders. One of the aims of this volume is to bring together both medical and surgical experts to cover the advances in both fields. We have been fortunate in obtaining world authorities in both areas. As Dr. Welch has so aptly stated in the Foreword . . ."it is time that hatchets should be buried and that the wisdom of both physicians and surgeons be available to all who are concerned with diseases of the esophagus."

Our own experience is based on evaluation of over 15,000 patients in the gastrointestinal laboratory. Our surgical experience covers over 2,000 procedures for benign esophageal disease and over 500 procedures for esophageal cancer. In addition, basic research regarding the anatomy and function of the esophagus, and in particular the gastroesophageal barrier to reflux, is ongoing. We have documented the role of the gastroesophageal valve as a powerful factor in the prevention of reflux. This has given us a better overall understanding of the antireflux mechanism and for the first time we are able to present a comprehensive view of the anatomy and physiology of the gastroesophageal junction.

All of the authors have brought to bear on their area the new technology and advances that have occurred with great rapidity in the past decade. The chapter on Barrett's esophagus, for example, presents the most comprehensive pathologic analysis coupled with flow cytometry studies to give us the clearest picture of this disorder that has yet been presented. The chapters on medical management, physiology, complications of gastroesophageal reflux, diagnosis, and function have likewise included the latest technology and the action of the newest drugs. The discussion of intraoperative manometry again stresses bringing the new technology to the surgical procedure itself to complement the pre- and postoperative use of these technologic advances.

Laser technology and sclerotherapy are recent advances that are reviewed with authority. The advances in fiberoptic endoscopy and new therapeutic balloons and catheters are presented in several of the chapters and represent an expanding field that will continue to enhance both the diagnosis and the therapy of esophageal disease.

In addition to the outstanding authors, this book would not have been possible without the efforts of many who have supported this work. The support of the board members of the Ryan Hill Research Foundation and of the members of the Howard Wright family has been crucial to the success of this work. The Howard Wright Fellows have done much of the basic and clinical research leading to the conclusions presented in this volume. They have returned to such diverse places as Australia, Chile, Canada, and Sweden, where they are teaching the principles presented here. The pathology departments of Virginia Mason and Swedish Medical Centers as well as of the University of Washington have been very helpful.

Our thanks must also go to Bette Glass, who has been indispensible in organizing and collating the manuscripts and getting them to the publisher on time. Our office staff and associates, including Brenda Adamcza, Wendy Cornell, Edward H. Morgan, M.D., Mary Jane Dake, and the members of the Gastroesophageal Laboratory, particularly Lillian Neal and Wendy Guidash, have helped us through the years. I am most grateful to my wife, Torrance, for her inspiration and help and for her editing of the manuscripts.

Our gratitude goes out to those many physicians and gastroenterologists with whom we have had the privilege of sharing the patients presented in these pages.

Our thanks also to the operating room staff and to a superb Department of Medical Illustration, particularly Joann Clifford, Taylor Ubben, Richard Schlag, John Boliver, and Robert Redlinger.

Dr. Claude Welch, one of the world's leading surgeons and a noted writer, kindly agreed to write the Foreword. This is most appropriate, since he discussed our first presentation before the American Surgical Association. Then, as now, his words pierce right to the heart of the matter and lend credence and clarity to the subject.

Our appreciation is also extended to Lisa McAllister, Bill Preston, and the entire staff at W.B. Saunders Company, who have done, as always, an outstanding job in putting together this volume.

Our ultimate aim in writing this volume is to present material that will aid physicians in helping patients with disorders of the esophagus.

Last, our thanks to the many patients suffering with esophageal disease who have allowed us to follow their course through the years.

Lucius Hill
Richard Kozarek
Richard McCallum
C. Dale Mercer

Contents

Color Plate I

Color Plate I. *A,* Five sutures are placed through the anterior and posterior phrenoesophageal bundles and carried through the preaortic fascia and median arcuate ligament. Instrument placed beneath the median arcuate ligament protects the celiac artery. *B,* Finger placed in the esophageal hiatus beneath the preaortic fascia allows for safer placement of sutures without dissection of the celiac artery. *C,* As sutures are tied with single throw of the knots, the barrier pressure is measured by passing the sidehole of a modified nasogastric tube through the barrier. *D,* Completed operation included anchoring of gastroesophageal junction permanently to the preaortic fascia with calibration of lower esophageal sphincter and restoration of the angle of His and the gastroesophageal valve.

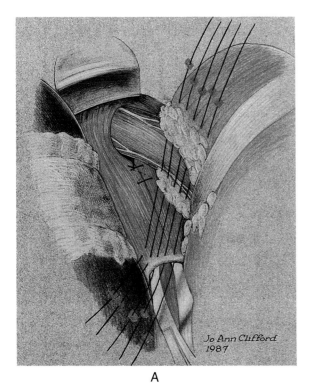

A

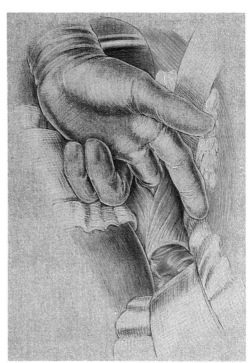

B

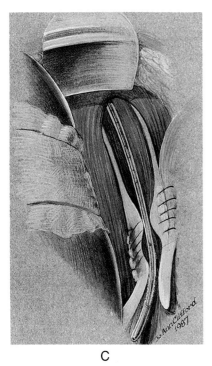

C

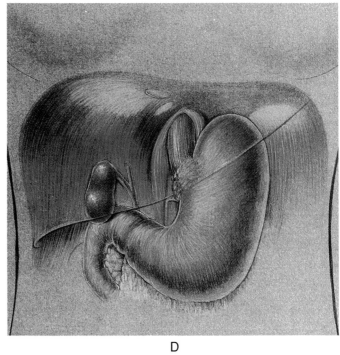

D

Plate I

Color Plate II. *A,* The gastroesophageal valve viewed through a gastrostomy. Probe is in the esophageal lumen, showing the valve to be 3 to 4 cm in length. *B,* The valve closes against the lesser curvature of the stomach so effectively that it may be difficult to find. If the hiatus is very large with atrophic crura, we perform a hiatoplasty with interrupted sutures and then research the median arcuate ligament. A Kocher guiding probe is put under the median arcuate ligament. *C* and *D,* First degree caustic burns of the distal esophagus; 48 hours after lye ingestion. *E* and *F,* Exudate, esophageal ulcerations one week after liquid lye ingestion.

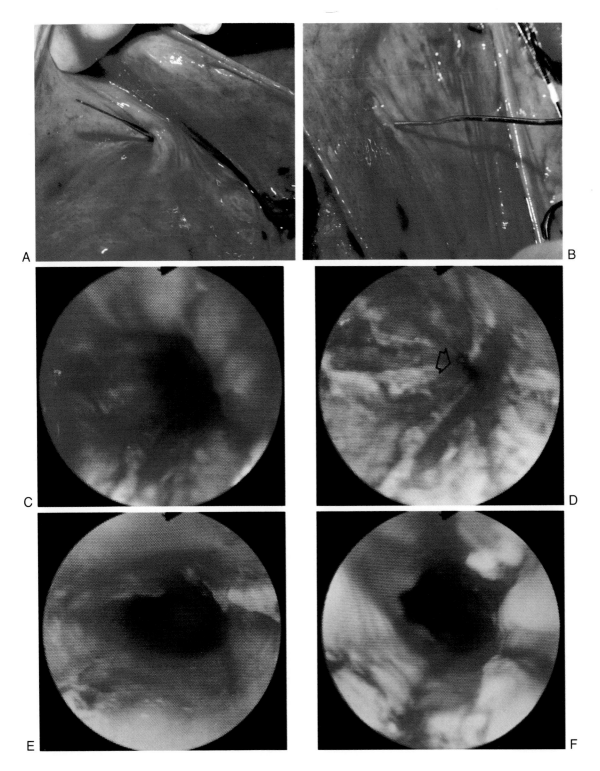

Plate II

Color Plate III

Color Plate III. *A*, Exudate, local hypopharyngeal ulcers 12 hours after granular alkali ingestion. *B*, Arrow depicts stricture of midesophagus related to KCl tablets. Note partially dissolved pull in lower aspect of photo. *C*, Bifid epiglottis following lye ingestion. *D*, Adhesive bands (arrows) at esophageal inlet 20 years after liquid alkali ingestion. *E*, Avulsed, ulcerated distal esophagus following sulfuric acid suicide attempt several weeks prior. *F*, De-epithelialized strictured esophagus resected for undilatable lye stenosis. Radiograph depicts lye stenosis.

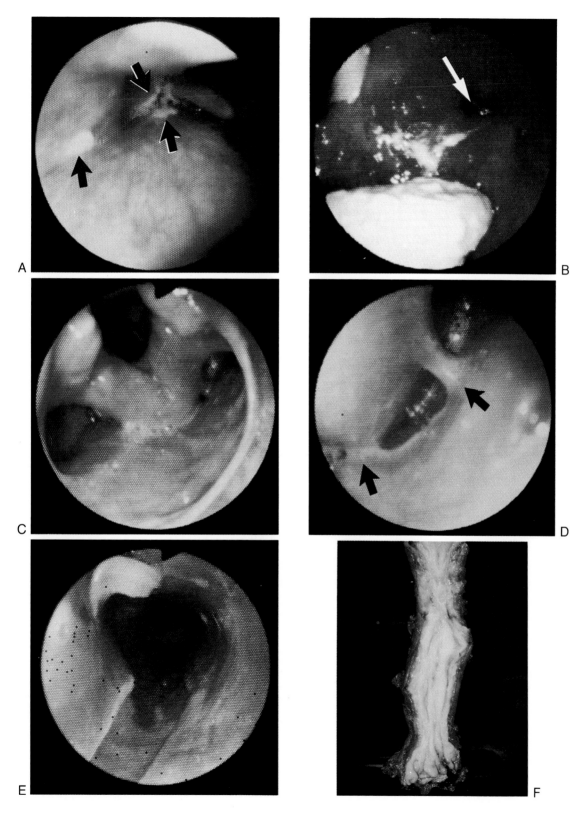

Plate III

Color Plate IV

Color Plate IV. *A*, Early intramural squamous cell cancer not seen on initial esophagography. *B*, Bulging varix (small arrow) after injection of 1 ml sodium tetradecyl. Note injection needle within varix (7 o'clock). *C*, Extensive esophageal ulceration, 7 to 9 o'clock, after sclerotherapy. Ulcers are commonly colonized by yeast. *D*, Probe demonstrates deep esophageal ulceration with free mediastinal perforation. *E*, Autopsy specimen demonstrates probe through patent portacaval anastomosis in a patient who died from bleeding gastric varices. Arrow shows portal vein clot propagated from left gastric veins after sclerotherapy. *F*, Sheath containing quartz fiber through which Nd-YAG laser is transmitted. Aiming beam (arrow) is a low power laser.

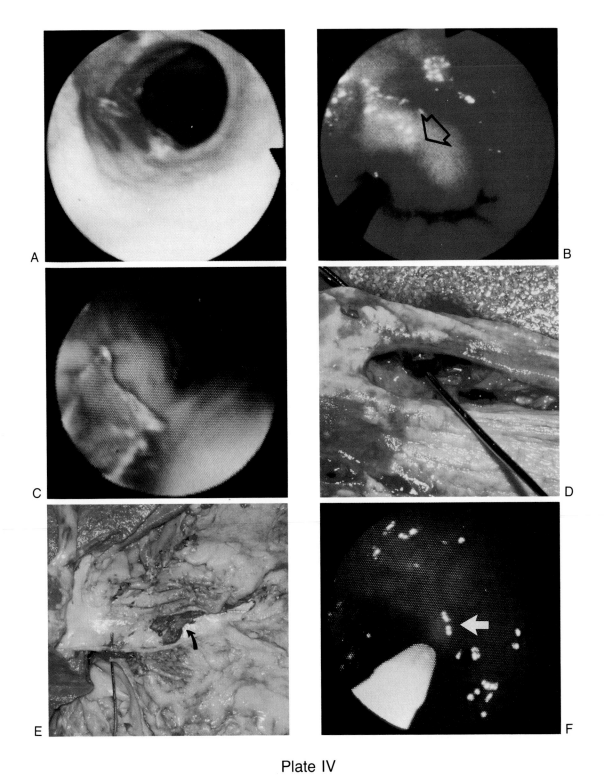

Plate IV

Color Plate V

Color Plate V. *A,* Laser-treated Mallory-Weiss tear of the gastroesophageal junction. Note edema and tissue blanching related to circumferential treatment of the laceration. *B,* Gastroesophageal junction neoplasm with 2 mm opening into stomach. *C,* Arrows delineate necrotic tissue after initial laser treatment of 4800 J. *D,* Gastroesophageal junction of patient depicted in V*B* and V*C* after second laser treatment. Note progressive increase in luminal size. Patient required two additional treatments to increase lumen to 15 mm. *E,* Chicken bone lodged in cervical esophagus. *F,* Polyp snare passed around impacted bone depicted in V*E*.

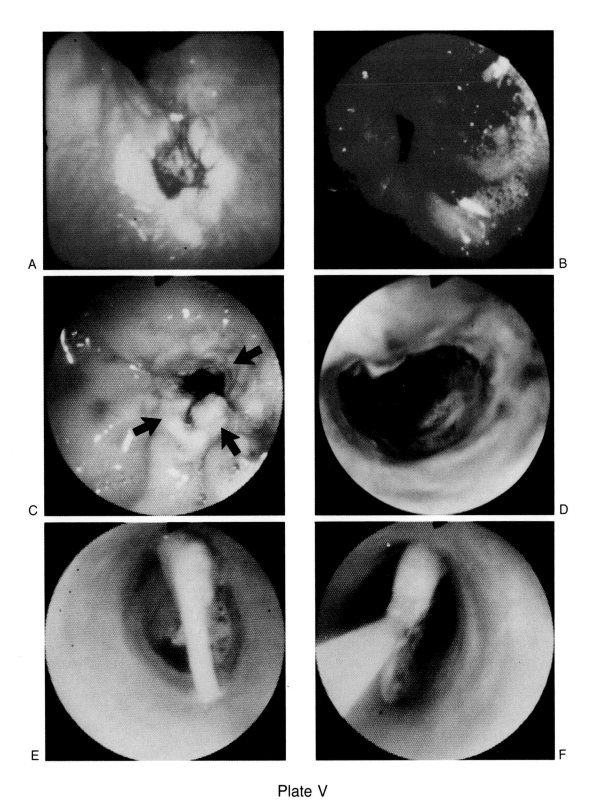

Plate V

Color Plate VI

Color Plate VI. *A*, Esophageal perforation following emergency room attempts to dislodge impacted food bolus with mercury bougie. This photograph is the per os view of mediastinum. *B*, Food bolus impacted gastroesophageal junction. Esophageal fluid has been endoscopically aspirated. *C*, Tight Schatzki's ring noted after endoscopic retrieval of food impaction depicted in VI*B*. Hiatal hernia can be seen distally.

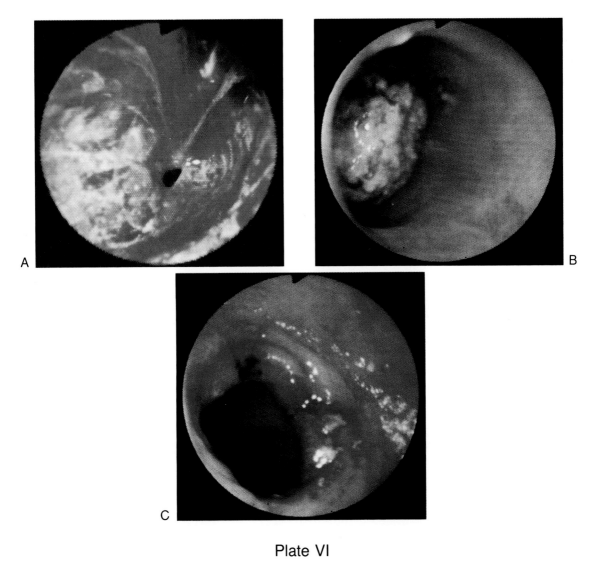

Plate VI

Historical Notes on Surgery of the Esophagus

Lyman A. Brewer III

The esophagus, because of its dangerous location in the deep cervical and thoracic planes, marginal blood supply, and lack of mesentery, was the nemesis of surgeons until the modern era. In 2500 BC surgery of the esophagus began with an isolated repair of the cervical esophagus described in the Smith Surgical Papyrus.[1] In spite of courageous attempts to operate upon the esophagus in the intervening years, the real progress had to wait for the development of abdominal surgery in the nineteenth century and of thoracic surgery in the twentieth.

To simplify the involved story of esophageal surgery within the limits of this chapter, five eras are delineated to clarify the understanding of the development of this slowly evolving segment of surgery: (1) ancient Egypt (Egypt of the pharaohs), (2) the progress from 2500 BC to the fifteenth century AD, (3) the seventeenth and eighteenth centuries, (4) the nineteenth century, and (5) the twentieth century.

■ *Ancient Egypt (2500 BC)*

In 1862 the American Egyptologist, Edwin Smith, discovered the document that became known as the "Smith Surgical Papyrus," the first written anatomic, physiologic, clinical, and pathologic observation recorded. It was not until 1930 that Henry Breasted made his classical translation, reporting 48 clinical cases.[1] All cases in the Smith Papyrus are classified as (1) "an ailment which I will treat" (believed curable), (2) "an ailment with which I will contend" (possibly curable), or (3) "an ailment which will not be treated" (incurable). Case 28, "a gaping wound of the throat penetrating the gullet," was called "an ailment with which I will contend." Under "Examination" the translation is as follows (Fig. 1–1):

> If thou examinest the man having a gaping wound in his throat piercing through to his gullet; if he drinks water he chokes; if it comes out of the mouth of the wound; is greatly inflamed so that develops fever from it; thou should draw together the wound with stitching.

This is the first very accurate description of an esophageal wound, and the first mention in medical literature of the suturing of a wound, a concept that was rediscovered again and again centuries later. Under "First Treatment" the translation states:

> Thou should bind it with fresh meat the first day. Thou should treat it afterwards with grease, honey, and lint every day until he recovers.

These medical nostrums persisted until the development of the modern understanding of sepsis, antisepsis, and wound care. The "Second Examination" states:

> If thou findest him continuing to have fever from the wound thou should give him the second treatment which includes thou shouldst apply for him dry lint in the mouth of the wound and 'moor him at his mooring stakes' until he recovers.

The latter statement of "mooring to the mooring

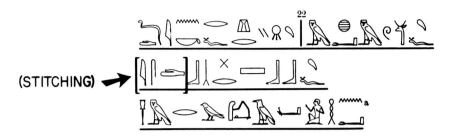

(STITCHING) ➤

Translation

Thou shouldst say concerning him : " One having a wound in his throat, piercing through to his gullet. An ailment with which I will contend."

Figure 1–1. The "diagnosis" describes the wound and states that the physician will "contend" or elect to treat the patient. The hieroglyphic symbol for stitching is the first record of wound suture.

stakes" (curiously) means that he should be fed by mouth. Allowing him to ingest food suggests successful healing of the wound. One cannot but be filled with the greatest admiration for this first recorded surgery of the esophagus and the apparent favorable outcome.

The Fifteenth Century

It is hard to believe that in some 2000 years no one attempted to dilate a stricture of the throat or perform surgery on the esophagus, yet not until the fifteenth century was there a definite report, which was made by Avenzoar,[2] an outstanding physician of the Western Caliphate, who reported that a silver or tin cannula should be placed in the throat of patients who are unable to swallow to permit the ingestion of liquids. Thus, we must conclude that the esophagus was a forbidden organ for surgery by the early surgeons.

Seventeenth and Eighteenth Century Advances

Prior to the Renaissance, dissection of the human body was forbidden. However, with the first anatomic dissections, there was a basic understanding of the anatomy. The planning and execution of surgical operations for the first time became practical. The cervical esophagus was the first site of surgery of the esophagus that could be carried out without the disastrous physiologic consequences of

invading the thorax. Making a giant leap from the days of the pharaohs, Richard Wiseman[3] in 1676 advised suturing the esophagus and placing the patient on a thin diet. This started a controversy over the treatment of wounds of the esophagus in the cervical region, with Purmann[4] in 1694 condemning surgery and Stoffel[5] recommending surgical treatment.

In 1701 John Baptiste Verduc[6] advised surgical removal of impacted foreign bodies through a neck wound. Verduc placed the patient in a sitting position in a chair with his head firmly in extension. Then, after performing a tracheostomy, a long incision was made in the cervical esophagus. In 1757, Goursaud and Roland[7] reported the successful removal of foreign bodies in the esophagus and cervical region as had been previously advised by Verduc. After the removal of foreign bodies, the esophagus was not sutured, healing spontaneously. Oral feedings were discontinued for six days and nourishing enemas were given. At the end of the century in 1786 Teranget[8] successfully opened the surgical esophagus for stricture. Sixteen months later the patient was still alive. Thus, at the end of the eighteenth century, a beginning had been made on surgery of the cervical esophagus, offering hope for the future.

The Nineteenth Century

This century was to see dramatic advances affecting surgery of the esophagus, which would be a springboard for the remarkable progress in the twentieth century. In 1805 Vigardonne[9] categorically stated that a correctly performed esophagotomy was not dangerous provided that the patient was nourished through a rubber feeding tube while the wound was healing. Probangs were devised to remove foreign bodies by the transoral approach. In 1857, Colegrove[10] by using a probang, extracted a coin from the lower esophagus just above the cardia. Esophagotomy for foreign bodies was championed by Cheever in 1867,[11] Arenlanos,[12] and Gross.[13] The fears of cervical thoracotomy voiced in the eighteenth century seemed to be allayed by these reports.

Strictures of the esophagus were first handled by passing dilators transorally into the gullet beginning with Vareliaud[14] in 1801. A more radical approach was that of Lannelonge,[15] who in 1867 devised an instrument with a cutting blade similar to a urethrotome, which he called an instrument for "internal esophagotomy." This was a radical advance over the simple dilating techniques, and it was not without fatalities. Von Bergmann[16] in 1883 was the first to employ retrodilatation performed through a gastrostomy. Abbe[17] in 1893 used a string to saw through the stricture. At the end of the century, Woolsey[18] was able to report 28 cases of esophageal dilatation, so this operation was becoming more commonplace.

Kussmaul[19] had the distinction of being the first surgeon to look inside the esophagus. In 1868 he passed a lighted tube through the entire length of the esophagus into the stomach with the patient being examined in a "sword-swallowing" position. Over a decade later (1881) MacKenzie[20] and Von Mickulicz[21] developed their own particular types of esophagoscopic instruments. Lesions of the esophagus could now be brought under the direct vision of the operator for biopsy or dilation of strictures without surgical exploration.

During the latter half of the nineteenth century certain general advances had a profound effect upon surgery of the esophagus. These included the introduction of anesthesia by Long[22] and Morton,[23] the discovery of pathogenic bacteria by Pasteur,[24] the recognition of advantages of antisepsis in surgery by Lister,[25] the introduction of diagnostic radiology by Roentgen,[26] and the development of gastrointestinal surgical techniques of the abdomen by Czerny,[27] Billroth,[28] and others.

The delineation of the anatomic changes in the esophagus were made possible by Walter B. Cannon[29] in 1897, when he was a freshman at Harvard Medical School (Fig. 1–2). He fed grain that had been covered with barium nitrate to a goose and radiographically followed the passage of this radiopaque material down the gullet of the goose to the stomach. This pioneering study was an important stimulus to radiologists to improve the technique and to delineate the various diseases of the

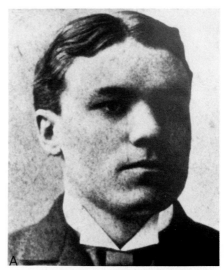

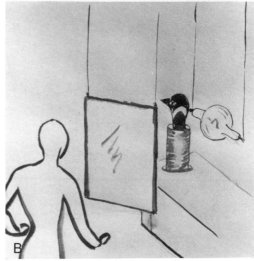

Figure 1–2. *A,* Walter B. Cannon as a medical student began physiologic studies on digestion in the laboratories of Dr. H. P. Bowditch, professor of physiology. In 1896, one year after Roentgen's discovery, Cannon was the first to study the passage of contrast medium down the long neck of a goose and so performed the first esophagogram. Subsequently, he made further major contributions to the mysteries of digestion. *B,* Cannon observes the passage of grain impregnated with barium down the gullet of a Canadian goose, suitably restrained in a box with a high collar. This imaginative demonstration proved to be the beginning of the development of the upper gastrointestinal series.

esophagus and those of the lower digestive track. In 1898 Bliss[30] used the roentgenogram to identify a radiopaque foreign body in the esophagus for the first time, which led to the successful removal of the foreign body (Fig. 1–3). Foreign bodies such as metal would readily show up on even the primitive radiologic instruments that were available at that time.

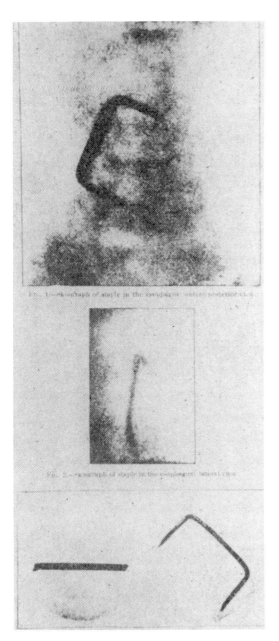

Figure 1–3. In 1898, three years after Roentgen's discovery of the x-ray, Bliss took this crude roentgenogram, clearly showing the presence and location of this metallic foreign body, which is shown in the lower portion of the illustration after its successful extraction from the esophagus.

■ *The Twentieth Century*

Surgery of the esophagus benefited from certain general measures that were introduced in the twentieth century: aseptic surgery by Halstead[31]; intratracheal anesthesia by Meltzer and Auer[32]; the un-

derstanding of the physiologic problems of the open pneumothorax by Graham and Bell[33]; the introduction of sulfonamides by Domagk[34]; and of antibiotics by Fleming[35] were important in the management of surgical patients.

■ WORLD WAR II: SURGICAL ADVANCES

During World War II the author was given the assignment by Colonel E. D. Churchill, Consultant Surgeon, Mediterranean Theater of Operations, of working out the immediate treatment of wounds of the thorax in the forward hospitals during the Italian Campaign. The primary treatment evolving from this study was the rapid restoration of the deranged cardiopulmonary physiology and minimized the role of the pleura, which had been the main concern in World War I. The therapeutic regimen included improved resuscitation,[36–41] better emergency measures, more accurate diagnoses, and a very sharp limitation of the indications for emergency thoracotomy, which were being performed in a rather wholesale manner by various surgeons in the front lines at that time. The identification and treatment of the "wet lung of trauma" by the author,[42,43] which is now called the respiratory distress syndrome (RDS), was a significant advance. I also devised the first machine for the production of intermittent positive pressure oxygen therapy which was used initially at Casino, Italy, in January 1944.[42,43] From this rather simple device have been developed elegant pressure- and volume-regulated respirators, which are now used in all major hospitals. The physiologically oriented regimen of therapy which resulted from this study was accepted as the official treatment first in the Mediterranean Theater of Operations, then by the U.S. Army Medical Corps. These principles were also followed in Korea and Viet Nam and have been proved again and again at the Los Angeles County University of Southern California Medical Center.

This development of an understanding of the basic physiologic derangements of the heart and the lungs in the surgery of war wounds, thoracotomies, and post-thoracotomy states and their management in World War II provided the basis for the explosive development of thoracic and cardiac surgery in the post-war era. An appreciation of these principles was fundamental to the introduction of total esophagectomy by the author, described later in this chapter.

Thoracic surgery also received a great impetus when it was rescued from the section of "septic surgery" in the United States Army Medical Corps and was given its deserved recognition as a specialty. This was started by Burford, Samson, and the author when they set up the first thoracic center in World War II on July 15, 1943, at Bizerte, Tunisia. Subsequently Harken developed a chest center in England where he pioneered the removal of foreign bodies from the chambers of the heart. Reintroduction of decortication of the lung, the first use of penicillin in infected thoracic wounds, and indications and techniques for the removal of intrathoracic foreign bodies were developed at the Bizerte chest center. These general advances in thoracic surgery facilitated the performance of major surgical operations on the esophagus.

As far as wounds of the esophagus were concerned, we confirmed the opinion that early diagnosis and repair of such wounds were mandatory. This will be discussed in greater detail later in the chapter.

■ THORACIC SURGERY IN THE MODERN ERA

The first thoracic surgery residency established by John Alexander in 1928 at the University of Michigan was a milestone in the development of the specialty. Alexander set very high standards, which were eventually adopted by the American Board of Thoracic Surgery two decades later. Other thoracic surgery residencies followed: Olive View Sanitorium outside Los Angeles, and Barnes Hospital in St. Louis under the direction of Evarts Graham. Under the stimulus of the advances in thoracic surgery gained in World War II, thoracic surgery residencies sprung up in all sections of the country. In 1948 the American Board of Thoracic Surgery was founded by not only the surgeons who had pioneered this specialty in the Army, but also by prominent senior members of the American Association for Thoracic Surgery. This was a very significant step forward in improving the quality of thoracic surgery in this country. In 1974 the author chaired a committee to study thoracic surgical manpower in this country.[44] For the first time the problems and the performance of thoracic surgery were evaluated on a nationwide scale. The large number of *non–board-certified* surgeons practicing thoracic surgery in this country was uncovered in this survey. Tightening requirements for hospital practice has decreased this number according to subsequent surveys made by the two major thoracic surgical societies.

Having discussed the general background for the history of the development of thoracic and esophageal surgery through and following World War II, we are in a position to examine the particular historical development of some of the diseases of the esophagus which offered great challenges to surgeons pioneering this specialty.

■ WOUNDS OF THE ESOPHAGUS

Beginning with the first repair of a wound of the esophagus in 2500 BC,[1] surgery for trauma of the esophagus was limited to the cervical region until the twentieth century. During the Civil War, penetrating wounds of the chest were sewn up tightly to obviate the problems of the open pneumothorax, with a resultant 60 per cent mortality rate. Patients with wounds of the thoracic esophagus probably all succumbed. Little if any attention was given to the wounds of the esophagus during World War I. In World War II, with the successful management of the open pneumothorax and improvement of the cardiorespiratory status, the opportunity for suture of thoracic esophageal wounds was made possible.

In World War II, however, because of simultaneous wounds of the heart, blood vessels, trachea, and bronchi, very few patients survived an external wound in which the esophagus was also involved. Among the 2267 critically wounded in nontransportable casualties for thoracic and abdominal wounds that were managed by the Second Auxiliary Surgical Group in World War II, there were only six patients with severe wounds in the esophagus who survived to reach the field hospital.[45] None of these patient recovered. In the group of less severely wounded patients there were three patients with esophageal wounds who survived and lived to reach the base hospital where they were treated with drainage and repair. Of the 24 late wounds of the esophagus treated at the Kennedy General Hospital in Memphis, Tennessee, six had fistulas or strictures, or both.[46] This is just a small sampling of the World War II experience.

Early exploration and repair were recommended ''on the slightest suspicion of esophageal perforation''[41] (Fig. 1–4). Ingestion of a very thin high-contrast medium such as Hypaque or Gastrografin will detect the perforation in most instances. In questionable cases esophagoscopy should be promptly carried out for further identification for a possible laceration. When the patient has been anaesthetized for repair, a quick, rigid esophagoscopic examination will help the surgeon decide the extent of the tear and condition of the esophageal mucosa. Because almost 30 per cent of esophageal perforations are secondary to esophagoscopy and 24 per cent occur following other endoscopy (gastroscopy and bronchoscopy), a very high index of suspicion must be accorded these procedures for possibility of esophageal perforation.

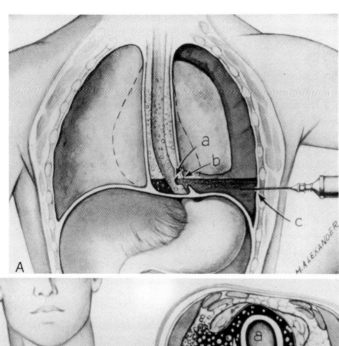

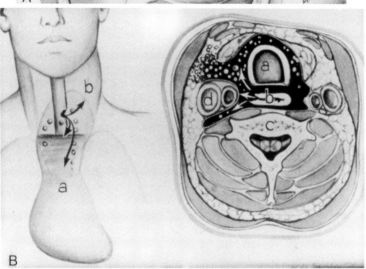

Figure 1–4. *A,* Perforation of the thoracic esophagus. (a) Wound of the esophagus permits escape of air and fluid, producing a hydropneumothorax; (b) rupture of mediastinal pleura; (c) aspiration of gastric fluid with a low pH confirms the diagnosis. *B,* Perforation of the cervical esophagus. Cross section drawing of spread of fluid and infection secondary to a wound of the cervical esophagus. (a) Trachea; (b) perforation of the esophagus—infection spreads in fascial planes to upper mediastinum; (c) sixth cervical vertebra; (d) carotid sheath. As developed by the author and associates in World War II.

The first notable advance in the management of spontaneous perforations of the esophagus since Boerhaave's original description in 1724* was made by Barrett in 1946 when he prognosticated that

> given these diagnoses I am convinced that surgeons will be able to save some of the patients combine the principles already established in the case of abdominal perforation with those relevant to thoracotomy.

But the ink on his article was scarcely dry when on March 7, 1946, he performed the first successful repair of a spontaneous rupture of the esophagus

---

*Boerhaave's report in Lud G., Batav. 1724, of a massive tear of the esophagus graphically described the patient's death from septic shock. When the mediastinum and pleura are subject to extensive contamination, repair is ill advised and the esophagus is isolated, as described later in this chapter. Of course, there was no chance of repair of the thoracic esophagus in the eighteenth century.

ten hours after the onset of symptoms. Since then there have been many such patients who have been operated on and saved by emergency surgery.

Following World War II, the introduction of powerful antibiotics and delayed referral patterns have shown us that there are a number of treatment options that are available. In an unpublished study of 90 patients with perforation of the esophagus, made by the author and associates, about one-half of the patients (43) were treated within the first 24 hours, 29 after 24 hours, and 15 patients with delayed referrals had no surgery whatsoever.[49] Thus, we must add to the preferred treatment (repair and drainage within the first 24 hours) the possibility the (1) performing drainage with an irrigating tube, (2) esophageal exclusion operations, (3) esophageal resection, and (4) nonoperative treatment.

With large thoracic perforations and those with gastric contents in the mediastinum and/or pleura, we now believe that isolation of the esophagus with

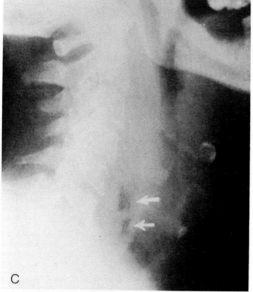

Figure 1–4 *Continued C,* Perforation of the cervical esophagus: lateral roentgenogram. Arrows point to widened prevertebral space with fluid and air, a classical finding in perforation of the cervical esophagus, in a World War II battle casualty. *D,* Perforation of the thoracic esophagus. Left. Chest roentgenogram. Contrast medium flows from esophagus into the pleural cavity with right hydropneumothorax. Right. Chest x-ray six weeks after delayed repair of esophagus and decortication of right lung, performed by author's group in World War II.

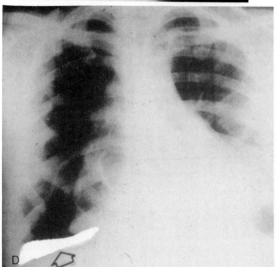

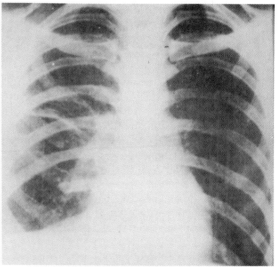

a cervical esophagostomy, occlusion of the cardia, and jejunostomy, along with hyperalimentation, are the procedures of choice. Small perforations need only irrigating tubes for drainage because they may frequently heal spontaneously without established infection. Nonoperative treatment with gastric suction and hyperalimentation was employed mostly in late referrals without evidence of significant infection. When the obstruction is present and the diagnosis is made early, whether the obstruction is benign or malignant, without the presence of established infection, esophageal resection is properly employed in these early cases.

■ REFLUX ESOPHAGITIS AND HIATAL HERNIA

Although it was as early as 1570 that Ambrose Paré[50] first described hiatal hernia, it was not until the third decade of the twentieth century that reflux esophagitis was recognized as the pathologic condition that made hiatal hernia symptomatic. The first successful repair of a hiatal hernia by the transthoracic approach was made by Postemski[51] in 1884. Within a year six cases had been reported from his clinic. The early writings of Hedbloom,[52] Harrington and Kirklin,[53] and others in this country based their main emphasis on repairing the anatomic defect. Thus, surgery had as its principal object the returning of the herniated stomach to the abdomen. Winkelstein[54] in 1930 was probably the first to point out that peptic esophagitis was secondary to reflux from hiatal hernia. In 1947 Bernstein[57] and more recently others have emphasized this fact. Hiatal hernia per se does not cause symptoms unless there is reflux esophagitis. Harrington[53] reported that over half of the patients undergoing laparotomy for other conditions could be shown to have a totally asymptomatic hiatal hernia. Hence, repair of the hiatal hernia is dependent upon severity of the esophagitis and response to medical treatment.

It is of historical interest that Kronecker and Meltzer[55] reported as early as 1883 the studies of acidity in the lower esophagus. These were revived by Kramer and Ingelfinger[56] in 1949 using modern equipment. Acidity studies in the lower esophagus were also carried out by Bernstein[57] and Bernstein and Baker[58] and others to make it possible to accurately determine the necessity for surgical correction. The propriety of surgery is frequently questioned without such objective studies. It also can be used following the operation to objectively evaluate the completeness of the surgical repair. All types of surgical repair rely on the prevention of esophageal reflux, which is probably most simply performed by placing a sufficient length of esophagus intrabdominally so that the increased abdominal pressure prevents the reflux.* The distal esophageal muscles and vagal fibers must be preserved.

There is no form of surgery in which the ingenuity of surgeons has produced such a variety of surgical operations, which in the main have been successful. The history of the modern surgical treatment of hiatal hernia may be likened to a type of periodic surgical Olympics in which the followers and the four main proponents of their own surgical operation (Fig. 1–5) (Belsey, Nissen, Collis, and Hill) have been the major contestants. Because the results in the majority of cases have been reasonably satisfactory with each of these methods, thoracic surgeons have had to use their own judgment in deciding which type of repair suits their surgical expertise. Subsequent chapters in this volume present an excellent discussion of this type of surgery.

■ ESOPHAGEAL ATRESIA AND TRACHEOESOPHAGEAL FISTULA

Esophagel atresia was one of the very earliest esophageal abnormalities to be reported in medical literature. The first observations were made by Durston in 1670.[59] In 1679 Gibson[60] recorded the first description of the esophagotracheal fistula. But

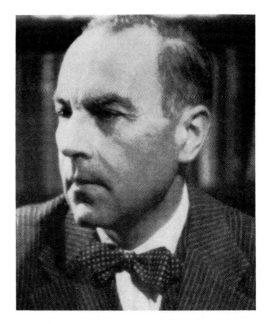

Figure 1–5. Rudolph Nissen, 1896–1983, assistant to Sauerbruch, Professor of Surgery in Istanbul, Turkey, and University of Basel, Switzerland; and pioneer thoracic surgeon, productive for four decades. In 1931 he performed the first pneumonectomy (two-stage procedure for bronchiectasis). Thirty years later he introduced "fundoplication" for hiatal hernia, an operation now widely performed, often in conjunction with other procedures. This photograph of Nissen was taken at the time of his 1931 pneumonectomy.

because of the difficulties of operating on tiny babies and because of the problems of open pneumothorax, tracheoesophageal fistula remained in the realm of anatomic curiosities for almost 300 years, until the first half of the twentieth century. As early as 1913, Richter[61] in Chicago transpleurally ligated an esophageal fistula and performed a gastrostomy. He used intratracheal anesthesia delivered by a homemade respirator, fabricated from a vacuum cleaner. Unfortunately, success was not to come to him. And likewise with Mixter[62] in 1929 at the Boston Children's Hospital. His patient met with the same fate. Mixter divided the tracheoesophageal fistula and exteriorized the distal esophagus segment out to the chest wall as a feeding "esophagogastrostomy." He moved to the Beth Israel Hospital soon after this and did not report another case.

In the late 30s and early 40s an interest in perfecting a one-stage operation became intense, and there was a spirited competition between four of the leading children's centers in this country. These centers were the Boston Children's Hospital (Ladd[63] and Lanman[64]), University of Michigan Hospital (Haight and Towsley[65,66]), in Dallas (Shaw[67]), and the University of Minnesota Hospital (Leven[68]). Lanman in 1936 to 1939 operated on

---

*The author devised a hiatal hernia repair consisting of transplanting the hiatus to the dome of the diaphragm so that there was a sufficient length of abdominal esophagus, which permitted the increased abdominal pressure to prevent reflux. Lack of objective pH tests prevented the authors from reporting this technique. It is most useful with a pronounced short esophagus.

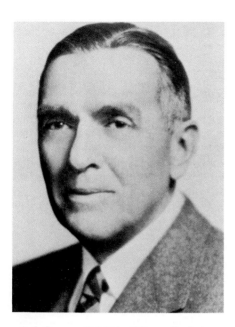

Figure 1–6. Cameron Haight in 1941 was the first surgeon to successfully close a congenital tracheoesophageal fistula with anastomosis of the ends of the esophagus as a single stage operation in a newborn infant. In 1932 he performed the first pneumonectomy (two stages) in this country for bronchiectasis.

four patients. Unfortunately, there were no long-term survivors. In 1938 Shaw[67] performed what was first seen to be a satisfactory anastomosis on the infant, but the patient died on the twelfth postoperative day.

On April 30, 1939, I assisted Dr. Cameron Haight at the University of Michigan Hospital when he performed his first primary anastomosis of the esophageal segments and division of fistula in a four-day-old infant. He used an extrapleural approach with 0.25 per cent pipericaine to provide local anesthesia. I remember vividly that we spent the entire night after the operation desperately trying to get the infant to breathe properly in an oxygen tent with intratracheal suction, also giving intravenous fluids and a blood transfusion. Unfortunately, our high hopes were shattered when the infant died 17 hours after surgery. At the autopsy it was shown that fetal (not acquired) atelectasis, bone marrow giant cell emboli to the lungs and liver, and overhydration (a common failing in those days) were the causes of death. Four more failures at the University of Michigan occurred before Haight became the first one to succeed in a one-stage operation on March 15, 1941 (Fig. 1–6).[65]

However, with another approach, Ladd[63] in Boston and Leven[68] in Minneapolis independently developed the multistage operation, using gastrostomy and ligation of the fistula in the thoracic esophagus followed by delayed esophageal substi-

tution. Both achieved recoveries in 1939, two years before Haight's one-stage successful case. Victory had finally crowned the efforts of these determined surgeons. One-stage procedures are now preferred, with certain specific exceptions.

■ ACHALASIA

Thomas Willis[69] (Fig. 1–7) first described this condition in 1679, making it one of the oldest recorded diseases of the esophagus. He reported as follows:

> . . . a certain man of Oxford, shew an almost perpetual vomiting by the shutting up of the left orifice (cardia). . . he languished away from hunger and every day was in danger of death. I deployed an instrument for him, a rod of whalebone with a little round button of sponge fixed to the top of it. . . . Putting it down the esophagus he could thrust it into the ventricle its orifice being opened and by this means he has daily taken his sustenance for 15 years.

This was obviously the description of a successful diagnosis and treatment of achalasia.

Two centuries after this remarkable description by Willis, C. J. Russell[70] of South Hampton, Eng-

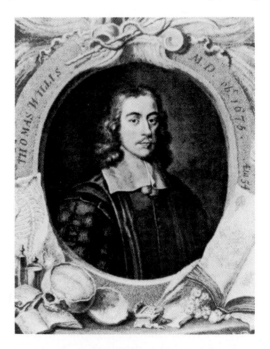

Figure 1–7. Thomas Willis in 1679 first diagnosed and treated a case of achalasia. By inserting transorally a whale bone and sponge dilator, he was able to periodically dilate the cardia so that his patient took sustenance for 15 years. (From Ellis FH, Olsen AM: Achalasia of the Esophagus. Philadelphia, W.B. Saunders Co., 1969.)

land, devised an inflatable rubber balloon covered with silk which he placed on the ends of a bougie and blew up to dilate the stricture. He reported five successful cases in which achalasia was treated in this manner. However, as with other conditions of the esophagus, surgical treatment was not developed until the twentieth century. Mikulicz in 1904[71] through an abdominal incision inserted a rubber sheathed forceps through a gastrostomy opening and dilated the cardia from below. It is interesting that in 1907, three years later, Risinger[72] used the transthoracic plication operation to reduce the size of the dilated esophagus, but this of course did not improve the swallowing.

A major advance in surgical treatment of achalasia was made by E. Heller[73] in 1913. He introduced an effective operation consisting of a vertical anterior myotomy extending from 2 cm above the constriction down over the cardia. This successful procedure, with minor variations, has stood the test of time. H. Plummer,[74] in 1908, used olive-tipped bougies over a swallowed string to open the tight cardia. Later he used a hydrostatic dilator[75] to effectively relieve the symptoms by rupturing the constricting circular muscle fibers in a manner somewhat like the Heller operation. This procedure could not be precisely controlled and resulted in a number of esophageal perforations.

Pathologic studies in 1925 by Rake[76] and Hurst in 1927[77] and others since then have described the degeneration of the ganglion cells of Auerbach's plexus as probably being the most likely cause of this condition. Why these changes occur is not known. Physiologic studies employing manometry, first reported by Kronecker and Meltzer in 1883,[55] were not duplicated for over half a century. Since World War II, there has been a physiologic approach with pressure studies by Kramer and Ingelfinger,[56] Pope,[78] Ellis,[79] and Code[80] who have shown the efficacy of the Heller operation.

■ SURGICAL TREATMENT OF CARCINOMA OF THE ESOPHAGUS

Because of the anatomic location of the esophagus as previously described, progress in treating esophageal cancer was slow, leaving the patients to be the most miserable of any cancer patients with death by slow starvation. In 1877 Czerny[27] successfully resected a carcinoma of the cervical esophagus after careful experimentation in animals. The patient lived for one year. In 1909 at Westminster Hospital in London, Arthur Evans[81] excised the pharynx, larynx, and cervical esophagus with a 24-year survival. The more accessible

cervical portion of the esophagus was the area where cancer was first attacked.

With the use of intratracheal anesthesia, Torek in 1913[82] was able to enter the chest and successfully resect the thoracic esophagus, pulling the cervical stump out onto the skin of the neck and performing the gastrostomy for feeding. Fourteen years later Grey Turner[83] resected the thoracic esophagus in a patient with carcinoma by the so-called cervicoabdominal approach, mobilizing the thoracic esophagus through cervical and abdominal incisions without opening the thorax. By connecting the cervical stump to the stomach with an anterothoracic skin tube, swallowing was achieved. This technique was revived by Orringer and Sloan[84] in 1978, an event which created quite a stir among thoracic surgeons. But it was the report of Adams and Phemister,[85] who resected the lower thoracic esophagus, replacing the esophagus with the stomach in 1938, that stirred up the most interest in this country. Unknown at that time was the fact that Oshawa[86] in 1933 had performed the same operation with survival in 8 out of 18 patients.

A great advance in the resection and replacement of the esophagus for cancer was the technique that was introduced by Richard Sweet[87] during World War II (Fig. 1–8). It had been repeatedly stated

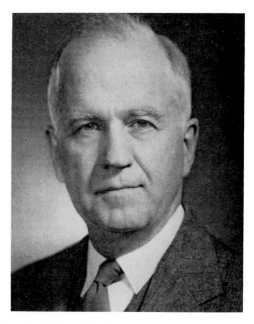

Figure 1–8. Richard H. Sweet was the first surgeon to divide the left gastric artery along with the short gastric vessels in order to mobilize the stomach as an esophageal replacement at the level of the arch of the aorta. At that time Garlock and others insisted that the stomach would die, as it was supplied by only the gastroepiploic vessels. Sweet opened the door to gastric replacement of the thoracic esophagus resected because of cancer. (From Churchill EC: J Thorac Cardiovasc Surg, 44:140, 1962.)

by Garloch and others that the division of the short gastric arteries and the left gastric artery of the stomach would not yield a viable stomach. However, Sweet showed that the stomach mobilized by the severing of the left gastric and short gastric arteries was viable, even when it was brought up to the arch of the aorta. Immediately after World War II, I had the privilege of studying this advanced technique under Dr. Sweet. In 1945 on returning to Southern California, I performed the first esophageal resections there with esophagogastrostomy and the first high thoracic gastric replacement.[88,89] Employing the Kocher Maneuver in 1947, I found it possible to mobilize the duodenum and place the stomach entirely in the chest.[90] Not until 1948, however, did I have a case referred to me of carcinoma of the cervical esophagus that lent itself to this procedure. In that year I performed a successful resection of the cervical and thoracic esophagus in a 66-year-old man with a subpharyngeal esophagogastrostomy.[91] This operation was the first in the West and certainly one of the first, if not the first, in this country. The patient recovered and swallowed well for 10 months following the procedure (Fig. 1–9A to D). This technique resulted in the removal of more cancer-bearing tissue than did the limited Wookey operation,[92] which did not include the resection of the thoracic esophagus and was prone to early recurrence. The one-stage replacement of the resected esophagus by the stomach was a great advance over the many-stage procedure and unsatisfactory results with antithoracic skin tubes.

Ivor Lewis[93] in 1946 introduced the right-sided thoracotomy to resect the thoracic esophagus and a laparotomy to free up the stomach for intrathoracic anastomosis. Ellis[94] reported a right-sided thoracic abdominal operation with gastric replacement. Both the small intestines and the large intestines have been used as esophageal replacement. Gastroesophagostomy has also been employed to bypass a nonresectable carcinoma to permit the patient to ingest food while the cancer is treated by radiation therapy.

Palliation of cancer of the esophagus is important because most of the patients are in the advanced stage when they are referred to the surgeon. Palliations must permit satisfactory ingestion of food for the patient with obstructing esophageal cancer, or it is not worth the effort. Gastrostomy dating back to the late 1800s merely prolonged the miserable existence and afforded poor palliation. The plastic Celestin tube[95] inserted through the obstructing carcinoma permits swallowing. We have found that this tube should be used only in the cardia, not in the cervical or upper thoracic portions, because of the danger of tracheal or bronchial perforation.[96] To improve the effects of external radiation in destroying cancerous tissue and permission of swallowing, we have combined this with the use of iridium-192 placed intraluminally with a specially constructed many-channeled tube.[87] Palliation from six to 48 months has been affected by this technique.

■ *Summary*

Progress of esophageal surgery, from the first successful repair of an esophagus in Egypt in 2500 BC until the end of the nineteenth century, was one of faltering steps. The more accessible cervical esophagus was attacked early in the seventeenth and eighteenth centuries for the removal of foreign bodies and repair of lacerations. However, it was the tremendous scientific progress in the nineteenth century that was the prolegomenon to the modern surgical approach to various esophageal diseases in the twentieth century. Both abdominal surgery and intrathoracic techniques, combatting the open pneumothorax, had to be mastered before the thoracic esophagus could be successfully treated. Rapid strides in World War II in thoracic surgery in general and esophageal surgery in particular paved the way for the advances made in the latter part of this century. Physiologic studies of the esophagus placed the surgery of this organ on a sound scientific basis. In replacing the resected esophagus, the stomach, with its excellent blood supply, was shown to be a very satisfactory substitute for the entire esophagus.

Thus, we have come full circle, and the esophagus without its mesentery and with its treacherous course in the mediastinum can now be attacked surgically, as were other portions of the gastrointestinal tract in the latter part of the nineteenth century. It has been the privilege of the author to have developed an interest in the treatment of esophageal diseases early in his career and so to have literally grown up with the development of surgery of the esophagus and thus had the opportunity to make modest contributions. The surgical historian has the responsibility of recording the salient achievements of the preceding ''toilers in the vineyard'' of surgery for the edification of present-day surgeons. Truly, we all have stood on the shoulders of giants. It is hoped that this brief résumé of the past will provide a meaningful historical background for the excellent chapters on surgery of the esophagus that follow.

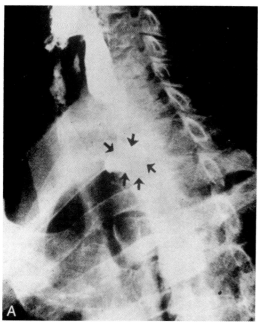

Figure 1–9. *A,* Cancer of the cervical esophagus as seen on a preoperative esophagogram, showing obstruction above the clavicles. The successful one stage total esophagotomy with subpharyngeal esophagogastrostomy performed by the author was the first in the West and possibly the first in the country. *B,* Author's technique. Left. Cervical incision anterior to the sternocleidomastoid muscle, and a thoracic incision over the sixth rib, for total resection of the esophagus for carcinoma of the cervical esophagus. Sterile draping of the left arm made it possible to move the arm to the most advantageous position for the cervical and thoracic exposures. Right. Exposure of upper mediastinum reveals an intrathoracic extension of the cervical esophagus—impossible to resect by the Wookey procedure, but readily excised by the combined exposure.

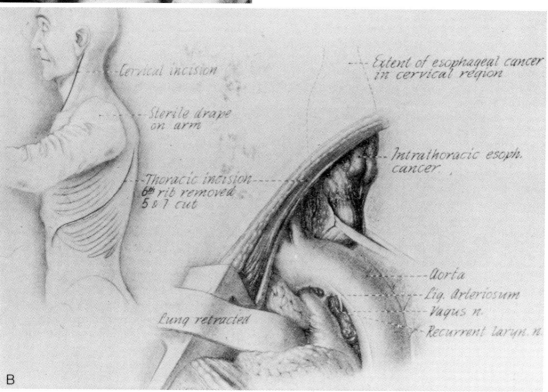

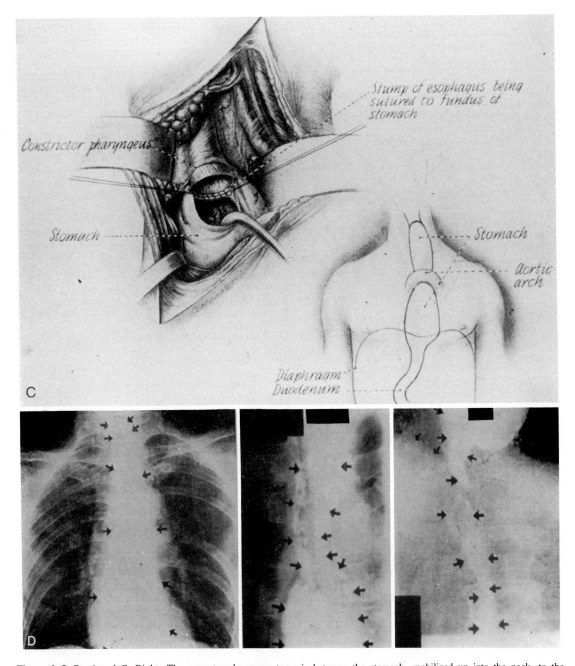

Figure 1–9 *Continued C,* Right. The open two layer anastomosis between the stomach, mobilized up into the neck, to the pharyngoesophageal junction in author's case. Left. Diagram of the esophageal replacement with the stomach nourished by the gastroepiploic vessels. The arch of the aorta may prevent some regurgitation from the stomach. Not shown is the Heineke-Mikulicz pyloroplasty. *D,* Left. Upper gastrointestinal roentgenograms following operation show wide open cervical anastomosis. Center. The arch of the aorta partially constricts the stomach. Right. The pylorus of the stomach lies in the chest. Excellent egress of barium from stomach to the duodenum is the result of a functioning pyloroplasty. By extensive mobilization of the Kocher maneuver, the duodenum is straight (author's case.)

■ REFERENCES

1. Breasted JH: The Edwin Smith Surgical Papyrus. Chicago, University of Chicago Press, 1930, pp 312–316.
2. Avenzoar (1162), quoted by Major RA in A History of Medicine. Springfield, Ill., Charles C Thomas, 1954, pp 252–254.
3. Wiseman R: Several chirurgical treatises. London, R. Royston, 1676.
4. Purmann MG: Chirurgia curiosa. London, D. Browne, R. Smith and T. Browne, 1706.
5. Stoffel, quoted by Hochberg LA in Thoracic Surgery before the 20th century. New York, Vantage Press, 1960.
6. Verduc JB: Traite des Operations de Chirurgie. Paris, L. d'Houry, 1701.
7. Goursaud and Roland: *In* Guattani: Essai sur l'oesophagotomie. Mem l'Acad Rou Chir, *3*:13, 1757.
8. Tevenget: Observations sur une maladie rare de l'oesophage. J Med Chir Pharm, *67*:254–257, 1786.
9. Vigardonne J: Quelques Propositions sur l'Oesophagotomie (thesis). Paris, 1805.
10. Colegrove BH: Extraction of a copper coin from the oesophagus. Boston Med Surg J, *56*:514–516, 1857.
11. Cheever DW: Two Cases of Oesophagotomy for Removal of Foreign Bodies with a History of the Operation. 2nd Ed. Boston, Jas. Campbell, 1868.
12. Arenlanos, Plater, quoted by Cheever DW: Oesophagotomy. First Med Surg Report, Boston City Hospital Medical and Surgical Reports, *1*:519–523, 1870.
13. Gross SD: American gastrostomy, oesophagostomy, internal oesophagotomy, combined oesophagotomy, oesophagectomy and retrograde divulsion in the treatment of stricture of the oesophagus. Am J Med Sci, *88*:58–69, 1884.
14. Variliaud: Observations sur un retrecissement de l'oesophage; et description d'un procede nouveau du citoyen boyer pour des sondes elastiques dans ce conduit. L'introduction. J Med Chir Pharm, *1*:139–150, 1801.
15. Lannelongue O: Observations avec quelques considerations pour servir a histoire de l'oesophagotomie interne. Mem Soc Chir Paris, *6*:547–560, 1867.
16. von Bergman E: Uber operationen am schlundrohre. Dtsch Med Wochenschr, *19*:605–621, 1833.
17. Abbe R: Relief of oesophageal stricture by a string saw. Ann Surg, *17*:489, 1893.
18. Woolsey G: The treatment of cicatricial strictures of the oesophagus by retrograde dilatation. Ann Surg, *21*:253, 1895.
19. Kussmaul A: Zur geschichte der oesophago und gastroskopie. Arch Klin Med, *6*:456, 1868.
20. MacKenzie M: A new oesophagoscope in disease of the gullet. Br Med J, *1*:813, 1881.
21. von Mikulicz J: Uber gastroskopie und oesophagoskopic. Wein Med Presse, *22*:1405, 1881.
22. Long C: An account of the first use of sulphuric ether as an anesthetic in surgical operations. South Med Surg, *5*:705–713, 1849.
23. Morton WTG: On the physiological effects of sulphuric ether and its superiority over chloroform. Boston, David Clapp, 1850.
24. Pasteur L: Etudes sur le vin. Paris, 1866.
25. Lister J: On the antiseptic principles in the practice of surgery. Lancet, *2*:353, 1867.
26. Roentgen K, quoted by Coolidge WD: A powerful roentgen ray tube with a pure electron discharge. Am J Roentgenol, *1*:115, 1913.
27. Czerny V: Neue operationen. Zentralb Chir, *4*:433–434, 1877.
28. Billroth T, quoted by Hurwitz A, Degenshein G in Milestones in Modern Surgery. New York, Paul B. Hoeber, 1958.
29. Cannon WB: The movements of the intestines studied by the means of roentgen rays. Am J Physiol, *6*:251, 1902.
30. Bliss AA: Foreign body (iron staple) in the oesophagus located by means of roentgen rays. Intern Med Mag, *6*:83, 1872.
31. Halsted WS: The treatment of wounds with a special reference to the value of the blood clot in the management of dead spaces. Johns Hopkins Hosp Rep, *2*:277, 1891.
32. Meltzer SJ, Auer J: Continuous respiration without respiratory movement. J Exp Med, *11*:622, 1909.
33. Graham EA, Bell RD: Open pneumothorax: Its relation to the treatment of acute empyema. Am J Med Sci, *156*:939, 1918.
34. Domagk G: Eine neue klasse von disinfektionsmitteln. Dtsch Med Wochenschr, *61*:829, 1935.
35. Flemming A: On the antibacterial action of cultures of penicillin with special reference to their use in the isolation of *B. influenzae*. Br J Exp Pathol, *10*:226. 1929.
36. Brewer LA III: Resuscitation and Preoperative Preparation. Surgery in World War II. Thoracic Surgery. Washington, DC, U.S. Government Printing Office, 1963, pp 237–259.
37. Brewer LA III: Emergency Measures. Surgery in World War II. Thoracic Surgery. Washington, DC, U.S. Government Printing Office, 1963, pp 213–218.
38. Brewer LA III: Diagnosis. Surgery in World War II. Thoracic Surgery. Washington, DC, U.S. Government Printing Office, 1963, pp 219–236.
39. Brewer LA III: Initial Wound Surgery. Surgery in World War II. Thoracic Surgery. Washington, DC, U.S. Government Printing Office, 1963, pp 269–297.
40. Brewer LA III: Long-term (1943–61) Follow-up Studies in Combat-incurred Thoracic Wounds. Surgery in World War II. Thoracic Surgery. Washington, DC, U.S. Government Printing Office, 1965, pp 441–527.
41. Brewer LA III, Burford TH: Special Types of Thoracic Wounds. Surgery in World War II. Thoracic Surgery. Washington, DC, U.S. Government Printing Office, 1963, pp 269–297.
42. Brewer LA III. The wet lung in war casualties. Ann Surg, *123*:343–361, 1946.
43. Brewer LA III: Respiration and respiratory treatment. A historical overview. Am J Surg, *138*:342, 1979.
44. Brewer LA III, Ferguson TB, Langston HT, Weiner JM: National Thoracic Surgery Manpower Study. Los Angeles, Cunningham Press, 1974.
45. Forward Surgery of the Severely Wounded. 2nd Auxiliary Surgical Group. 1942–1946. Report to the Surgeon General of United States Army Medical Corps.
46. Kay EB: Surgical lesions of the esophagus seen in an army thoracic surgery center. J Thorac Surg, *16*:207, 1947.
47. Barrett NR: Spontaneous perforation of the oesophagus: A review of the literature and report of three cases. Thorax, *1*:48–70, 1946.
48. Barrett NR: Report of a case of spontaneous perforation of the eosophagus successfully treated by operation. Br J Surg, *35*:216, 1947.
49. Brewer LA III, Mulder GA, Stiles QR, Carter R: Unpublished data.
50. Paré A (1580), cited by Harrington SW: Diaphragmatic hernia. Part 2. Arch Surg, *16*:386–415, 1928.
51. Potempski P: Nuovo processo operativo per la riduzione cruenta della ernie diaframmatiche de trauma e per la suture delle ferite del diaframma. Bull Reale Accad Med Roma, *15*:191–192, 1889.
52. Hedbloom CA: Diaphragmatic hernia. Ann Intern Med, *8*:156–176, 1934.
53. Harrington SW, Kirklin BR: Clinical and radiological man-

ifestations and surgical treatment of diaphragmatic hernia with a review of 13 cases. Radiology, *30*:147, 1938.

54. Winklestein A: Peptic esophagitis (a new clinical entity). JAMA, *104*:906, 1935.

55. Kronecker H, Meltzer S: Der Schluckmechanismus, seine Erregung und seine Hemmung. Arch F. Physiol Suppl, 328–362, 1883.

56. Kramer P, Ingelfinger FJ II: Cardiospasm, a generalized disorder of esophageal motility. Am J Med, *7*:174–179, 1949.

57. Bernstein A: Hiatal hernia—a frequent and clinically important condition. Univ W Ont M5. *17*:159, 1947.

58. Bernstein LM, Baker LA: A clinical test for esophagitis. Gastroenterology, *34*:1, 1961.

59. Durston W: A narrative of a monstrous birth in Plymouth, October 22, 1670; together with the anatomical observations, taken thereupon by William Durston, Doctor in Physick, and communicated to Dr. Tim Cler. Philos Trans (Lond), *5*:2096–2098, 1670.

60. Gibson T: Anatomy of Humane Bodies Epitomized. 5th ed. London, printed by T. W. for Awnsham and John Churchill at the Black Swan in Peter-Noster-Row, and sold by Timothy Childe at the White-Hart, the West end of St. Paul's Church Yard, 1697.

61. Richter HM: Congenital atresia of the oesophagus: An operation designed for its cure, with a report of two cases operated upon by the author. Surg Gynecol Obstet, *17*:397–402, 1913.

62. Mixter CG, quoted by Gage M, Ochsner A: The surgical treatment of tracheoesophageal fistula in the newborn. Ann Surg, *103*:725, 1936.

63. Ladd WE: The surgical treatment of esophageal atresia and tracheoesophageal fistulas. N Engl J Med, *230*:625–637, 1944.

64. Lanman TH: Congenital atresia of the esophagus: A study of thirty-two cases. Arch Surg, *41*:1060–1083, 1940.

65. Haight C, Towsley HA: Congenital atresia of the esophagus with tracheoesophageal fistula: Extrapleural ligation of fistula and end-to-end anastomosis of esophageal segments. Surg Gynecol Obstet, *76*:672–688, 1943.

66. Haight C: Some observations on esophageal atresia and tracheoesophageal atresia of congenital origin. J Thorac Surg, *34*:141, 1957.

67. Shaw R: Surgical correction of congenital atresia of the esophagus with tracheosophageal fistula. J Thorac Surg, *9*:213–219, 1939.

68. Leven NL: Congenital atresia of the esophagus with tracheoesophageal fistula: Report of successful extrapleural ligation of fistulous communication and cervical esophagostomy. J Thorac Surg, 10:648–657, 1941.

69. Willis T: Pharmaceutic Rationalis: Sive Diatriba de Medicamentorum; Operationibus in Humano Corpore. London, Hagae-Comitis, 1974.

70. Russell JC: Diagnosis and treatment of spasmodic stricture of the oesophagus. Br Med J, *1*:1450–1451, 1898.

71. von Mikulicz J: Zur pathologie und therapie des cardiospasmus. Dtsch Med Wochenschr, *30*:17–19, 50–54, 1904.

72. Reisinger G: Ueber die operative behandlung der erweitrung des oesophagus. Verh Dtsch Ges Chir, *36*:86–88, 1907.

73. Heller E: Extramukose cardioplatik beim chronischen cardiospasmus mit dilation des oesophagus. Mitt Grenz Med Chir, *27*:141–149, 1914.

74. Plummer HS: Cardiospasm with a report of forty cases. JAMA, *51*:549–554, 1908.

75. Plummer HS: Diffuse dilatation of the esophagus without anatomic stenosis (cardiospasm): A report of 91 cases. JAMA, *58*:3013, 1912.

76. Rake GW: Annular muscular hypertrophy of oesophagus: Achalasia of cardia without oesophageal dilatation. Guy's Hosp Rep, *76*:145–152, 1926.

77. Hurst AF, Rake GW: Achalasia of the cardia (so-called cardiospasm). Q J Med, *23*:491–508, 1930.

78. Pope CE II: A dynamic test of sphincter strength: Its application to the lower esophageal sphincter. Gastroenterology, *52*:779–786, 1967.

79. Ellis FH, Olsen AM: Achalasia of the esophagus. Philadelphia, W.B. Saunders, 1969, p 45.

80. Code CF: Physiological studies. *In* Ellis FH Jr, Olsen AM (Eds.): Achalasia of the Esophagus. Philadelphia, W.B. Saunders, 1969, p 45.

81. Evans A: Rubber oesophagus. Br J Surg, *20*:388, 1933.

82. Torek F: The first successful case of resection of the thoracic portion of the oesophagus for carcinoma. Surg Gynecol Obstet, *16*:614–617, 1913.

83. Turner GG: The Esophagus. London, Cassell and Company, 1946, pp 81–82.

84. Orringer MB, Sloan H: Esophagectomy without thoracotomy. J Thorac Cardiovasc Surg, *76*:643–654, 1978.

85. Adams WE, Phemister DB: Carcinoma of the lower esophagus. Report of a successful resection and esophagogastrostomy. J Thoracic Surg, *7*:621–632, 1938.

86. Oshawa T: The surgery of the oesophagus. Jap Chir, *10*:604–695, 1933.

87. Sweet RH: Surgical management of cancer of the midesophagus. Preliminary report. N Engl J Med, *233*:1–7, 1945.

88. Brewer LA III, Dolley FS: The surgical treatment of carcinoma of the thoracic esophagus. The technique of transthoracic thoracolaparotomy with esophageal resection and high esophagogastrostomy. West J Surg Obstet Gynecol, *56*:517–528, 1948.

89. Brewer LA III, Dolley FS: Carcinoma of the thoracic esophagus: A discussion of early diagnosis and surgical treatment. Calif Med, *71*:1–6, 1949.

90. Brewer LA III: Surgical treatment of carcinoma of the cervical and upper thoracic esophagus. West J Surg Obstet Gynecol, *60*:1–12, 1952.

91. Brewer LA III: One-stage resection of carcinoma of the cervical esophagus with subpharyngeal esophagogastrostomy. Ann Surg, *130*:9–20, 1949.

92. Wookey H: The surgical treatment of carcinoma of the hypopharynx and the oesophagus. Br J Surg, *35*:255–266, 1948.

93. Lewis I: The surgical treatment of carcinoma of the oesophagus with special reference to a new operation for growths in the middle third. Br J Surg, *34*:18–31, 1946.

94. Ellis FH Jr: Treatment of carcinoma of the esophagus and cardia. Mayo Clin Proc, *35*:653–663, 1960.

95. Celestine LR: Permanent intubation in inoperable cancer of the oesophagus and cardia: A new tube. Ann R Coll Surg Engl, *25*:165–170, 1959.

96. Carter PR, Hinshaw DB: Use of the celestin indwelling plastic tube for inoperable carcinoma of esophagus and cardia. Surg Gynecol Obstet, *117*:641–644, 1963.

97. George FW III: Radiation management in esophageal cancer. With review of intraesophageal radioactive iridium treatment in 24 patients. Am J Surg, *139*:796–809, 1980.

2

Anatomy of the Esophagus

C. Dale Mercer ■ Lucius D. Hill

The primary functions of the esophagus are propelling food and fluid into the stomach while preventing reflux of gastric juice. The esophagus also allows for belching, regurgitation, and vomiting. A discussion of the anatomic features which are important to these functions forms the basis of this chapter.

The important anatomic structures which allow the esophagus to perform its work are (1) the upper esophageal sphincter, (2) the musculature of the body of the esophagus, (3) the lower esophageal sphincter, (4) the gastroesophageal valve at the angle of His, and (5) the posterior fixation of the esophagus.

A basic review of the relationships of the esophagus as well as the blood supply and innervation is essential to the understanding of the organ. This information is included in this chapter.

The esophagus is a musculomucosal canal extending from the pharynx to the stomach. It begins as a continuation of the pharynx at the lower border of the cricoid cartilage, which is marked by the lower border of the cricopharyngeus muscle and lies at the level of the sixth cervical vertebra. The esophagus descends along the front of the vertebral column through the superior and posterior mediastinum, passing through the diaphragm and entering the abdomen to end at the lower esophageal sphincter opposite the eleventh thoracic vertebra. The squamocolumnar junction does not mark the termination of the esophagus, for this junction can migrate in pathologic conditions, such as Barrett's esophagus. The esophagus is indented during its course by several landmarks familiar to the endoscopist: (1) the cricopharyngeus muscle or upper esophageal sphincter and the cricoid cartilage marking the esophageal inlet, the narrowest portion of the esophagus, (2) the aortic arch indenting the esophagus on its left side at the level of the third or fourth vertebra, (3) the left mainstem bronchus, and (4) the lower esophageal sphincter. The esophagus is a midline structure deviating to the left at the thoracic inlet, then returning to midline. The lower esophagus inclines again to the left, entering the esophageal hiatus of the diaphragm.

The esophagus may be divided conveniently into the cervical, thoracic, and abdominal portions. The cervical esophagus lies posterior to the membranous portion of the trachea. In the neck the esophagus projects to the left in relation to the thyroid gland; posteriorly it rests on the longus colli musculature and the fascia overlying the vertebral column; laterally the common carotid arteries are present. The recurrent laryngeal nerves lie in the groove between the trachea and esophagus bilaterally. The thoracic esophagus continues in contact with the prevertebral fascia posteriorly and the membranous portion of the trachea anteriorly to the level of the tracheal bifurcation at the fifth thoracic vertebra.

At this level the left mainstem bronchus crosses in front of the esophagus and indents it, as does the aortic arch passing over the mainstem bronchus. The esophagus descends on the right side of the aorta to the level of the eighth or ninth thoracic vertebra, where it passes in front of the aorta, reaching the esophageal hiatus at the level of the tenth vertebra. In the posterior mediastinum it is related to the pericardium anteriorly and the prevertebral fascia posteriorly. On the left side in the superior mediastinum lie the left subclavian artery, aortic arch, thoracic duct, and the left parietal pleura. On the right side, it is in relation to the parietal pleura and azygos vein. The vagus nerves disperse below the tracheal bifurcation, forming the esophageal plexus, giving branches to the esophagus and tracheobronchial tree. The right posterior and left anterior vagus nerves coalesce from this plexus and descend along the esophagus to the cardia of the stomach.

Included in the thoracic segment of the esophagus are the ampulla and vestibule, which initially were described in 1950. In our 50 cadaver dissections the ampulla is identified when the esophagus and stomach are distended with alcohol, saline, or formalin as a dilatation of the terminal part of the esophagus. It can also be demonstrated in the living human with fluoroscopy during a barium swallow. The ampulla is 2 to 3 cm in length and varies in shape but is intimately related to the lower esophageal sphincter. The gastroesophageal vestibule is also easily seen in the distended esophagus, and in the normal subject it lies in the diaphragmatic hiatus, being limited superiorly by the lower esophageal sphincter (Fig. 2–1).

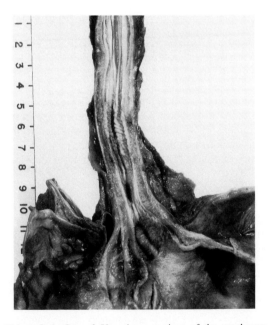

Figure 2–1. One of 50 cadaver sections of the esophagus: stomach, phrenoesophageal fascial complex, and diaphragm are removed in toto. This shows the relationship of the gastroesophageal vestibule, lower esophageal sphincter, and squamocolumnar junction. Note that the vestibule is visible as a dilatation of the distal esophagus and that the sphincter is two to three times thicker than the musculature of the esophagus.

The short segment of esophagus present within the abdomen extends from below the diaphragm to the junction of the esophagus and stomach. The abdominal esophagus lies posterior to the left lobe of the liver and anterior to the crura of the diaphragm. On the left side the medial aspect of the spleen may be in close proximity to the esophagus. This segment of esophagus has received a good deal of attention because it is the only portion of the esophagus surrounded by a positive intra-abdominal pressure; this is in contrast to the thoracic esophagus, which is surrounded by negative intrathoracic pressure. The positive intra-abdominal pressure is said to augment closing of the sphincter and maintaining the abdominal portion of the esophagus in a closed state except during deglutition. More experimentation is needed to clarify the role of the intra-abdominal esophagus. Careful examination of the intra-abdominal esophagus shows it to be very short, 1.5 cm. There is no convincing objective measurement in the living human that the intra-abdominal esophagus plays a role in the antireflux mechanism.

■ *Upper Esophageal Sphincter*

The muscle fibers of the upper esophageal sphincter have been of interest clinically because of the occurrence of pharyngoesophageal diverticula but have been difficult to study physiologically because of the rapidity with which contraction and relaxation occur. The pharyngoesophageal segment is the junction of the pharynx and cervical esophagus and is marked by the cricopharyngeal muscle which is the inferior part of the lower constrictor of the pharynx. The cricopharyngeus originates at the posterolateral sides of the cricoid cartilage covering the posterior aspect of the pharyngoesophageal junction. Unlike the pharyngeal constrictors above, this muscle forms a continuous muscle band without a median raphe. The location of this bundle of fibers can be recognized, both externally and at the time of esophagoscopy, but inferiorly its fibers blend in with the esophageal wall.[2] The muscle is of great importance for the normal functioning of the esophagus, as it constitutes the upper esophageal sphincter.

Relaxation and contraction of the upper sphincter occur with normal deglutition and initiate the primary peristaltic wave in the esophagus. Between the ascending oblique muscle fibers in the upper end of the esophagus, a weak area exists posteriorly, Killian's triangle.[3] This weak area proximal to the cricopharyngeus muscle is the site of origin of pharyngoesophageal diverticula.

■ *Body of the Esophagus*

The musculature of the body of the esophagus is responsible for esophageal peristalsis and, most important, for clearance of gastric content from the esophagus when reflux occurs. The longitudinal muscle fibers originate from the cricoesophageal tendon. In the upper third of the esophagus or 4 to 8 cm from the cricopharyngeus, the musculature is striated. At around 8 cm the musculature is mixed, and the lower third of the esophagus contains only smooth muscle.

The muscle fibers do not follow the axis of the esophagus. It should be recalled that the esophagus rotates, as the stomach does, 90 degrees to the right so that the musculature is spiral.[4] The longitudinal muscles interdigitate with the inner circular and elliptical muscle fibers and in fact interdigitate with fibers from the trachea, the left mainstem bronchus, and the pleura.

The inner muscle layer of the esophagus is thicker than the outer layer, and although it is often designated as circular, it in essence is mainly elliptical and forms a syncytium rather than a regular or orderly inner circular layer. It is this elliptical musculature that forms a syncytium of fibers that is responsible for peristalsis of the esophagus. Lerche[1] and Laimer[5] both noted that the circular muscle fibers vary in their arrangement in different segments of the esophagus. The musculature is elliptical in the upper third, with the highest point of the ellipse being posterior. They become truly circular in the middle portion of the esophagus and in the lower portion of the esophagus the musculature again becomes elliptical, with the highest point being anterior. Particularly in the lower third, where the musculature is thicker, the inner layer is truly a syncytium of muscle bundles that run elliptically, obliquely, and occasionally longitudinally. At the gastroesophageal junction, bracket-like fibers have been described by Lerche and confirmed by Liebermann-Meffert et al.[6]

Kaufman et al.[4] found three types of muscle fiber arrangement: spiral, winding, and screw-like. It is this elliptical and screw-like arrangement that has been cited as giving the esophagus its power to produce strong peristaltic waves that propel food aborally.

■ *The Gastroesophageal Junction*

Esophageal Hiatus ■ Numerous studies have clarified the anatomy of the esophageal hiatus.[7–9]

Eleven different anatomic arrangements of the musculature of the hiatus have been identified, but the two most common types account for 80 per cent of the variants.[17] In the first type the right crus contributes all the fibers that form the esophageal hiatus. The right margin of the hiatus is formed by the right crus rising from the anterolateral aspect of the second to the fourth lumbar vertebrae and passing separately anteriorly to insert in the central tendon. The left margin is formed by muscles with similar origins which pass posteriorly and superiorly to the right bundle, circle the esophagus on its left, and insert into the central tendon. The second type is virtually identical to the first except that a small bit of muscle arises from the left crus of the diaphragm and passes posterior to the esophagus and inserts indefinitely into the posterior aspect of the muscle forming the right margin of the hiatus. The other variations occur in patients with a more prominent left crus of the diaphragm and variable participation in the anatomy of the esophageal hiatus.

The esophageal hiatus is innervated by both phrenic nerves. Even though the left margin of the hiatus most commonly originates from the right crus, it is innervated by the left or ipsilateral phrenic nerve. The left inferior phrenic artery lies 1.5 to 2 cm from the hiatal rim. The right inferior phrenic artery lies at a greater distance from the hiatus beneath the foramen of the inferior vena cava.

Aortic Hiatus, Median Arcuate Ligament, Preaortic Fascia, and Phrenoesophageal Ligaments ■ The area about the preaortic fascia and the median arcuate ligament is seldom visualized by surgeons. In fact, it is possible for experienced surgeons to perform a large amount of upper abdominal surgery without dissecting and identifying the median arcuate ligament. Indeed, some surgeons state that the median arcuate ligament does not exist.

In some dissections, the median arcuate ligament appears entirely muscular, but if the muscular fibers of the crura of the diaphragm are dissected away, there is a tough plate of fibrous tissue lying anterior to the aorta and extending upward into the thorax. The aortic hiatus, lying at the level of the twelfth thoracic vertebra, is formed by the crura of the diaphragm and the ligamentous continuation of the crura which blend with the anterior spinal ligaments of the vertebral column. The right crus is larger and longer than the left and arises from the anterior surfaces of the bodies of the intervetebral fibrocartilage of the upper three lumbar vertebrae, and the left crus arises from the corresponding part of the upper two only. The medial tendinous margins of the crura pass forward and medially and meet in the midline, forming an arch across the front of the aorta. This creates an osseoaponeurotic aortic hiatus lying between the vertebral column and the diaphragm. The left celiac ganglion is formed about the celiac trunk within the aortic hiatus and is attached to the diaphragm as well as the celiac artery and the aorta, thus filling the aortic hiatus.

When both the extensive lymphatic network and the sympathetic and parasympathetic nerves are dissected away, the anterior margin of the aortic hiatus, termed the median arcuate ligament, is identified as a well-defined, exceedingly tough structure. A finger placed beneath the aortic hiatus and passed upward demonstrates clearly that the preaortic fascia extends behind the hiatus and continues into the thorax for a variable distance above the diaphragm (Fig. 2–2).

The inferior phrenic arteries arise from the lateral aspect of the aorta and pass into the diaphragm within the aortic hiatus. These small arteries should be borne in mind because they may produce troublesome bleeding if divided within the aortic hiatus. There are usually no arterial branches off the anterior aorta in the midline, so dissection in this plane can be performed without the hazard of disrupting important blood vessels or any other structures.

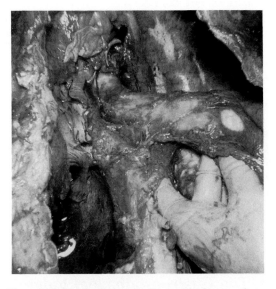

Figure 2–2. The median arcuate ligament is shown as the anterior margin of the aortic hiatus. Note the celiac axis at the level of the aortic hiatus. The posterior phrenoesophageal ligament is tacked to the median arcuate ligament and the preaortic fascia as it would be in the posterior fixation and sphincter calibration antireflux procedure (Hill repair). The esophagus is visualized with the anterior and lateral portions of the diaphragm cut away with only the posterior attachment holding it in place.

■ *Posterior Fixation of the Esophagus*

A review of the embryology of the gastrointestinal tract shows that the entire gut is fixed posteriorly by a dorsal mesentery. This is equally true for the esophagus, which in the normal patient is fixed to the preaortic phrenoesophageal ligament. This maintains the intra-abdominal position of the gastroesophageal junction and gives a segment of intra-abdominal esophagus as well as fixing the lower esophageal sphincter beneath the diaphragm. This posterior fixation represents the prime attachment for the esophagogastric junction. It is this ligament alone that maintains the esophagogastric junction in its usual intra-abdominal position in patients with true paraesophageal hernias in which the entire stomach may be rolled up into the mediastinum. In this setting the anterolateral phrenoesophageal compartments are grossly attenuated and form the sac of the hernia. pH and hydrostatic esophageal pressure studies show normal fixation and normal function of the lower esophageal sphincter in these individuals.

Other structures have been identified by various authors as fixators of the esophagogastric junction. The left gastric vascular pedicle has been termed a "tether of the stomach."[10] However, cadaver dissections demonstrate clearly that division of the left gastric pedicle plus the mesentery of the lesser curvature of the stomach does not allow herniation of the stomach through the diaphragmatic hiatus. The right gastric artery and pyloric fixation have also been proposed as fixation points of the esophagogastric junction.[10] Similar cadaver work reveals that fixation about the pylorus is exceedingly mobile and does not prevent herniation. The posterior aspect of the left lobe of the liver is closely opposed to the anterior wall of the abdominal segment of the esophagus and has been credited in maintaining the esophagus in position. However, there are no attachments of this "liver tunnel" to the esophagus and this also does not contribute to esophageal fixation. Removal of all these factors allows for only a slight increase in mobility of the esophagus because the only remaining structure, the phrenoesophageal fascial complex, firmly fixes the esophagus posteriorly to the preaortic fascia.

Laimer, in 1883, was one of the first to draw attention to the "fixation apparatus" of the esophagus and diaphragm.[5] More recent descriptions of the phrenoesophageal membrane have drawn attention to the importance of this membrane and the role it plays in the formation of hiatal hernia.[11–14]

■ *Phrenoesophageal Membrane*

The phrenoesophageal membrane is a complex structure consisting of peritoneal reflections from the undersurface of the diaphragm. These reflections form a gastrophrenic ligament to the left of the esophagus and are continuous to the right of the esophagus with the gastrohepatic ligament. Posteriorly the peritoneum is continued directly onto the crura of the diaphragm. External to the peritoneum is a varying amount of preperitoneal fat. Deep in the preperitoneal fat lies the phrenoesophageal ligament, which is a continuation of the transversalis fascia from the undersurface of the diaphragm. In the hiatus, this structure contains numerous elastic fibers, especially in younger individuals. From its reflection off the undersurface of the diaphragm, this ligament divides into ascending and descending fibers extending upward for varying lengths, enmeshing in the wall of the esophagus and becoming anchored among the muscle layers. The elastic fibers of the descending part of the membrane extend downward, enmeshing the fat globules within the phrenoesophageal membrane in what is referred to as the subdiaphragmatic fat ring surrounding the esophagus at the hiatus.[1,13] These fibers then pass onto the lower portion of the abdominal esophagus and the cardia of the stomach, anchoring to the muscle fibers of the esophagus and the cardia.

The anterior and lateral parts of the phrenoesophageal complex are thin and mobile. Indeed, when all the phrenoesophageal complex except the posterior aspect is cut away and the diaphragm removed entirely, the esophagogastric junction and cardia of the stomach remain anchored posteriorly by fibroelastic bands passing from the esophageal wall to the preaortic fascia and the median arcuate ligament. Cadaver dissections and clinical demonstrations indicate that the principal point of attachment of the esophagus is posterior.[15] However, when the posterior portion of the membrane fails and becomes attenuated, the patient then has a true sliding hiatus hernia that is analogous to the failure of the transversalis fascia in an inguinal hernia. The pleural reflections form the superior or cephalad portion of the phrenoesophageal membrane passing from the diaphragm to the esophagus.

Lower Esophageal Sphincter ■ The existence of an anatomic sphincter in the terminal esophagus has been debated for the past 50 years. Studies denying the existence of this sphincter,[10,16,17] when scrutinized carefully, are poorly documented, and in fact one author[16] describes the anatomic presence of the sphincter and then discounts it entirely. Studies indicating that the sphincter exists have been published,[18–21] but that of Lerche[1] carefully documents with anatomic dissections the musculature of the terminal esophagus. We have performed 50 cadaver dissections examining the esophagus in both fresh and fixed states as well as collapsed and distended specimens. In all specimens, carefully examined both with a dissecting microscope and by conventional light microscopy, we were able to demonstrate the presence of an anatomic sphincter. This sphincter is unlike the pyloric sphincter in that it is not a short, thick contraction ring but is rather an elongated fusiform thickening of the terminal esophagus above the vestibule. Below this there is a slight thinning of the circular musculature within the vestibule itself and again a thickened ring at the cardioesophageal junction below.

It is exceedingly difficult to include all this thickening on a single microscopic field. Only by coiling the gastroesophageal junction can the entire area be included in a single field[16]; otherwise, the thickening of the circular musculature goes unappreciated, and the observer does not have circular musculature of the body of the esophagus for comparison. Our work and that of others[22] leaves no doubt as to the presence of an anatomic sphincter, which can be seen grossly as an increase in the circular musculature extending over 2.5 to 3 cm of the distal esophagus.

The meticulous dissections of Liebermann-Meffert et al.[6] show clearly the presence of a gastroesophageal ring (GER). This GER is the site of maximal thickness of the muscularis and is located at the fold transition line where the longitudinal esophageal folds meet the gastric folds. The muscle fibers composing the GER are not circular; rather, they are semicircular on the lesser curvature. At the greater curve the semicircular fibers of the GER interlace within the oblique gastric fibers which make up the collar sling. Our findings support the presence of the GER, but in addition, our cadaver dissections support the presence of a thickening of the musculature of the distal esophagus. These fibers may be expected to contract in a circular manner. There is ample physiologic evidence to support the efficiency of this sphincter, which will be discussed in Chapter 9.

■ *The Gastroesophageal Valve and Angle of His*

The valve created by the angle of His on the greater curvature side of the esophagogastric junction has been the subject of much research and discussion. As early as 1951 Allison[23] believed that the value was important in preventing reflux. Dornhorst et al.,[24] Lortat-Jacob et al.,[25] and Guiseffi et al. in 1954,[26] along with Barrett,[27] all demonstrated that there is a valve enhanced by the collar-sling muscle fibers of the stomach. Other workers since then have been unable to demonstrate a flap valve at the gastroesophageal (GE) junction. In the textbook *Surgery of the Esophagus,* Postlethwaite concludes the discussion on the flap valve and angle of His by stating, ''there is no convincing evidence to support the role of a flap valve in antireflux operations.''

We have demonstrated in cadavers[28] with no esophageal disease that there is a measurable pressure gradient across the GE junction which requires 7 to 15 cm of water pressure in the stomach before reflux occurs. By depressing the fundus of the stomach to approximately 45 degrees, the angle of His becomes obtuse, the valve is eliminated, and the introitus of the esophagus is converted into a funnel. Upon elimination of the valve, reflux occurs, and the gradient across the GE junction is eliminated. Because there is no sphincter action in the cadaver, the valve appears to be the only mechanism responsible for the demonstrable gradient across the GE junction in cadavers.

When viewed through the wall of the stomach with an endoscope or through a gastrostomy in the living patient, the valve is seen as a flat mucosal leaf that closes against the lesser curvature. By depressing the fundus in the living patient, the valve can be eliminated. Division of the posterior attachment of the GE junction in the cadaver allows the sphincter to slide into the posterior mediastinum and eliminates the gastroesophageal angle. This also eliminates the gradient across the GE junction and allows reflux.

Whereas many workers have indicated that the sphincter is the only barrier to reflux, others have stressed the role of the valve; McLaren in 1963 could demonstrate no relation between gastroesophageal reflux and sphincter pressure. Others, including Clark and Haddad, and our laboratory, have found a definite correlation between resting sphincter pressure and reflux. The sphincter generates pressures up to 100 mm Hg. The barrier can withstand pressures much greater than this. Indeed, under normal conditions a 72 kg person can stand on the abdomen of another person without inducing reflux!

While controversy rages between the group favoring the valve mechanism and those who favor the sphincter, the mature view appears to be that both the sphincter and the valve, along with the phrenoesophageal membrane and the diaphragm, all play a role in maintaining gastroesophageal competence. We, along with others, have shown

clearly that elimination of the valve by depression of the cardia produces reflux in the cadaver. If the posterior attachment of the gastroesophageal junction is lost, the gastroesophageal junction is displaced into the posterior mediastinum and the gastroesophageal valve is lost, which allows reflux. In the paraesophageal hernia, and even in a patient with a large hiatal hernia, if there is a paraesophageal component with maintenance of the valve, the gastroesophageal junction may remain competent.

Current antireflux operations appear to both raise the sphincter pressure and recreate the flap valve. The Hill procedure produces a demonstrable flap valve that can be shown radiographically and can be seen with retroflexion of the endoscope. This is clearly demonstrated in the chapter on surgery of hiatal hernia. The modern concept therefore is shown in the composite illustration showing both the gastroesophageal valve and the musculature at the GE junction, which creates both the anatomic and physiologic sphincter demonstrable in the living human as the high pressure zone at the junction of the esophagus and stomach (Fig. 2–3). This composite anatomic and physiologic view of the GE junction brings together the voluminous work done to demonstrate both the valve and the sphincter. Our studies indicate that the loss of either the sphincter or the valve impairs the competence of the GE junction against the reflux. A new operation

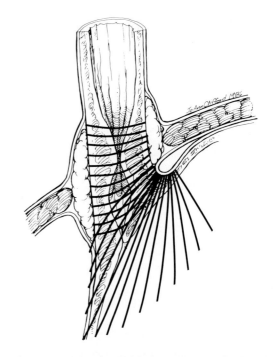

Figure 2–3. Synthesis. The gastroesophageal valve and the lower esophageal sphincter complex together with the posterior attachment of the gastroesophageal junction and the phrenoesophageal membrane make up the antireflux barrier.

based on fixing the valve described in Chapter 9 for hiatal hernia and esophagitis has been highly successful in selected cases in preventing reflux.

■ Arterial Blood Supply of the Esophagus

The esophagus receives a variable but segmental blood supply but with extensive collateralization.[28] The arteries to the cervical esophagus are fairly constant and consist of branches from the inferior thyroid artery, a branch of the subclavian artery. Other accessory vessels may rarely be derived from the common carotid, subclavian, vertebral, ascending pharyngeal, superficial cervical, and costocervical trunks.

The intrathoracic portion of the esophagus receives branches from (1) the aorta, (2) bronchial arteries, (3) the aortic arch, (4) intercostal arteries, (5) the internal mammary artery, and (6) the carotid artery. Aortic branches are variable, consisting of two unpaired vessels entering the esophagus posteriorly and dividing into ascending and descending branches which anastomose with branches from the inferior thyroid and bronchial arteries. One to three unpaired bronchial arteries supply the esophagus by entering at the tracheal bifurcation. Additional collateral branches arise from the aortic arch, intercostal arteries, internal mammary artery, and carotid arteries so that the nutrient arteries are not end vessels.

The abdominal esophagus receives its blood supply principally from branches of the left gastric and left inferior phrenic arteries. These latter vessels arise from the aorta, supplying the crura of the diaphragm and then entering the abdominal portion of the esophagus, anastomosing with the left hepatic or splenic arteries and occasionally directly from the celiac axis.

The segmental nature of the arterial blood supply to the esophagus suggests that extensive surgical mobilization of the esophagus without regard to its blood supply may result in ischemic complications. Cadaver injection studies confirm these findings.[30]

■ Venous Drainage of the Esophagus

Similar to the arterial supply, the venous drainage of the esophagus is also variable. Venous drainage commences as an intrinsic submucosal plexus of veins dispersed through the esophagus. Branches from this plexus pierce the muscle layers and form a venous plexus on the external surface of the esophagus (extrinsic veins).[31] Tributaries from this plexus drain in the neck, into the inferior thyroid vein, and then the innominate vein. In the thoracic esophagus the venous plexus empties into the azygos system, the vertebral veins, and the hemiazygos, and in the upper portion into the innominate veins. The tributaries from the abdominal portion of the esophagus drain into the inferior phrenic and left gastric veins. The left gastric branch drains into the portal system, whereas the inferior phrenic branches communicate freely with both the portal system and the inferior vena cava.

Communication between the portal system and the esophageal venous plexus by way of the inferior phrenic and coronary vessels represents a collateral of the portal venous system which in the event of portal obstruction allows the increased pressure to be reflected into the esophageal plexus. The elevated pressure on the submucosal plexus of veins, especially in the distal esophagus, produces varicosities.

■ Lymphatic Drainage of the Esophagus

Contrary to the arterial supply and venous drainage of the esophagus, the lymphatic drainage is not segmental.[32] A dense network of lymphatic vessels present in the mucosa and submucosa coalesces forming a lymphatic plexus. The forward lymph flow, as shown with injection of contrast medium, is seen to be about six times that of transverse spread and is predominantly longitudinal. In addition to the mucosal and submucosal plexus, there are a few vessels in the muscular layers as well as following vessels on the outside of the esophagus.

Owing to extensive collaterals, there may be considerable variation in the eventual drainage points for the esophageal lymphatics. The primary drainage of the cervical esophagus is by way of the cervical lymph nodes, which drain the trachea and esophagus and empty into the internal jugular nodes and then directly into the thoracic duct. The thoracic esophagus is drained by both superior mediastinal, peribronchial, hilar, and paraesophageal nodes. The lymphatics of the abdominal esophagus drain into left gastric nodes of the stomach and then into the celiac nodes. These nodes in turn empty into the cisterna chyli of the thoracic duct. The free communication of all these nodal groups with posterior mediastinal, intercostal, and internal mammary nodes and those about the trachea, bronchi, and pericardium allows passage of tumor cells to areas remote from the esophagus. Thus, the surgical importance of lymphatic drainage of the esophagus is quite apparent.

▪ Innervation of the Esophagus

The esophagus is supplied by both the vagus parasympathetic and sympathetic nerves. The vagus parasympathetic supply is of primary importance. The vagus fibers intercommunicate with filaments from the paravertebral sympathetic trunk and its branches, making innervation of the esophagus mixed sympathetic and parasympathetic in nature. The vagus nerves descend into the superior mediastinum, giving branches to the esophagus at the tracheal bifurcation. The vagus nerves arborize to form the esophageal plexus. This plexus gives off branches to the tracheobronchial tree and surrounding viscera, ultimately coalescing at a variable distance above the hiatus into the two major vagal trunks—the left anterior vagus and the right posterior vagus. The posterior branch passes down in the posterior part of the hiatus to the celiac plexus. The anterior branches pass along the stomach innervating the fundus, cardia, and antrum and supplying a large hepatic branch to the liver.

The cervical esophagus receives innervation from the recurrent laryngeal nerves in addition to variable elements from the main vagus nerves. In the thorax, the upper third of the esophagus receives filaments from the recurrent nerves and from both vagus nerves.

The intrinsic innervation of the esophagus is effected through the enteric plexuses similar to the remainder of the gastrointestinal tract. These are composed of ganglion cells lying between the layers of the muscular coats (Auerbach's plexus) and the submucosa (Meissner's plexus), but they have fewer ganglion cells than any other portion of the gastrointestinal tract.

The contribution of the sympathetic nerves to the function of the esophagus is not well understood and appears to play a minor role. The pharyngeal plexus supplies the uppermost part of the esophagus while the stellate ganglia supply the upper thoracic and lower cervical esophagus. The remainder of the thoracic esophagus is provided by the thoracic aortic plexus, sympathetic chain, and splanchnic nerves. The abdominal portion of the esophagus is supplied from the celiac ganglion by fibers passing to the esophagus around the left gastric artery and inferior phrenic artery. The celiac ganglion is identified during posterior fixation and sphincter calibration (Hill antireflux repair) underlying the median arcuate ligament. Division of this ganglion is infrequently required for adequate exposure of the ligament but if performed in the midline this does not result in any significant gastrointestinal symptoms because of the decussation of fibers in the midline.

▪ Histology of the Esophagus

The esophagus contains no serosal coat. The bulk of the wall of the esophagus consists of two muscle layers, an outer longitudinal and an inner circular layer, which assume an oblique or elliptical course in the esophagus.[1] The longitudinal fibers commence as three fascicles, one in front from the cricoid cartilage and the other two on each side arising continuously from the muscular fibers of the lower pharyngeal constrictor. As they descend, the fascicles blend together and form a vertical layer covering the surface of the esophagus. The longitudinal fibers course in an elongated spiral around one quarter of the esophageal circumference with fibers arranged in an elliptical fashion. The inner circular layer is usually thinner than the longitudinal layer. This inner layer ends approximately 1 to 2 cm above the diaphragm at the vestibule. It is at this point that the musculature of the esophagus thickens to form the lower esophageal sphincter or gastroesophageal ring.

The mucosa consists of noncornified, stratified squamous epithelium as a continuation of the epithelial lining of the pharynx. Within the esophageal vestibule this squamous epithelium is replaced by columnar epithelium. One to three cm of esophagus is lined by columnar epithelium. This varies considerably and may be highly irregular in the presence of hiatal hernia of other abnormalities such as reflux. In the normal individual, the squamocolumnar junction is relatively constant in the vestibule but may vary widely. Uncommonly the entire esophagus may be lined by columnar epithelium. The muscularis mucosa, a continuation of the pharyngeal aponeurosis, changes from fibrous tissue to muscle at the level of the cricoid cartilage.

The submucosa of the esophagus is dense and contains both elastic and collagen fibers and a number of lymphocytes. In the submucosa lies Meissner's nerve plexus along with arterial and venous channels. The myenteric plexus of Auerbach lies between the two muscle layers comprising the muscular coat of the esophagus. The adventitia of the esophagus consist of loose fibroelastic connective tissue extending from the esophagus to surrounding structures. Posteriorly this is quite dense and attaches the esophagus to the preaortic fascia or the aorta itself. The strands firmly anchor the esophagus posteriorly all the way from the celiac axis to the thoracic inlet.

Two types of glands are present in the esophageal mucosa. The esophageal or deep glands present throughout the esophagus are compound glands which penetrate the muscularis mucosa and extend into the submucosa, at which point they arborize and branch. The superficial cardiac glands extend only as far as the muscularis mucosa, resembling the cardiac glands of the stomach. These are found at both ends of the esophagus. In the normal individual neither of these types of glands contains parietal cells. Occasionally parietal cells may be seen in the esophagus as high as the aortic arch. There has been a great deal of controversy as to how these cells arrive as high as the aortic arch.[10] Studies have indicated that these parietal cells are capable of secreting small amounts of acid. Barrett's description of gastric mucosa in the esophagus is well documented. This type of epithelium may occur at any level in the esophagus and is distinctly abnormal. This will be discussed in Chapter 12.

■ REFERENCES

1. Lerche W: The Esophagus and Pharynx in Action: A Study of Structure in Relation to Function. Springfield, Ill., Charles C Thomas, 1950.
2. Zaino C, Jacobson HG, Lepaw H, Ozturk CH: Pharyngoesophageal Sphincter. Springfield, Ill., Charles C Thomas, 1950.
3. Killian G: La baudre de l'oesophage. Ann Mal Oreille Larynx, 34:1; 1908. (Cited by Moersch and Judd: Surg Gynecol Obstet, 58:781, 1934.)
4. Kaufmann P, Lierse W, Stark J, Stelzner F: Die Muskelanordnung in der Speiserohre (Mensch, Rheususaffe, Kaninchen, Maus Ratte, Seehund). Ergebn Anat Entwickl-Gesch, 40:3–33, 1968.
5. Laimer F: Beitrag zur Anatomie des Oesophagus. Med Jahrbucher, pp 333–338, 1883.
6. Liebermann-Meffert D, Allgower M, Schmid P, Math SD, Blum AL: Muscular equivalent of the lower esophageal sphincter. Gastroenterology, 76:31–38, 1978.
7. Listerud MB, Harkins HW: Anatomy of the esophageal hiatus. Arch Surg, 76:835–842, 1958.
8. Collis JL, Strachwell LM, Abrams CD: Nerve supply of the crura of the diaphragm. Thorax, 9:22, 1954.
9. Carey JM, Hollinshead WH: Anatomy of the esophageal hiatus related to repair of hiatal hernia. Proc Staff Mayo Clin, 30:223–226, 1955.
10. Barrett NR, Franklin RN: Concerning the unfavorable results of certain operations performed in the treatment of cardiospasm. Br J Surg, 37:194, 1949.
11. Dillard D: Personal communication.
12. Ciceri C: Morfolgia e struttura della diaframmatico esofageo. Monit Zool Ital, 40:501–505, 1929.
13. Anders HE, Bahrmann E: Uber die sogennten Hiatushernien des Ziverchfells in hoheren alter und ihre Genese. Zeitchshr F Klin Med, 122:736–796, 1932.
14. Fulde E: Uber die Anatomie und Physiologie des unteren Speiserohrenabschnittes. Deutsch Zeitschr F Chir, 242:380–589, 1934.
15. Nauta J: The closing mechanism between the esophagus and the stomach. Gastroenterologia, 86:219, 1956.
16. Peters PM: Closure mechanisms at the cardia with special reference to the diaphragmatico-oesophageal elastic ligament. Thorax, 10:27, 1955.
17. Ledrum FC: The Anatomical Features of the Cardiac Orifice of the Stomach. Graduate Thesis, University of Minnesota, 1934, p 122.
18. Mosher HP: The lower end of the oesophagus at birth and in the adult. J Laryngol Otol, 45:161, 1930.
19. Byrnes CK, Pisko-Dubienski ZA: An anatomical sphincter of the oesophago-gastric junction. Bull Soc Internat Chir, 22:62, 1963.
20. Hurst AF: Les sphincters du canal alimentaire et leur signification clinique. Arch Mal App Dig, 15:1, 1925.
21. Pisko-Dubienski ZA, Harkins HN: Anatomy of sliding hiatal hernia. In Myhus LM, Condon R, eds: Hernia. Philadelphia, J.B. Lippincott, 1964, p 434.
22. Bombeck CT, Dillard DH, Nyhus LM: Muscular anatomy of the gastroesophageal junction and the role of the phrenoesophageal ligament. Ann Surg, 164:643–654, 1966.
23. Allison PR: Reflux esophagitis, sliding hiatal hernia, and anatomy of repair. Surg Gynecol Obstet, 92:419–431, 1951.
24. Dornhorst AC, Harrison K, Pierce JW: Observations on the normal esophagus and cardia. Lancet, 1:695, 1954.
25. Lortat-Jacob JL, Parma A, Riberi A: Recent knowledge in the pathology of esophageal hiatus: the malposition of the cardiac tuberosity. (Recenti acquisizioni nella patalogia dello iato esofageo: Le malposizioni cardi-tuberositarie.) Arch Ital Mal App Dig, 20:247, 1954.
26. Guiseffi VJ, Grindlay JH, Schmidt HW: Canine esophagitis following experimentally produced esophageal hiatal hernia. Proc Staff Meet Mayo Clin, 29:399, 1954.
27. Barrett NR: Hiatus hernia: a review of some controversial points. Br J Surg, 42:231, 1954.
28. Thor KBA, Hill LD, Mercer CD, Kozarek RA: Reappraisal of the flap valve mechanism. A study of a new valvuloplasty procedure in cadavers. Acta Chir Scand, 153:25–28, 1987.
29. Demel R: The blood supply of the esophagus: a study of surgery of the esophagus. (Die Gefassversorgung der Speiserahre. Ein Beitrag zur Oesophaguschirurgie.) Arch Klin Chir, 128:453, 1924.
30. Hermann JD, Murugasu JJ: The blood supply of the oesophagus in relation to oesophageal surgery. Aust NZ J Surg, 35:195, 1966.
31. Butler H: The veins of the eosophagus. Thorax, 6:276, 1951.
32. Sakata K: On the lymphatics of the esophagus and on the regional lymph nodes with consideration of metastasis of the carcinoma. (Ueber die Lymphgefasse des Oesophagus und uber seine regionaren Lymphdrusen mit Berucksichtigung der Verbreitung des Carcinoms.) Mitt Grezgeb Med Chir, 11:634, 1903.

3

Physiology

Donald O. Castell

The esophagus is a muscular tube that is usually closed at both ends by a circular muscle segment forming a functional sphincter. Pressure relationships in and adjacent to the esophagus, including the sphincters, are illustrated in Figure 3–1. Intraesophageal pressure, reflecting intrathoracic pressure, is negative in relation to that in the pharynx and the stomach. Thus, tonically closed circular smooth muscle segments (sphincters) are necessary to control movement of inspired air or gastric contents into the esophagus. Obviously, these sphincters must open with appropriate timing during swallowing to allow antegrade movement of ingested material. Available information on normal function of these two sphincters and that segment of the hollow digestive tube (the esophagus) which they define will be discussed in this chapter.

■ *Upper Esophageal Sphincter*

The upper esophageal sphincter (UES) maintains closure to seal off the esophagus to the external environment. This striated muscle segment is maintained in a state of contraction at rest by constant discharge of motor action potentials.[1] During swallowing these action potentials are abolished and relaxation occurs.[2]

Radial Asymmetry ■ The resting pressures, as measured by intraluminal manometry, vary depending on the orientation of the recording office. Winans first demonstrated that pressures in the hu-

man UES are asymmetric, being greater in the anterior and posterior orientations (100 mm Hg) than in the right or left lateral (30 mm Hg) orientation.[3] These observations have since been confirmed by Gerhardt et al., as shown in Table 3–1.[4] The directional difference in recorded pressures is referred to as the radial asymmetry of the UES.

Axial Asymmetry ■ The peak pressures for the anterior and posterior orientations do not occur at the same level in the pull-through. Peak anterior pressures occur on the average 0.5 cm more proximal than peak posterior pressures. This corresponds with anatomic findings that the inferior border of the cricopharyngeus muscle lies 0.5 cm below that of the cricoid cartilage. This difference in location of peak pressures is referred to as the axial asymmetry of the UES.[5] Following laryngectomy (larynx, supporting muscles, and hyoid bone), both the radial and axial asymmetry disappear.[5]

Resting Pressure ■ High resting UES pressure is important because the average pressure in the esophageal body is approximately 5 mm Hg lower than normal atmospheric pressure. Thus, the UES prevents the esophagus from filling with air during the normal respiratory cycle. During the voluntary act of initiating a swallow, UES relaxation occurs in a coordinated sequence as forceful pharyngeal contractions move ingested material from the pharynx into the upper esophagus. Respiration is inhibited during this process.

Upper esophageal sphincter pressures increase significantly over resting pressures in response to

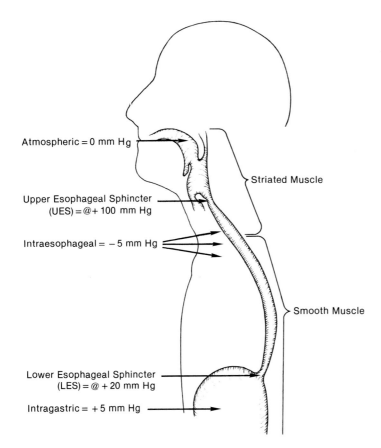

Atmospheric = 0 mm Hg

Striated Muscle

Upper Esophageal Sphincter
(UES) = @+ 100 mm Hg

Intraesophageal = − 5 mm Hg

Smooth Muscle

Lower Esophageal Sphincter
(LES) = @ + 20 mm Hg

Intragastric = + 5 mm Hg

Figure 3–1. Schematic representation of important functional physiologic and anatomic relationships in the pharynx and the esophagus, including representative pressure levels in the esophageal segments, sphincters, and adjacent areas of the pharynx and stomach. The area of transition from striated to smooth muscle is also identified.

an intraluminal fluid bolus (saline) infused below the UES or to intraesophageal balloon distention.[4,6] At present, two different types of stimuli appear to be involved in this response, namely volume and acid. Volume, whether it be fluid or a balloon distention, results in increased UES pressure. Infusion of 0.1 N HCl results in a greater stimulatory effect on UES pressures than does saline alone. The closer to the UES the fluid is perfused, the greater is the response. These studies suggest a protective role of the UES in prevention of regurgitation of esophageal contents into the pharynx with possible resultant aspiration.

Sphincter Relaxation ■ Relaxation of the UES is produced by inhibition of tonic contraction of the cricopharyngeus muscle and possibly of the

Table 3–1. RESTING UPPER ESOPHAGEAL SPHINCTER PRESSURE (mm Hg)*

Orientation	Mean	Range
Posterior	101	60–142
Anterior	84	55–123
Lateral	48	30–65

*Data from 20 normal subjects. (From Gerhardt D, et al: Human upper esophageal sphincter. Gastroenterology, 75:268, 1978.

inferior pharyngeal constrictor as well.[1] Forward displacement of the larynx by the geniohyoid muscle may also play a role in relaxation. The normal sphincter always relaxes prior to the arrival of the pharyngeal peristaltic contraction. The UES resting pressure falls abruptly within 0.2 to 0.3 s of a swallow to pharyngeal or baseline pressure, and the sphincter remains relaxed for 0.5 to 1.2 s.[7] The relaxation is followed by a peristaltic wave which propels the bolus through the pharynx and through the UES into the esophagus.

Neural Control ■ The sequential action of the onset of peristalsis in the pharynx and UES relaxation is finely coordinated through the swallowing center located in the medulla. This mechanism involves impulses transmitted over five cranial nerves: V, VII, IX, X, and XII. Therefore, a variety of lesions in the CNS or cranial nerves can produce abnormalities in the pharyngeal and upper esophageal swallowing mechanism.

There is little information on the effect of drugs on the upper esophageal sphincter in humans, but a few animal studies suggest that relaxation is mediated by a cholinergic, nicotinic-mediated mechanism. The UES and upper esophagus are innervated by the vagus nerve and others, and require integrity of the central nervous system. If the vagus nerves are intact, peristalsis will progress normally, even after complete esophageal transection.

■ Lower Esophageal Sphincter

The lower esophageal sphincter (LES) is a high-pressure zone separating the gastric cavity from the esophageal lumen. A specific smooth muscle sphincter at the esophagogastric junction has been difficult to demonstrate in humans, but there is no question that a functional sphincteric mechanism exists in this location. The sphincteric segment can be demonstrated radiographically and consists of a muscular ring at the proximal border, an ampulla or vestibule in the middle, and a mucosal ring at the squamocolumnar junction.

The LES is innervated by efferent fibers from the autonomic nervous system. The vagus nerves and the thoracic greater splanchnic nerve provide the parasympathetic and sympathetic input, respectively. An extensive network of connections in the esophageal wall (enteric nervous system) provides the ultimate control.

The LES serves two main functions: it prevents reflux of gastric contents into a lower esophagus, and it relaxes during swallowing to allow the passage of ingested material from the esophagus into the stomach.[8] Abnormalities of either of these functions are major causes of esophageal disease or symptoms. Changes in the antireflux pressure barrier result in gastroesophageal reflux and its complications. Ineffective relaxation of the sphincter results in dysphagia. The physiologic function of this sphincter is regulated by a complex interaction of three factors: sphincteric smooth muscle, autonomic and enteric innervation, and gastrointestinal hormones and peptides. Tables 3–2 and 3–3 include many substances that have been shown experimentally to change LES resting pressure. The LES remains closed except during swallowing to allow transport of the bolus from the esophagus into the stomach. It also opens during vomiting and belching. This zone of increased pressure ranges from 2 to 4 cm in length. Using current low compliance manometric systems, the normal pressure range for the LES in many laboratories is 10 to 40 mm Hg.

Radial Asymmetry ■ Pressures recorded within the LES vary to some degree according to the orientation of the recording orifice within the sphincter. Pressure asymmetry of the LES was first described by Kaye and Showalter.[9] Subsequently, Winans showed that pressures in the LES were higher in the left (33 mm Hg) and left posterior

Table 3–2. AGENTS PRODUCING INCREASED LOWER ESOPHAGEAL SPHINCTER PRESSURE

Hormones/peptides
Gastrin
Motilin
Substance P
Bombesin
Vasopressin
Angiotensin

Neurotransmitters
Alpha-adrenergic agonists (noradrenaline, phenylephrine)
Beta-adrenergic antagonists
Cholinergic drugs (bethanechol)
Anticholinesterase (edrophonium)

Other Agents
Histamine
Antacids
Metoclopramide
Domperidone
Protein meals
Prostaglandin F_{2a}
Indomethacin
Coffee

Table 3–3. AGENTS PRODUCING DECREASED LOWER ESOPHAGEAL SPHINCTER PRESSURE

Hormones
Secretin
Cholecystokinin
Glucagon
Gastric inhibitory polypeptide (GIP)
Vasoactive intestinal polypeptide (VIP)
Neurotensin
Progesterone

Neurotransmitters
Beta-adrenergic agonist (isoproterenol)
Alpha-adrenergic antagonist (phentolamine)
Dopamine
Anticholinergics (atropine)

Foods
Fat
Chocolate
Ethanol
Peppermint

Other Agents
Theophylline
Caffeine
Gastric acidification
Smoking
Diazepam
Pethidine/morphine
Prostaglandins E_1, E_2, A_2, I_2
Nitroprusside
Calcium-blocking agents
Lidocaine
Hypothyroidism

(34 mm Hg) than in the other six directions (14.5 to 23.5 mm Hg).[10]

The LES has been shown to contract in response to transient increases in abdominal pressure such as abdominal compression and the Valsalva maneuver.[11] This would appear to be an important mechanism in the antireflux competence of the sphincter. Although LES pressure is only one of several factors proposed to be important in preventing reflux, recent studies have supported its crucial role. When intraesophageal pH and LES pressure were monitored overnight, reflux was closely associated with decreases in LES pressure.[12]

Three factors are potentially important in controlling LES pressure: muscle, nerves, and hormones. A major problem in determining the relative importance of these factors has been the variation in response found in different animal species, making it difficult to interpret some of the data.

Sphincter Smooth Muscle ■ Intrinsic tonic myogenic activity of the smooth muscle of the LES itself contributes to the resting sphincter pressure.[13] It has been suggested that LES tone might even be primarily due to myogenic factors. The membrane potential of the LES smooth muscle is lower than that of the adjacent stomach or esophageal smooth muscle.

Sphincter smooth muscle has been shown to be very dependent on available calcium. Decreased tone in muscle strips from the sphincteric region of the opossum esophagus occurs during immersion in calcium-free solution.[14] Calcium channel-blocking agents have also been shown to cause a fall in LES pressure in animals and humans.[15–17]

Neural Control ■ Neurogenic regulation appears to be mediated through both inhibitory and excitatory autonomic nerves. Alpha-adrenergic neurotransmitters increase LES pressure and alpha blockers decrease it, while beta stimulation lowers LES pressure and beta blockers raise it. Tetrodotoxin, a neural poison, does not lower resting LES tones in the opossum, indicating that neural control is not an important mechanism in maintaining basal LES tone in that animal.[13] Cholinergic mechanisms would appear to maintain some of the resting LES pressure in humans, however, since atropine and other anticholinergic agents have been shown to decrease the pressure.[18]

Lower esophageal sphincter relaxation in the opossum is controlled by nerves carried within the vagus, since stimulation of the distal end of the vagus sectioned in the neck produced reduced LES pressure. This relaxation is not inhibited by cholinergic or by adrenergic blockade, but is abolished by the nonspecific neurotoxin tetrodotoxin.[15] The specific neurotransmitter for this nonadrenergic inhibition has remained a mystery. Once thought to be "purinergic," recent evidence suggests that neither ATP nor adenosine appear to be the inhibitory neurotransmitter for LES relaxation, thus seeming to rule out a "purinergic" mechanism. Vasoactive intestinal polypeptide (VIP) has been proposed as the possible neurotransmitter.[19]

Hormonal Regulation ■ The actions of hormones on the LES have been studied in detail. Castell and Harris first postulated a stimulatory effect of endogenous gastrin on the LES when they alkalinized the gastric contents in human volunteers and noted increases in LES pressure, although they did not measure endogenous gastrin levels.[20] This effect was later shown to be related to the gastric alkalinization per se and not to significant increases in serum gastrin.[21] Marked increases in LES pressure do occur, however, in normal subjects following injection of exogenous pentagastrin.[20] When endogenous gastrin is released from the antrum after feeding meat extracts, sphincter pressures are increased. Furthermore, the LES response to alkali and protein can be inhibited by somatostatin, suggesting a definite hormonal effect.[22] The true physiologic role, if any, of endogenous gastrin in regulating LES pressure remains a controversial issue.

Secretin has been shown to inhibit the effect of gastrin on LES pressure, presumably by noncompetitive inhibition of the sphincter.[23] In normal volunteers, fat ingestion reduces LES pressures, suggesting an effect of endogenous cholecystokinin (CCK) on the LES.[24] The other members of the secretin family of hormones—glucagon, gastric inhibitory peptide, and vasoactive intestinal peptide (VIP)—have also been shown to lower LES pressure in humans and in animals. As noted above, VIP is currently a strong candidate as chemical mediator of the nonadrenergic, noncholinergic pathway for LES relaxation. Siegel et al. compared the effects of VIP, glucagon, and secretin on LES pressures in awake baboons and found VIP to be much more potent in lowering both resting pressure and LES pressure response to pentagastrin.[25] Cells stained with immunofluorescent antibody to VIP are found in heavy concentration in the ganglion area of the lower esophageal sphincter.[26] Neurotensin is another peptide which has recently been shown to produce decreased LES pressure. Infusions of this peptide in human volunteers significantly lowered sphincter pressures when plasma neurotensin-like immunoreactivity was below a level obtained after a meal or ingestion of fat.[27]

Hormones or peptides known to change LES pressure are listed in Tables 3–2 and 3–3. Many peptides (hormones?) from the gastrointestinal tract have been proposed as possible physiologic regulators of the LES. Which of these are producing pharmacologic responses and which are physiologic regulators remains to be elucidated. Motilin is a strong candidate for a possible physiologic regulator of LES pressure owing to its proposed role in the migrating motor complex (MMC). This rhythmic organized muscle contraction pattern of the gastrointestinal tract has been shown to occur in both animals and humans. In humans, the MMC propagates distally along the small intestine about every 90 to 100 min during fasting. There is now evidence that motilin may be important in initiating MMC activity and that phasic increases in LES pressure seen during fasting correspond with fluctuations in plasma motilin levels and MMC phases.[28]

Other Effects ■ A great variety of factors (foods, drugs) produce changes in LES pressure under normal conditions. The pressure should be regarded as quite dynamic and subject to many changes throughout the day. Some of these agents are listed in Tables 3–2 and 3–3.

Thus, there clearly are multiple factors responsible for the maintenance of the sustained contraction or resting tone of the LES. The lower esophageal sphincter is not a static barrier but responds to a variety of stimuli with changes in the force of its closure (Fig. 3–2). In the resting state, intraluminal pressure is greater in the LES than in the stomach. High-protein meals increase LES pressure, and high-fat meals decrease LES pressure without changing intragastric pressure. Increased intra-abdominal pressure results in an immediate rise in LES pressure, usually greatly exceeding the rise in abdominal pressure and thus maintaining the effectiveness of the antireflux barrier. This response is believed to be a vagovagal reflex. Gastric distention initiates sphincter relaxation, thus facilitat-

ing eructation. The LES is a dynamic barrier indeed!

The two esophageal sphincters provide excellent examples of the role of sphincters in the GI tract. They maintain a *resting tone* sufficient to appropriately separate the adjacent segments and they *relax* transiently during swallowing to allow ingested material to pass down the GI tract.

■ *Mechanism of Swallowing*

Swallowing has been traditionally divided into three stages: the voluntary or oral stage, the pharyngeal or involuntary stage, and the esophageal stage. The frequency of this important function varies greatly during the day. Normal subjects swallow approximately 70 times per hour while awake and only seven times per hour during sleep. During eating the swallowing frequency increases to approximately 190 to 200 swallows per hour.

The *voluntary (oral) stage* of swallowing is initiated by processes occurring in the mouth. Food is voluntarily moved to the posterior part of the mouth where the tongue forces the food bolus back into the pharynx by pushing backward and upward against the palate. The posterior portion of the tongue is forced posteriorly to the pharyngeal wall by the styloglossus and hyoglossus muscles. The soft palate is elevated by the veli palatini muscles, closing the nasopharynx. The middle and inferior pharyngeal constrictors narrow the hypopharynx as the epiglottis closes over the ascending larynx. It is at this point that the process is no longer voluntary and continues by reflex.

In the *pharyngeal stage*, food is transferred from the pharynx into the esophagus. The bolus in the

Figure 3–2. Examples of pressure relationships between intragastric pressure (G) and lower esophageal sphincter (LES) pressure (S) during a variety of common occurrences. The relative increases and decreases of sphincter pressure (S) and gastric pressure (G) that occur throughout the day may account for reflux episodes at different times.

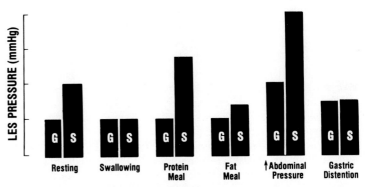

LES IS A DYNAMIC BARRIER

G = intragastric pressure
S = LES pressure

pharynx stimulates afferent receptors around the opening of the pharynx to send impulses to the swallowing center in the brain stem. This area, located in the medulla and pons, controls the involuntary sequences of swallowing and simultaneously stops respiration by inhibiting the respiratory center in the medulla. The CNS areas initiate a series of involuntary responses. The soft palate extends upward, closing the posterior nares, and preventing expulsion of food through the nose. The palatopharyngeal folds are pulled medially, limiting the opening through the pharynx and preventing the passage of large boluses. The vocal cords are closed and the epiglottis swings backward and downward to close the pharynx. The larynx is pulled upwards and forward by muscles attached to the hyoid bone, stretching the opening of the esophagus. At this point the upper esophageal sphincter relaxes and contraction of the superior constrictor muscle of the pharynx initiates a peristaltic wave, propelling food into the esophagus.

The *esophageal stage* is characterized by transport of the bolus by normal peristalsis the length of the esophagus. In normal subjects, this transit takes approximately 7 to 10 s. A normal contraction wave initiated by a swallow, which progresses down the esophagus, is considered primary peristalsis. Secondary peristalsis is a similar wave that originates in the esophagus, being initiated by esophageal distention produced by an ingested bolus or by gastroesophageal reflux. This phenomenon can be readily demonstrated by distending a balloon within the esophagus. It is a major mechanism for clearing swallowed food or reflux gastric contents. Tertiary contractions are nonperistaltic contraction waves which may occur spontaneously or after swallowing.

■ *Esophageal Peristalsis*

In Vitro Responses ■ Three distinct responses have been described by Christensen and Lund from muscle segments of opossum esophagus during in vitro studies with electrical field stimulation.[29] During stimulation of the outer longitudinal muscle layer the muscle contracts, shortening the segment for the duration of the electrical response. This *"duration response,"* which also involves the muscularis mucosa, can be blocked by atropine and the general nerve poison tetrodotoxin and, therefore, is thought to be caused by excitatory cholinergic nerves.

Two responses of the circular muscle to similar stimulation were seen: *"on response"* and the *"off response."* The brief *on response* is a short contraction accompanied by a burst of action potentials proximal to the point of stimulation or stretch. This is not blocked by tetrodotoxin, suggesting mediation by non-neural pathways. The *off response* is a larger contraction of the circular muscle layer which occurs after the stimulus has ended. This contraction is inhibited by tetrodotoxin, but not by any of the known neurohormonal autonomic antagonists. Thus, the specific neurotransmitter is unknown. These responses are summarized in Table 3–4. The *off response* was also characterized by a delay in the onset of contraction after termination of the stimulus, i.e., a latency period. The duration of the latency was shown to increase with distance down the esophagus, producing what has been called a "latency gradient."

Unifying Concept ■ The in vitro studies described above have led to an integrated "unifying concept" as an hypothesis for the mechanism of peristalsis. One could propose that the primary neural discharge to the esophagus from the CNS is primarily of an inhibitory nature. The LES, being chronically contracted, responds with an appropriate relaxation immediately following the initiation of the swallow. The esophageal body shows two responses. The longitudinal muscle contracts and shortens the esophagus for the duration of the peristaltic wave (i.e., the duration response). The circular muscle shows no immediate response to the swallow. It is only after the stimulus is withdrawn that the circular smooth muscle of the esophageal body contracts, consistent with the off response. Because of the gradient of latency period down the esophagus, the peristaltic wave occurs progressively later following the initial inhibitory stimulus. Finally, it is only after the peristaltic contraction has reached the distal end of the esophagus that the LES contracts to its normal tonic resting pressure.

Neural and Hormonal Effects ■ There are definite cholinergic controls to human esophageal peristalsis. Cholinergic agents edrophonium and bethanechol increase peristaltic amplitudes in the distal esophagus,[30] and peristaltic pressures are lower in the distal esophagus after atropine.[18] The effect of the dopamine antagonist metoclopramide is controversial and there is no clear evidence that it increases peristaltic pressures. Adrenergic nerves have not been shown to be very important in the motor function of the esophageal body. There are no known hormonal effects on esophageal peristalsis, but not many hormones have been studied. Neither glucagon nor gastrin seem to affect peristalsis, despite their strong effects on the lower esophageal sphincter.[31,32]

Pressure Profiles ■ Peristaltic pressures in the distal portion of the human esophagus are higher

Table 3–4. ESOPHAGEAL SMOOTH MUSCLE RESPONSES (IN VITRO OPOSSUM MUSCLE)

Response	Muscle Involved	Antagonist	Timing
"Duration"	Longitudinal	Atropine; tetrodotoxin	Throughout stimulus
"On"	Circular	None identified	Onset of stimulus
"Off"	Circular	Only tetrodotoxin	After stimulus

than those in the more proximal esophagus. Pressures in the esophagus are symmetrical at each level.[33] Pressure recordings throughout the human esophagus indicate that there is a pressure trough, or low pressure zone, located about 4 to 6 cm below the upper esophageal sphincter and about 2 to 3 cm in length. Pressure in this area in many subjects is below 20 mm Hg.[34] This low pressure zone seems to correspond to the region of the esophagus where the striated and smooth portions are approximately equal in amount (the "transition" zone).

The average speed at which the peristaltic waves move through the proximal esophagus is 3.0 to 3.5 cm/s. The peristaltic velocity seems to increase somewhat as the wave approaches the lower third of the esophagus, slowing down to 2.0 cm/s in the distal 2 to 3 cm.[34]

Bolus Effects ■ Characteristics of the swallowed bolus affect the peristaltic response to swallowing. "Dry" swallows result in lower amplitude waves that are not very reproducible. Liquid boluses greater than 2 ml give more reproducible waves of higher amplitude.[35] The temperature of the bolus has been shown to be important. Single cold water swallows (0.5 to 3.0°C) markedly decrease the frequency of peristalsis in the esophagus, slow the speed of peristalsis throughout the esophagus, and prolong the duration of the peristaltic wave in the distal esophagus. On the other hand, hot water (58 to 61°C) slightly increases the peristaltic frequency in the proximal esophagus, accelerates peristalsis throughout the esophagus, and shortens the contraction duration throughout the esophagus.[36] Repeated swallows of ice water (0 to 3°C) and soft ice creams (−5°C) lower peristaltic frequency and amplitude throughout the esophagus, most markedly in the midesophagus.[37] Ingestion of ice water or cold barium causes esophageal dilatation with loss of the peristaltic waves after repeated swallows.[37,38] Normal subjects can induce chest pain if they swallow cold liquids rapidly enough. In most cases, the chest pain is associated with a normal electrocardiogram, a dilated esophagus, and aperistalsis.

"Deglutitive Inhibition" ■ When several swallows are performed in rapid sequence (less than 10 s between swallows), many swallows are not followed by peristalsis. This phenomenon, called "deglutitive inhibition," has been proposed for many years to be due to a stimulus of inhibition that precedes the peristaltic wave. Recent studies of this phenomenon indicate that it is also partially due to esophageal muscle refractoriness.[39]

■ REFERENCES

1. Asoh R, Goyal R: Manometry and electromyography of the upper esophageal sphincter in the opossum. Gastroenterology, 74:514–520, 1978.
2. Carr A, Roman C: L'activité spontanée du sphincter oseophagien superieur chez le mouton. J Physiol (Paris), 62:505–511, 1970.
3. Winans CS: The pharyngoesophageal closure mechanisms: a manometric study. Gastroenterology, 63:68–77, 1972.
4. Gerhardt DC, Shuck TJ, Bordeaux RA, Winship DH: Human upper esophageal sphincter. Gastroenterology, 75:268–274, 1978.
5. Welch RW, Luckman K, Ricks PM, Drake ST, Gates GA: Manometry of the normal upper esophageal sphincter and its alterations in laryngectomy. J Clin Invest, 63:1036–1041, 1979.
6. Creamer B, Schlegel J: Motor responses of the esophagus to distention. J Appl Physiol, 10:498–504, 1957.
7. Ingelfinger FJ: Esophageal motility. Physiol Rev, 38:533–584, 1958.
8. Castell DO: The lower esophageal sphincter: Physiologic and clinical aspects. Ann Intern Med, 83:390–401, 1975.
9. Kaye MD, Showalter JP: Manometric configuration of the lower esophageal sphincter in normal human subjects. Gastroenterology, 61:213–223, 1971.
10. Winans CS: Manometric asymmetry of the lower esophageal high pressure zone. Am J Dig Dis, 22:348–354, 1977.
11. Cohen S, Harris LD: The lower esophageal sphincter. Gastroenterology, 63:1066–1073, 1972.
12. Dodds WJ, Dent J, Hogan WJ, et al: Mechanisms of gastroesophageal reflux in patients with reflux esophagitis. N Engl J Med, 307:1547–1552, 1982.
13. Goyal RK, Rattan S: Genesis of basal sphincter pressure: Effect of tetrodotoxin on the lower esophageal sphincter in opossum in vivo. Gastroenterology, 71:62–67, 1976.
14. Fox JE, Daniel EE: Role of Ca++ in the genesis of lower esophageal sphincter tone and other active contractions. Am J Physiol, 237:E163–171, 1979.
15. Goyal RK, Rattan S: Effects of sodium nitroprusside and verapamil on lower esophageal sphincter. Am J Physiol, 238:640–641, 1980.
16. Richter JE, Sinar DR, Cordova CM, Castell DO: Verapamil—a potent inhibitory of esophageal function in baboon. Gastroenterology, 82:882–886, 1982.
17. Richter JE, Spurling TJ, Cordova CM, Castell DO: Effects of oral calcium blocker, diltiazem, an esophageal contractions. Dig Dis Sci, 29:649–656, 1984.
18. Dodds WJ, Dent J, Hogan WJ, Arndorfer RC: Effect of atropine on esophageal motor function in humans. Am J Physiol, 240:G290–296, 1981.
19. Goyal RK, Rattan S, Said SI: VIP as a possible neuro-

transmitter of non-cholinergic non-adrenergic inhibitory neurons. Nature, *288*:370–380, 1980.

20. Castell DO, Harris LD: Hormonal control of gastroesophageal sphincter strength. N Engl J Med, *282*:886–892, 1970.

21. Higgs RH, Smyth RD, Castell DO: Gastric alkalinization effect on lower esophageal sphincter pressure and serum gastrin. N Engl J Med, *291*:486–490, 1974.

22. Bybee DE, Brown FC, Georges LP, Castell DO, McGuigan JE: Somatostatin effects on lower esophageal sphincter function. Am J Physiol, *237*:E77–81, 1979.

23. Cohen S, Lipshutz W: Hormonal regulation of human lower esophageal sphincter competence: Interaction of gastrin and secretin. J Clin Invest, *50*:449–454, 1971.

24. Nebel OT, Castell DO: Lower esophageal sphincter pressure changes after food ingestion. Gastroenterology, *63*:778–783, 1972.

25. Siegel SR, Brown FC, Castell DO, Johnson LF, Said SI: Effects of vasoactive intestinal polypeptide (VIP) on lower esophageal sphincter in awake baboons. Dig Dis Sci, *24*:354–349, 1979.

26. Uddman R, Aluments J, Edvinsson L, Hakanson R, Sundler F: Peptidergic (VIP) innervaton of the esophagus. Gastroenterology, *75*:5–8, 1978.

27. Rosell S, Thor K, Rokaeus A, Nyquist O, Lewenhaupt A, Kager L, Folkers K: Plasma concentration of neurotensin-like immunoreactivity and lower esophageal sphincter pressure in man following infusion of neurotensin. Acta Physiol Scand, *109*:369–375, 1980.

28. Holloway RH, Blank E, Takahashi I, Dodds WJ, Laymen RD: Motilin: A mechanism incorporating the opossum lower esophageal sphincter into the migrating motor complex. Gastroenterology, *89*:507–515, 1985.

29. Christensen J, Lund GF: Esophageal responses to distention and electrical stimulation. J Clin Invest, *48*:408–419, 1969.

30. Hollis JB, Castell DO: Effects of cholinergic stimulation of human esophageal peristalsis. J Appl Physiol, *40*:40–43, 1976.

31. Hogan WJ, Dodds WJ, Hoke SE, Reid DP, Kalkhoff RK, Arndorfer RC: Effect of glucagon on esophageal motor function. Gastroenterology, *69*:160–165, 1975.

32. Hollis JB, Levine SM, Castell DO: Differential sensitivity of the human esophagus to pentagastrin. Am J Physiol, *222*:870–874, 1972.

33. Dodds WJ, Stef JJ, Hogan WJ, Hoke SE, Stewart ET, Arndorfer RC: Radial distribution of esophageal peristaltic pressure in normal subjects and patients with esophageal diverticulum. Gastroenterology, *69*:584–590, 1975.

34. Humphries TJ, Castell DO: Pressure profile of esophageal peristalsis in normal humans as measured by direct intraesophageal transducers. Am J Dig Dis, *22*:641–645, 1977.

35. Hollis JB, Castell DO: Effect of dry swallows and wet swallows of different volumes on esophageal peristalsis. J Appl Physiol, *38*:1161–1164, 1975.

36. Winship DH, Viegas deAndrade SR, Zboralske FF: Influence of bolus temperature on human esophageal motor function. J Clin Invest, *49*:243–250, 1970.

37. Meyer GW, Castell DO: Human esophageal response during chest pain induced by swallowing cold liquids. JAMA, *246*:2057–2059, 1981.

38. Ott DJ, Kelly RJ, Gelfand DW: Radiographic effects of cold barium suspension on esophageal motility. Radiology, *140*:830–838, 1981.

39. Meyer GW, Gerhardt DC, Castell DO: Human esophageal response to rapid swallowing: Muscle refractory period of neural inhibition? Am J Physiol, *241*:G129–G136, 1981.

4

Symptoms of Esophageal Disease

Colin O.H. Russell

The functions of the esophagus can be grouped into three general categories:

1. Transport of nutrients to and retention within the digestive system
2. A barrier between digestive and respiratory tracts
3. A vent (socially acceptable) for gaseous material either ingested or manufactured in the proximal GI tract.

Esophageal disease can lead to disturbances of any of these functions, and the symptoms that can arise will be presented in this chapter under these three categories.

■ *Transport and Retention of Nutrients*

The esophagus is a hollow muscular tube with a sphincter mechanism at each end. These three parts act in synchrony to permit and to promote smooth progression of a bolus from mouth to stomach. Obstruction of the tube itself (internal or external) or malfunction of sphincters or muscular propulsion (peristalsis) along the tube can all result in failure of transport. The predominant clinical manifestation is, of course, dysphagia. *Dysphagia* is by common usage best described as the sensation of the bolus ''lodging''at any part on its downward course through the esophagus. This should not be confused with *odynophagia*, which is the awareness of the bolus traversing the esophagus, de-

scribed as either pain or discomfort after swallowing, and is analogous to the dysuria of urinary tract infection. A careful clinical history of the features of dysphagia can suggest which of the two basic mechanisms—luminal obstruction or functional (motility) disorder—is more likely to be present.

Luminal obstruction is associated with the following features:

- Short, often progressive, history of dysphagia for solids initially; then, if the obstruction increases, softer foods and even liquids become affected.
- Marked weight loss favors a diagnosis of malignancy.
- Associated symptoms of gastroesophageal reflux (GER) preceding the dysphagia raise the possibility of a peptic stricture.
- Sudden onset of persisting and total dysphagia immediately after ingestion of a solid bolus (usually meat) suggests bolus impaction has occurred.

Motility disorder is associated with these findings:

- Intermittent history of dysphagia for solids and liquids from the onset (i.e., bolus size and consistency do not predict symptoms). The problem often is not progressive in severity, and close questioning often reveals that milder symptoms have been present for several years.
- Weight loss, if present, is usually mild.
- Associated symptoms of chest pain are present in a large proportion of patients with motility disorders.

Although it is intellectually satisfying to reach the correct clinical diagnosis by means of the history alone, the sensitivity and specificity of this method most certainly do not reach 100 per cent. It is therefore dangerous to assume a diagnosis achieved in this manner. A protocol of investigation (as in Chap. 6) will minimize the chances of a clinically unsuspected malignancy at a potentially more curable stage going undetected. The level of bolus obstruction as suggested by the patient is unreliable, except in one instance. When the patient states the bolus lodges in the neck immediately on swallowing and this is accompanied by coughing or spluttering (symptoms of aspiration), then the problem is proximal (most commonly pharyngeal or upper esophageal sphincter). Dysphagia, however, is not the sole manifestation of transport abnormalities. Hiccoughs after swallowing and without any associated sensation of the bolus having lodged can be the sole symptom of a transport problem. Similarly, chest pain, during or after food ingestion, can carry the same implication.

This section would be incomplete without some discussion on globus. *Globus* is best defined as a *constant* sensation of a lump in the throat during waking hours. It is further described as like a piece of food being lodged. This resulting discomfort may be exacerbated by further swallowing, but on close questioning the examiner may find that there is no actual impedance to swallowed boluses. Globus, although it may persist for months or even years, is generally self-limiting. It is said to be more prevalent in patients with GER or motility disorders and to respond to treatment appropriate for these conditions.

The preceding statements assume that symptoms will invariably accompany transport abnormalities. This is incorrect, for many patients with proven motility disorders have no symptoms. This is particularly well documented in patients with systemic disorders affecting esophageal motility (e.g., diabetes, scleroderma). Our own studies have shown dysphagia to be a poor marker for esophageal dysfunction.[1] An equation is therefore proposed:

Transport disorder + perception = symptoms.

There is some indirect evidence to support this concept. Our studies[2] on the incidence of esophageal motor dysfunction in GER detected an abnormality in 15 of 29 patients before antireflux surgery. These abnormalities were found not only in the patients with severe and mild dysphagia but also in some patients who did not complain of dysphagia. Three months after surgery (successful by objective parameters) all but 1 of 12 patients with esophageal dysfunction and dysphagia had lost their dysphagia. On testing, however, all 12 patients had retained their esophageal dysfunction. Perhaps the mucosal changes secondary to reflux allowed perception of the arrested bolus (dysphagia) and when the mucosal changes were reversed by control of the reflux, the dysphagia disappeared.

■ RETENTION OF NUTRIENTS

Retention refers to the normal mechanisms that control gastroesophageal reflux and modify its effects on the esophagus. Failure of those mechanisms may give rise to sympathetic GER. Unfortunately, pathologic reflux may be asymptomatic and may be detected only when the patient presents with complications, such as peptic stricture or iron deficiency anemia. This suggests that perception is again a factor.

The classic symptoms of GER are heartburn and regurgitation; however, heartburn means many things to many people, and it should not be assumed that when patients use the term "heartburn" they are referring to symptoms of reflux. True heartburn is a retrosternal burning pain that commences inferiorly in the epigastrium and proceeds upward often as far as the throat. No other description is acceptable. It most often occurs within 30 to 45 min after a meal. It may also be induced by changes in posture—lying down or stooping. Regurgitation, which is the spontaneous and retrograde passage of esophageal or gastric contents into the pharynx or mouth, will often occur: this is felt as an unpleasant sour or bitter tasting fluid in the mouth. (This has also been termed "water brash.")

Earlier in this chapter I alluded to the symptom of odynophagia and its occasional confusion with dysphagia. Unfortunately, these two clinical entities are not always readily discernible from a careful clinical history. Odynophagia is likened to the sensation expected when swallowing an object with sharp edges. Odynophagia occurs in the presence of inflammatory changes in the esophageal mucosa, either macroscopic or microscopic. Reflux esophagitis is but one cause of esophagitis; others include monilial and herpetic infections and the chemical irritation caused by some drugs (e.g., doxycycline).

When a patient presents with a history of heartburn and regurgitation of gastric contents and when these symptoms generally occur within the hour following a meal and are exacerbated by lying down or stooping but are relieved by antacids, the diagnosis of gastroesophageal reflux can be made with confidence. Alternatively, the entire clinical presentation may be atypical. Such atypical symptoms include dysphagia, anemia, globus, and respiratory symptoms and are dealt with elsewhere in this chapter.

■ *Barrier Between Digestive and Respiratory Tracts*

About 10 per cent of the referrals to our esophageal service who subsequently are found to have significant motility disorders come from respiratory physicians. They have often had problems of recurrent bronchopulmonary infection, nocturnal aspiration, paroxysmal nocturnal coughing, obstructive airways disease, or hoarseness. Careful questioning of all patients with esophageal motility disorders or reflux problems will raise this prevalence of respiratory disorders (especially nocturnal aspiration and hoarseness). One study using 24-hour pH monitoring in a group of patients with reflux and symptoms suggesting aspiration found evidence of aspiration in only 17 per cent.[3] Others, using radionuclide scanning techniques, have demonstrated actual aspiration of regurgitated fluid in up to 50 per cent of patients with chronic lung disease suspected to be secondary to reflux.[4] In support of this concept of the esophagus being a barrier between digestive and respiratory tracts is the measured improvement in respiratory symptoms after antireflux surgery in carefully selected patients with chronic lung disease and documented reflux.[3,5] Similar benefits have been demonstrated after correction of esophageal motility disorders (especially achalasia).

When a patient with pulmonary problems says that he or she wakes at night with retrosternal burning pain, coughing, and spluttering and describes the bed pillow as being drenched with bile-stained fluid, the presence of reflux-induced pulmonary disease can be inferred. Such a classic history is, however, uncommon, and a history suggestive of esophageal dysfunction is not always obtainable in patients with esophageal-derived respiratory disease. Clinicians must be alert to the fact that unexplained respiratory disease just might be secondary to esophageal disease. Unfortunately, objective evidence of aspiration into the respiratory tract is more elusive than some workers claim.

A recent study has documented objective evidence of inflammatory lesions of the posterior larynx in patients with GER. This was clinically manifested by sore throats, especially on rising in the morning, and intermittent hoarseness.

■ *Vent from the Gastrointestinal Tract*

The esophagus might also be compared to a factory chimney that allows escape of unwanted gaseous products. The lower esophageal sphincter, possibly under control of vagal efferents, responds to gaseous distention, and by transient relaxation allows escape of gaseous products. Recent (as yet unpublished) studies by Martin and Dent suggest that perhaps belching and other nonspecific symptoms such as postprandial bloating may be secondary to lower esophageal sphincter dysfunction. It is already well known that when fundoplication is used to control reflux, postprandial gas bloat is an unpleasant side effect. This hitherto poorly recognized aspect of esophageal function needs further investigation.

This chapter could be described as imprecise in that the actual prevalence of the many symptoms in specific esophageal disorders is not listed. The omission is intentional. There is such a considerable overlap in symptoms between disorders that such a listing, although possibly of academic interest, has no real clinical value.

■ REFERENCES

1. Russell C, Gannan R, Coatsworth J, et al: Relationship among esophageal dysfunction, diabetic gastroenteropathy, and peripheral neuropathy. Dig Dis Sci, *28*:289–293, 1983.
2. Russell C, Pope C, Gannan R, et al. Does surgery correct esophageal motor dysfunction in gastroesophageal reflux? Ann Surg, *194*:290–296, 1981.
3. Pellegini C, De Meester T, Johnson L, et al: Gastroesophageal reflux and pulmonary aspiration: Incidence, functional abnormality and results of surgical therapy. Surgery, *26*:110–119, 1979.
4. Chernow B, Johnson L, Janowitz W, et al. Pulmonary aspiration as a consequence of gastroesophageal reflux: A diagnostic approach. Dig Dis Sci, *24*:839–844, 1979.
5. Larrain A, Garasco J, Golleguillos J, et al: Reflux treatment improves lung function in patients with intrinsic asthma (abstract). Gastroenterology, *80*:1204, 1981.

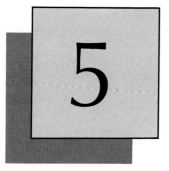

5

Functional Evaluation of the Esophagus

Colin O.H. Russell

The esophagus is a hollow muscular tube with a sphincter mechanism at each end. These three parts (sphincters and muscle) must act in concert to provide the two main functions of the esophagus: (1) transport and (2) control of reflux. Although these functions do overlap, each will be discussed separately in this chapter.

■ Transport

We must first consider the development and true value of the techniques currently employed in the evaluation of esophageal transport (or transit). The clinical history was and remains the initial screening test for dysfunction. By the end of the nineteenth century many of the classical features of the clinical history of esophageal motility disorders were well described. Auscultation over the chest during the swallowing of a fluid bolus was used to detect the noise of turbulence associated with dysfunction. Sounds (bougies) were often passed to assess the patency of the esophageal lumen. This assessment of luminal patency was much improved by the development of endoscopic techniques by Kussmaul in 1868. Esophageal manometry began in 1883 when Kronecker and Meltzer used balloons to study intraluminal pressure changes. In 1897 Walter Cannon initiated radiology of the esophagus when he observed the passage of bismuth subnitrate down the esophagus of a goose.

■ ESOPHAGEAL MANOMETRY

In 1940 the open-tipped catheter system was introduced by Body and gradually replaced balloon manometry. Perfusion of the catheters was later suggested, but it was not till 1970 that Pope demonstrated that only perfused systems accurately predicted pressure changes under experimental conditions.[1] The nonperfused systems constantly underestimated the pressures. The rate of perfusion was found to be critical when the pressures to be recorded were changing rapidly. In these experiments a syringe pump provided the constant perfusion, and this system of manometry was in use for many years. In 1977 Dodds and his group proved that infusion rates in excess of 6 ml/min per catheter were necessary to achieve an accurate measure of esophageal peristaltic pressure.[2] With a three catheter assembly (minimal requirement for esophageal manometry) this would have meant 18 ml of water entering the esophageal lumen each minute. This causes some patients to gag and swallow continuously. These high perfusion rates were necessary to overcome the intrinsic high compliance of syringe pumps. They overcame this problem by developing a pneumohydraulic capillary perfusion system with very low compliance, giving a flow rate of only 0.5 ml/min per catheter.

Manometry systems contain a pressure tranducer in series with the catheter but at some distance from the esophageal lumen. This means any pressure wave generated in the lumen must traverse the column of fluid in the catheter before it reaches the pressure measuring system. Such a system is inefficient owing to damping of the pressure wave. A more accurate system actually places the strain gauge in the esophageal lumen (see below).

Dodds and his coworkers used this latter method to study the peristaltic wave form.[2] They employed wave spectrum analysis to compare the wave forms obtained by the traditional perfused catheter–distant transducer system and this intraluminal strain gauge method. The former showed variable damping of the pressure wave. This damping was a product of the length of the catheter and its internal diameter (ID). If a catheter of 0.8 mm ID exceeded a length of 1 m, then significant damping occurred. The manometry systems in general use today are a product of this research and give high fidelity recordings with pressure responses of 200 mm Hg per second or greater. The slow infusion rates and miniaturization of catheter assemblies within acceptable limits of damping have led to the construction of eight lumen assemblies with a total outside diameter (OD) of only 6 mm. Dodds et al. have shown that these multicatheter systems are a most efficient method for studying esophageal function by manometry.[3]

Despite the advances already mentioned there is still some inherent compliance and damping within perfused catheter manometry systems. This is because the pressure wave still has to be transmitted via a column of fluid to a distant transducer. Manometry systems comprising three or four miniature pressure transducers built into a flexible catheter of acceptable dimensions are now commercially available. There is no doubt such systems have superior frequency and dynamic responses, but their relative bulk, high costs, and fragility are adverse features that limit their use.

Manometry by the usual continuous perfusion side hole catheter system outlined above relies on occlusion of the side hole, producing a pressure rise within the system. Occlusion is provided by the esophageal mucosa during peristalsis. Assuming total occlusion and noncompliance, the pressure within the catheter assembly will rise until it equals the occluding pressure and flow will resume. This occlusive force is a circumferential squeeze only. When a multiple catheter system with side holes at measured intervals is used, then the velocity of the pressure wave down the esophagus can be calculated. The transducer converts the pressure response to electrical energy, which then undergoes linear amplification. A recording system (e.g., pen and ink) traces the changes in pressure on paper moving at a constant velocity (Fig. 5–1). Therefore, the duration of the peristaltic pressure wave, its amplitude, and its velocity can be measured. A manometry tracing from a normal subject is shown in Fig. 5–1.

The esophageal musculature has a complex structure. The longitudinal muscle is arranged as a longitudinal spiral and the circular muscle is arranged in ellipses of varying inclination.[4] Electromyography suggests the longitudinal component is first to contract.[5] When these anatomic and functional observations are combined, it seems likely that peristalsis is more akin to a "wringing" motion than a simple propagated squeeze along the length of the esophagus. We should therefore consider the force of peristalsis as having two vectors—a circumferential force or squeeze and a downward or aboral force. Manometry only estimates one of these vectors—squeeze. Pope used an intraluminal strain gauge to measure the two forces—aboral and squeeze—simultaneously.[6] Some patients with dysphagia had a normal squeeze, but the aboral force was weak: i.e., there was not a constant correlation between the peristaltic amplitude and the force that drives the bolus in an aboral direction. This suggests that absolute measures of the amplitude of the peristaltic wave as recorded by manometry may have limited value.

My own studies of peristaltic values measured in a group of normal volunteers and using modern low-compliance, high-fidelity manometry equipment confirm the lack of usefulness of absolute values. There was a large interindividual variation in the amplitude, duration, and velocity of the peristaltic wave despite all measurements being made at a similar level in the esophagus. Analysis of variance showed that this interindividual variation was the major source of variance ($f = 48.1$; $P < .001$). This wide normal variation must further limit the usefulness of these absolute manometric values for assessing esophageal function. In contrast, the small intraindividual variation at a constant site does mean that these absolute values as measured by manometry can be used to assess the effect of drugs, or other pharmacologic agents, on esophageal peristalsis. This is, however, valid only when each subject is used as his or her own control and only when measurements of amplitude, velocity, and duration are made at the same level before and after therapeutic manipulation are compared.

The study of esophageal function includes assessment of its upper and lower sphincters. Magendie in 1813 first described the ring of contracted muscle at the gastroesophageal (GE) junction known as the lower esophageal sphincter (LES). Since then there has been much debate about how to assess LES pressure (LESP) and the true value of any such isolated measurements of LESP. A review of the problems and variables inherent in the assessment of LESP is important. The most

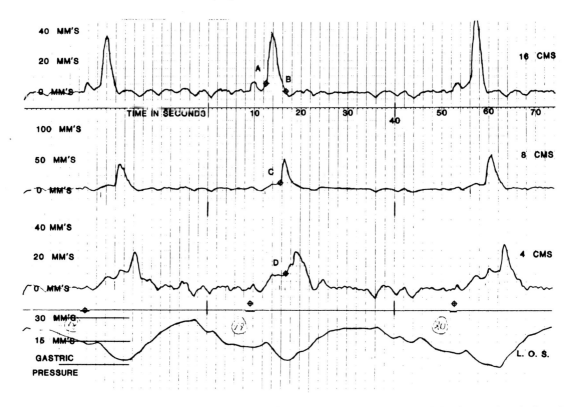

Figure 5–1. Manometry tracing from normal volunteer (amplitude in mm Hg on vertical axes and time in seconds on horizontal axes). From top to bottom are seen the pressure events at 16 cm, 8 cm, and 4 cm above the lower esophageal sphincter (LES) and at the LES itself. Points A and B are the onset and completion, respectively, of a peristaltic wave measured at 16 cm. Points C and D are the onset of that same wave seen more distally at 8 cm and 4 cm, respectively.

common method of measuring LESP has been to pull a side-hole catheter assembly across the LES and record the resulting pressure rise. The pressure rise differs greatly, depending on whether the side-hole catheter assemblies are uninfused[7] or infused[8] and again vary with the method of infusion. Both the diameter of the catheter assembly and the rate at which it traverses the GE junction are significant. Rapid pull-through measurements appear to vary most.[9] Another factor is the actual part of the manometric pressure profile used to read pressure. This can be the point of respiratory reversal at the end of expiration, at the end of inspiration, or indeed at any other point. Radial asymmetry of the pressure profile can produce variations in pressure of as much as 68 per cent.[9]

In 1974 it was shown that although side-hole catheter manometry might be adequate for assessing peristalsis, it was inappropriate for prolonged continuous studies of LES function. The considerable vertical movement (up to 2 cm) of the esophagus and its lower sphincter over the fixed side-hole catheter system during respiration and swallowing creates movement artifact and is a major source of error.[10] Dent came independently to a similar conclusion and developed the "sleeve"

sensor.[11] This 6-cm long infused sleeve responds to the maximal pressure exerted at any point along it and limits the outflow of the infused fluid. This resistance is transmitted to an external pressure transducer in exactly the same way as the side-hole system. When the midpoint of the 6-cm sleeve is placed within the LES, the normal range of vertical movement will not displace it from the LES, and a fall in pressure can be stated to be due to relaxation rather than to movement artifact. Prolonged measurements of LESP were therefore made possible. Studies demonstrated not only a large interindividual variation but also a large intraindividual variation with time. It therefore seems that isolated measures of absolute values of LESP are of limited value.

In the upper esophageal sphincter (UES) there is greater vertical movement than in the LES, and pressure changes occur more rapidly. The response rate of the "sleeve" system has been thought to be too slow to accurately record these rapid changes in pressures. Recent data in abstract form suggests that this is not the case and that sleeve manometry may be the method of choice for studying UES function.

The preceding paragraphs have highlighted the

weaknesses of manometry; however, manometry is a valid measure of esophageal function provided that these limitations are borne in mind. What, then, constitutes a normal manometric examination? My criteria for a normal manometric examination are as follows:

- A pressure wave should be seen to pass down the entire length of the esophagus in response to at least 90 per cent of wet or dry swallows.
- The LES should be seen to relax in response to these swallows.
- The amplitude of the peristaltic waves at any level should not exceed 200 mm Hg, and the velocity should be within the range of 1 to 5 cm/sec. The duration of the wave at any level should not exceed 7 sec.
- LESP should probably be in the range of 8 to 30 mm Hg, but the diagnostic significance of absolute values beyond this range is questionable.

■ RADIOLOGY

The discovery of a new type of radiation by Roentgen in 1895 led to a rapid perception of its potential in diagnostic medicine. By 1898 barium had been selected from the metallic salts as being the safest and most appropriate contrast medium. By 1921 the radiologic features of normal esophageal peristalsis were well documented, as were the motility disorders of achalasia and esophageal spasm. Developments in the field of electronics have greatly improved image enhancement and reduced the problems of radiation exposure.

Studies of normal subjects in the supine position (to overcome gravity) show that a liquid bolus of barium rapidly enters the esophagus and spreads distally, creating a long radiopaque column of barium. This shortens and passes distally into the stomach. The initial rapid dissemination of the bolus along the esophagus, and the subsequent shortening and distal passage are caused by pharyngeal contraction and esophageal peristalsis, respectively. This means that these two phases of deglutition can to some degree be studied separately. The transit of barium and associated events occur so rapidly (especially within the pharynx) that very careful attention by the radiologist during fluoroscopy is necessary. The interpretation of events is highly subjective and fleeting in nature. If a permanent record of events is obtained, as by cineradiology, repeated playback at slower speeds greatly enhances assessment. This method is expensive and time-consuming and is employed infrequently.

The volume of the swallowed bolus has been shown to be a significant factor in the manometric evaluation of esophageal function, but it seems there is little attempt by radiologists to use a constant volume bolus. Barium tablets maintain a constant form and are used to study esophageal transport. Normal individuals, however, may require more than one swallow for the tablet to reach the stomach, rendering this an insensitive method of discriminating normal from abnormal transport. Even with advances in technology the radiation exposure associated with adequate assessment of esophageal transport is significant (6 to 8 rad). This precludes its use during pregnancy and when repeated studies over a short time period are necessary.

Despite these apparent drawbacks, radiology, with its ability to detect mechanical obstruction (particularly that due to malignancy), must remain the first stage in the investigation of dysphagia. Two clinical studies of systemic disorders known to affect esophageal function compared manometry and cineradiology. These studies showed that cineradiology performed by an enthusiastic expert has a sensitivity for detection of esophageal dysfunction close to that of manometry. Cineradiology is not now in general use, and the more generally used fluoroscopic imaging methods could not have a similar sensitivity. It therefore seems that radiology lacks the sensitivity necessary to detect subtle abnormalities of esophageal motor function.

■ NUCLEAR MEDICINE

The development of nuclear medicine has been made possible by a careful integration of nuclear physics, engineering, computer science, chemistry, pharmacology, and physiology. The first recorded use of nuclear medicine in the study of esophageal disorders was reported in 1972 by Kazem.[12] He used a radionuclide bolus to measure esophageal clearance in normal volunteers and patients with obstructing lesions of the esophagus. The first real attempt to use nuclear medicine techniques to study the functional disorder of the esophagus was described by Tolin et al. in 1979.[13] In this study they measured percentage clearance of an ingested standard volume (15 ml) bolus of water and technetium sulfur colloid (TcSC) from the esophagus in patients with motility disorders and in normal volunteers. After the initial swallow to ingest the bolus, "dry" swallows occurred every 15 sec for a total of 10 min. A temporal analysis of esophageal clearance was performed. This demonstrated that normal individuals emptied the esophagus in <15 sec (i.e., with one swallow), whereas patients with scleroderma, achalasia, and diffuse esophageal spasm (DES) required >15 sec (i.e., more swallows). The emptying rate of patients with DES appeared significantly different from that of achalasia and scleroderma, but separation of the last two was not possible on this basis. Tolin's method therefore assessed esophageal clearance and, although sensitive, it was not specific as to cause. In addition, there were two major potential sources of error:

1. If the entire bolus was not ingested with the first swallow, the subsequent dry swallows would increment the radioactivity within the esophagus.
2. Retrograde flow of radionuclide from the stomach—gastroesophageal reflux—would also increment esophageal radioactivity.

Both of these situations would lead to a false positive diagnosis of impaired esophageal clearance.

Tolin's paper, however, inspired further efforts to develop the concept toward a more dynamic and specific test of transit. We have developed the following technique, which has been well described elsewhere:[10]

■ Radionuclide Transit—Technique

- Patient lies supine over a gamma camera linked to a minicomputer and is positioned to record events in the mouth, entire esophagus, and stomach.
- A radioactive marker is placed alongside the cricoid cartilage to denote the proximal boundary of the esophagus.
- A 10-ml homogeneous bolus of water and 400 μCi TcSC is introduced to the mouth by a syringe, and this radionuclide bolus is then ingested with a single swallow.
- The swallowing sequence is recorded by the minicomputer for a total of 30 sec. The events can be replayed, and the cricoid and gastroesophageal junction are identified.
- With a lightpen, regions of interest representing mouth and pharynx; proximal, middle and distal esophagus; and stomach can be delineated (Fig. 5–2).

The actual passage of the bolus through each area is plotted graphically using radioactivity representing volume on the vertical axis and time in seconds on the horizontal axis (Fig. 5–3).

The radionuclide transit (RT) graph from a normal volunteer is shown in Figure 5–3. It is our practice to record the transit of three boluses: these are recorded in the supine position, but if a transit abnormality is detected, then the last swallow is performed in the sitting (upright) position. Transit is defined as normal where there is smooth passage

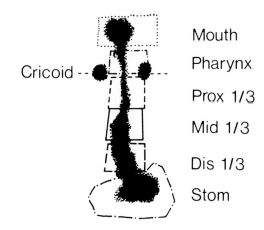

Figure 5–2. Composite image from radionuclide transit study. Six regions of interest—mouth; pharynx; proximal, middle, and distal thirds of esophagus; and stomach—have been created. The cricoid markers are easily seen.

of the bolus in an aboral direction with <5 per cent residual radioactivity within the esophagus at 15 sec (Fig. 5–3). The following transit abnormalities are described:

Adynamic transit (Fig. 5–4)—complete loss of the normal distinct and sequential peaks of activity indicating lack of distal bolus progression. If the study is repeated in the sitting position and the entire bolus, or the major portion of it, still remains in the esophagus, then in the absence of other forms of mechanical obstruction one would assume failure of relaxation of the LES.

Incoordination (Fig. 5–5)—multiple peaks of activity showing disorganized bolus transit with periods of retrograde bolus movement.

Prolonged transit—three sequential peaks indicating smooth passage of the bolus in an aboral direction are present, but transit time exceeds 15 sec.

Gastroesophageal reflux (Fig. 5–6)—transit appears normal but is followed by activity peaks in the esophagus corresponding to a fall in gastric radioactivity.

In addition, monitoring radioactivity in the mouth and pharynx will indicate if the entire bolus was ingested.

In the initial validation studies the technique (RT) was applied to two groups—normal volunteers and patients with obvious motility disorders, as demonstrated by manometry and radiology. This suggested RT has a sensitivity of 100 per cent for detecting an abnormality.[14] In addition, it provided some information as to the possible type of abnormality present. Because RT tests esophageal function in a totally different manner from manometry, assessment of specificity according to a clas-

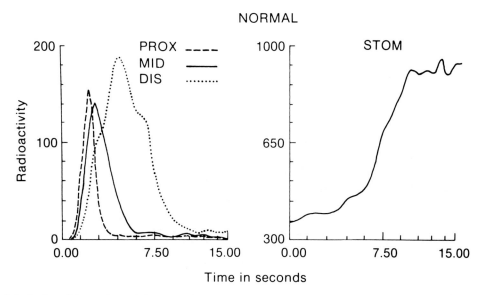

Figure 5–3. Radionuclide transit graph from normal volunteer. Vertical axes represent the radioactivity in each region, and the horizontal axes measure the time in seconds. Note sequential peaks in proximal, middle, and distal esophagus, indicating smooth passage of the bolus in an aboral direction with early and complete entry into the stomach.

sification of abnormality based on manometric values is not appropriate. Adynamic transit, however, equates with aperistalsis. When the technique was applied to a group of patients with a primary complaint of dysphagia but who had normal manometric findings and no radiologic evidence of obstruction, 64 per cent were found to have a transit disorder. Although this latter study was biased in favor of RT, it did indicate that the method was capable of detecting dysfunction where conventional methods—manometry and radiology—had failed. A further study to test the correlation between results of assessment of esophageal function by manometry and by RT was performed in a population group known to have a high prevalence of esophageal dysfunction—diabetes mellitus. This

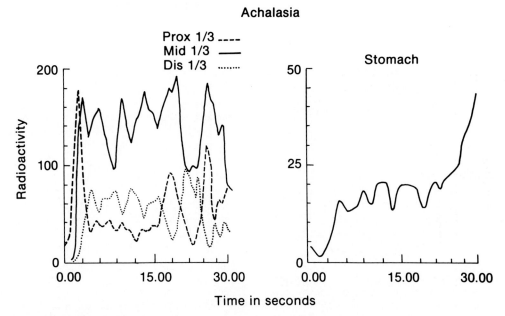

Figure 5–4. Radionuclide transit graphs from patients with achalasia. The vertical axes and horizontal axes measure radioactivity and time (in seconds), respectively. Note the failure of the bolus to progress beyond the mid segment at 30 sec. This is an adynamic pattern. Very little of the bolus enters the stomach.

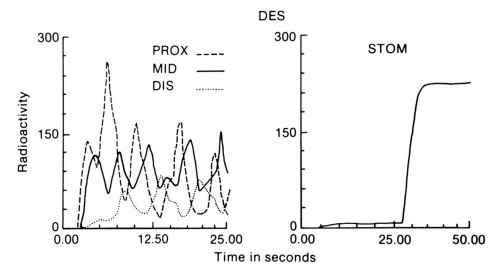

Figure 5–5. Radionuclide transit graphs for a patient with diffuse esophageal spasm. Vertical axes and horizontal axes show radioactivity and time (in seconds), respectively. Note multiple peaks of activity representing disorganized bolus transit. Some of the bolus, however, reached the stomach within the 30 sec period.

demonstrated a strong positive association between the results obtained by both methods (P = 0.003).[15]

We can therefore conclude that RT is a valid test for esophageal dysfunction with a sensitivity possibly greater than, but at least equal to that of manometry. When region of interest analysis is used, artifacts due to reflux and anomalies of ingestion can be excluded. Some qualitative information regarding peristalsis is also gained. By varying the posture, achalasia can be confidently discriminated

from other forms of aperistalsis. Where facilities exist, RT may be best used as a screening test for esophageal dysfunction or where manometry and radiology have failed to detect abnormal esophageal motor function.

RT with solid boluses has been tested, but because normal subjects can have abnormalities of solid bolus transit this method is felt to be unreliable. Perhaps the use of semisolid or viscous substances will overcome this problem. Already, advances in RT analysis allow us to measure bolus

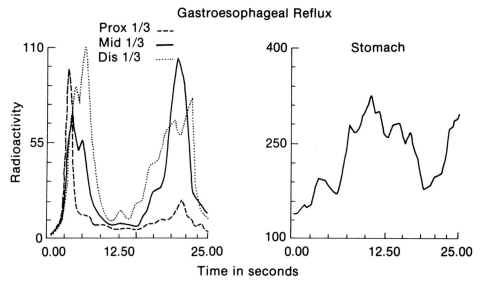

Figure 5–6. Radionuclide transit graph from patient with known gastroesophageal reflux. Vertical axes and horizontal axes show radioactivity and time (in seconds), respectively. Note initial "normal" transit and then second activity peaks in esophagus coinciding with marked fall in gastric radioactivity.

velocity, but the clinical relevance, if any, of such advances has yet to be assessed.

■ AN APPROACH TO THE CLINICAL EVALUATION OF ESOPHAGEAL TRANSIT

Transport abnormalities are usually manifested clinically as dysphagia and occasionally as odynophagia. Transport of nutrients to the digestive system can be considered in two phases.

Phase I—preparation of the bolus and the events preceding its entry into the esophageal lumen.

Phase II—transport within and exit from the esophagus into the stomach.

Phase I ■ The physical characteristics of a nutrient bolus may be unsuitable for ingestion. The grinding action of a good set of teeth and lubrication by saliva will facilitate bolus passage. The bolus must then be swallowed. *Swallowing* is a cascade of action of different muscle groups—lingual, palatal, and pharyngeal—and relaxation of the upper esophageal sphincter. In the normal state this efficient mechanism will propel a 10-ml liquid bolus into the proximal esophageal lumen at a velocity of 40 mm/sec or even faster.[16]

If the history suggests a disorder of phase I, evaluation must include examination of the cranial nerves responsible for deglutition and the patient should be observed during the act of swallowing in order to ascertain whether aspiration occurs. The single most useful method of studying phase I is by barium swallow. The passage of a number of boluses of barium should be observed fluoroscopically *by the clinician*. There are two main abnormalities seen—oropharyngeal weakness and cricopharyngeal incoordination. When the cricopharyngeus fails to relax, barium is seen to strike a bar in the distal pharynx and rebound (often into the nasopharynx) and may even enter the trachea.

Esophageal manometry will detect pharyngeal contraction, but events are so rapid that the response rate of perfusion manometry is inadequate for obtaining meaningful values of contractile force. Even the electronic manometry systems (e.g., Honeywell probe) may be inadequate. As discussed earlier, the rapidity of events in the UES and its considerable vertical movement during swallowing have raised doubts about its suitability for study by manometry; however, a Dent sleeve catheter may well overcome these problems.

Phase II ■ My personal scheme of investigation after taking the clinical history is outlined by the algorithm shown in Table 5–1. I feel that today endoscopy is a mandatory adjunct to radiology to exclude mechanical obstruction, especially malig-

nancy. It is also well known that motility disorders can be secondary to malignancy. When a motility disorder is suspected at radiology, any further evaluation requires manometry. If, however, barium swallow and endoscopy find no cause for the dysphagia and symptoms persist, then radionuclide transit is a good screening test for abnormality. In our experience and others it is extremely unusual for RT to be normal in the presence of genuine manometric abnormality. Therefore, it is generally unnecessary to further evaluate a patient with normal RT. Where RT is abnormal and where further classification of the disorder will assist management, then manometry should be performed.

It must always be remembered that some motility disorders are present only intermittently, and evaluation will be more liable to detect abnormality when symptoms are present. The topic of provocation is discussed below.

■ PROVOCATIVE TESTS IN CHEST PAIN OF UNKNOWN ETIOLOGY

The intermittent nature of some esophageal motility disorders may render diagnosis difficult. In such cases a definitive diagnosis may be obtained only when the patient is studied while symptomatic. This could be achieved by detaining the patient in the hospital and having staff available 24 hours per day seven days per week to study the patient as soon as symptoms developed. An alternative and more acceptable approach would be to use a provocative agent that could reliably unmask any pre-existing, but quiescent, motility disorder and reproduce the patient's symptoms. Such attempts to provoke abnormality have been used most commonly in the investigation of patients with noncardiac chest pain.

It has long been accepted that gastroesophageal reflux and esophageal motility disorders can be a source of chest pain indistinguishable from cardiac pain. This has led to the common practice in many centers of referring all patients with chest pain, but no evidence of cardiac disease, for esophageal function studies and an esophageal stress test. Various provocative agents have been used: ice water swallows, intraluminal acid, bethanecol. (There is, however, no good evidence that ice water swallows provoke motility disorders.)

Acid infusion: Infusing acid into the esophagus (the Bernstein test), in addition to reproducing the heartburn of reflux, can also reproduce chest pain if it is an atypical symptom of reflux. In my own unpublished study of 60 consecutive patients with noncardiac chest pain, acid infusion reproduced the

Table 5–1.

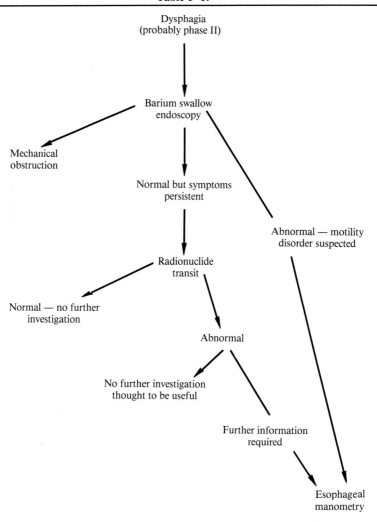

pain in only one patient (1.5 per cent), and the clinical history predicted that reflux was the most likely cause of that patient's symptoms. Mellow et al. demonstrated that esophageal acid infusion can produce electrocardiographic evidence of myocardial ischemia in some patients with known coronary artery disease.[17] This suggests that a positive Bernstein test cannot safely implicate reflux and exclude cardiac disease as a cause for chest pain unless blood pressure, heart rate, and multiple lead electrocardiography have been assessed simultaneously. I no longer perform the Bernstein test and prefer to use prolonged pH monitoring if I suspect gastroesophageal reflux might be the potential cause of pain.

Drug provocation: Bethanecol and pentagastrin have been shown to amplify some motility abnormalities but have not been effective in provoking quiescent abnormalities. Ergonovine can produce chest pain in association with abnormal esophageal contractions in patients with unexplained chest pain. There have as yet been no studies using this drug in normal volunteers, so the true sensitivity and specificity of this method of provocation must remain in doubt. Normal studies have not been performed, as the cardiac risks of this drug are such that it should be used only while monitoring patients in the catheter laboratory and during coronary angiography.[18] Fortunately, most patients who develop abnormal esophageal contractions in response to ergonovine will respond in a similar manner to edrophonium, which is a much safer drug. Edrophonium is currently the best tolerated and most effective provocative agent available. It has been shown to have increased the pick-up of esophageal abnormalities by 18 per cent in one group of patients with chest pain suspected of being of esophageal origin.[19]

Pope has set the ground rules for adjudging whether the esophagus is determined as the site of chest pain. An absolute verdict of esophageal abnormality can be reached only if the patient experiences pain during manometry and this coincides with either objective evidence of abnormality on the manometry tracing or a documented episode of reflux as measured by a pH probe. Of course, to be technically accurate, one must note that unless one *simultaneously* measures all structures that can cause chest pain, then some doubt must remain!

■ *Control of Reflux*

It is now concluded by most workers that reduced LES pressure is the sine qua non for reflux leading to esophagitis, whether this reflux occurs continuously across a persistently low resting LES pressure or whether it occurs because of transient relaxation of the LES.[20] Reflux has also been shown to be a physiologic event, especially after meals. What may render reflux pathologic—with esophagitis and reflux symptoms—is the duration of contact between the esophageal mucosa and the refluxed gastric contents. Esophageal peristalsis is the main mechanism for obtaining clearance of such contents. Any evaluation of a patient suspected of having pathologic gastroesophageal reflux (GER) must therefore include assessment of LES function and esophageal peristalsis.

Because GER is a physiologic event, some quantitative measure of actual reflux must be used to separate normal from abnormal. The methods used in this regard are discussed below:

Dye markers can be instilled into the stomach and the esophageal contents sampled regularly via an indwelling catheter. This method is inefficient, tedious, and not much used.

Reflux of barium as seen on fluoroscopy has been the most common method used in clinical practice. This method may be relatively specific but it lacks sensitivity.

Radiation exposure limits the duration of any fluoroscopic studies of barium reflux. More recently, *radionuclides* have been used as markers of reflux and this has overcome this problem.[21] Both the original authors[21] and more recently Velasco claim this method is sensitive and specific. In contrast to barium studies, this radionuclide method allows quantification as well as assessment of the duration of reflux episodes, i.e., information on the length of exposure of the esophageal mucosa to reflux. Velasco was able to demonstrate a correlation between this duration of reflux and the severity of esophagitis as seen at endoscopy.

Despite such advances in assessing GER, *pH monitoring* in the distal esophageal lumen (approximately 5 cm above the LES) remains the "gold standard." This method is really specific only for detecting acid reflux, and a reflux episode is said to have occurred when the pH falls below 4 and remains so for longer than 30 sec. These pH changes are continuously recorded on moving paper, and a chart similar to a manometry tracing is obtained. This allows calculations of the frequency and duration of reflux episodes over a prolonged period of time. Helm et al.[22] introduced a word of caution regarding measures of duration with this technique. He demonstrated that acid remaining on the surface of the pH probe did not always indicate that a significant volume had remained in contact with the esophageal mucosa.

Advances in the electronics industry reduced the size of pH sensitive probes and increased their reliability. Radiotelemetry capsules have been developed and have been shown to be as reliable. The computer industry has facilitated the subsequent analysis of the large volume of data from prolonged studies. This has meant the patient can be studied in the home environment and under the conditions in which symptoms are normally experienced.

De Meester et al. have championed 24-hour monitoring of distal esophageal pH. They developed an elaborate scoring system that appears to give a 90 per cent sensitivity and specificity for detecting or excluding acid reflux.[23] In contrast to prolonged monitoring in the natural environment is the brief monitoring under laboratory conditions of the standard acid reflux test (SART). This short-term study can be scored as follows:

0—No reflux despite acid loading of the stomach and provocative maneuvers, e.g., Valsalva maneuver.

1—Reflux only after acid loading with provocative maneuvers.

2—Reflux present after acid loading of the stomach without such maneuvers.

3—Reflux present with provocative maneuvers; no acid loading necessary.

4—Reflux present without acid loading or maneuvers; can be cleared by repeated swallowing.

5—Free reflux throughout the study.

If a patient scores 4 or 5, then pathologic reflux is likely; but a score of less than 4 is not diagnostic in either a positive or a negative sense.

There is little doubt in my mind that prolonged monitoring of distal esophageal pH is still the best method for detecting pathologic reflux. However, the duration of the monitoring period necessary may be considerably less than the 24 hours proposed by De Meester. A study of 6 hours' duration may be adequate in many cases. Prolonged monitoring also allows investigators to study the correlation between a patient's symptoms and reflux episodes. This can be achieved by patients maintaining an accurate diary of symptoms or by activating an event signal that is recorded synchronously with the pH data.

Regarding control of reflux, we can now answer what I feel are the important questions: (1) is (pathological) reflux present? (2) Is reflux the cause of the symptoms? (3) Is esophageal function normal? (4) Is LES function abnormal? The only remaining question (Has the mucosa been damaged?) is best answered with endoscopy and biopsy.

■ REFERENCES

1. Pope CE: Effect of infusion on force of closure measurements in the human esophagus. Gastroenterology, 58:616–624, 1970.
2. Arndorfer R, Stef J, Dodds W, et al. Improved infusion system for intraluminal oesophageal manometry. Gastroenterology, 73:23–27, 1977.
3. Dodds W, Hogan W, Arndorfer R, et al: Efficient manometric techniques for accurate regional measurement of esophageal body water activity. Am J Gastro, 70:21–24, 1978.
4. Kaufmann PO, Liese W, Stark J, et al.: Die Muskelanordung in der Speiserohre. Ergebn Arat Entwickl Gersch, 44:3–33, 1968.
5. Helemans J, Vantrappen G, Valembois P, et al: Electrical activity of striated and smooth muscle of the oesophagus. Am J Dig Dis, 13:320–334, 1968.
6. Pope C, Horton P: Intraluminal force transducer measurements of human oesophageal peristalsis. Gut, 13:464–470, 1977.
7. Stanciu C, Hoare R, Bennett J: Correlation between manometric and pH tests for gastroesophageal reflux. Gut, 18:536–540, 1977.
8. Pope C: A dynamic test of sphincter strength: Its application to the lower esophageal sphincter. Gastroenterology, 52:779–786, 1967.
9. Welch R, Drake S: Normal lower esophageal sphincter pressure: A comparison of rapid vs. slow pullthrough techniques. Gastroenterology, 78:1446–1451, 1980.
10. Lyda S, Dodds W, Hogan W, et al: The effect of manometric assembly diameter on intraluminal esophageal recording. Dig Dis Sci, 209:968–970, 1975.
11. Dent J: A new technique for continuous sphincter pressure measurement. Gastroenterology, 71:263–267, 1976.
12. Kazen I: A new scintigraphic technique for the study of the oesophagus. Am J Roentgen, 115:681–688, 1972.
13. Tolin R, Malmud L, Rullery J, et al: Esophageal scintigraphy to quantitate esophageal transit. Gastroenterology, 76:1402–1408, 1979.
14. Russell C, Hill L, Holmes E, et al. Radionuclide transit: A sensitive screening test for esophageal dysfunction. Gastroenterology, 80:887, 1981.
15. Russell C: Relationship among esophageal dysfunction, diabetic gastroenteropathy and peripheral neuropathy. Dig Dis Sci, 28:289–293, 1983.
16. Fisher M, Henrix T, Hunt J, et al: Relation between volume swallowed and velocity of the bolus ejected from the pharynx into the esophagus. Gastroenterology, 74:1238–1240, 1978.
17. Mellow M, Simpson A, Watt L, et al. Esophageal acid perfusion in coronary artery disease. Gastroenterology, 85:306–312, 1983.
18. Gravino F, Perloff J, Yeatman L, et al: Coronary artery spasm versus esophageal spasm. Am J Med, 70:1293–1296, 1981.
19. Benjamin S, Richter J, Cardova C, et al: Prospective manometric evaluation with pharmacological provocation of patients with suspected esophageal motility dysfunction. Gastroenterology, 84:813–901, 1983.
20. Dent J, Dodds W, Friedman R, et al: Mechanism of gastroesophageal reflux in recumbent asymptomatic human subjects. J Clin Invest, 65:256–267, 1980.
21. Fisher RS, Malmud LS, Roberts GS, et al. Gastroesophageal scintiscanning to detect and quantitate GE reflux. Gastroenterology, 70:301–308, 1976.
22. Helm J, Dodds W, Pelc L, et al. Mechanisms of esophageal acid clearance in supine normal subjects: A unifying hypothesis. Gastroenterology, 80:1171A, 1981.
23. De Meester T, Wang C, Wernly J, et al: Technique, indications and clinical use of twenty four hour esophageal pH monitoring. J Thorac Cardiovasc Surg, 656–670, 1980.

6

Esophageal Endoscopy, Dilation, and Intraesophageal Prosthetic Devices

Donald E. Low ▪ Richard A. Kozarek

▪ *Endoscopy*

History ▪ Upper gastrointestinal endoscopy is an invasive diagnostic and therapeutic modality which has seen ever-increasing utilization over the past several decades. The fiberoptic instruments have virtually replaced rigid endoscopy in all but the rarest cases. Recently video endoscopes have appeared, although the ultimate utilization of this new technology is still being assessed.

The first semiflexible gastroscope was introduced by Schindler in 1932. This instrument allowed visualization of 75 per cent of the gastric mucosa and could be attached to a camera or used as a biopsy conduit. In 1958, Hirschowitz introduced the first fiberoptic gastroscope which extended the field of observation to include a greater portion of the cardia and the duodenum.

Currently, the scopes being utilized for most esophageal endoscopic examinations are 8 to 12 mm in width and have a working length of approximately 1 m. They contain anywhere from 20,000 to 30,000 integrated fibers which are coated with a light refractive glass that prevents light from diffusing outward and allows it to be bent at acute angles without distortion. The scopes also contain wire controls which allow integrated multidirectional movement enabling the tip of the scope to undergo flexion to at least 180 degrees. Within the tube are accessory channels which allow for air insufflation, suction, and water irrigation as well as the passage of biopsy and fulguration instruments. Through these same channels can be passed

various other instruments, including spray catheters, flexible-tip dilatation wires, laser beam catheters, and polypectomy snare wires.

Preparation ▪ Patients undergoing routine diagnostic upper GI endoscopy are maintained on nothing by mouth for a period usually ranging from 6 to 8 hours. This time period may be increased for patients with strictures or gastric outlet obstructions. Patient tolerance during the endoscopic procedure often depends on how well informed the patient is about the technical aspects of the procedure. This should include a working knowledge of the progression of expected events before the procedure is actually begun. Along with this reassurance, the ease of the procedure can be augmented by utilizing various oral and intravenous medications. Topical pharyngeal anesthetics which may include 2 per cent viscous xylocaine, Cetacaine, or Hurricaine can be utilized to minimize gagging with the introduction of the scope. These compounds should be utilized carefully in heavily sedated patients or patients with large fluid collections in the stomach or esophagus. Oral simethicone can be used to decrease the amount of foam and bubbles encountered, and IV anticholinergics, usually atropine, can be used to decrease oral secretions and gastric motility. The effectiveness of these last two compounds is controversial, and anticholinergic agents should not be utilized in patients with severe dysmotility problems or a history of tachyarrhythmias.

The most commonly used combination of premedications is IV meperidine with one of the various benzodiazepine agents. Both of these drugs should be administered in a dosage which will vary according to a patient's age, weight, medical condition, and degree of apprehension. Meperidine can be given intravenously up to a dosage of 1 mg/kg of body weight, and its action can be quickly and effectively reversed should the need arise.

Examination ■ It should be noted that examination of the esophagus is rarely done in isolation. Whenever possible, it should be done in conjunction with a full examination of the upper gastrointestinal tract which should extend from the hypopharynx to the third portion of the duodenum.

The examination itself usually is done with the patient in the left lateral decubitus position. The scope can be introduced under direct vision, or a controlled blind intubation with the patient swallowing the scope can be done. However, regardless of how the scope is inserted, the hypopharynx should be examined routinely during either insertion or removal of the scope. This examination should include visualizing the vocal cords, piriform sinus, posterior cricoid cartilage, and glottis.

As a general principle, the scope should never be advanced unless the lumen is visualized, and diagnostic and therapeutic manipulations should always wait until the entire general examination is completed. Whenever the situation is appropriate, areas of stricture, ulceration, and suspected columnar metaplasia can be biopsied. This can be done with brushings for cytologic examination or forceps or suction biopsies. The accuracy of cytologic brushings varies considerably according to the level of experience of the cytologist. Forceps biopsy is quick and easy and all these specimens should be completely sectioned. Accuracy can be increased with multiple biopsies, which are especially important when dealing with presumed submucosal lesions. Suction biopsies tend to take a deeper sampling of tissue and are particularly effective when a large number of biopsies are being taken.

A great deal of controversy has arisen concerning the role of endoscopy versus upper gastrointestinal barium studies with respect to initial examinations for patients with upper GI symptoms. Multiple studies have been done which demonstrate that endoscopy has a significantly greater sensitivity than upper GI series in identifying esophageal and other upper gastrointestinal disease.[1-3] In addition, endoscopy is gaining increasing acceptance as an initial assessment of patients with dyspepsia refractory to initial medical therapy.[4] Experience has shown that patient acceptance to endoscopy versus upper GI barium series is equivalent[5,6] and that prior knowledge of previous x-ray results does not alter subsequent endoscopic findings.[1] Histor-

ically, barium studies have been identified as being less expensive; however, recently even this has been challenged.[7]

Almost all patients undergoing routine diagnostic upper endoscopy can be examined as outpatients in either the office, clinic, or hospital outpatient setting. This can be extended to selected patient populations undergoing certain therapeutic procedures including biopsy, dilatation, obliterative sclerotherapy, and even laser therapy. In addition, even sick and heavily monitored patients can undergo examination. The portability of endoscopy allows the procedure to be done effectively in both the intensive care unit and the operating room setting.

Indications ■ Symptomatically, the three most common esophageal symptoms which may ultimately lead to endoscopic examination are dysphagia, heartburn, and odynophagia. Although each of these symptoms can be suitably assessed initially by barium swallows, many of these examinations will show abnormalities that require further assessment by endoscopy (Figs. 6–1 to 6–3).

Initial barium studies done in a patient with dysphagia will often show a filling defect, ulceration, or stricture. Endoscopy and biopsy often will be required to rule out the presence of cancer or Barrett's esophagus. Other radiologic abnormalities associated with dysphagia which do not require immediate endoscopic evaluation include diverticula, Schatzki's ring, and motility patterns suggestive of diffuse esophageal spasm; however, surveillance endoscopy may be recommended for some clinical entities associated with dysphagia which have shown an increased risk for the development of carcinoma. These include the hy-

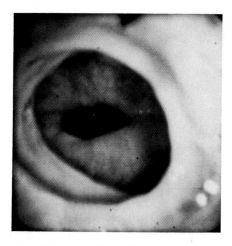

Figure 6–1. Tight Schatzki's ring in a patient with solid food dysphagia. Hiatal hernia can be seen distally. (See Color Plate I*A*.)

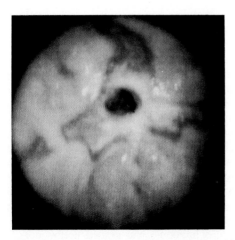

Figure 6–2. Circumferential ulceration in association with reflux strictures of the esophagus. (See Color Plate I*B*.)

popharyngeal web of Plummer-Vinson syndrome, achalasia, and lye stricture.

Endoscopic examination of a patient with heartburn should be undertaken if a significant abnormality is noted on barium swallow or if the patient is refractory to medical therapy and antireflux surgery is planned. Many patients with severe reflux may benefit from initial endoscopic assessment because the severity of symptoms does not always correlate with the severity of esophagitis. Patients with minimal symptoms and normal-appearing esophageal mucosa on radiologic examination may show endoscopic signs of friability, erosion, and polymorphonuclear infiltration of the lamina propria on biopsy.

Odynophagia usually indicates that the esophagus is obstructed, inflamed, or undergoing periodic spasm. Diagnosis of opportunistic infections such as candidiasis, herpes simplex, cytomegalovirus,

histoplasmosis, and tuberculosis in immunosuppressed patients requires biopsy and brushings. Suspected candidal plaques can be confirmed at the time of endoscopy by brushing the white plaques and smearing them on a glass slide. After allowing this to dry and applying 10 per cent potassium hydroxide, the slide can be immediately examined for the classic branched hyphae and budding yeast.

Endoscopy should be used routinely to diagnose the etiology, pinpoint location, and when appropriate, control the source of upper gastrointestinal bleeding. This can be accomplished using heater probes, laser, or either mono- or bipolar (multipolar) electrocoagulation. Monopolar electrocoagulation requires a remotely situated grounding plate and has been shown to be successful at controlling bleeding.[8] There has been a suggestion that this treatment method may help avoid rebleeding in patients with nonbleeding ulcers but a visible vessel.[9] Bipolar electrocoagulation requires no grounding plate and is more limited with respect to its depth of tissue injury. The multipolar electrode is an effective method of controlling bleeding and is generally considered to be easier to use then either the mono- or the bipolar electrode. Lasers have also been used to control upper gastrointestinal bleeding, the most common varieties being the gas-assisted argon laser or the neodymium YAG laser. Both systems have been shown to be effective in controlling bleeding; however, the YAG laser has been associated with a somewhat deeper tissue penetration, and therefore, the advantage of increased hemostatic efficiency must be balanced by an increased risk of perforation.

Other therapeutic applications of endoscopy include acute and obliterative variceal sclerotherapy for bleeding varices; snare polypectomy of esophageal polyps; foreign body extraction utilizing snares, baskets, and overtubes; and long-term follow-up of patients at increased cancer risk due to documented Barrett's esophagus, lye stricture, or achalasia. In addition, the endoscope has provided an invaluable adjunct to many of the new techniques now being utilized for esophageal dilatation and placement of esophageal stents.

Complications and Risks ∎ Simply stated, there are no absolute contraindications to endoscopy. In experienced hands, it can be done in almost any clinical setting, in the presence of significant inflammatory and obstructive conditions of the esophagus, and even following surgery to the head, neck, esophagus, and stomach in the appropriate clinical situation.

Medication reactions are among the most common complications associated with endoscopy. These can be in the form of allergic reactions but are more commonly respiratory depression due to

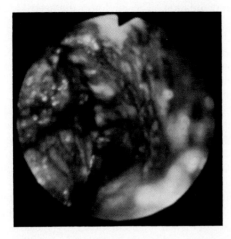

Figure 6–3. Polypoid, ulcerated squamous cell carcinoma of distal esophagus. (See Color Plate I*C*.)

the overzealous use of IV narcotics and benzodiazepines. Cardiopulmonary failure can occur secondary to laryngospasm as a result of endoscopic intubation or reflux and aspiration during the procedure. The risk of aspiration is increased in patients with significant obstructive or stenotic lesions in the esophagus or pylorus or in patients who are obtunded or who have actively bleeding esophageal lesions. In addition, myocardial infarction and tachyarrhythmias can be stimulated by intraesophageal manipulation and biopsy, electrocoagulation, or laser therapy to neoplastic or inflammatory lesions which may be adherent to the pericardium. As a result, full cardiopulmonary resuscitation apparatus should always be immediately available in the endoscopy suite. ECG and blood pressure monitoring should be utilized routinely in all patients who have had a documented or suspected myocardial infarction within the last six months or who have a history of atrial or ventricular tachyarrhythmias.

Bleeding, perforation, and infection are other problems that have been associated with endoscopy. Bleeding may be secondary to intubation or to biopsy of inflammatory, vascular, or extremely sessile lesions. In the absence of major coagulation defects, bleeding problems are usually self-limited. The incidence of perforation is increased in uncooperative patients in the presence of unrecognized epiphrenic and Zenker's diverticulum, cases of active esophageal hemorrhage following surgery to the esophagus or stomach, following caustic ingestion, or in the hands of inexperienced endoscopists. In general, the cervical esophagus is at greatest risk; however, most perforations occur in association with therapeutic maneuvers in the presence of inflammatory or neoplastic conditions.

Systemic bacteremia associated with endoscopic manipulation and biopsy has been documented. The incidence of this problem can be decreased with a more vigorous and uniform training of personnel with respect to cleaning endoscopic equipment.[10] However, patients at increased risk for bacterial endocarditis should still have preprocedural antibiotic coverage.

■ Esophageal Dilation

Esophageal dilation for benign and malignant strictures and various motility disorders predates Thomas Willis' sixteenth century description of using a cork-tipped whalebone to treat a patient with presumed achalasia.[11] The nineteenth century saw increasing utilization of various techniques of bougienage beginning with Hildreth's report in

1821. A major advance, introduced at the turn of the century, was the technique of dilation over a previously placed wire or string. This development coincided with an immediate decrease in the incidence of dilation-related complications. Subsequent developments included the introduction of various woven silk, Teflon, and elastic gum dilators which could be directed through rigid endoscopes.[12] Mercury-filled rubber bougies and eventually the Puestow system of graded metal dilators passed over a fluoroscopically placed wire were introduced in the 1950s.[13,14] This evolutionary process continued to include retrograde esophageal bougienage through a gastrostomy, stepped high-density polymer dilators, variable diameter polyethylene balloons, and graded hollow-core polyvinyl dilators (Fig. 6–4).

These developments were paralleled by other less well known or experimental alternatives, including direct dilation with graded or tapered endoscopes or the use of various sized endoscopic oversheaths or balloons fitted over a pediatric endoscope or bronchoscope.[15–20] Other mechanical dilators have been proposed which have the ability to continuously monitor the width and force of dilatation during the procedure (Table 6–1).[21]

It should be recognized, however, that the development of these new techniques did not take place in isolation. They occurred concomitantly with the development of other therapeutic modalities including the Nd YAG laser, bicap tumor probes, and various types of esophageal stents. The treatment of the various types of esophageal obstructive problems is therefore an assimilation of all these various technologies.

The vast array of dilators currently available has arisen not so much from dissatisfaction with any one method but from the recognition of the variety of pathologic situations in the esophagus which will require dilation. The etiology, diameter, length, and angulation of various esophageal strictures as well as the maintenance costs of the various dilator systems will all figure in the choice of bougienage apparatus. However, certain techniques have been identified as particularly suitable for specific anatomic situations.

Long angulated or eccentric strictures, whether benign or malignant, are best handled with guidewire technology using endoscopic or fluoroscopic control, and often both.[22] Short, pliable, and mild (luminal diameter >13 mm) strictures, including webs and Schatzki's rings, can be managed with a single pass of a 48 to 54 French Maloney bougie following a six-hour fast and aided by pharyngeal anesthesia when required. Generally speaking, restoring the esophageal lumen to at least a 44 French diameter will relieve dysphagia. Historically, phy-

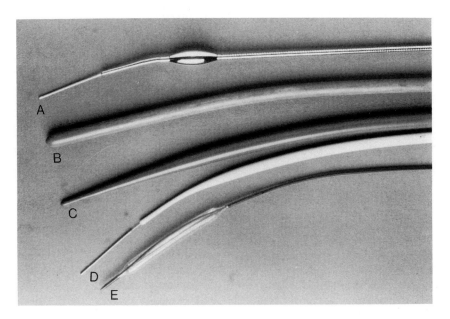

Figure 6–4. Currently available esophageal dilators. (A) Eder-Puestow dilator utilizing sequentially sized metal olives, guidewire. (B) Blunt tip mercury dilator (Hurst). (C) Tapered tip mercury dilator (Maloney). (D) Polyvinyl dilator, which utilizes guidewire technology (American). (E) Grüntzig type hydrostatic balloon.

sicians have utilized sequential dilations over days or weeks to increase luminal diameter by increments of no more than 2 mm (6 French).[23] This is unnecessary in most rings, webs, and some reflux and postsclerotherapy strictures.[24,25]

Maloney and Hurst dilations are cost effective ($40 to $80 per session in our institution) and can be carried out by the patient at home when indicated.[26] This usually necessitates several physician-supervised dilations in the office prior to independent home bougienage. Generally speaking, however, mercury dilators do not have the rigidity required in most cervical strictures or cases of severe stenosis.[27] Fluoroscopic guidance is therefore a necessity when dilation is contemplated in eccentric strictures and stenoses with pseudodiverticula.

Patients with severe (<7mm) or complex moderate (7 to 13 mm) strictures require an overnight fast along with an initial endoscopic examination to assess the proximal stricture and may require fluoroscopically controlled placement of a guidewire through the stricture. Biopsies, when required, are routinely delayed until after dilation is complete because of reported increased perforation and bleeding risk. The Puestow dilation system has historically been the most commonly utilized technique in this situation.[22,28] This employs sequential passage of 16 to 45 French metal olives over the previously situated guidewire and is often followed by subsequent mercury bougie dilations.[14] As indicated by stricture complexity, chronicity, and patient tolerance, the Puestow dilations are often spread out over a period of days to weeks.

Combined Puestow-Maloney dilations of complex strictures has demonstrated a 70 to 100 per cent improvement rate in over 850 patients in combined series.[22,28] In this same patient population, the complications included perforations (16), major bleeding (5), aspiration (2), and death (1). The proven efficiency and relative safety of this technique has led to increased support for reports indicating that some chronic reflux strictures can be managed primarily with a trial of dilation and medical antireflux therapy.[29–41] However, repeated dilations may cause an increase in rigidity and loss of mobility based on enhanced reflux postdilation, which can ultimately compromise surgical results.[69] When dilation provides only temporary symptomatic relief (2 to 3 weeks), then surgery

Table 6–1. ESOPHAGEAL DILATORS

Mercury-filled dilators
  Hurst
  Maloney

Guidewire directed dilators
  Metal olives: Eder-Puestow, Jackson-Plummer
  Neoplex "stepped": Celestin
  Polyvinyl: American, Savary-Gillard

Polyethylene balloons
  Miscellaneous
  Woven silk
  Graded plastic oversheath
  Tapered-tip endoscope
  Balloon or tape affixed to endoscope shaft

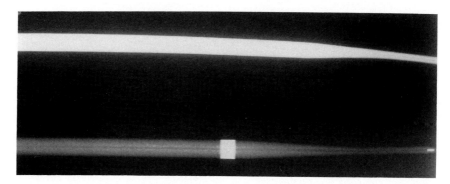

Figure 6–5. American (top) versus Savary-Gillard polyvinyl dilators. The former is radiopaque and shorter; the latter has a more gradual dilating section.

should be considered before resection becomes the only recourse.

Alternative guidewire-directed techniques include the Celestin and hollow core polyvinyl dilating systems.[42–44] The Celestin dilator consists of two neoplex graded dilators with a 10-cm tapered tip, reaching a maximum diameter of 12 to 18 mm, respectively. Although equally effective as the Puestow system in dilating both benign and malignant strictures, this must be weighed against reported perforation rates as high as 10 per cent.[42]

The safest and most efficient method for dilating tight or complex esophageal strictures is currently the hollow-core polyvinyl dilator, for example, American (CR Bard, Inc.) and Savary-Gillard (Wilson-Cook, Inc.) (Fig. 6–5). These systems require fluoroscopic or endoscopic placement of a guidewire across the stricture and can be done with pharyngeal or IV sedation. The Savary-Gillard, like the Celestin system, has a log tapered tip and requires one loop of guidewire completely within the stomach to prevent impaction of the dilator tip on the guidewire (Fig. 6–6). Care must be exercised not to attempt too aggressive a progression of dilations based on the ease with which these dilators can be passed through tight, irregular strictures. Dilations which increase luminal size in increments of 10 to 12 French can sometimes be acceptable as long as patient discomfort is minimal, dilation is done under fluoroscopic control, and the force required for dilation is not excessive. Although there is only minimal objective data currently available concerning efficiency and complication rates of the polyvinyl dilating systems, such systems will undoubtedly see increasing utilization in the years ahead.

Endoscopically placed guidewires with fluoroscopic control can also be used to position hydrostatic or pneumatic balloon dilators.[45–50] The TTS (through the scope) balloon dilating system can also be inserted under direct vision through the endoscope itself (Fig. 6–7). The balloon dilators are comparatively easy to position and offer the advantage of dilating the stricture using radial rather than vector force. These dilators would seem to offer a safe and effective mechanism for managing difficult strictures, although long-term experience is limited. In a survey conducted through 3000 ASGE members, 89 per cent of patients were reported to have acute relief of dysphagia with a complication rate of 2.1 per cent.[51] Some of these complications may have been related to the dilator tip (subsequently modified) and too rapid dilation of fixed chronic strictures.

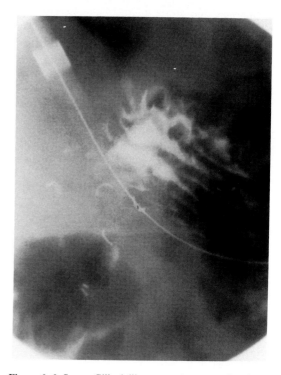

Figure 6–6. Savary-Gillard dilator passed over a spring-tipped piano style guidewire.

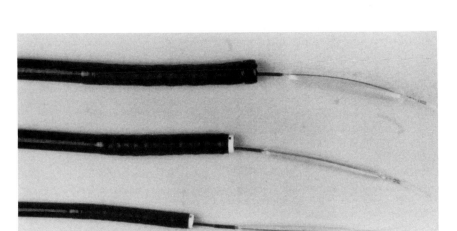

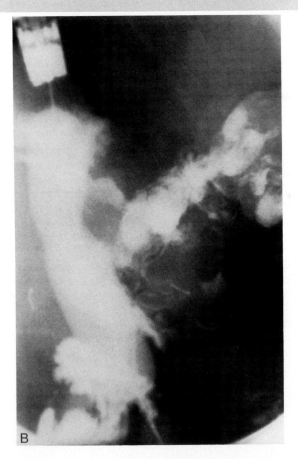

Figure 6–7. *A,* Variable sizes of through the scope (TTS) hydrostatic balloons that can be used to dilate esophageal, gastric, and colonic stenoses. *B,* TTS balloon used to dilate tight esophageal junction following antireflux surgery. Contrast material in gut. Note the balloon "waist."

Unfortunately, the TTS balloons have a life span of only one to four procedures; therefore, their utilization will continue to be limited to portions of the gastrointestinal tract not accessible to more conventional dilators (for example, bile duct, pylorus, and colon).[52] The obvious exception is the Grüntzig balloon used in pneumatic dilation of the LES in achalasia. Technically achalasia and other types of hydrostatic and pneumatic balloons require endoscopic guidewire placement and fluoroscopic control to assure balloon waist obliteration and thus an effective dilation. Balloon dilation of strictures may see increased utilization at the expense of mercury bougies. However, before this occurs, preliminary reports of lower complication rates will have to be verified, and the cost of balloon dilation (approximately $600 per episode in our institution) must be more in line with the costs of conventional methods.[53]

■ *Esophageal Stents*

The current alternatives available for the management of the 50 per cent of patients who present with nonresectable esophageal carcinoma include surgical bypass, radiation therapy, periodic bougienage, thermal methods of neolumen formation (Nd YAG laser and bicap tumor probe), and esophageal prosthesis insertion.[54] Symmonds inserted the first reported prosthesis in 1885.[55] Gootstein improved design with the introduction of the proximal funnel and distal rim to decrease the incidence of migration.[64] The Celestin tube, which has been the most commonly utilized esophageal prosthesis over the past 20 years, originally required traction insertion through an anterior gastrostomy.[56] However, further technical advances have seen ever-increasing utilization of endoscopically placed stents for obstructing tumors of the esophagus, stomach, lung, and mediastinum.[56–63] They have also been inserted for malignant fistulas, iatrogenic

Table 6–2. INDICATIONS FOR ESOPHAGEAL PROSTHESES

Tracheoesophageal fistula
Obstructive malignancy not responsive to conventional treatment
Esophageal
Gastric
Mediastinum
Reported uses, benign disease
Acute caustic ingestion
Iatrogenic perforation

perforations, and prevention of stricturing following caustic ingestion (Table 6–2).[23,64,65]

Prior to the insertion of these devices, the esophageal lumen must be dilated to a size at least 2 to 4 French larger than the diameter of the proposed prosthesis. This dilation process often requires several days; once it is complete appropriate length and luminal diameter prostheses can be chosen from several commercially available alternatives. These stents are constructed or reinforced to be relatively resistant to kinking and occlusion.

The Atkinson tube comes in three lengths and two diameters (Key Med, Inc.) and is inserted with a special introducer following dilation and endoscopic or fluoroscopic wire placement. The Nottingham introducer holds the prosthesis in place with an expandable metal olive at its tip (Fig. 6–8). The introducer is inserted orally over the wire, and the prosthesis is positioned fluoroscopically with the funnel and flange located proximal and distal to the tumor respectively.[64] The metal olive is then released and the introducer withdrawn while using the pushing tube to stabilize the prosthesis. A Gastrografin swallow verifies position and checks for evidence of perforation (Fig. 6–9). The Atkinson tube offers the advantage of allowing repositioning of the prosthesis by reinserting the introducer and re-expanding the olive if necessary.

An alternative placement system utilizes a polyvinyl dilator passed over a piano wire. The Savary system (CR Bard or Wilson-Cook, Inc.) uses a guidewire, pusher tube, and 33 French polyvinyl

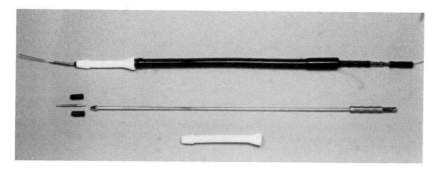

Figure 6–8. Nottingham introducer and stent placement kit. Introducer has an expandable metal olive.

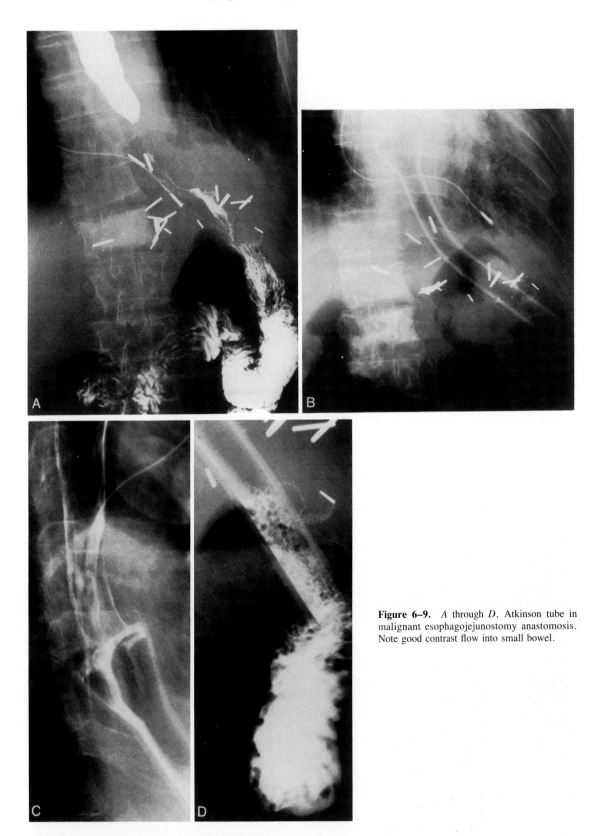

Figure 6–9. *A* through *D*, Atkinson tube in malignant esophagojejunostomy anastomosis. Note good contrast flow into small bowel.

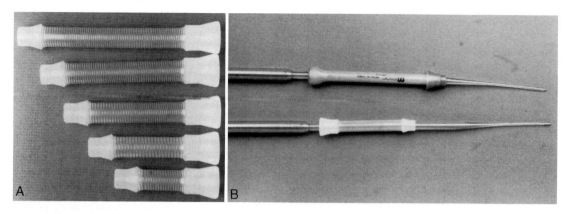

Figure 6–10. *A*, Commercially available esophageal prostheses. Note variable lengths and central spring core. *B*, Polyvinyl prosthesis insertion setups available from C.R. Bard (top) and Wilson-Cook (bottom).

dilator as an introducer (Fig. 6–10). These systems differ primarily in the length, diameter, and composition of the stents themselves.

Both systems require initial bougienage to restore esophageal luminal diameter to a size of at least 2 to 4 French larger than the prosthesis which can then be positioned using the dilator and pusher tube over the guidewire. The funnel of the stent should be situated just proximal to the tumor (Fig. 6–11). If a prosthesis is improperly situated using this technique, various methods of tube retrieval have been used. These include threading a double length of 0 silk through the side of the funnel por-

tion of the prosthesis. This can then be used to retrieve or reposition the tube if necessary and can be easily removed when position is correct. Other methods include using rats-tooth forceps or a Foley catheter inflated inside the stent to facilitate repositioning or removal. Occasionally the stent has to be pushed right into the stomach and then retrieved flange end first using a snare or long rats-tooth forceps.

To date, at lest 1670 of these stents have been reported.[54,56–63,65,66] Successful intubations have been achieved in 96.6 per cent of instances; however, this has been associated with an alarmingly

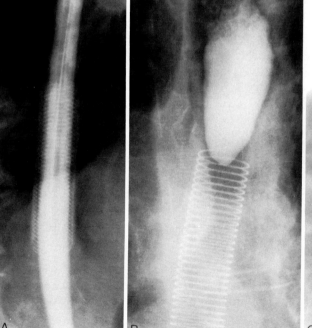

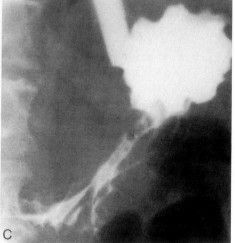

Figure 6–11. *A*, Stent placement using a pusher tube to push prosthesis over American dilator, through tumor obstruction. *B*, Prosthesis in proper position after dilator removal. *C*, Gastrografin swallow demonstrating significant linitis plastica of fundus.

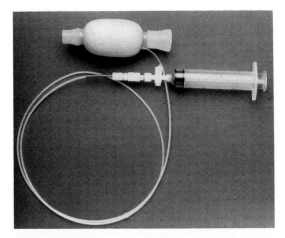

Figure 6–12. Balloon stent designed to occlude tracheoesophageal fistula. Theoretically, it has been designed to obviate need for tumor shelf.

high acute complication rate (17.8 per cent) and mortality rate (8.6 per cent). Acute procedure-related complications vary in frequency, depending on patient selection, insertion technique, and reporting variables. These factors include bleeding, perforation, dyspnea secondary to tracheal compression, prosthesis occlusion or migration, and postintubation fever. These complications may individually involve a spectrum of severity, an example being a small, localized esophageal perforation noted in association with a properly positioned prosthesis. The majority of these will spontaneously seal with simple conservative management including limiting oral intake and broad-spectrum parenteral antibiotics.

Late complications may include tube migration or erosion with bleeding or perforation, tumor overgrowth of the proximal funnel, tube obstruction with food, or chronic aspiration.[59] To minimize these problems, these patients must be maintained on soft or even liquid diets and should sleep with the head of the bed elevated at least 30 degrees.

Earlam and Cunha-Melo reported 8489 patients from 49 series who underwent irradiation for esophageal cancer.[67] They reported that only 50 per cent of these patients required additional therapy, in most cases entailing simple bougienage only. This data is supported by other investigators who believe that radiation with or without dilation alone gives adequate palliation without the significant and often fatal complications associated with stent placement.[68]

Additional support for this approach has come from the increasing utilization of palliative laser photoablation in treatment of patients with malignant esophageal obstruction. The combination of increasing specificity of modern therapeutic radia-

tion and further developments in the field of esophageal dilation, laser therapy, and bicap tumor probes will be associated with a further decline in stent use.

Currently accepted indications for prosthesis placement include tracheoesophageal fistula formation in conjunction with significant aspiration, extremely long (>10 cm) neoplasms, particularly those in which 5 to 6 cm of fundus is involved, or neoplasms that rapidly reclose after successful bougienage or apparently successful laser therapy.[54,68] In addition, lesions causing esophageal obstruction which are primarily extrinsic or extraluminal may also require stent insertions. Contraindications for stent insertion include severely angulated stenoses that cannot be dilated adequately, neoplasms that do not have a proximal shelf in which to seat the prosthesis, or a tumor that is so extensive that the distal end of the stent abuts directly against additional tumor or gastric wall. Recently, an esophageal prosthesis has been developed which may allow occlusion of an esophagobronchial fistula despite the absence of a proximal tumor shelf (Fig. 6–12). This prosthesis, which is currently undergoing further investigation, has a firm central core and a soft outer balloon sheath that can be variably inflated with a removable catheter. However, further data is required before comment can be made on this tube's ultimate efficiency, especially with respect to tube migration.

■ REFERENCES

1. Martin TR, Vennes JA, Silvis SF, Ansel HT: A comparison of upper gastrointestinal endoscopy and radiography. J Clin Gastroenterol, 2:21–25, 1980.
2. Dooley CP, Larson AW, Stace NH, et al: Double-contrast barium meal and upper gastrointestinal endoscopy: A comparative study. Ann Intern Med 101:538–545, 1984.
3. Schuman BM: The gastroscopic yield from the negative upper gastrointestinal series. Gastrointest Endos, 19:79–80, 1972.
4. Health and Public Policy Committee, American College of Physicians: Endoscopy in the evaluation of dyspepsia. Ann Intern Med, 102:266–269, 1985.
5. Lichtenstein FL, Feinstein AR, Suzio KD, Deluca VA, Spiro HM: The effectiveness of panendoscopy in diagnostic and therapeutic decisions about chronic abdominal pain. J Clin Gastroenterol, 2:31–36, 1980.
6. Dooley CP, Weiner JM, Larson AW: Endoscopy or radiography? The patient's choice. Prospective comparative survey of patient acceptability of upper gastrointestinal endoscopy and radiography. Am J Med, 80:203–207, 1986.
7. Overholt BF, Hargrove RL, Farris RK, Porter FR. Primary panendoscopy. Gastrointest Endosc, 33:1–3, 1987.
8. Gaisford WD: Endoscopic electrohemostasis of active upper gastrointestinal bleeding. Am J Surg, 137:47–53, 1979.
9. Papp JP: Endoscopic electrocoagulation of the nonbleeding visible ulcer vessel (abstract). Gastrointest Endosc, 25:45, 1979.

10. Mellow MH, Lewis RJ: Endoscopy-related bacteremia. Arch Intern Med, *136*:667–669, 1976.

11. Earlan R, Cunha-Melo JR: Benign esophageal strictures: Historical and technical aspects of dilatation. Br J Surg, *68*:829–836, 1981.

12. Sawyer R: Treatment of upper esophageal strictures. Otolaryngol, *93*:379–384, 1985.

13. Goldberg RI, Manten HO, Barkin JS: Esophageal bougienage with triple metal dilators. Gastrointest Endosc, *32*:226–228, 1986.

14. Puestow KL: Conservative treatment of stenosing diseases of the esophagus. Postgrad Med, *18*:6–14, 1955.

15. Aste H, Munizzi F, Saccomanno S, Pugliese V: "Splitting" and stretching dilation of esophageal strictures. Endoscopy, *15*:41–43, 1983.

16. Buess G, Thon J, Hutterer F: A multidiameter bougie fitted over a small-caliber fiberscope. Endoscopy, *15*:53–54, 1983.

17. Buess G, Thon J, Schellong H, et al: The endoscopic multidiameter bougie: Clinical results after one year of application. Endoscopy, *15*:337–341, 1983.

18. Huchzermeyer H, Freise J, Becker H: Dilatation of benign esophageal strictures by peroral fiberoendoscopic bougienage. Endoscopy, *9*:207–211, 1977.

19. Lehman GA, O'Connor KW: Endoscopic tape dilator—A simple and inexpensive method to dilate upper gastrointestinal strictures. J Clin Gastroenterol, *7*:208–210, 1985.

20. Rockman S, Morrissey JF, Koizumi H: A simple approach to narrow esophageal strictures. Gastrointest Endosc, *16*:212, 1970.

21. Frimberger E: Endoscopic treatment of benign esophageal stricture. Endoscopy, *15*:199–202, 1983.

22. Tulman AB, Boyce HW: Complications of esophageal dilation and guidelines for their prevention. Gastrointest Endosc, *27*:320–324, 1981.

23. Toledo-Pereyra LH, Michel H, Manifacio G, Humphrey EW: Management of acid-peptic esophageal strictures. J Thorac Cardiovasc Surg, *72*:518–524, 1976.

24. Eastridge CE, Pate JW, Mann JA: Lower esophageal ring: Experiences in treatment of 88 patients. Ann Thorac Surg, *37*:103–107, 1984.

25. Lifton LJ: Multiple esophageal dilations at a single session. Gastrointestinal Endosc, *31*:114–115, 1983.

26. Grobe JL, Kozarek RA, Sanowski RA: Self-bougienage in the treatment of benign esophageal stricture. J Clin Gastroenterol, *6*:109–112, 1984.

27. Kozarek RA: Proximal strictures of the esophagus. J Clin Gastroenterol, *6*:505–511, 1984.

28. Silvis SE, Nebel O, Rogers G, et al: Endoscopic complications: Results of the 1974 American Society of Gastrointestinal Endoscopy Survey. JAMA, *235*:928, 1976.

29. Barrett NR: Benign stricture in the lower esophagus. J Thorac Cardiovasc Surg, *43*:703–715, 1962.

30. Benedict EB: Peptic stenosis of the esophagus. A study of 223 patients treated with bougienage, surgery, or both. Am J Dig Dis, *11*:761–770, 1966.

31. Bolstad DS: The management of strictures of the esophagus. Ann Otol Rhinol Laryngol, *75*:1019–1028, 1966.

32. Buchin PS, Spiro HM: Therapy of esophageal stricture: A review of 84 patients. J Clin Gastroenterol, *3*:121–128, 1981.

33. Flood CA: Bougienage therapy for constrictive esophagitis. Gastrointest Endosc, *25*:130–132, 1979.

34. Glick ME: Clinical course of esophageal stricture managed by bougienage. Dig Dis Sci, *27*:884–888, 1982.

35. Henderson RD: Management of the patient with benign esophageal stricture. Surg Clin North Am, *63*:885–903, 1983.

36. Luna LL: Endoscopic therapy of benign esophageal stricture. Endoscopy, *15*:203–206, 1983.

37. Palmer ED: The hiatus hernia-esophagitis-esophageal stricture complex. Twenty year prospective study. Am J Med, *44*:566–579, 1968.

38. Patterson DJ, Graham DY, Smith JL, et al: Natural history of benign esophageal stricture treated by dilation. Gastroenterology, *85*:346–350, 1983.

39. Raptis S, Milne DM: A review of the management of 100 cases of benign stricture of the oesophagus. Thorax, *27*:599–603, 1972.

40. Starlinger M, Appel WH, Schemper M, et al. Long-term treatment of peptic esophageal stenosis with dilatation and cimetidine: Factors influencing clinical result. Eur Surg Res, *17*:207–214, 1985.

41. Stoddard CJ, Simms JM: Dilatation of benign oesophageal strictures in the outpatient department. Br J Surg, *71*:752–753, 1984.

42. Aste H, Munizzi F, Martines H, Pugliese V: Esophageal dilation in malignant dysphagia. Cancer, *56*:2713–2715, 1985.

43. Celestin LR, Campbell WB: A new and safe system for oesophageal dilatation. Lancet, *1*:74–75, 1981.

44. Hine KR, Hawkey CJ, Atkinson M, Holmes GKT: Comparison of the Eder-Puestow and Celestin technique for dilating benign oesophageal stricture. Gut, *25*:1100, 1984.

45. Johnsen A, Jensen LI, Mauritzen K: Balloon dilation of esophageal strictures in children. Pediatr Radiol, *16*:388–391, 1986.

46. Lindor KD, Ott BJ, Hughes RW: Balloon dilatation of upper digestive tract strictures. Gastroenterology, *89*:345–348, 1985.

47. London RL, Trotman BW, DiMarino AJ, et al.: Dilation of severe esophageal strictures by an inflatable balloon catheter. Gastroenterology, *89*:545–548, 1985.

48. Rogers BHG: Hydrostatic dilation of upper gastrointestinal strictures with endoscopic control. Gastrointest Endosc, *31*:343–346, 1985.

49. Taub S, Rodan BA, Bean WJ, et al: Balloon dilatation of esophageal strictures. Am J Gastroenterol, *81*:14–18, 1986.

50. Webb WA: Balloon dilatation of esophageal strictures. Gastrointest Endosc, *31*:224–225, 1985.

51. Kozarek RA: Hydrostatic balloon dilation of gastrointestinal stenoses. A national survey. Gastrointest Endosc, *32*:15–19, 1986.

52. Kozarek RA: Endoscopic Grüntzig balloon dilation of gastrointestinal stenosis. J Clin Gastroenterol, *6*:401–407, 1984.

53. Graham DY, Smith JL: Balloon dilatation of benign and malignant esophageal strictures. Blind retrograde balloon dilatation. Gastrointest Endosc, *31*:171–174, 1985.

54. Lux G, Groitl H, Ell C: Tumor stenoses of the upper gastrointestinal tract—therapeutic alternative to laser therapy. Endoscopy, *18*:37–43, 1986.

55. Peura DA, Johnson LF: Treatment of esophageal obstruction. *In* Castell DO, Johnson CF (Eds): Esophageal Function in Health and Disease. New York, Elsevier Publishing Co., 1983, pp 306–22.

56. Granström L, Backman L: Malignant stenosis of the esophagus treated with dilation or intubation. Acta Chir Scand, *520*:33–36, 1984.

57. Angorn IB, Hegarty MM: Palliative pulsion intubation in oesophageal carcinoma. Ann R Coll Surg Engl, *61*:212–214, 1979.

58. Chisholm RJ, Stoller JL, Carpenter CM, Burhenne HJ: Radiologic dilatation preceding palliative surgical tube placement for esophageal cancer. Am J Surg, *151*:397–399, 1986.

59. DenHartog Jager FCA, Bartlesman JFWM, Tylgat CNJ: Palliative treatment of obstructing esophagogastric malignancy by endoscopic positioning of a plastic prosthesis. Gastroenterology, 77:1008–1124, 1979.

60. Jones DB, Davies PS, Smith PM: Endoscopic insertion of palliative oesophageal tubes in oesophagogastric neoplasms. Br J Surg, 68:197–198, 1981.

61. O'Connor T, Watson R, Lepley D, et el. Esophageal prosthesis for palliative intubation. Arch Surg, 87:105–108, 1963.

62. Palmer ED: Peroral prosthesis for the management of incurable esophageal carcinoma. Am J Gastroenterol, 59:487–498, 1973.

63. Peura DA, Het HA, Johnson LF, et al.: Esophageal prosthesis in cancer. Am J Dig Dis, 23:796–800, 1978.

64. Ghazi A, Nussbaum M: A new approach to the management of malignant esophageal obstruction and esophagorespiratory fistula. Ann Thorac Surg, 4:531–534, 1986.

65. Palmer ED: Experiences with management of malignant esophagorespiratory fistula by peroral esophageal prosthesis. Gastrointest Endosc, 17:12–16, 1970.

66. Atkinson M, Ferguson R: Fiberoptic endoscopic palliative intubation of inoperable oesophagogastric neoplasms. Br J Surg, 63:947–948, 1976.

67. Earlan R, Cunha-Melo JR: Oesophageal squamous cell carcinoma II: A critical review of radiotherapy. Br J Surg, 67:457–461, 1980.

68. Graham DY, Dobbs SM, Zubler M: What is the role of prosthesis insertion in esophageal carcinoma? Gastrointest Endosc, 29:1–5, 1983.

69. Mercer CD, Hill LD: Surgical management of peptic esophageal strictures. J Thorac Cardiovasc Surg, 91:371–378, 1986.

7

Complications of Gastroesophageal Reflux

Charles E. Pope, II

This chapter will cover some of the complications of gastroesophageal reflux disease (GERD). Long-term monitoring in control subjects demonstrates that reflux occurs in all such patients so investigated. Symptomatic reflux (heartburn, regurgitation) is an extremely common condition. Although severe pyrosis or chest pain due to reflux can drive the patient to the physician, it is the onset of complications which can convert GERD from a minor annoyance to a morbid or life-threatening condition. Columnar epithelial and pulmonary complications of reflux will be covered later in this chapter; esophageal strictures, esophageal ulcers, and esophageal hemorrhage will be reviewed first.

■ *Esophageal Stricture*

■ ETIOLOGY AND PATHOPHYSIOLOGY

The most common reason for an esophageal stricture is damage from refluxed gastric contents. Presumably, the reflux has continued for a prolonged length of time, has caused circumferential injury to the esophageal wall, and has caused transmural damage. In one series, patients with esophageal strictures were found to be older and to have a longer history of heartburn than did a control group of patients who complained of reflux but did not have an esophageal stricture.[1] The patients with

stricture had values of lower esophageal sphincter (LES) pressure lower than patients without a stricture. This decrease in LES pressure was not confirmed in another study, although those with strictures tended to have pressures in the lower range for that particular laboratory.[2]

It would seem possible that patients destined to develop peptic strictures might have a defect in the ability to clear refluxed acid or bile from the esophagus, which allows more prolonged contact time. Abnormalities of peristalsis have been demonstrated in those with strictures,[1] although it is difficult to know whether these changes preceded the stricture or were a result of its presence. One clinical observation bearing on the etiology of reflux strictures is that patients with strictures usually present to the physician with the stricture already present. It is distinctly unusual to follow a patient with reflux symptoms for years and suddenly find the patient develops a stricture when it had not been present before. This would seem to indicate that the degree of reflux damage noted by x-ray or by endoscopy is not the predominant factor in the pathogenesis of stricture formation, as patients with severe endoscopic esophagitis can be followed for years without developing a stricture.

Another fact incriminating free reflux in the genesis of stricture is that strictures will disappear when reflux is corrected surgically, even without concomitant dilatation. As will be mentioned below, the medical treatment of acid production with H_2-blockers seems to be ineffective in the treatment of peptic strictures. It will be of interest to study the effect of omeprazole, which completely blocks the output of gastric acid.

Not all peptic strictures are heralded by preceding symptoms of reflux. Occasionally, a patient will present with dysphagia and be shown to have a stricture, even though there has been no history of heartburn or regurgitation. Many of these patients will have endoscopic and pH evidence for esophageal reflux. It is almost as if they did not have an early warning system which would force them to take action to alleviate symptoms of reflux.

Other factors exist which might explain the occurrence of strictures in patients without an antecedent history of reflux. Two studies have now shown that patients with strictures have much more likelihood of a history of ingestion of nonsteroidal anti-inflammatory drugs within the preceding year than that found in control subjects from the same environment.[3,4] Other compounds will also cause corrosive damage to the esophageal wall with subsequent stricture formation. Clinitest tablets,[5] vitamin C tablets,[6] and quinidine tablets[7] have all been implicated in stricture formation.

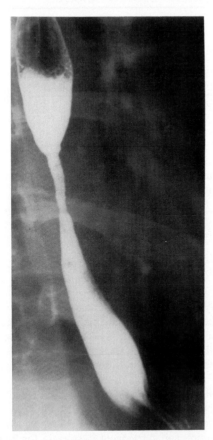

Figure 7–1. Herpetic stricture. A high stricture with proximal dilation of the esophagus following circumferential ulceration. Squamous epithelium was found both above and below the stricture. (Courtesy of George B. McDonald, M.D.)

Infections of the esophagus have also been associated with stricture formation. Rarely, tuberculosis[8,9] and syphilis[10] have been shown to cause stricture formation. Viral infections can also cause esophageal narrowing. Figure 7–1 shows the stricture that resulted from a severe herpetic infection in an immunocompromised host. During the acute illness, endoscopy showed severe circumferential ulceration of the esophageal mucosa. Nuclear inclusion bodies were shown in biopsies from the ulcerated area, and herpesvirus was grown from the biopsy material. Three months later, repeat endoscopy performed after the barium swallow was obtained showed an intact mucosa with squamous epithelium above and below the stricture.

Iatrogenic esophageal strictures can result from variceal sclerosis through the endoscope.[11] It seems likely that paravariceal rather than intravariceal injections will cause such a sequel. Stricture following repair for esophageal atresia can result either from relative ischemia at the suture line or from the postoperative reflux often found in these patients.[12] In the latter, stricture formation is undoubtedly aided by the defect in acid clearing produced by the motor abnormality of the esophagus found in these patients.

Radiation to the esophagus, especially when combined with surgical dissection around the gullet, has been blamed for producing stenosis.[13] This is common when patients receive radiation after head and neck dissections; the strictures are located high in the esophagus, an unusual location for ordinary peptic strictures.

Another clearly acquired type of esophageal stricture is that following the onset of chronic graft-versus-host (GVH) disease in patients who have received a bone marrow transplant.[14] The earliest lesion seems to be a desquamative process involving the upper and middle portions of the esophageal mucosa. In some patients it progresses to form a lumen-narrowing stenosing web or stricture[15] (Fig. 7–2). This process can also be complicated by ordinary gastroesophageal reflux, which may superimpose changes on the affected mucosa. The relative sparing of the distal esophagus mitigates against reflux as a primary inciting factor in this process. Caution was advised in the endoscopic examination and bougienage therapy of this condition, as perforation was encountered in two of the eight reported patients.

Another relatively rare cause of stenosis of the esophagus is the disease process known as diffuse intramural esophageal pseudodiverticulosis.[16] This illness has a characteristic radiographic apearance (Fig. 7–3). Numerous small flask-shaped outpouchings are seen, often appearing throughout the length of the esophagus or restricted to an area of

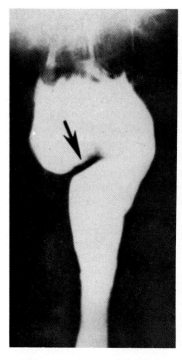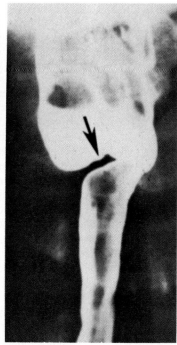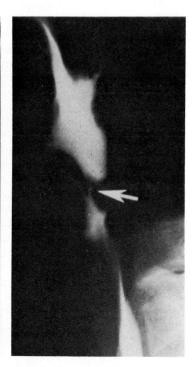

Figure 7–2. Graft-versus-host stricture: A high stricture is seen in a patient who has survived the acute graft-versus-host reaction. (From McDonald GB, Sullivan KM, Schuffler MD, et al: Gastroenterology, *80*:914, 1981.)

narrowing that tends to be located in the upper esophagus. *Candida albicans* has been retrieved from approximately half of the reported patients; *Candida* is probably not the causative agent in this condition but rather a passing pathogen.

Epidermolysis bullosa, a hereditary skin condition characterized by bullae and erosions, also has an esophageal manifestation which can lead to esophageal stenosis.[17] The fragility of the external skin is mirrored in the squamous epithelium of the esophageal mucosa, and even the minimal trauma of eating solid food can lead to bullous formation, scarring, and an eventual esophageal stricture. The strictures again tend to involve the upper and middle esophagus in contrast to ordinary peptic strictures. Squamous cell epithelium is found both above and below the stricture, a characteristic of nonpeptic strictures.

Scattered case reports present uncommon but well-documented reasons for esophageal stenosis. A very rare congenital cause for stenosis was presented in a two-month-old female infant who was found to have a stenotic area in the midesophagus.[18] Pathologic examination showed that the narrowing was caused by a failure of development of the circular layer of esophageal musculature. A 46-year-old woman who suffered from severe rheumatoid arthritis was found to have a midesophageal stricture with squamous cell epithelium above and be-

low it. This eventually required resection and was found to have been caused by severe rheumatoid arteritis accompanied by rheumatoid granulomas.[19] Finally, for collectors of medical trivia, there is Kindler's syndrome, a combination of epidermolysis bullosa, poikiloderma congenitale, and photosensitivity.[20] This extremely rare condition has been associated with both esophageal and urethral strictures.

■ SYMPTOMS

The primary clinical manifestation of an esophageal stricture is dysphagia. This is usually much more marked for solid food than for liquids. It usually begins insidiously, and becomes more marked as the luminal diameter of the strictured area decreases. Poor dentition and rapid eating habits will increase the dysphagia. Spongy foods such as meat and bread are often the prime offenders. If the patient complains of dysphagia for liquids as well, then an associated motor disorder must be suspected. Alternatively, a solid bolus may have wedged itself in a stricture, producing esophageal obstruction and subsequent dysphagia for liquids.

Another relatively characteristic clinical feature of dysphagia produced by a stricture or other mechanical narrowing of the esophageal lumen is the

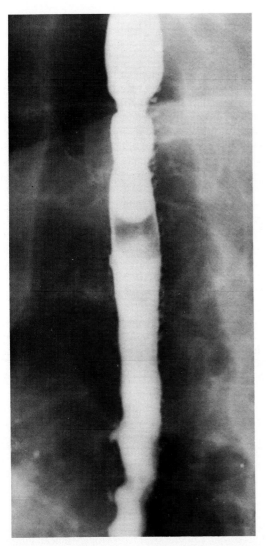

Figure 7–3. Intramural pseudodiverticulosis: A short stricture is seen at the upper end of the esophagus. In this strictured area and below are seen numerous small outpouchings. (From Sleisenger MH, Fordtran JS (Eds): Gastrointestinal Disease—Pathophysiology, Diagnosis, Management. Philadelphia, W.B. Saunders Co., 1983.)

need to regurgitate the offending bolus before swallowing can be resumed. Attempts to aid the passage of an impacted bolus by drinking fluids will some times work, but more often, the fluid will be regurgitated back into the mouth because of the esophageal obstruction.

If the stricture is indeed tight, the food intake of the patient may become so restricted as to cause weight loss and malnutrition. Strictures may also cause great difficulties in the ingestion of tablets and capsules. This can be a problem if medication is relied on for the management or amelioration of esophageal strictures.

■ DIAGNOSIS

When the presence of a stricture is suspected on clinical grounds, the first step in confirming the clinical impression should be a barium examination of the esophagus. This examination is easily obtained, is atraumatic for the patient, and can provide a road map in case endoscopic evaluation becomes necessary. The sensitivity of barium examination is quite high, and especially if double contrast techniques are employed with an effervescent powder, accurate delineation of the luminal diameter and extent of a stricture is possible.[21] Certain modifications of radiologic technique are of great importance. Especially if only single contrast techniques are employed, it is essential to distend the wall of the esophagus fully, or a stricture which does not markedly narrow the lumen can be missed completely. If a high-grade stricture exists, then the passage of barium through the stricture can be retarded and the esophageal wall below the stricture will not be expanded. This will cause an overestimation of the length of the stricture. This can be remedied by placing the patient in the Trendelenburg position and causing the barium to reflux up to the lower extent of the stricture, thus outlining it.

Another important aid in the delineation of subtle strictures is the use of a bolus impregnated with barium. Marshmallows have been suggested, but bread, chewed up with a small portion of barium and then swallowed before complete mastication, is usually more easily available and is equally effective. If marshmallows are to be used, the large size is more useful than the small marshmallow, which will detect only a very tight stricture. Arrest of a bolus in a single location should direct added radiologic attention or even endoscopic attention to this particular area.

Endoscopy not only allows the recognition of the presence and extent of a stricture but also allows an evaluation of the cause of the stricture. The advent of modern fiberoptic endoscopy, especially the smaller caliber endoscopes, has been a large step forward in the evaluation (and treatment) of esophageal strictures.[22] The appearance of a peptic stricture on endoscopy can vary widely. A stricture in which acute damage from continued reflux is absent will appear as a fixed narrowing which will not distend when air is insufflated. A stricture without much luminal compromise can easily be missed with a small caliber endoscope which will pass right through the narrowed area. In such a case, prior x-ray evaluation or the arrest in the strictured area of a large caliber dilator passed subsequently will reveal the true state of affairs.

Strictures of peptic origin in which the reflux

process is very active will present as an ulcerated friable narrowing of the esophageal lumen. Visual differentiation between reflux stricture, a carcinoma of the esophagus with narrowing, and an infectious stricture can be extremely difficult and often requires biopsy or cytologic examination to help in this differentiation. If a stricture with a very active looking epithelium is encountered, then both grasp biopsies and brush cytologic specimens can be obtained in order to differentiate what type of process is present. Biopsies should be taken of the edge of ulcerated areas, as well as blindly from the depths of the stricture in order to rule out a carcinoma that is producing surrounding inflammation. Similarly, brush cytologic samples can be taken both in visible areas of abnormal mucosa and from deep within the strictured zone. Since the advent of small flexible endoscopes with directed brush cytologic examination, exfoliative cytology screening for malignancy has fallen into disuse. If used, the tube collecting the exfoliative cytologic specimen must be passed through the strictured area to make certain that all areas are sampled by the exfoliative fluid.

Other diagnostic methods have only a limited place in the diagnosis and definition of esophageal strictures. Occasionally a wide stricture will be detected by noting that a portion of the wall of the esophagus does not contract during esophageal manometry. Computed tomography and magnetic resonance imaging examination of the esophageal wall and surrounding mediastinal nodes have only a limited role in the delineation and understanding of strictures.[23]

■ THERAPY

Most effective methods of treating a stricture require some form of invasive intervention. Yet a great deal can be done by improving the individual's dental apparatus and by counseling in terms of dietary therapy. Occasionally patients with very tight strictures, which by x-ray seem to have an effective diameter of only 2 to 3 mm, can survive without other therapy by chewing the food very thoroughly and by eating slowly.

If the stricture is on the basis of reflux, how effective is medical treatment of reflux in controlling peptic stricture? In and of itself, medical treatment is not very effective, according to a trial which employed the H_2-receptor blocker, cimetidine, in a double-blind crossover trial. Neither dysphagia nor the need for esophageal dilatation was reduced during the time of treatment with the active compound, although the gross appearance of the mucosa improved during treatment with active

drug.[24] Whether more efficient acid-suppressing drugs such as omeprazole will improve primary medical therapy of strictures remains to be determined.

There are a large number of different techniques which can be applied to the dilatation of an esophageal stricture. Most depend on the gradual increase in diameter obtained by passing various types of dilators sequentially through the stricture. Dilatation can be done either antegrade by means of dilators passed through a gastrostomy and pulled up into the esophagus over a swallowed string, or prograde by several different devices. Graded dilators can be passed through a rigid endoscope, passed without guidance perorally as is done with Hurst and Maloney dilators (Fig. 7–4), or passed over a previously introduced guidewire, as in the case of Puestow dilators.[25] The use of fixed-expansion balloons has recently been introduced in the treatment of strictures, and this seems to be quite effective.[26,27]

The choice of the type of dilator to be used is made by personal preference of the operator, by the characteristics of the stricture to be dilated, and sometimes by the personal preference or past dilatation history of the patient undergoing the procedure. Dilatation with mercury-filled dilators such as the Hurst seem to work best when the stricture is short in length and within the longitudinal axis of the esophagus. If the stricture is angulated, long, or next to a diverticulum, then dilatation over an intraluminal guidewire would seem to be a better choice. Guidewires can be placed through an endoscope or can be gently passed under fluoroscopic guidance. Dilating balloons can be passed under direct vision by using an endoscope or by passing the balloon catheter over a previously placed guidewire.

When graded dilators such as the Hurst or Puestow dilators are being used, a fair amount of judgment is required to select the initial size of dilator and the rate of dilator size increase to be followed. My personal preference is to pass either three or four dilators at a sitting. The initial size is determined by either the past history of dilation, by a rough estimate of luminal size obtained by a recent barium examination, or by interpretation of the patient's symptoms. If the first dilator passes through without any sense of hesitation and without producing any pain or blood on the dilator, it is generally safe to skip the next size of dilator. When resistance is felt, then dilatation should be done by utilizing the next size of dilator. If there is unusual pain or more than just a little blood tinging the surface of the dilator, or if an unusual amount of force is required to pass the dilator, then the procedure is terminated for the day. Only pharyngeal

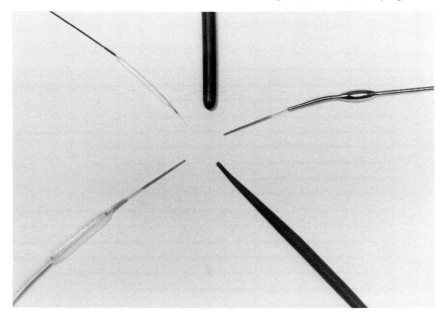

Figure 7–4. Esophageal dilators: Clockwise from the top, a Hurst bougie, an Eder-Peustow dilator with its guidewire, a Maloney tapered dilator, a fixed-expansion balloon dilator, and another fixed-expansion dilator, which can be passed through the channel of an endoscope.

anesthesia is used; marked sedation interferes with careful monitoring of the patient's reaction to the dilatation.

If possible, I prefer to dilate patients in the sitting position, preferably under fluoroscopic control, which is useful for nonendoscopic placement of guidewires and allows the observation of the depth to which the dilator has reached. Experienced patients who require the placement of a guidewire under endoscopic control can often remain sitting without receiving intravenous injections of diazepam.

Dilatation is continued during a number of sessions until the desired esophageal diameter is attained or until the patience and fortitude of the patient is exhausted. Most patients will be able to swallow if a 35 French dilator can be passed. I usually continue the dilatation until a dilator of 43 to 45 French diameter will pass. Although larger dilators are available, it is not certain that added benefit will be obtained by employing them. The fixed-diameter dilating balloons avoid a series of dilatations; one intraluminal inflation will allow the desired diameter to be attained. Presumably, a safety factor is the fact that the expanding forces are applied radially instead of with a shearing force along the long axis of the esophagus.

Balloon dilatation can be performed under direct fluoroscopic control. After the balloon is centered in the general area of the stricture, water with a small amount of contrast material is slowly injected until the impression of the stricture is seen on the walls of the balloon. If the catheter is not well centered, then the balloon is deflated and repositioned. During actual dilatation, the impression of the stricture on the balloon is observed until it is seen to widen. Dilatation can then be stopped.

The results from several large series suggest that adequate esophageal patency can be maintained with repeated dilatation in from 80 to 90 per cent of patients with strictures.[28-30] Some patients seem to require only one course of dilatation; others will require more frequent series of dilatations. It is not known what determines whether multiple courses will be necessary. The wide range in need for dilatation is shown in Figure 7–5. There is a suggestion that the addition of cimetidine to a regimen of dilatation allows less frequent dilatation, although this was not studied in an organized fashion.[31]

Bougienage of the esophagus can produce complications. The most obvious complication would be perforation. In a large survey done approximately 10 years ago the perforation rate ranged from 4 to 6 per 1000.[32] There is a tendency for bad news to be underreported, so the true rate may be somewhat higher. Intramural hematomas[33] and bacteremia[34] have also been reported; neither seems to be as much of a problem as perforation. Whether the new balloons will be much safer remains to be determined when they enter into wider use.

■ **SURGICAL THERAPY**

If patients require frequent bougienage to maintain luminal patency, if the act of dilatation is un-

Months Follow-up

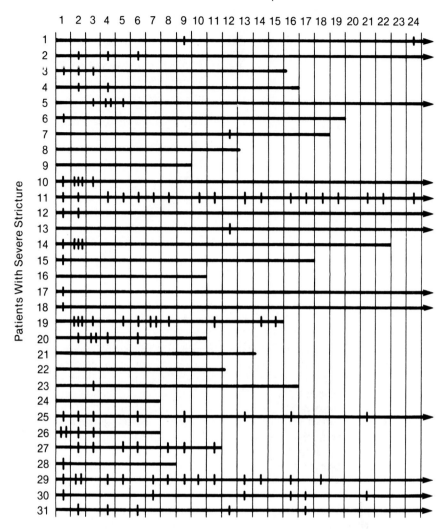

Figure 7–5. Dilatation results: Course of 31 patients with severe strictures. Each tick represents esophageal dilatation performed on that patient. (From Lanza FL, Graham DY: Bougienage is effective therapy for most benign esophageal strictures. JAMA *240*:844, 1978.)

acceptable to the patient, or if other symptoms of reflux cannot be controlled, then a surgical approach can be considered. Attempts to resect the stricture directly often lead to renewed stricture formation or anastomotic leaks. Currently, the two main surgical approaches to peptic stricture are surgical correction of reflux with or without attention directly to the stricture or replacement of the esophagus with another organ.

Surgical correction of reflux with intraoperative dilatation of the esophagus was first popularized by Hill and his colleagues.[35] This approach has had its advocates,[36,37] and it has been suggested that an adequate antireflux operation will cause the stricture to vanish even without dilatation.[38] The advantage of this approach is that it does not require

the resection of the esophagus with the possible attendant problems of suture-line leak. The disadvantage is that reflux must be controlled by the operation. Failure to do so results in recurrence of the stricture.[36]

The other main approach is the resection of the esophagus and its replacement with another viscus in order to restore continuity. Colon, jejunum, and stomach have all been used; colon seems to offer the most satisfactory long-term results.[39] These are large operations with significant mortality and morbidity rates. Often the coexisting cardiopulmonary problems of the patients with esophageal strictures makes this approach too hazardous. In an attempt to avoid both thoracotomy and an intrathoracic anastomosis, the technique of esophagectomy without thoracotomy has been applied to the correction of complicated strictures.[40] However, before a resection it seems wise to just do an antireflux procedure and, if that is not satisfactory, a resection.

■ SUMMARY

Strictures of the esophagus usually arise in patients with severe reflux and represent one of the most troublesome complications of this disease. They present with dysphagia and are best recognized and evaluated with a combination of x-ray and endoscopy. Medical management alone is rarely adequate to maintain luminal patency, and either dilatation or surgery is required. Surgery either tries to eliminate reflux or else replaces the scarred esophagus with another organ substitute.

■ *Esophageal Ulcer*

Ulceration of the esophagus as a manifestation of gastroesophageal reflux damage is not uncommon. This ulceration can be on a microscopic level or can present as longitudinal, very shallow ulcers that can be appreciated endoscopically much more easily than by radiology. A much more uncommon type of ulcer, with which this section will be concerned, is a deep ulceration which can be seen easily by x-ray techniques. Although an uncommon manifestation of GERD, it can produce striking and occasionally even fatal consequences.

■ PATHOPHYSIOLOGY

Ulcers deep enough to be appreciated on a routine barium meal are usually located in columnar (Barrett's) epithelium. They can be located at the stricture, which usually marks the junction between the columnar and squamous epithelium, although more commonly the ulcer is found in the distal portion of the esophagus with columnar epithelium well above the level of the ulcer.[41] The factors which select the site for ulceration remain unknown. It is not clear whether the ulceration is found in specialized epithelium or whether columnar epithelium bearing parietal or chief cells is necessary for ulceration to occur. As is true with peptic ulceration in other locations, removal of acid and pepsin from the luminal contents by either medical or surgical methods will lead to healing of the ulceration.

Another type of esophageal ulceration is caused by a chemical burn from an ingested capsule. Doxycycline is one of the most common offenders,[42] although vitamin C and other medications have also been implicated. Since transient arrest of capsules is seen in normal control subjects, it is surprising that chemical burns from tablets are not even more common than reported.

Another possible mechanism for the production of ulceration might be through infection of the esophagus. Viral involvement by herpes simplex virus has been reported, although the depth of ulceration was not mentioned in this report.[43] Perhaps the combination of an initial ulcerative process caused by infection with subsequent reflux damage might lead to deep ulceration, although this sequence has not yet been demonstrated.

■ SYMPTOMS

Pain is the most common symptom that signals the presence of an esophageal ulcer. The pain is constant and severe, and is usually not relieved by the ingestion of antacids. The pain may be felt either anteriorly or in the interscapular area. It may be aggravated by the ingestion of solid food.

Hemorrhage may be the other manifestation of such an ulcer. This may be very brisk indeed, which suggests that the ulcer has eroded either into an artery located in the wall of the esophagus, or has involved a contiguous structure such as the aorta or the atrium.[44]

■ DIAGNOSIS

By definition, the type of ulceration under discussion is one that can be appreciated on an ordinary examination of the esophagus by barium. The ulcer is usually seen projecting outside the lumen of the esophagus (Fig. 7–6). It may also be demonstrated as a retained collection of barium within the lumen of the esophagus. It is sometimes rather difficult to differentiate an ulcer of the esophagus from a wide-mouthed diverticulum of the esophageal wall. The absence of pain favors the diagnosis of a diverticulum, but occasionally endoscopy must be employed to differentiate between these two conditions.

Esophagoscopy will show a classic peptic ulcer which is usually located in noninflamed red mucosa, which can be shown to be columnar on biopsy. The bed of the ulcer is usually clean and white; biopsy will show only necrosis and sheets of polymorphonuclear leukocytes. The edge of the ulcer may be slightly raised, but there is usually little difficulty in differentiation from a malignant

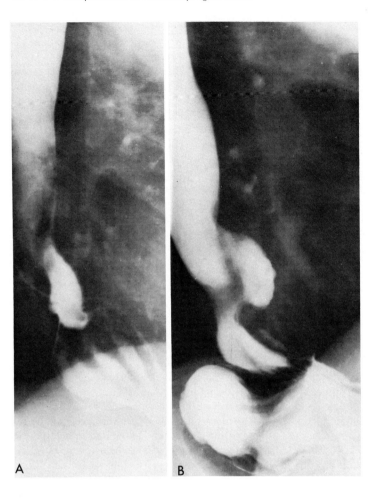

Figure 7–6. Esophageal ulcer. Two views of a deep esophageal ulcer. The standard view on the left (A) does not show the ulcer as well as the view on the right (B), which was obtained by rotating the patient slightly. (From Sleisenger MH, Fordtran JS (Eds): Gastrointestinal Disease—Pathophysiology, Diagnosis, Management. Philadelphia, W.B. Saunders Co., 1983.)

process. To eliminate the possibility of an ulcerated neoplasm, biopsy of the edge of the ulcer should be employed.

■ THERAPY

The methods employed in the treatment of less complicated forms of reflux can be tried. There has been a report documenting healing of esophageal ulcers after treatment with cimetidine, an H$_2$-blocker.[45] No large series exist of such ulcers. Before the advent of such drugs, I was able to effect healing of a large esophageal ulcer in a patient who was paraplegic, and thus a difficult operative risk, by employing a course of gastric radiation.[46] The patient had not responded to intensive antacid therapy, but following 1500 rads of gastric radiation, the pain of the ulcer promptly subsided, the x-ray became normal, and the patient has done well for the subsequent seven years without recurrence. Presumably, a good antireflux operation would be an effective form of therapy for this complication.

■ *Hemorrhage*

Bleeding from the esophagus as a result of reflux damage is not an uncommon event. In most cases, brisk hemorrhage requiring urgent blood replacement is distinctly unusual; hemorrhage is manifested by occult blood in the stool or in unexplained iron deficiency anemia. In a series collected before the advent of flexible fiber endoscopy, 72 of a group of 269 patients undergoing endoscopy because of bleeding were found to have peptic esophagitis.[47] In the same series, bleeding from an esophageal ulcer was seen in four patients.

Symptoms of the hemorrhage will depend on the rapidity of the bleeding. Some patients whose bleeding source is later defined to be from reflux damage of the esophageal mucosa will have no ancillary symptoms of reflux disease such as heartburn or dysphagia.

Diagnosis should be by means of endoscopy. Because oozing can occur from very shallow microulcers of the esophageal mucosa, x-ray should not be depended upon as a diagnostic modality.

Endoscopy will allow the location and extent of the bleeding problem to be defined. It also will allow the recognition of associated gastric and duodenal disorders to be made.

Therapy should depend on the urgency of the situation. Patients with iron deficiency anemia or occult blood should undergo standard antireflux therapy as outlined in the appropriate chapter. More brisk hemorrhage from severe reflux esophagitis represents a difficult therapeutic challenge. Ice water lavage has been recommended.[47] Emergent antireflux surgery was reported to be efficacious in a series of seven patients who had not responded to conservative therapy.[48] A case report details the use of angiography followed by arterial embolization to control bleeding from an esophageal ulcer.[49]

■ REFERENCES

1. Ahtaridis G, Snape WJ, Cohen S: Clinical and manometric findings in benign peptic strictures of the esophagus. Dig Dis Sci, 24:858, 1979.
2. Lobello R, Stekelman M, Edwards DAW: Lower oesophageal sphincter tone in patients with peptic stricture. Thorax, 33:574, 1978.
3. Heller SR, Fellows IW, Ogilvie AL, et al: Non-steroidal anti-inflammatory drugs and benign oesophageal stricture. Br Med J, 285:167, 1982.
4. Wilkins WE, Ridley MG, Pozniak AL: Benign stricture of the oesophagus: Role of non-steroidal anti-inflammatory drugs. Gut, 25:478, 1984.
5. Genieser NB, Becker MH: "Clinitest Strictures" of the esophagus. Clin Ped, 8:17A, 1969.
6. Walta D, Giddens JD, Johnson LF, et al: Localized proximal esophagitis secondary to ascorbic acid ingestion and esophageal motor disorder. Gastroenterology, 70:766, 1976.
7. Teplick JG, Teplick SK, Ominsky, et al: Esophagitis caused by oral medication. Radiology, 134:23, 1980.
8. Fahmy AR, Guindi R, Farid A: Tuberculosis of the oesophagus. Thorax, 24:254, 1969.
9. Dow CS: Oesophageal tuberculosis: Four cases. Gut, 22:234, 1981.
10. Stone S, Friedberg SA: Obstructive syphilitic esophagitis. JAMA, 177:147, 1961.
11. Sorensen T, Burcharth F, Pederson ML, et al: Oesophageal stricture and dysphagia after endoscopic sclerotherapy for bleeding varices. Gut, 25:473, 1984.
12. Hicks LM, Christie DL, Hall DG, et al: Surgical treatment of esophageal stricture secondary to gastroesophageal reflux. J Pediatr Surg, 15:863, 1980.
13. Kozarek RA: Proximal strictures of the esophagus. J Clin Gastroenterol, 6:505, 1984.
14. McDonald GB, Sullivan KM, Schuffler MD, et al: Esophageal abnormalities in chronic graft-vs-host disease in humans. Gastroenterology, 80:914, 1981.
15. McDonald GB, Sullivan KM, Plumley TF: Radiographic features of esophageal involvement in chronic graft-vs-host disease. AJR, 142:501, 1984.
16. Castillo S, Aburashed A, Kimmelman S, et al: Diffuse intramural esophageal pseudodiverticulosis. Gastroenterology, 72:541, 1977.
17. Orlando RC, Bozymski EM, Briggaman RA, et al: Epi-

dermolysis bullosa: Gastrointestinal manifestations. Ann Intern Med, 81:203, 1974.
18. Groote AD, Laurini RN, Polman HA: A case of congenital esophageal stenosis. Human Path, 16:1170, 1985.
19. John V, Stirling AS, Matthews HR: Rheumatoid stricture of oesophagus. Br Med J, 1(611):479, 1978.
20. Alper SC, Badem HP, Goldsmith LA: Kindler's syndrome. Arch Dermatol, 114:457, 1978.
21. Ott DS, Gelfand DW, Lane TG, et al: Radiologic detection and spectrum of appearances of peptic esophageal strictures. J Clin Gastroenterol, 4:11, 1982.
22. Ott DS, Chen YM, Wu WC, et al: Endoscopic sensitivity in the detection of esophageal strictures. J Clin Gastroenterol, 7:121, 1985.
23. Quint LE, Glazer GM, Orringer MB: Esophageal imaging by MR and CT: Study of normal anatomy and neoplasms. Radiology, 156:727, 1985.
24. Ferguson R, Dronfield MW, Atkinson M: Cimetidine in treatment of reflux oesophagitis with peptic stricture. Br Med J, 2(628):472, 1979.
25. Hine KR, Haw Key CJ, Atkinson M, et al: Comparison of the Eder-Puestow and Celestin techniques for dilating benign oesophageal strictures. Gut, 25:1100, 1984.
26. Starck E, Paolucci V, Herzer M, et al: Esophageal stenosis: Treatment with balloon catheters. Radiology, 153:637, 1984.
27. Dawson L, Mueller PR, Ferrucci JT, et al: Severe esophageal strictures: Indications for balloon catheter dilatation. Radiology, 153:631, 1984.
28. Lanza FL, Graham DY: Bougienage is effective therapy for most benign esophageal strictures. JAMA, 240:844, 1978.
29. Glick ME: Clinical course of esophageal stricture managed by bougienage. Dig Dis Sci, 27:884, 1982.
30. Wesdorp ICE, Bartelsman JFWM, den Hartog FCA, et al: Results of conservative treatment of benign esophageal strictures: A follow-up study in 100 patients. Gastroenterology, 82:487, 1982.
31. Starlinger M, Appel WH, Schemper M, et al: Long-term treatment of peptic esophageal stenosis with dilatation and cimetidine: Factors influencing clinical results. Eur Surg Res, 17:207, 1985.
32. Mandelstam P, Sugawa C, Siluis SE, et al: Complications associated with esophagogastroduodenoscopy and with esophageal dilatation. Gastroenterol Endosc, 23:16, 1976.
33. Bradley JL, Han SY: Intramural hematoma (incomplete perforation) of the esophagus associated with esophageal dilatation. Radiology, 130:59, 1979.
34. Welsh JD, Griffiths WJ, McKee J, et al: Bacteremia associated with esophageal dilatation. J Clin Gastroenterol, 5:109, 1983.
35. Hill LD, Gelfand M, Bauermeister D: Simplified management of reflux esophagitis with stricture. Ann Surg, 172:638, 1970.
36. Gatzinsky P, Bergh P, Lof BA: Hiatal hernia complicated by oesophageal stricture. Acta Chir Scand, 145:149, 1979.
37. Moghissi K: Conservative surgery in reflux stricture of the oesophagus associated with hiatal hernia. Br J Surg, 66:221, 1979.
38. Larrain A, Csendes A, Pope CE II: Surgical correction of reflux. Gastroenterology, 69:578, 1975.
39. Orringer MB, Kirsh MM, Sloan H: Esophageal reconstruction for benign disease. J Thorac Cardiovasc Surg, 73:807, 1977.
40. Orringer MB, Sloan H: Esophagectomy without thoracotomy. J Thorac Cardiovasc Surg, 76:643, 1978.
41. Chen YM, Galfand DW, Ott DS, et al: Barrett esophagus as an extension of severe esophagitis. AJR, 145:275, 1985.

42. Schneider R: Doxycycline esophageal ulcer. Am J Dig Dis, 22:805, 1977.
43. Matsumoto S, Sumiyoshi A: Herpes simplex esophagitis—a study in autopsy series. Am J Clin Path, 84:96, 1985.
44. Cunnane K: Esophago-atrial fistula. Can J Surg, 21:466, 1978.
45. Kothari T, Mangla SC, Kalra TMS: Barrett's ulcer and treatment with cimetidine. Arch Intern Med, 140:475, 1980.
46. Cooper JN, Gelzayd EA, Kirsner JB: Mild gastric fundal

47. Palmer ED: The hiatus hernia-esophagitis-esophageal stricture complex. Am J Med, 44:566, 1968.
48. Safaie-Shirazi S, Hardy BM. Treatment of reflux esophagitis resulting in massive esophageal bleeding. Arch Surg, 111:365, 1976.
49. Michal JA, Brody WR, Walter S, et al: Transcatheter embolization of an esophageal artery for treatment of a bleeding esophageal ulcer. Radiology, 134:246, 1980.

irradiation in the treatment of peptic esophagitis. Gastrointest Endosc, 14:222, 1968.

RESPIRATORY COMPLICATIONS OF GASTROESOPHAGEAL REFLUX

Augusto Larrain • Charles E. Pope, II

During early development of the human embryo, the lungs arise as a diverticulum of the foregut, which in turn gives rise to the esophagus. In later life, the functions of the lungs and esophagus are separate. However, reflux into the esophagus can in certain cases produce pulmonary symptoms. This chapter will outline the relationships currently recognized between gastroesophageal reflux and pulmonary symptoms and will discuss recognition and the management of this problem.

Many respiratory complications have been associated more or less firmly with gastroesophageal reflux. These include massive aspiration (Mendelson's syndrome),[1,2] aspiration pneumonia,[3] bronchiectasis,[4] bronchial asthma,[5,6] chronic bronchitis,[7] irritative cough,[8] nocturnal shortness of breath,[9] glottic spasm,[10] diffuse pulmonary fibrosis,[11] and sudden death syndrome.[12] There are laryngeal lesions such as posterior laryngitis,[13] and contact ulcer[14] which may produce specific symptoms of their own in addition to coexisting with symptoms of the more distal respiratory tree. This chapter will devote itself mainly to reactive airway disease (intrinsic asthma, acute recurrent bronchitis). In addition, laryngeal lesions due to reflux will receive attention not only because of their intrinsic interest but also because such lesions may serve as markers for reflux which is producing respiratory symptoms.

■ *Asthma*

■ DEFINITION

Asthma has been defined by the American Thoracic Society as a syndrome whose primary char-

acteristic is an increased responsiveness of the trachea and bronchi (bronchial hyperreactivity) to various stimuli. It is manifested by widespread intermittent narrowing of the airways which change either spontaneously or as a result of therapy. Asthma may be further subdivided into extrinsic and intrinsic asthma. *Extrinsic asthma* can be characterized by a strong relationship to atopy, strong family history, induction by specific pollens and irritants, a tendency to display eosinophilia, high concentrations of IgE, and a relatively young age of onset. *Intrinsic asthma*, with which we feel reflux is most strongly associated, tends to have a relatively late age of onset, no family history, negative skin tests for allergens, and normal levels of IgE. Failure to consider these two subdivisions of asthma may have led to some current confusion in the literature.

■ PATHOPHYSIOLOGY

There are three possible mechanisms by which gastroesophageal reflux might produce acute reversible airway obstruction, or asthma. These mechanisms are aspiration of gastric contents into the trachea and bronchi, reflex bronchoconstriction from laryngeal irritation, and bronchoconstriction resulting from esophageal reflux.

Aspiration of Gastric Contents ■ The most obvious mechanism for pulmonary disease is by direct transfer of gastric contents into the upper and lower airways. Such transfer has been easily recognized in cases of aspiration secondary to the induction of anesthesia (Mendelson's syndrome).[1] In some patients with severe reflux, it is possible to obtain a history of large-scale aspiration at night with the patient awakening suddenly with stridor and a mouthful of regurgitated gastric contents. However, such a history is not often obtained in patients with asthma secondary to reflux disease. Microaspiration may be much more common. Normal individuals can be shown to aspirate small quantities of fluid materials if a radioactive tracer is placed in the posterior pharynx during sleep.[15] Therefore, it is not difficult to understand that if small quantities of fluid could reach the posterior pharynx after gastroesophageal reflux, then the fluid could pass into the tracheobronchial tree by the same mechanisms present in normal subjects. We have noted that patients shown to have pulmonary disease associated with reflux have a less sensitive pharynx than do control subjects, as shown by their ability to tolerate an infused manometric catheter located in the hypopharynx without coughing. A similar location of an infused catheter in a control subject usually produces instantaneous coughing and laryngospasm.

Evidence for such microaspiration in adults is rather sparse. In one study utilizing a radioactive marker placed in the stomach upon retiring, radioactive material was found by scanning the lungs the next morning in three of six patients tested.[16] Other investigators have not been able to reproduce this finding.[17] In 10 patients in whom the probability of pulmonary aspiration seemed high on clinical grounds, we were unable to document such nocturnal reflux into the lungs with a radioactive fluid placed in the stomach.

Laryngeal Irritation ▪ Stimulation of the larynx with dust particles[18] or sulfur dioxide[19] in experimental animals produces bronchoconstriction, even when the larynx is surgically isolated from the remainder of the respiratory tract so that there could be no direct transfer of irritants. This bronchoconstriction is vagally mediated. It can be blocked by atropine or by cooling the cervical vagal trunks. Zimmerman has shown that proteolytic enzymes placed in the larynx can cause increased reactivity of the lower airways when stimulated by acetylcholine.[20] Other reports by the same authors stress the importance of the larynx as a "trigger zone" in asthma.[21]

As will be mentioned below, there is some evidence that the larynx in patients with respiratory symptoms due to reflux shows gross morphologic and histologic evidence that gastric contents have reached this area. This is true even though the patient may not report any symptoms of laryngeal stridor.

Reflex Bronchoconstriction Secondary to Esophageal Irritation ▪ Although aspiration of gastric contents into the respiratory tree would seem to be the most likely cause of reflux-produced respiratory symptoms, it may not be necessary for the refluxed material to travel any further than the esophagus to produce changes in pulmonary airflow. Several studies in humans have demonstrated that perfusion of the esophageal mucosa with hydrochloric acid will produce reflex bronchoconstriction, even though care is taken to ensure that none of the perfused acid spills over into the respiratory tree.[22-24] Such reflex bronchoconstriction is not found in normal individuals or in patients with reflux who have no respiratory symptoms.[25] In another experiment, indwelling esophageal catheters were placed in asthmatic children in whom the esophagus was perfused with acid or saline during sleep.[26] There was no response to either solution at midnight, but perfusion of acid at 4 AM produced a typical attack of asthma. The timing is of special interest because early morning is the period during which asthma attacks are most commonly experienced.[27]

In patients with reactive airway disease, ingestion of weakly acidic beverages (colas) causes no acute change in pulmonary function.[28] However, when the response to inhaled histamine is measured, those who have taken acid drinks will show much more bronchospasm than those who have downed a beverage with a neutral pH.

Could the medications that many patients with asthma and other pulmonary diseases take actually predispose them toward reflux? A study in normal individuals showed that therapeutic levels of theophylline decreased sphincter pressure and led to reflux in 62 per cent of those tested.[29] However, the same group of investigators found that 24-hour monitoring of pH in both asthmatic and normal subjects did not reveal an increased incidence of reflux when therapeutic levels of theophylline and metaproterenol were reached.[30] In another study of children with nocturnal asthma, there was no correlation between theophylline levels and episodes of nocturnal reflux.[31]

▪ CLINICAL DESCRIPTION

The first reported associations between reflux and pulmonary symptoms were case reports[5,6] or papers dealing with severe gastrointestinal problems and bronchiectasis, pneumonia and lung abscess.[4,32] One of us (A.L.) became interested in this subject when his patients undergoing antireflux surgery for more conventional indications kept reporting that they had noted improvement in their respiratory function as well. Our subsequent experience suggests that patients with pulmonary problems associated with reflux often have very subtle manifestations of reflux disease. Heartburn and regurgitation may be present but rarely cause the patient to seek medical help for these manifestations of reflux. The pulmonary symptoms far overshadow the symptoms of reflux. Other surgeons had also noted the beneficial effects of antireflux surgery in patients with both respiratory and reflux symptoms.[33,34]

One of the problems in discovering whether there is a relationship between reflux and respiratory symptoms is that in adults, reflux is common, as is smoking and respiratory disease. Therefore, we decided to investigate a group in which smoking was not a confounding variable. It was shown that reflux or a low sphincter pressure could be demonstrated in a group of children presenting with recurrent bouts of wheezing unassociated with pulmonary infiltrates.[35] Furthermore, treatment by postural and dietary modifications aimed at decreasing reflux led to marked improvement in pulmonary symptoms.

Subsequently, we selected a group of individuals in whom reflux might be responsible for pulmonary symptoms.[36] These were patients with adult-onset asthma who had no family histories of asthma or atopy. Investigation by x-ray or pH probe demonstrated a 90 per cent prevalence of reflux. It should again be emphasized that symptoms of reflux in this group were minimal, and had not led to medical consultation for these reflux symptoms. Nocturnal or early morning wheezing was very common, but actual awareness of esophageal regurgitation was uncommon. Symptoms of laryngeal irritation such as a hoarse voice, especially in the morning; a sensation of a foreign body in the neck; and the need to clear the throat repeatedly were common in this group of patients.

A more alarming manifestation of esophageal reflux is apnea which can be observed in infants. First suspected clinically,[12] this association was later proved by simultaneous monitoring of respiratory rate and intraesophageal pH.[37] The episodes of reflux immediately preceded the spells of apnea. Control of reflux by medical or surgical means led to disappearance of apnea.

■ DIAGNOSIS

Pulmonary disease can be diagnosed and quantified by means of pulmonary function tests; reflux can be measured by x-ray, pH probe, and scintigraphy. The major problem is establishing a causal relationship between reflux and pulmonary disease. Reflux can produce pulmonary disease, and pulmonary disease can produce reflux. Therefore, the mere demonstration of an association does not prove causality. The effect of removal of reflux on pulmonary function is the other main method of proving a direct relationship. Barium studies of esophageal function in children have been of some help in detecting a relationship between gastrointestinal and pulmonary function. A prevalence of hiatus hernia (often associated with reflux in young children) of 48 per cent was found in patients with chronic unremitting asthma in contrast to a prevalence of 13 per cent in patients without asthma.[38] When children with radiographic evidence of pulmonary disease such as recurrent pneumonias were examined, 68 per cent were found to have radiologic evidence of esophageal reflux.[39] Radiographic reflux was demonstrated in 54 per cent of patients with idiopathic pulmonary fibrosis compared to a 9 per cent incidence of reflux in controls.[11] The same group showed that in severe adult-onset asthmatics, radiologic reflux could be found in 46 per cent.[40]

pH studies using a microelectrode are a more sensitive way of demonstrating esophageal reflux than is the use of barium. In infants, the prevalence of reflux in those with recurrent chest problems was shown to be high.[35] This was confirmed by other authors who found a prevalence of reflux ranging from 63[41] to 100 per cent[42] when infants with severe pulmonary disease were studied. In an older group of patients with presumably extrinsic asthma, the prevalence of reflux was 47 per cent.[43]

In adults, pH testing in a group with predominantly adult-onset asthma showed that 92 per cent were pH positive.[9] This would agree with our own findings in a similar group of patients.[36] More important, correlation of symptoms with results from pH testing can allow an estimation of cause or effect to be made. In a study of patients shown to be refluxers by 24-hour monitoring, eight of 100 patients were demonstrated to develop wheezing and asthma after an episode of reflux (Fig. 7–7).[44] Conversely, five subjects with primary respiratory disease were shown to develop reflux only after bouts of coughing (Fig. 7–8).

One method of proving an association between esophageal reflux and pulmonary disease is to demonstrate some component of gastric contents in the pulmonary tree. In infants, this has been accomplished by finding components of ingested milk, either fat globules[45] or lactose,[46] in the sputum. The use of radioactive tracers placed in the stomach and later detected over the pulmonary area has been employed. Although this technique will show some positive results in patients whose reflux has led to pulmonary infiltrates,[16] it has been less successful when tried in adults presenting with asthmatic attacks.[17] We, too, have not had success in a series of 10 patients in whom aspiration seemed likely on clinical grounds. There may be several reasons

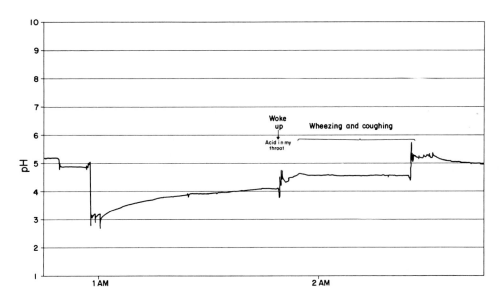

Figure 7–7. A portion of a 24-hour esophageal pH monitoring record from an aspirator. Note the delayed clearance in the supine position (the patient was asleep), followed by the sensation of acid taste in the mouth upon awakening and the onset of asthma, which lasted 35 min. (From Pellegrini CA et al: Gastroesophageal reflux and pulmonary aspiration. Surgery, *86*:112, 1979.)

for failure to demonstrate reflux by this technique. In two of our patients, hourly scans of the gastric area showed that most of the radioactive technetium solution had emptied from the stomach during the first 90 min after ingestion. Therefore, fluid which might have refluxed later in the evening or early the next morning would not have been labeled and could not show in a pulmonary scan. Perhaps patients demonstrating reflux into the lungs fall into the subset of patients who suffer from delayed emptying of fluids and solids. We have also had no success in analyzing the sputum of suspected aspirators for pepsinogen, even though pepsinogen added to the sputum can be identified by radioim-

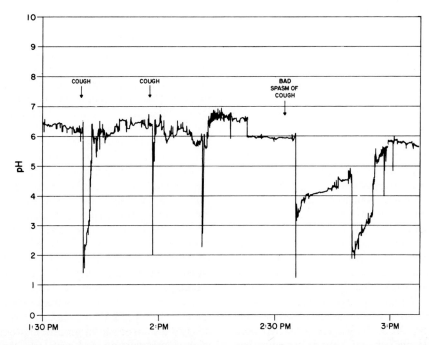

Figure 7–8. A portion of a 24-hour esophageal pH monitoring record from a patient with a primary respiratory disorder. Note the time relationship between cough and the drop in esophageal pH as well as the rapid clearance of acid. (From Pellegrini CA, et al: Gastroesophageal reflux and pulmonary aspiration. Surgery, *86*:114, 1979.)

munoassay. Clearly, a more sensitive test to demonstrate transfer of material from stomach to lung needs to be developed.

In the present state of knowledge it is difficult to recommend a truly satisfactory diagnostic approach to the patient with pulmonary disease in whom reflux is suspected to play a causal role. Demonstration of reflux or mucosal changes of reflux proves only that the gastric contents have reached the esophagus. If the facilities are available, prolonged pH monitoring, especially during sleep, will be useful if it can be shown that reflux immediately precedes an attack of pulmonary symptoms. The advent of portable 24-hour pH monitors will allow such studies to be performed without requiring hospitalization.

If there is strong clinical suspicion of such a relationship and prolonged monitoring facilities are not available, then it might be well worth considering a radioisotopic scan. The technique of Chernow et al. would seem to be a practical one.[16] Ten millicuries of technetium-99m sulfur colloid in 10 ml of water can be instilled into the stomach at bedtime. The nasogastric tube used to instill the fluid can be washed with another 30 ml of fluid. If the patient has not required additional fluid to assist the passage of the tube, then another 30 ml of fluid should be added down the tube to give a final intragastric volume of 70 ml. The next morning, the pulmonary fields can be scanned by a gamma camera. Normally, no counts will be found in the pulmonary area of interest. It should be remembered that only a positive scan will be of use because the sensitivity of this test is not very high. Often a therapeutic trial will be necessary as a final diagnostic test.

■ THERAPY

The choice of type of therapy depends on the age of the patient, the manifestation of reflux, and presence of coexisting morbid conditions. Reflux in infants will often respond to postural and dietary maneuvers.[35] However, if the reflux has produced episodes of apnea; if the manifestations of reflux in the infant include recurrent pulmonary aspirations with pneumonia, bronchiectasis, or pulmonary abscess; or if there are other significant manifestations of reflux, such as failure to grow or iron deficiency anemia, then a surgical approach should be considered. In a mixed series of infants and young children, 26 of 30 patients who had been operated upon because of recurrent pneumonia were free from further attacks of pneumonia.[47] In the same paper, 14 of 17 children with severe bronchial asthma had relief from such attacks postoperatively.

The results of medical treatment in older children is not well documented. In a small series of patients with steroid-dependent asthma who had been treated for three weeks with postural methods and antacids, no beneficial effect on pulmonary function or clinical symptoms could be demonstrated.[43] In another series of very young children with severe gastrointestinal and pulmonary symptoms of reflux, 7 of 17 patients responded to dietary and positional management; the remainder required surgery.[48]

Jolly et al. have suggested that a prophylactic fundoplication be added to a feeding gastrostomy in young children who are unable to maintain oral alimentation.[49] These children were found to have significant reflux preoperatively, and many had congenital abnormalities as well as poor esophageal function. In similar patients in whom fundoplication was not done at the time of gastrostomy, postoperative reflux became a severe problem leading to a fundoplication in several cases.

Medical therapy in carefully chosen adults appears reasonable. In a group of patients identified to have both reflux symptoms and pulmonary complaints, a six-week course of postural therapy and alginic acid–antacid mixture caused improvement of gastrointestinal symptoms in most patients.[50] Unfortunately, only 50 per cent showed improvement in their pulmonary status. There were no changes whatsoever in pulmonary function tests between the treated and untreated patients. In an important study, 18 patients treated with either cimetidine or a placebo in a double-blind crossover study showed improvement in reflux symptoms and nocturnal wheezing during the active phase of treatment.[51] Pulmonary function tests improved during the period of active treatment, but the improvement did not reach a statistically significant level. Fourteen of the 18 patients felt that their pulmonary symptoms were better while on cimetidine.

As part of a randomized trial of medical versus surgical therapy of reflux-induced respiratory symptoms, we were able to compare the effect of cimetidine, 300 mg qid, to placebo.[36] Twenty of 27 patients on cimetidine noted improvement in respiratory symptoms; only 10 of 28 placebo patients improved. Eleven of the cimetidine-treated patients were totally asymptomatic for the six-month period of treatment; only one of the placebo patients became totally asymptomatic. In the cimetidine group, FEV_1 and midexpiratory flow rates showed a statistically significant improvement. No such changes were noted in the placebo group.

In adults, earlier reports of the results of surgery were limited to small series[5,6,52] or did not contain objective measurement of pulmonary function.[34,53,54] In a more recent series of patients with intrinsic asthma who were steroid dependent, corrective surgery led to marked improvement in 31 of 50 patients undergoing antireflux surgery.[55]

In our own randomized series, surgery led to improvement in respiratory function in 20 of 26 patients operated upon. Nine of the surgical patients became totally asymptomatic from a pulmonary point of view. Interestingly, 8 of 11 patients who had been on steroids preoperatively were able to discontinue steroids completely postoperatively. Only 2 of 13 patients on cimetidine and none of the placebo-treated patients were able to discontinue steroid therapy.

This experience suggests to us that both medical and surgical therapy may play a role in treating selected patients with both reflux and pulmonary disease. However, there is a problem in choosing the best forms of therapy. Certainly, a drug trial in an individual patient can be tried and discontinued if not found to be efficacious. Offering surgery, however, is a much more invasive step and cannot so easily be undone. Therefore, one of us (A.L.) has reviewed other patients not in the series above who suffer from both reflux and pulmonary symptoms and who have undergone antireflux surgery for varying indications. This review would suggest that patients with extrinsic asthma operated on either because of severe problems of gastroesophageal reflux or in the hope of improving the asthma did not benefit greatly from the operation. Patients with intrinsic asthma who were operated upon for esophageal indications similarly did not fare well. On the other hand, patients with intrinsic asthma who had early onset of their asthma in childhood or who noted the onset of pulmonary and esophageal symptoms simultaneously had good results as far as lung disease was concerned after antireflux surgery. These initial impressions will have to be tested in formal trials and can be offered only as tentative guidelines. We still feel that antireflux surgery for pulmonary indications needs to be employed sparingly and with a great deal of preoperative investigation.

In summary the decision for selecting treatment in patients with potential problems of reflux causing pulmonary disease is a difficult one. It will depend on the age of the patient, the type of pulmonary problem, the certainty of the relationship between reflux and the pulmonary disease, the skill of the antireflux surgeon, and many other factors. This area is under active investigation. The number of good studies is limited. Decisions made at the present time will be based on insufficient evidence, which should lead to a cautious approach. It is hoped that further investigations and newer forms of diagnostic and therapeutic modalities will place this area on a more solid footing.

■ The Larynx and Reflux

The larynx, as the most proximal portion of the respiratory tree, is in a favored position to be affected by refluxed material. Since the early 1970s it has been recognized that reflux can produce various manifestations in and on the larynx. Granulomas,[56] contact ulcers,[14] and subglottic stenosis[57,58] have all been reported. The most common lesion due to reflux damage of the larynx is posterior laryngitis (acid laryngitis, pachydermia).[13] Posterior laryngitis not only has its own characteristic set of symptoms which in themselves may cause discomfort, but also posterior laryngitis serves as an important clue to the presence of significant esophageal reflux.

■ CLINICAL MANIFESTATIONS

Hoarseness is the most common presentation of posterior laryngitis. The hoarseness is usually worse in the early morning. There is a compulsion to clear the throat repeatedly. There also is a sensation of a deep pressure at the base of the neck. This is hard to describe in words. Some patients who are labeled as globus hystericus undoubtedly have posterior laryngitis. Many of these patients are not aware of aspiration of gastric contents into the pharynx at night. There may be associated wheezing if the more distal respiratory tree is also involved.

■ PATHOPHYSIOLOGY

Chronic irritation of the respiratory epithelium of the posterior portion of the larynx leads to metaplasia and transformation of the epithelium to a stratified squamous epithelium which resembles the esophageal mucosa. Presumably, even further irritation can lead to granuloma formation or to ulceration.

■ DIAGNOSIS

The condition can be diagnosed easily by indirect laryngoscopy using a hand mirror. The earliest changes are small white patches on the posterior larynx which become confluent, elevated, and eventually wrinkled. Associated reflux in patients with such laryngeal lesions was suggested during acid barium studies.[13] We have sought the presence of reflux in 65 consecutive patients with posterior laryngitis consulting an ENT physician, and have demonstrated pH proven reflux in 64 of them. We first encountered this lesion when we were evaluating patients with pulmonary symptoms and reflux and hoped that this lesion would serve as a useful marker for pulmonary disease due to reflux. However, investigation of another group of patients with reflux but no pulmonary symptoms showed that 75 per cent had lesions of posterior laryngitis present.[59] Although posterior laryngitis is not specific for pulmonary disease due to reflux, it is reassuring to find the lesion in a specific patient in whom the association is being sought.

■ THERAPY

There is little published data on medical or surgical treatment of reflux and its effect on posterior laryngitis. Voice therapy, thought to be effective in treating contact ulcers of the larynx, does not seem to be very effective. Most of our patients undergoing corrective antireflux surgery for other reasons note that the symptoms of posterior laryngitis vanish. The early lesions also tend to regress when examined with a mirror, but the elevated wrinkled lesions of advanced posterior laryngitis tend to persist even though the reflux has been corrected.

Laryngeal irritation by refluxed gastric contents can lead to symptoms of hoarseness, a foreign body sensation, or even aphonia. White plaques on the posterior larynx mark this condition. Such posterior laryngitis may not only explain symptoms but may also serve as a marker for the presence of significant reflux. Surgical correction of reflux can produce symptomatic improvement in posterior laryngitis but may not always return the gross or microscopic appearance of the larynx to a normal one.

■ REFERENCES

1. Mendelson CL: The aspiration of stomach contents into the lung during obstetric anesthesia. Am J Obstet Gynecol, 52:191, 1946.
2. Richman H, Abramson SF: Mendelson's syndrome. Am J Surg, 120:531, 1970.
3. Cameron JL, Zuidema GD: Aspiration pneumonia. JAMA, 219:194, 1972.
4. Belsey R: The pulmonary complications of oesophageal disease. Br J Dis Chest, 54:342, 1960.
5. Overholt RH, Ashraf MM: Esophageal reflux as trigger in asthma. NY State J Med, 66:3030, 1966.
6. Babb RR, Notarangelo J, Smith VM: Wheezing: A clue to

gastroesophageal reflux. Am J Gastroenterol, 53:230, 1970.
7. David P, Denis P, Nouvet G, et al: Lung function and gastroesophageal reflux during chronic bronchitis. Bull Eur Physiopathol Respir, 18:81, 1982.
8. Hallewell JD, Boyce CT: Isolated head and neck symptoms due to hiatus hernia. Arch Otolaryngol, 92:499, 1970.
9. Perrin-Fayolle M, Bel A, Kofman J, et al: Asthme et reflux gastro-oesophagien. Poumon-Coeur, 36:225, 1980.
10. Chodosh PL: Gastro-esophageal-pharyngeal reflux. Laryngoscope, 87:1418, 1977.
11. Mays EE, Dubois JJ, Hamilton GB: Pulmonary fibrosis associated with tracheobronchial aspiration. Chest, 69:512, 1976.
12. Leape LL, Holder TM, Franklin JD: Respiratory arrest in infants secondary to gastroesophageal reflux. Pediatrics, 60:924, 1977.
13. Delahunty JE: Acid laryngitis. J Laryngol Otol, 86:335, 1972.
14. Cherry J, Margulies SI: Contact ulcer of the larynx. Laryngoscope, 78:1937, 1968.
15. Huxley EJ, Viroslav J, Gray WR, et al: Pharyngeal aspiration in normal adults and patients with depressed consciousness. Am J Med, 64:564, 1978.
16. Chernow B, Johnson LF, Janowitz WR, et al: Pulmonary aspiration as a consequence of gastroesophageal reflux. Dig Dis Sci, 24:839, 1979.
17. Ghaed N, Stein MR: Assessment of a technique for scintigraphic monitoring of pulmonary aspiration of gastric contents in asthmatics with gastroesophageal reflux. Ann Allergy, 42:306, 1979.
18. Widdicombe JG, Kent DC, Nadel JA: Mechanism of bronchoconstriction during inhalation of dust. J Appl Physiol, 17:613, 1962.
19. Nadel JA, Salem H, Tamplin B, et al: Mechanism of bronchoconstriction during inhalation of sulfur dioxide. J Appl Physiol, 20:164, 1965.
20. Zimmerman I, Haxhiu MA, Bugalho de Almeida AA, et al: Localization of the changes of the sensitivity of the airways by proteolytic enzymes (Pronase) against acetylcholine. Respiration, 38:249, 1979.
21. Zimmerman I, Bugalho de Almeida AA, Ulmer WT: The site of action of a β_2-receptor stimulating drug (Fenoterol) on antigen-induced bronchoconstriction. Lung, 158:15, 1980.
22. Mansfield LE, Stein MR: Gastroesophageal reflux and asthma: A possible reflux mechanism. Ann Allergy, 41:224, 1978.
23. Kjellen G, Tibbling L, Wranne B: Bronchial obstruction after esophageal acid perfusion in asthmatics. Eur J Respir Dis, 1:285, 1981.
24. Spaulding HS, Mansfield LE, Stein MR, et al: Further investigation of the association between gastroesophageal reflux and bronchoconstriction. J Allergy Clin Immunol, 69:516, 1982.
25. Jakes ME, Agran P, Khing SO: Does gastroesophageal reflux (GER) or low pH in the lower esophagus (LE) cause bronchoconstriction? Chest, 82:246, 1982.
26. Davis RS, Larsen GL, Grunstein MM: Respiratory response to intraesophageal acid infusion in asthmatic children during sleep. J Allergy Clin Immunol, 72:393, 1983.
27. Li JCT, Reed CE: Nocturnal asthma and timing of treatment. Am J Med, 79(suppl 6A):10, 1985.
28. Wilson NM, Charette L, Thomson AH, et al: Gastroesophageal reflux and childhood asthma: The acid test. Thorax, 40:592, 1985.
29. Berquist WE, Rachelefsky GS, Kadden M, et al. Effect of theophylline on gastroesophageal reflux in normal adults. J Allergy Clin Immunol, 67:407, 1981.

30. Berquist WE, Rachelefsky GS, Rowshan N, et al: Quantitative gastroesophageal reflux and pulmonary function in asthmatic children and normal adults receiving placebo, theophylline, and metaproterenol sulfate therapy. J Allergy Clin Immunol, 73:253, 1984.

31. Martin ME, Grunstein MM, Larsen GL: The relationship of gastroesophageal reflux to nocturnal wheezing in children with asthma. Ann Allergy, 49:318, 1982.

32. Davis MV, Fiuzat J: Application of the Belsey hiatal hernia repair to infants and children with recurrent bronchitis, bronchiolitis, and pneumonitis due to regurgitation and aspiration. Ann Thor Surg, 3:99, 1967.

33. Urschel HC, Paulson DL: Gastroesophageal reflux and hiatal hernia. J Thorac Cardiovasc Surg, 53:21, 1967.

34. Henderson RD, Woolfe CR: Aspiration and gastroesophageal reflux. Can J Surg, 21:352, 1978.

35. Danus O, Casar C, Larrain A, et al: Esophageal reflux—an unrecognized cause of recurrent obstructive bronchitis in children. J Pediatr, 89:220, 1976.

36. Larrain A, Carrasco J, Galleguillos J, et al: Reflux treatment improves lung function in patients with intrinsic asthma. Gastroenterology, 80:1204, 1981.

37. Herbst JJ, Minton SD, Book LS: Gastroesophageal reflux causing respiratory distress and apnea in newborn infants. J Pediatr, 95:763, 1979.

38. Freidland GW, Yamate M, Marinkovich VA: Hiatal hernia and chronic unremitting asthma. Pediatr Radiol, 1:156, 1973.

39. Darling DB, McCauley RGK, Leonidas JC, et al: Gastroesophageal reflux in infants and children: Correlation of radiological severity and pulmonary pathology. Radiology, 127:735, 1978.

40. Mays EE: Intrinsic asthma in adults. JAMA, 236:2626, 1976.

41. Euler AR, Byrne WJ, Ament ME, et al: Recurrent pulmonary disease in children: a complication of gastroesophageal reflux. Pediatrics, 63:47, 1979.

42. Christie DL, O'Grady LR, Mack DV: Incompetent lower esophageal sphincter and gastroesophageal reflux in recurrent acute pulmonary disease of infancy and childhood. J Pediatr, 93:23, 1978.

43. Shapiro GG, Christie DL: Gastroesophageal reflux in steroid-dependent asthmatic youths. Pediatrics, 63:207, 1979.

44. Pellegrini CA, DeMeester TR, Johnson LF: Gastroesophageal reflux and pulmonary aspiration: Incidence, functional abnormality, and results of surgical therapy. Surgery, 86:110, 1979.

45. Williams HE, Freeman M: Milk inhalation pneumonia—the significance of fat filled macrophages in tracheal secretion. Aust Paediatr J, 9:286, 1973.

46. Hopper AO, Kwong LK, Stevenson DK: Detection of gastric contents of tracheal fluid of infants by lactose assay. J Pediatr, 102:415, 1983.

47. Foglia RP, Fonkalsrud EW, Ament ME, et al: Gastroesophageal fundoplication for the management of chronic pulmonary disease in children. Am J Surg, 140:72, 1980.

48. Jolley SG, Herbst JJ, Johnson DG, et al: Esophageal pH monitoring during sleep identifies children with respiratory symptoms from gastroesophageal reflux. Gastroenterology, 80:1501, 1981.

49. Jolley SG, Smith EI, Tunell WP: Protective antireflux operation with feeding gastrostomy. Ann Surg, 201:736, 1985.

50. Kjellen G, Tibbling L, Wranne B: Effect of conservative treatment of oesophageal dysfunction on bronchial asthma. Eur J Respir Dis, 62:190, 1981.

51. Goodall RJR, Earis JE, Cooper DN, et al: Relationship between asthma and gastro-oesophageal reflux. Thorax, 36:116, 1981.

52. Klotz SD, Moeller RK: Hiatal hernia and intractable bronchial asthma. Ann Allergy, 29:325, 1971.

53. Iverson LIG, May IA, Samson PC: Pulmonary complications in benign esophageal disease. Am J Surg, 126:222, 1973.

54. Lomasney TL: Hiatus hernia and the respiratory tract. Ann Thorac Surg, 24:448, 1977.

55. Perrin-Fayolle M, Bel A, Braillon G, et al: Asthme et reflux gastro-oesophagien. Poumon-Coeur, 36:231, 1980.

56. Goldberg M, Noyek AM, Pritzker KPH: Laryngeal granuloma secondary to gastro-esophageal reflux. J Otolaryngol, 7:196, 1978.

57. Bain WM, Harrington JW, Thomas LE, et al: Head and neck manifestations of gastroesophageal reflux. Laryngoscope, 93:175, 1983.

58. Little FB, Koufman JA, Kohut RI: Effect of gastric acid on the pathogenesis of subglottic stenosis. Ann Otol Rhinol Laryngol, 94:516, 1985.

59. Larrain A, Lira E, Otero M, et al: Posterior laryngitis—a useful marker of esophageal reflux. Gastroenterology, 80:1204, 1981.

8

The Medical Approach to the Treatment of Gastroesophageal Reflux

John M. Petersen ▪ Richard W. McCallum

Gastroesophageal reflux (GER) is an extremely common problem. It is endemic in the population, representing the major reason why people take ad lib antacids, such as Tums and Rolaids. Its frequency is such that in the largely referral practice of a gastroenterologist in this country, GER and irritable bowel rank variably as the first and second most commonly seen problems. It has considerable associated morbidity, the pathophysiology of which has been better elucidated in the last decade. Reflux disease encompasses a wide spectrum of clinical presentation. At one extreme, it may present with more typical symptoms of heartburn, regurgitation, or chest pain and may respond to standard forms of therapy. At the other, it may masquerade under the guise of disorders attributed to a cardiac, pulmonary, peptic, or gallbladder origin, or it may be resistant to the most aggressive medical therapy.

There have been several recent reviews of GER,[1–4] and our aim here will be to discuss the pathophysiology and methods of investigation in GER and examine the approaches and outcomes of medical therapy.

▪ *Pathophysiology*

The mechanism of GER has a multifactorial basis, all of which are important to understand in that they form the foundation and rationale for basing

medical and surgical therapeutic decisions (Fig. 8–1).

▪ LOWER ESOPHAGEAL SPHINCTER COMPETENCE

The lower esophageal sphincter (LES) is not morphologically identifiable in humans, although it is functionally distinct from the adjacent smooth muscle in the body of the esophagus. As judged by its physiologic and pharmacologic responses and by the intrinsic properties of its muscle, the LES creates a positive pressure gradient between the abdomen and thorax. The increase in gradient that may occur during exercise, coughing, and abdominal compression has been attributed to the contributions of some less clearly defined extrinsic anatomic factors, such as the phrenoesophageal membrane, the gastric sling fibers, the right diaphragmatic crus, and others that create a "valve" or pinchcock at the esophageal hiatus. These extrinsic factors have been downplayed in recent years, particularly because of the observation that many patients with hiatal hernia are not refluxers. However, the loss of support that accompanies displacement of the LES into the thorax when an hiatal hernia develops does result in a hernia sac with positive intra-abdominal pressure located above the diaphragm and immediately below the LES.[5] Could this situation contribute to the pathophysiology of GER disease? Gastric acid could be secreted by

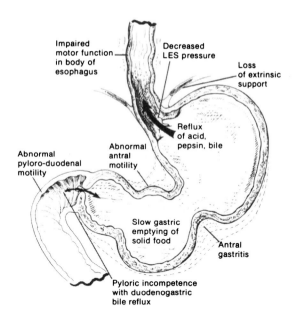

Figure 8-1. The physiologic basis for gastroesophageal reflux.

parietal cells in the hiatal hernia, and reflux into the esophagus could occur during a swallow, when the LES is relaxed. In addition, the hiatal hernia could interfere with acid clearance mechanisms because the hernia sac could be a site of pooling when refluxed gastric contents are attempted to be cleared from the esophagus by swallowing. The positive pressure in the hernia sac could promote orad movement of acid out of the sac when the LES is relaxed during a swallow. These mechanisms and questions are attempts to invoke a role for hiatus hernia, and more studies are still required.

Intrinsic LES tone appears to be the major mechanism that prevents GER. Mean basal LES pressures in GER patients are lower than in control subjects, although considerable overlap is observed.[6] The LES maintains a high pressure zone during resting conditions that relaxes with swallowing, esophageal distention, and vagal stimulation, all of which are independent of the diaphragm and persist even when the LES is located in the chest, as in patients with hiatal hernia.

Current evidence suggests that the LES in humans is innervated by both inhibitory and excitatory autonomic nerves, and the major role of the inhibitory nerves is in mediating sphincter relaxation during swallowing. The preganglionic transmission to the LES is cholinergic, and the postganglionic messenger is probably peptidergic, namely, vasoactive intestinal peptide (VIP). The inhibitory transmission is not blocked by atropine or adrenergic blockers, and the excitatory innervation that can be induced with cervical vagal stimulation is blocked by atropine.

In humans, in addition to a primary myogenic mechanism, a cholinergic neural, paracrine, or neuroendocrine (substance P) messenger may contribute to LES tone and hence the barrier to gastric reflux.[7] There is experimental evidence in the cat to show that reflux-induced inflammatory changes may themselves induce LES dysfunction,[8] possibly by interfering with calcium handling mechanisms of LES smooth muscle.[10] However, there are data in humans showing that the cholinergic response of the LES in normal subjects and reflux patients with the same LES pressure is similar, providing evidence against an esophagitis-induced change in LES muscle tone or contractile properties.[9] These latter observations would suggest that previous findings of absolute LES hypotension in 30 per cent or so of symptomatic GER patients could be explained by hypothesizing that a certain percentage of people may be born with a low normal or absolutely decreased LES pressure and are at risk to later develop symptoms of esophagitis.[9] This is consistent with observations that the LES hypotension persists even after resolution or improvement of the histologic esophagitis.[11] Young, asymptomatic normal volunteers with decreased LES pressure may be symptomatic refluxers in their fifth, sixth, or seventh decades, the age when most GER patients present to major medical centers, because it is thought that GER symptoms do increase with age.

As Dodds et al.[3] have shown, with the aid of the sleeve method of LES pressure recording, simultaneous pH monitoring, as well as manometric recording of body motor activity and swallowing, normal subjects and GER patients often reflux even when their basal LES pressure is normal. Dodds et al. found a temporal correlation between LES pressure, GER, motor activity of the body, and swallowing. Some GER episodes were noted in patients with transient LES relaxation, while some accompanied a transient increase in intra-abdominal pressure, and others occurred as spontaneous free reflux. All normal subjects and many refluxers had normal LES pressure ($\geqslant 10$ mm Hg) and reflex occurred primarily during a transient LES relaxation, whereas the subgroup with low basal LES pressure initially had reflux with increased abdominal pressure or spontaneously. Episodes of transient LES relaxation offer an explanation of why GER may occur in subjects with normal LES tone. Similarly, when LES pressure is $\geqslant 10$ to 15 mm Hg, even vigorous stress maneuvers fail to induce reflux unless a transient LES relaxation occurs.

What causes this transient LES relaxation? One possibility is that gastric distention accompanying eating initiates a "gastrosphincteric reflex" resulting in transient relaxations.[12] In other situations, a cholinergic neural contribution may be impaired, or there exists some functional or morphologic dysfunction of the LES smooth muscle (e.g., atrophy of the LES in scleroderma). Could swallows, esophageal distention, or receptors in the pharynx, esophageal body, or stomach interact with the CNS and stimulate inhibitory motor pathways to the LES and cause relaxation without exciting a peristaltic sequence? It is known that a threshold inhibitory stimulus to the pharynx can be elicited through the vagus and the recurrent laryngeal nerve without causing an esophageal motor sequence of contractions. LES relaxation could, therefore, occur without observing a peristaltic sequence, and this could be one explanation for the term "transient" LES relaxation.[13] These questions deserve careful study.

Among these questions are whether or not GER develops during a transient LES relaxation, the duration of the event, the efficiency of peristalsis, patient position, gastric volume and pressure, and normal gastric emptying. The latter concept is particularly relevant. Slow or delayed gastric emptying (an observation already reported in >50 per cent of GER patients) could result in prolonged gastric distention, and a greater gastric volume may also reflux with each relaxation. These latter possibilities are relevant because recent studies from our laboratory in normal subjects and reflux patients have suggested that gastric distention results in significant transient LES relaxation and may be a major mechanism for the postprandial increase in gastroesophageal reflux.[12] In both study groups, the increase in LES relaxation was volume-related and the reflux patients had a significantly higher percentage of complete relaxations (87 per cent) than did the normal subjects (P ≤0.01). The well-documented delay in gastric emptying in refluxers (to be discussed later in this chapter) may result in prolonged gastric distention, thereby provoking more LES relaxations and reflux.

■ Esophageal Clearance

Once reflux has occurred and the esophagus is exposed to gastric acid or alkaline contents, mechanisms of acid clearance play important roles in preventing pathologic esophagitis. Helms et al.[14] noted the importance of swallow-induced peristaltic sequence in clearing the bulk of esophageal refluxate. Saliva stimulation improved acid clearance while oral aspiration of saliva abolished the stepwise increase in esophageal pH. The bulk of refluxed material appears to be emptied by the first peristaltic wave and the residual acid enters an "unstirred" mucous layer coating the esophagus

that is later neutralized by sequential swallows of saliva.

Prompt esophageal clearance by primary and secondary peristalsis is important in reducing contact time between the refluxed material and the esophageal mucosa. Stanciu and Bennett[15] showed a positive correlation between acid clearing, the duration of reflux, and the degree of histologic esophagitis. More recently, with the aid of a radioisotope method, an accurate assessment of esophageal clearance can be obtained. Although orderly clearance is determined by gravity, esophageal motor activity, and salivation, refluxers will often elicit a series of segmental secondary contractions that are nonperistaltic and markedly delayed during sleep when primary peristalsis and salivation nearly stops. Salivation is vital not only in its elicitation of swallow but in its dilution and HCO_3 buffering as well.[16] It is interesting, however, that in Sjögren's syndrome esophagitis is not epidemic. Perhaps, however, acid secretion is very low due to accompanying evidence of atrophic gastritis. It is also relevant that saliva volume decreases with age in normal subjects. However, in 50-year-old GER patients saliva volume was not less than in age-matched normal subjects.[17]

Acid clearance time between reflux patients and control subjects shows considerable overlap. The majority of subjects with GER have normal primary peristalsis when studied with an infused catheter system, and only in a very small subgroup can abnormal clearance be attributed to a motility disturbance (which may be secondary), resulting in a series of repetitive, nonperistaltic contractions in the distal esophagus. Recent work supports the concept that peristalsis, once initiated, is not altered by the level of consciousness. Whether acid, pepsin, or bile in the esophagus can alter peristalsis or contraction amplitudes has been debated. Increased salivary flow is seen with the presence of acid in the distal esophagus, and esophageal peristalsis is an important factor in delivering the saliva bolus and clearing acid from the distal esophagus.[16] Finally, there may be a role for hiatal hernia as discussed previously. We have isotopic documentation of orad movement of acid during swallowing to clear acid during a standard acid clearance test. Only GER patients with a hernia demonstrated this, and it accompanied a swallow-induced LES relaxation.[18] These data are consistent with the report of Johnson et al.[19] regarding the impairment of acid clearance due to the mechanical effects related to a hernia.

■ POTENCY OF REFLUXED MATERIAL

The composition of the material refluxed into the esophagus is an important factor in determining the presence and severity of GER. Acid and pepsin in small amounts play key roles in generating esophagitis. As expected, when Zollinger-Ellison patients develop esophagitis, the injury may be so severe as to cause stricture, bleeding, or even perforation.[20] Bile and pancreatic secretions (especially after gastric surgery) have an alkaline corrosive effect. At an acid pH, conjugated bile salts can increase the permeability of the esophageal mucosa to hydrogen ion.[21] However, there are no studies documenting the presence of bile acids in the esophagus during reflux episodes, and it is suggested that no bile accompanies an acid reflux event. The term "alkaline reflux" should be reserved for postoperative gastric surgery of pernicious anemia patients until investigation has clarified whether there is a role for bile in the "typical" refluxer.

■ GASTRIC VOLUME AND EMPTYING

The occurrence of GER depends on an available reservoir of intragastric fluid. Alterations in gastric volume and composition, the rate of secretion, the frequency of volume of duodenogastric reflux, and gastric emptying play the major roles in determining reflux. Recently, studies from our laboratory have reported up to 57 per cent of patients with symptomatic GER as having delayed gastric emptying of a solid meal, implying an antral motility disturbance.[22,49] Some patients with GER complain of vomiting that may be related to gastric retention and distention. Certainly most GER patients complain of bloating, fullness, postprandial satiety, and epigastric discomfort, all of which are explained by delayed gastric emptying. Smoking and high-fat meals also further delay gastric emptying, and both also provoke reflux symptoms. We have recently reported that antral gastritis may be the explanation for the antral motility disorder that predisposes to gastric stasis.[23] The investigation has shown that 78 per cent of refluxers had histologic gastritis versus 10 per cent of control subjects, thereby possibly explaining this markedly delayed gastric emptying in reflux patients.[23] We also hypothesized that pyloric sphincter incompetence could accompany this gastric slowing and perhaps predispose to duodenogastric (bile) reflux, and this duodenogastric reflux, in turn, induces gastritis. In summary, the gastric emptying research in GER has emphasized the fact that GER is much more than a disease of the distal 3 cm of the esophagus (the LES). More important, it is a diffuse motility disturbance of the upper gastrointestinal tract, and events occurring distal to the LES may indeed be the instigators of the reflux events, with the LES more of a "victim."

■ TISSUE RESISTANCE

The esophageal epithelium has a capacity to resist injury from refluxed gastric material, and this varies among individuals. Normal squamous epithelium is impermeable, but back diffusion of H^+ and its subsequent protein denaturization is potentiated by bile, pepsin, and alcohol.[24] Some workers believe that nerve endings in elongated papillae that are present as a manifestation of chronic inflammation are brought closer to the lumen by desquamation of the surface epithelial cells and may thereby elicit heartburn.[19] The prostaglandins and sucralfate, with their proven cytoprotective actions in the stomach and duodenum, may have a role in maintaining esophageal mucosal integrity, but this is yet to be proved. In addition, there may be other factors that promote healing or delay fibrosis and stricture formation, as well as possibly preventing Barrett's epithelium and its consequences.

In summary, reflux esophagitis is a multifactorial process dependent upon a mixture of LES incompetence, gastric volume and emptying, esophageal acid clearance, and tissue resistance. As shown in Figure 8-1, therapy should be directed toward increasing LES pressure, improving gastric emptying, suppressing gastric acidity, enhancing esophageal clearance or promoting salivation, and perhaps, decreasing these transient LES relaxations. These observations up to now of the possible pathophysiologic changes of GER also emphasize the need to look upon GER patients as a heterogeneous group as far as their individual problems are concerned. Although they may all present with heartburn and degrees of regurgitation, their individual predominant pathophysiologic changes will vary, and this must be appreciated in order to instigate appropriate tests to identify the abnormalities in each individual and also initiate therapy that will be "tailor made" for an individual.

■ *Diagnostic Approach to GER*

The diagnosis of GER is usually clinical. However, in a small number of patients, the judicious use of a few diagnostic tests may be necessary. Clinically, GER patients present with heartburn and regurgitation and many times chest pain that can be substernal, associated with diaphoresis, shortness of breath, and anginal type radiation. Dysphagia or odynophagia may indicate a stricture, severe mucosal inflammation, or an associated esophageal motility problem. Concordant with the high frequency of disordered gastric emptying in refluxers, postprandial nausea, bloating, and emesis may also occur.

The barium swallow is helpful in defining strictures, ulcers with reflux, or Barrett's and can be used to initially evaluate dysphagia and to rule out other upper GI disease. Eighty to 95 per cent of symptomatic GER patients have a hiatal hernia. Evidence suggests that at least 40 per cent of patients asymptomatic for GER and over the age of 50 will have a hiatal hernia. Additionally, GER at the time of cine-esophagography had a sensitivity of only 40 per cent, and reflux damage to esophageal mucosa is rarely detected by standard radiographic techniques. In the presence of a hiatal hernia, it is very difficult to evaluate LES competency.[25]

Since Fyke's description of the LES manometrically, there has been much controversy about the value of this measurement.[26] It is clear that a single LES pressure, unless extreme (≤6 mm Hg), provides little discrimination to suggest reflux. However, demonstration of esophageal spasm, ''nutcracker'' or hypercontracting esophagus, or disruption of normal peristalsis may help explain the atypical chest pain or dysphagia in the absence of mechanical obstruction.

Acid perfusion (Bernstein) testing represents a safe, simple, reproducible, and quite sensitive technique of identifying an esophagus sensitive to acid, yet a negative test does not exonerate the esophagus.

The reproduction of pain correlates best with symptoms. Positive tests are seen in approximately 85 per cent of patients with symptoms but in up to 15 per cent of asymptomatic subjects. It appears that relief of pain from acid infusion by saline is not a sensitive indicator of a positive Bernstein test. Work from our laboratory has shown that 52 per cent of GER patients failed to obtain relief following saline instillation, and elevation of esophageal pH to ≥4 or the use of antacids did not influence the outcome of pain relief in refluxers.[27] In the setting of chest pain that has a mixture of heartburn and/or pressure and squeezing, and a negative cardiac evaluation, the Bernstein test may be invaluable.

Endoscopy has shown us that up to 50 per cent of patients with objective criteria for GER have *no* macroscopic evidence of esophagitis. At the time of endoscopy, characteristic changes seen with esophagitis include erythema, friability, erosions, exudate, ulceration, stricture, and in some of the subjects, Barrett's columnar-lined esophagus.[28] With the aid of the Crosby capsule or Quinton

suction biopsy, specimens from 2.5 to 10 cm above the manometrically determined LES can be easily obtained. Data from our laboratory indicate that suction biopsies in normal subjects will show GER changes in only 5 per cent; therefore, finding biopsy changes in symptomatic patients is very significant. Routine endoscopic biopsies do not include the lamina propria, and they are also smaller, more fragmented, and difficult to orientate. However, the endoscopic biopsy specimens from the newer endoscopes with large biopsy channels (10 F) are adequate and will likely replace the more arduous suction biopsy technique. Although neutrophils can be observed, the lack of a true esophagitis in man biopsies is one of the reasons behind the change in terminology from reflux esophagitis to gastroesophageal reflux disease. Finally, intraepithelial eosinophils reported to be helpful in the diagnosis of GER in infants do not seem to suggest GER in adults. Intraepithelial eosinophils were present in 30 per cent of biopsies from pH-proven refluxers and 33 per cent of biopsies from asymptomatic normal control subjects.[29]

The standard acid reflux test (SART) introduced by Tuttle and Grossman in 1958[30] is an unphysiologic technique that requires intragastric instillations of acid followed by various artificial maneuvers to raise intragastric pressure. The false positive rate may be as high as 40 per cent and has lost favor in esophageal pH measurement. Our group has carried out a postprandial acid reflux test on patients with symptoms of GER and a positive SART.[27] Reflux was evaluated basally and postprandially in both the sitting (1 hour) and lying (2 hours) positions. Subjects ingest an egg-salad sandwich and 250 ml of milk, and esophageal pH is measured without maneuvers or acid infusion. The mean three-hour postprandial reflux time was 44.6 ± 6.7 min in refluxers as compared to 4.0 ± 1.2 min in normal subjects. It is important that a number of patients with GER had postprandial reflux times greater than the maximal reflux time demonstrated in normal subjects. The value of this exaggerated reflux time may not be appreciated under basal or in nonphysiologic settings, and we feel that postprandial pH monitoring is an accurate method that is attractive to both patient and investigator.

The acid clearance test introduced by Booth in 1968[31] is based on the concept that acid-induced changes in the esophagus lead to disordered peristalsis, which in turn results in impaired clearance of refluxed acid. Esophageal pH is measured 5 cm above the manometrically defined LES, and following ingestion of 15 ml of 0.1 N HCl, the number of swallows required to raise the esophageal pH to 5 or above is determined. Normally, less than 12 swallows are required. The rate of positive tests in symptomatic patients ranges from 53 to 100 per cent.[15] Patients with esophageal motility disorders will have false positive results, and manometry should be done on all study subjects.

The most recent application of esophageal pH measurements, 24-hour monitoring, has emphasized the importance of nighttime reflux with episodes of long duration and the concept of upright and supine GER. Despite the sensitivity of prolonged pH monitoring for detecting acid reflux, false negative findings range from 10 to 20 per cent, some of which may be bile reflux or may simply represent the artificial settings of hospitalization, which has been the usual method of studying patients up to now. The future in this area may involve ambulatory monitoring, with a device similar to a Holter monitor or telemetry, which would allow the patient to lead a normal life while obtaining important reflux information.

Data from our laboratory[32] reveal that, when compared to 24-hour pH recordings, the postprandial results pH <4.0 for three hours after breakfast and lunch and four hours after dinner, the sensitivity was 77 per cent and specificity was 96 per cent, yielding a positive predictive value of 79 per cent. When a single postprandial time period was compared to 24-hour testing as a diagnostic test, there was a sensitivity of 77 per cent and a specificity of 95 per cent. Therefore, postprandial pH testing is far more practical, being less time-consuming for patient and physician, less expensive, and better tolerated as a measure of esophageal pH.

The role for the radionuclide diagnosis of GER needs to be reviewed. In this procedure, 200 to 300 μCi ^{99m}Tc sulfur colloids are swallowed in the form of an isotope-labeled liquid meal, and interval counts are measured with a gamma camera over the area of the esophagus and stomach. The technique is simple, quick, and uniformly sensitive in 75 to 85 per cent of patients with symptoms. There are data to show a strong correlation with severity of GER and endoscopic esophagitis, and studies after medical or surgical therapy demonstrated significant reduction in radionuclide activity that corresponds closely to the clinical degree of reflux.[33,34] However, we and others[22,35] have been unable to reproduce these data. We have been impressed by the method's failure to detect any evidence of esophageal counts at times when a simultaneous pH recording in the distal esophagus has documented acid reflux. Emphasis in this field will be directed toward defining the contribution of esophageal scintigraphy when used with other esophageal function studies and to demonstrate this test's reproducibility in a number of research laboratories. While it may diagnose more severe and obvious forms of GER, as does the barium swallow, is it able to detect milder cases?

Blue et al.[36] demonstrated esophageal reflux with a DISIDA scan in a patient with a Billroth II anastomosis, indicating that bile reflux may have been the cause of the esophagitis and epigastric pain. In addition, earlier studies from our laboratory demonstrated that patients with pernicious anemia (PA) had delayed solid meal gastric emptying.[37] Orlando and Bozynski found that PA patients with betazole-fast achlorhydria may still have bilious heartburn and regurgitation with endoscopic and histologic esophagitis despite the absence of acid.[38]

In summary, we and others have found that the combination of a thorough history and physical examination, endoscopy with suction biopsy, Bernstein testing, and postprandial pH measurements provides the most accurate means of investigating the patient with reflux symptoms.

■ *Medical Therapy of GER*

Simple changes in lifestyle can play a major role in the medical treatment of GER (Fig. 8–2). Studies with overnight pH monitoring have shown a decrease in esophageal acid exposure with elevation of the head of the bed 6 to 8 inches.[30] Refluxers should avoid lying down soon after meals, as reflux is greatly increased during this time period. Weight reduction with fatty food avoidance or measures to reduce intra-abdominal pressure may reduce symptoms. Foods that lower LES tone, such as chocolate, fat, carminatives (peppermint, spearmint), and coffee, are to be avoided, while cigarettes, with their nicotine receptor effect, must be eliminated.[39] As shown in Table 8–1, a variety of commonly used drugs and hormones decrease LES pressure and slow gastric emptying. In addition, smaller, semisolid meals are emphasized.

We will now discuss the current therapeutic approaches emphasizing that the rationale for choosing an individual treatment rests with attempting to address the pathophysiology already discussed (see Fig. 8–1).

■ ANTACIDS

There are no published placebo-controlled trials examining antacids alone in the treatment of GER, yet antacids neutralize acid, blind bile acids, and cause small rises in LES pressure.[40] Behar et al.[41] found only 19 per cent of patients treated with antacids obtained symptomatic relief. Whether ant-

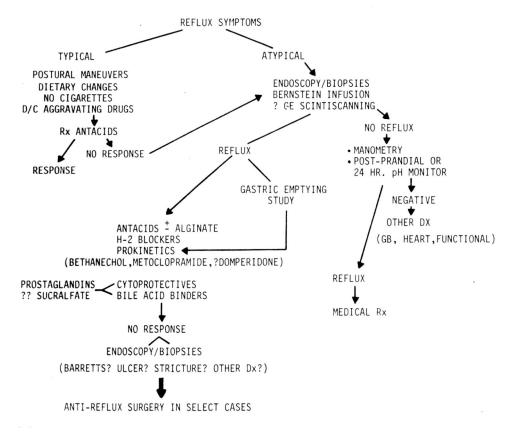

Figure 8–2. An algorithm for the approach to the medical management of gastroesophageal reflux.

Table 8–1. AGENTS THAT DECREASE LES PRESSURE OR SLOW GASTRIC EMPTYING

Foods
  Fat
  Chocolate
  Peppermint

Drugs
  Anticholinergics
Nitrates
  Theophyllines
  Nicotine (smoking)
  Alpha blockers
  Calcium channel blockers
  Levodopa
  Narcotics

Hormones, Miscellaneous
  Progesterone
  Estrogen
  Cholecystokinin
  Somatostatin
  Beta agonists
  Prostaglandins E_1, E_2

acid control of mild to moderate symptoms in GER is true pharmacologic efficacy or a placebo response remains to be proved. A recent controlled study showed them to be no more effective than placebo in controlling episodes of heartburn or pain induced by Bernstein infusion, and symptom relief did not correlate with intra-esophageal pH.[42] However, relief with either antacid (30 ml) or placebo was good. It appears that relief of heartburn pain, once it has occurred, by antacids is dependent on other factors, such as esophageal acid clearance and lavage of damaged mucosa. In addition, Stanciu and Bennett[43] studied Gaviscon, antacid minus the alginate, and placebo and found no significant differences in relief of symptoms among the three groups. Graham et al.[44] conducted a double-blind trial using prophylactically administered regimens and found symptom relief and healing of esophagitis when antacids were compared with alginate. Meyer et al.[42] showed that 7 oz antacid per day (one-half hour and 1 hour after meals and before bed) was no better than placebo in relief of heartburn and regurgitation, both resulting in a 30 per cent improvement, in patients referred to a university center. Although antacids are still referred to as the "mainstay" of medical therapy for GER, one should use them knowing that they are probably no better than placebo, which amounts to swallowing a volume of liquid, being erect, and having a series of saliva-related swallows associated with peristalsis.

■ H₂ ANTAGONISTS

Gastric acid secretion is not generally increased in GER subjects. The H₂-blockers have no effect on LES tone, esophageal peristalsis, or gastric emptying, yet cimetidine has consistently been shown to control reflux symptoms and improve esophagitis as compared to placebo. However, only a third of the studies to date have displayed healing of esophagitis during therapy.[11] Prolonged therapy is often necessary, and the side effects of mental confusion, transaminase elevation, mild renal impairment, gynecomastia, and oligospermia, along with drug interactions with the warfarins, beta-blockers, phenytoin, theophyllines, and benzodiazepines must be considered.

In recent multicenter trials patients with subjective and objective GER were studied with ranitidine (150 mg bid) in a six-week, randomized, placebo-controlled, double-blind trail. Patients achieved significant (P <.001) clinical remission, clinical improvement, and less day- and nighttime heartburn as compared to placebo.[45,46] The ranitidine increased the healing rate of endoscopic esophagitis, and its long-lasting inhibitory effect on gastric acid secretion indicates it is valuable in reducing nocturnal symptoms of GER. Because GER disease is a chronic, intermittently relapsing, life-long problem, maintenance therapy is a very important consideration. The long-acting inhibitors of acid are attractive, at least nocturnally in this regard, and more powerful and longer acting ones can be expected.

■ *Drugs That Increase LES Tone*

Bethanechol was the first smooth muscle stimulant to be used in GER. It increases LES pressure and esophageal clearance but does nothing to augment gastric emptying, and the drug may be no more effective than high-dose antacids overall.[47]

Recent investigations into the pathophysiology of gastroesophageal reflux have focused on the role of the gastric volume available to reflux into the esophagus, and specifically on the rate of gastric emptying of a meal. A study addressing antral function in patients with gastroesophageal reflux measured antral contractility with perfused catheters.[48]

Patients with reflux esophagitis had less activity than normal subjects, and oral metoclopramide increased the number of antral contractions and the cumulative antral activity index. However, gastric emptying using an isotope-labeled liquid meal was similar in reflux patients and an age-matched group of normal control subjects. A study by McCallum et al.[22] using an isotope-labeled mixed solid-liquid meal indicated that up to 41 per cent of patients with gastroesophageal reflux have a delay in gastric emptying, which is usually symptomatically latent. A recent study combining isotopic labeling of solid and liquid components of a meal defined the abnormality in gastric emptying as specific for the solid-food component, implying an impairment of antral motility. Slow gastric emptying of the solid component of the meal (isotope-labeled chicken liver) was observed in 57 per cent of the reflux poulation studied.[49] It is apparent that the motility abnormality present in gastroesophageal reflux is not confined to the LES and esophageal body, but extends distally to related parts of the upper gastrointestinal tract.

Previous investigations from our laboratory indicate that metoclopramide, both parenterally and orally, increased the rate of gastric emptying in gastroesophageal reflux patients in whom it was delayed. On the other hand, bethanechol, an agent commonly proposed for the treatment of reflux esophagitis, did not result in a significant improvement in gastric retention in the same patients at the parenteral dose used. In patients with symptomatic reflux and decreased LES pressure, 20 mg metoclopramide produced a greater increase in sphincter pressure than 25 mg bethanechol, whereas responses to 10 mg metoclopramide and 25 mg bethanechol were similar.[50] Metoclopramide does not increase gastric acid secretion nor stimulate endogenous gastrin release, and this is a theoretical advantage over bethanechol.

Metoclopramide, a procainamide derivative, stimulates gastrointestinal smooth muscle in animals and humans. It increases both LES pressure and the amplitude of esophageal contractions as well as accelerates gastric emptying in retention states and improves small bowel transit.[51] The exact mechanism of these effects on gastrointestinal smooth muscle is not precisely defined but is partially explained through dopamine antagonism. Although dopamine is regarded as an inhibitory neurotransmitter, the actual existence of dopaminergic neurons in the gastrointestinal tract has not been clearly established in humans. Metoclopramide also augments acetylcholine release from postganglionic cholinergic nerve terminals and sensitizes muscarinic receptors of gastrointestinal smooth muscle.[52] It may have a direct stimulating effect on smooth muscle, as suggested by its effect on opossum LES, which is not abolished by tetrodotoxin or atropine. Metoclopramide may have the ability to not only stimulate the gastrointestinal smooth muscle but to coordinate gastric, pyloric, and duodenal motor activity to result in net aboral movement.[52] This property is incompletely understood, but may differentiate its action from the nonspecific cholinergic effects of bethanechol and may help explain the observed differences of metaclopramide and bethanechol on gastric emptying.

We have observed that metoclopramide significantly enhanced gastric emptying in the subgroups of GER patients with slow as well as normal emptying rates.[53] The improvement in the group of normal emptying esophagitis patients was greater than that reported by Metzger et al.[54] in normal volunteers using the same test meal. Our result was obtained in a larger population and, although significant, the mean decrement of 10.8 per cent, 90 minutes after the meal, was only half the improvement achieved with metoclopramide in the slow emptying reflux patients (20.3 per cent). For a given patient, this improved emptying rate, although still in the "normal" range, may be clinically important by reducing the residual gastric volume available to reflux, particularly when combined with the purported reduction in duodenogastric reflux attributed to metoclopramide. These effects, augmented by the accompanying increase in LES pressure, may promote less gastroesophageal reflux.

Academically, and from a pathophysiologic point of view, investigations of gastric emptying remain an important aspect of research in GER patients. Such endeavors have already identified the gastric emptying abnormality as specific for the solid food component, and this forms the basis for advising a diet that stresses smaller, semisolid, or soft meals for those patients.[53] The usual recommendation for adherence to a low-fat diet in the management of reflux esophagitis is based not only on the ability of fat to decrease LES pressure but also to markedly inhibit gastric emptying. Methodology for gastric emptying can be easily adopted by nuclear medicine sections at both university and community hospital settings. From a patient management approach, a trial of a gastric "prokinetic" agent such as metoclopramide in GER is warranted and is not limited by the status of the patient's gastric emptying. If a gastric emptying test is not readily available, our findings support initiating therapy and monitoring the patient's clinical parameters. A double-blind study showed that metoclopramide significantly reduced day- and nighttime heartburn and regurgitation, as well as decreasing need for antacid use.[55] In addition, the

magnitude of increase in LES pressure after metoclopramide did not predict symptomatic response, indicating that the clinical response to this prokinetic compound is more related to enhanced gastric emptying and decreased duodenogastric reflux, thus facilitating acid removal from the lower esophagus.

Guslandi[56] randomly treated 45 patients with symptomatic GER and confirmed histologic esophagitis with either metoclopramide (10 mg tid) or ranitidine (150 mg bid). During the six-week trial, both drugs were effective in producing symptomatic and endoscopic improvement. More recently, metoclopramide was shown to provide symptom relief in patients not already adequately improved by cimetidine.[57] Metoclopramide (Reglan) is the only absorbed agent currently approved by the FDA for treatment of GER. The dose is 10 mg 30 min before meals and at night, but starting at a smaller dose, e.g., 5 mg, is recommended to minimize side effects, particularly in the older patient. The agent is very attractive for long-term maintenance use. It is FDA approved for use before large meals and activities known to provoke reflux. Clearly during the day when eating, a promotility agent can accelerate emptying of food and acid from the stomach, thus minimizing the role of gastric distention in inducing transient LES relaxations (as already discussed) and simultaneously increasing LES pressure and decreasing duodenogastric reflux.

In patients with ulcerative esophagitis or in those likely to be acid hypersecretors (e.g., patients with a history of duodenal ulcers), in patients with Barrett's esophagus in which cell turnover from ongoing acid reflux is incriminated in the complication of adenocarcinoma, and in patients awaking at night with heartburn or pulmonary symptoms, e.g., asthma, an initial trial of ranitidine is appropriate. In the remaining patients with or without symptoms suggestive of gastric stasis, and with or without objective evidence of slow gastric emptying, metoclopramide would be a more appropriate initial choice. Usually one month is enough to judge the effectiveness of a drug. In patients with severe day and night symptoms, the optimal treatment for now is Reglan, 10 mg before meals and at night (and increasing the dose as tolerated), and ranitidine 150 mg at night or bid. Maintenance dosage could be Reglan, 20 mg for the larger evening meal, and Zantac at night.

Domperidone, a patient dopamine antagonist without blood-brain barrier penetration and void of these CNS effects, has shown itself to be very effective in Europe, and controlled clinical trials in the United States are in progress. Its major indication for now may be in patients who cannot tolerate Reglan therapy because of side effects. Domperidone's only side effects are prolactin-related ones.

■ ESOPHAGEAL "CYTOPROTECTION"

Sucralfate is an aluminum salt of a sulfated disaccharide released in 1968 for the treatment of peptic ulcer. It adheres avidly to positively charged proteins in the ulcer base and may also serve as a surface barrier to acid, pepsin, and bile at the site of its cytoprotective coagulum. The efficacy of sucralfate in the healing of duodenal ulcer and gastric ulcer versus placebo and cimetidine is well reported, and there is recent evidence that it may heal esophageal ulcers associated with endoscopic sclerotherapy.[58] What role does sucralfate play in the treatment of GER mucosal disease? Schweitzer et al.[59] perfused the rabbit esophagus with acid, pepsin, and hydrochloric acid. When sucralfate was added, a significant reduction in gross and microscopic esophagitis was seen. In addition, mucosal permeability by pepsin was also reduced. Other studies have shown that sucralfate, when studied in double-blind controlled fashion, is effective, and it may act to increase tissue electrical resistance and prevent H^+ permeation into damaged mucosa.[60,61] A suspension form has now been developed and the results of controlled clinical trials will be awaited.

The antacid–alginic acid combination Gaviscon has been shown in pH-monitoring studies to reduce the duration of GER.[62] However, rationale for its more widespread use is lacking. It is now used as an antacid, and it is assumed that chewing and swallowing related to this compound promotes salivation and stimulates peristalsis. It is also thought to form a foam surface in the stomach and to coat the distal esophagus.

Finally, prostaglandins (E_2 especially) have received recent attention. If there is such an entity as "cytoprotection" of esophageal mucosa and the need for a more resistant esophageal mucosa, then prostaglandins may have a role. They are currently being evaluated in double-blind trials in which doses are both acid inhibitory and cytoprotective, making interpretation difficult. Nevertheless, it does make one consider tissue resistance factors and why some patients have different healing characteristics. At one point it was actually felt that prostaglandins released from the inflammatory esophagitis tissue may inhibit smooth muscle in the distal esophagus and perpetuate the GER cycle. However, treating GER with indomethacin (the prostaglandin inhibitor) did not gain enthusiasm and the wheel has turned full circle to now suggest that at least topical prostaglandins in the esophageal lumen help maintain esophageal mucosal integrity.

In summary, reflux esophagitis patients are a heterogeneous group. It should be remembered that GER is endemic in the population, is the commonest reason for ad lib antacid use, and is the commonest problem, along with irritable bowel syndrome, seen in gastroenterology practice. Several pathogenetic mechanisms may be operative, including decreased lower esophageal sphincter pressure, decreased esophageal acid clearance, delayed gastric emptying, duodenogastric reflux, hyperacidity, and esophageal mucosal barrier factors. Most patients with reflux have typical symptoms such as heartburn, substernal chest pain, and regurgitation and respond to medical treatment. However, a small number of patients require more sophisticated investigation to determine the diagnosis and extent of disease and some with severe symptoms require multidrug regimens for relief. Finally, antireflux surgery, to be discussed in the next chapter, has a prominent role in the management of refractory or complicated reflux esophagitis.

The future goals in medical therapy in GER lie in accepting the fact that it is a chronic remitting and relapsing disease. We should treat the acute relapses intensively but try to minimize their frequency and severity by devising a maintenance treatment plan. The goal in maintenance therapy is to treat with the minimal effective dose of an agent that addresses the particular pathophysiologic change in the individual patient, thus minimizing drug side effects. Since GER is an endemic problem in the population, treatment strategies are very important.

■ REFERENCES

1. Richter JE, Castell DO: Gastroesophageal reflux. Ann Intern Med, 97:93–103, 1982.
2. Dodds WJ, Hogan WJ, Helm JF, Dent J: Pathogenesis of reflux esophagitis. Gastroenterology, 81:276–291, 1981.
3. Dodds WJ, Dent J, Hogan EJ, et al: Mechanisms of gastroesophageal reflux in patients with reflux esophagitis. N Engl J Med, 307:1547–1552, 1982.
4. Holloway RH, Winnan G, McCallum RW: Upper gastrointestinal motility. Part I. The pathophysiologic approach to the management of reflux esophagitis. Am J Gastro, 76:280–290, 1981.
5. DeMeester TR, LaFontaine E, Joelson BE, Skinner DB, et al: Relationship of a hiatal hernia to the function of the body of the esophagus and the gastroesophageal junction. J Thor Cardiovasc Surg, 82:547–558, 1981.
6. Dodds WJ, Hogan WJ, Miller WN: Reflux esophagitis. Dig Dis, 21:49–67, 1976.
7. Reynolds JC, Ouyang A, Cotten S: A lower esophageal sphincter index involving substance P. Am J Physiol 246:G346–349, 1984.

8. Welch RW, Luckman K, Ricks P, et al: Later esophageal sphincter pressure in histologic esophagitis. Dig Dis Sci, 25:420–426, 1980.

9. Hongo M, McCallum RW: Cholinergic effects on esophageal function in man. Comparison between normal subjects and gastroesophageal reflux patients. Dig Dis Sci (in press).

10. Biancani P, Barwick K, Selling J, McCallum RW: Effects of acute experimental esophagitis on mechanical properties of the lower esophageal sphincter. Gastroenterology, 87:8–12, 1984.

11. Wesdorp E, Bartelsman J, Dekker W, Pape K, Tytgat GN: Oral cimetidine in reflux esophagitis: A double-blind controlled trial. Gastroenterology, 74:821–824, 1978.

12. Holloway RH, Hongo M, Berger K, McCallum RW: Gastric distention: A mechanism for post-prandial gastroesophageal reflux. Gastroenterology, 86:1115, 1984 (abstract).

13. Gidda JS, Goyal RK: Swallow-evoked potential in vagal preganglionic efferents. J Neurophysiol, 52:1169–1180, 1984.

14. Helms JF, Dodds WJ, Palmer DW, Hogan WJ, Teeter BC: Effect of esophageal emptying and saliva on clearance of acid from the esophagus. N Engl J Med, 310:284–288, 1984.

15. Stanciu C, Bennett JR: Oesophageal clearings: One factor in the production of reflux esophagitis. Gut, 15:852–857, 1974.

16. Orr WC, Johnson LF, Robinson MC: Effect of sleep on swallowing, esophageal peristalsis, and acid clearance. Gastroenterology, 86:814–819, 1984.

17. Sonnenberg A, Steinkamp U, Weise A, et al: Salivary secretion in reflux esophagitis. Gastroenterology, 83:889–895, 1981.

18. Mittal RK, Lange RC, Magyar L, McCallum RW: Identification of an acid clearance abnormality in patients with hiatal hernia (HH). Gastroenterology, 88:1503, 1985 (abstract).

19. Johnson LF, DeMeester TR, Haggitt RC: Esophageal epithelial responses to gastroesophageal reflux. A quantitative study. Am J Dig Dis, 23:498–509, 1978.

20. Dodds WJ, Dehn JG, Hogan WJ, et al: Severe peptic esophagitis in a patient with Zollinger-Ellison syndrome. Am J Roentgenol, 113:237–240, 1971.

21. Safaie-Shirazi S, Denbesten L, Zike WL: Effect of bile salts on the ionic permeability of the esophageal mucosa and their role in the production of esophagitis. Gastroenterology, 68:728–733, 1975.

22. McCallum RW, Berkowitz DM, Lerner E: Gastric emptying in patients with gastroesophageal reflux. Gastroenterology, 80:285–291, 1981.

23. Fink SM, Barwick KW, DeLuca V, Saunders FJ, Kandathil M, McCallum RW: The association of histologic gastritis with gastroesophageal reflux and delayed gastric emptying. J Clin Gastroenterol, 6:301–305, 1984.

24. Harmon JW, Johnson LF, Mayodonovitch CL: Effects of acid and bile salts on the rabbit esophageal mucosa. Dig Dis Sci, 26:65–72, 1981.

25. Neumann CH, Forster CF: Gastroesophageal reflux: Reassessment of the value of fluoroscopy based on manometric evaluation of the lower esophageal segment. Am J Gastroenterol, 78:776–780, 1983.

26. Fyke FE Jr, Code CF, Schlegal JF: The esophageal sphincter in healthy human beings. Gastroenterologia, 86:135–150, 1956.

27. Holloway RH, McCallum RW: New diagnostic techniques in esophageal disease. In Cohen S, Soloway RD (Eds): Diseases of the Esophagus. New York, Churchill Livingstone, 1982, pp 75–95.

28. Knuff TE, Benjamin SB, Worsham F, Castell DO: Histologic evaluation of chronic gastroesophageal reflux: An evaluation of biopsy methods and diagnostic criteria. Dig Dis Sci, 29:194–198, 1984.

29. Tummala V, Sontag S, Vlahcevic R, Barwick K, McCallum RW: Are intraepithelial eosinophils helpful in the histological diagnosis of gastroesophageal reflux? Gastroenterology, 88:1619, 1985 (abstract).

30. Tuttle SG, Grossman MI: Detection of gastroesophageal reflux by simultaneous measurements of intraluminal pressure and pH. Proc Soc Exp Biol Med, 98:225–227, 1958.

31. Booth DJ, Kemmerer WT, Skinner DB: Acid clearing from the distal esophagus. Arch Surg, 96:731–734, 1968.

32. Fink SM, McCallum RW: The role of prolonged pH monitoring in the diagnosis of gastroesophageal reflux. JAMA, 252:1160–1164, 1984.

33. Fisher RS, Malmud LS, Robert GS, et al: Gastroesophageal scintiscanning to detect and quantitate gastroesophageal reflux. Gastroenterology, 70:301–308, 1976.

34. Menin RA, Malmud LS, Pedersen RP, et al: Gastroesophageal scintigraphy to assess the severity of gastroesophageal reflux disease. Arch Surg, 191:66–71, 1980.

35. Jenkins AF, Cowan RJ, Richter JE: Gastroesophageal scintigraphy: It is a sensitive clinical test? Gastroenterology, 86:175, 1984 (abstract).

36. Blue PW, Jackson JW, Ghaed N: Duodenogastroesophageal reflux demonstration with ^{99m}Tc-DISIDA imaging. Clin Nuc Med, 9:238–240, 1984.

37. Frank EB, Lange RC, McCallum RW: Abnormal gastric emptying in patients with atrophic gastritis with or without pernicious anemia. Gastroenterology, 80:1551, 1981 (abstract).

38. Orlando RC, Bozynski EM: Heartburn in pernicious anemia—a consequence of bile reflux. N Engl J Med, 289:522–523, 1973.

39. Price SF, Smithson KW, Castell DO: Food sensitivity in reflux esophagitis. Gastroenterology, 75:240–243, 1978.

40. Holloway RH, McCallum RW: A practical approach to gastroesophageal reflux. Drug Ther, 151–160, March 1983.

41. Behar J, Sheahan DG, Biancani P, Spiro HM, Storer EH: Medical and surgical management of reflux esophagitis. A 38-month report on a prospective clinical trial. N Engl J Med, 293:263–268, 1975.

42. Meyer CT, Berenzweig H, McCallum RW: A controlled trial of antacid and placebo in the relief of heartburn. Gastroenterology, 76:1201, 1982 (abstract).

43. Stanciu C, Bennett JR: Alginate/antacid in the reduction of gastroesophageal reflux. Lancet, 1:109–111, 1974.

44. Graham DY, Lanzar F, Dorsch ER: Symptomatic reflux esophagitis: A double-blind controlled comparison of antacids and alginate. Curr Ther Res, 22:653–658, 1977.

45. Wesdorp KC, Dekker W, Klinkenberg-Knol EC: Treatment of reflux oesophagitis with ranitidine. Gut, 24:921–924, 1983.

46. Hune KR, Holmes GKT, Mehkian V, et al: Ranitidine in reflux eosophagitis. A double-blind placebo-controlled study. Digestion, 29:119–125, 1984.

47. Saco LS, Orlando RC, Levinson SL, et al: Double-blind controlled trial of bethanechol and antacid versus placebo and antacid in the treatment of erosive esophagitis. Gastroenterology, 82:1367–1375, 1982.

48. Behar J, Ramsby G: Gastric emptying and antral motility in reflux esophagitis. Gastroenterology, 74:253–256, 1978.

49. McCallum RW, Mensh R, Lange R: Definition of the gastric emptying abnormality present in gastroesophageal reflux patients. In Weinbeck M (Ed): Motility of the Digestive Tract. New York, Raven Press, 1982, pp 355–362.

50. McCallum RW, Kline MM, Curry N, Sturdevant RAL: Comparative effects of metoclopramide and bethanechol

on lower esophageal sphincter pressure in reflux patients. Gastroenterology, 68:1114–1118, 1975.

51. Albibi R, McCallum RW: Metoclopramide: Pharmacology and clinical application. Ann Intern Med, 98:86–95, 1983.

52. Eisner M: Gastrointestinal effects of metoclopramide in man. *In vivo* experiments with human smooth muscle preparation. Br Med J, 4:679–680, 1968.

53. Fink SM, Lange RC, McCallum RW: Effect of metoclopramide on normal and delayed gastric emptying in gastroesophageal reflux patients. Dig Dis Sci, 28:1057–1061, 1983.

54. Metzger WH, Cano R, Sturdevant RAL: Effects of metoclopramide in chronic gastric retention after gastric surgery. Gastroenterology, 71:30–32, 1976.

55. McCallum RW, Ippolitti AF, Cooney C, Sturdevant RAL: A controlled trial of metoclopramide in symptomatic gastroesophageal reflux. N Engl J Med, 296:354–357, 1977.

56. Guslandi M, Testoni PA, Passaretti S, et al: Ranitidine vs. metoclopramide in the medical treatment of reflux esophagitis. Hepato-Gastroenterology, 30:96–99, 1983.

57. Lieberman DA, Keefe EB. Double-blind controlled trial of metoclopramide and cimetidine versus placebo and cimetidine in the treatment of severe reflux esophagitis. Gastroenterology, 88:1476, 1985 (abstract).

58. Roark G: Treatment of post-sclerotherapy ulcers with Sucralfate. Gastroint Endosc, 39:9–10, 1984.

59. Schweitzer EF, Bass BL, Johnson LF, Harmon JW: Sucralfate blocks pepsin induced esophageal injury in rabbits. Gastroenterology, 86:1241, 1984 (abstract).

60. Weiss W, Brunner H, Buttner GR, et al: Therapie der refluxosophagits mit Sucralfat. Dtsch Med Wschr, 108:1706–1711, 1983.

61. Orlando RC, Powell DW: Effect of Sucralfate on esophageal epithelial resistance in the rabbit. Gastroenterology, 86:1201, 1984 (abstract).

62. Johnson LF, DeMeester TR: Evaluation of elevation of the head of the bed, bethanechol, antacid foam tablets on gastroesophageal reflux. Dig Dis Sci, 26:673–680, 1981.

9

Surgery for Hiatal Hernia and Esophagitis

Lucius D. Hill ▪ *Kjell Thor*
C. Dale Mercer

One of the most common abnormalities of the upper gastrointestinal tract is a malfunctioning gastroesophageal (GE) junction with its attendant esophagitis, heartburn, and dysphagia. The high frequency of GE reflux calls for strict indications for surgery. Operations should be founded on sound rationale and aided by modern technology to be effective.

Prior to the recognition of reflux as the cause of esophagitis, surgeons focused attention primarily on herniation of the stomach through the esophageal hiatus. Hiatal hernia was first clearly described by Bright of England in 1836.[1] In 1853, Bowditch[2] in the United States not only clearly described hiatal hernia but suggested that surgery for this condition could be lifesaving.

Because of the inability to study the underlying abnormalities, surgery for GE reflux developed slowly. Scudder was the first to perform a deliberate repair of sliding hiatal hernia in 1911.[3] In 1951, Allison[4] introduced a technique that was based on a somewhat better understanding of the underlying anatomy. The operation had an unacceptably high failure rate. In 1956, Rudolph Nissen[5] described the principle of fundoplication based on his observation of a patient who had excision of the cardia followed by wrapping of the stomach around the esophagus. In 1952, Ronald Belsey of England developed the Mark IV transthoracic repair, which included anchoring the GE junction to the anterior part of the undersurface of the diaphragm, thereby creating an anterior flap value aimed at the control of reflux.[6] In 1963 Andre Toupet from France described a semifundoplication to be used in hiatal hernia repair and as a complement to Heller myotomy in order to avoid "l'incapacité d'eructation."[7] In 1967, our group reported a procedure consisting of posterior fixation of the GE junction with calibration of the lower esophageal sphincter.[8] The posterior fixation recreates the GE valve. The goal of this procedure is restoration of the function and anatomy of the GE junction to as near normal as possible. To understand the rationale of the operation it is well to recount the important features of the normal antireflux barrier, for these components must be restored by an antireflux operation.

▪ Components of the Antireflux Barrier

The GE junction is a highly efficient and complex mechanism which allows for swallowing of a bolus and yet maintains a resting pressure that prevents reflux of gastric contents. The GE junction distinguishes between gas and liquid and allows for belching and vomiting but not for continuous bathing of the esophageal mucosa by gastric juice. When reflux, belching, or vomiting (normal phenomena) do occur, the esophagus clears the gastric juice rapidly and efficiently. The main components of this complex mechanism that can be assessed by objective measurements are (1) the lower esophageal sphincter, (2) the GE value created by the angle of His, (3) esophageal clearance, and (4) posterior fixation by the dorsal mesentery. The diaphragm needs further study to determine its importance. Failure of any of these components can impair the antireflux barrier. A brief discussion of these important features is warranted.

The Lower Esophageal Sphincter ■ Fyke et al. in 1956,[9] demonstrated an intraluminal, high-pressure zone (HPZ) at the distal end of the esophagus. Numerous studies have since provided evidence for a physiologic sphincter that maintains a resting pressure higher than the pressure in the adjacent body of the esophagus or the stomach. Other studies have also confirmed the presence of an anatomic sphincter (see Chapter 2 on anatomy). The anatomic sphincter or GE ring is located at the HPZ seen on manometric studies of the GE junction. This resting pressure is entirely independent of the respiratory excursions of the diaphragm. The sphincter relaxes in response to swallowing and permits belching, vomiting, and relaxation in response to esophageal distention and vagal stimulation.

With the development of esophageal manometry, the importance of the lower esophageal sphincter became apparent. Our laboratory was among the first to couple pH and pressure measurements in order to measure the gastroesophageal barrier pressure (GEBP) and the presence or absence of reflux.[10] This work represented the first use of pH and manometry pre- and postoperatively in 103 patients to assess the effect of therapy on the gastroesophageal barrier. This study conclusively demonstrated that raising the GEBP correlated directly with the correction of reflux. It emphasized the importance of preserving the lower esophageal sphincter by surgical means.

Mechanical stimuli increase the resting pressure in the lower esophageal sphincter (LES) over and above intragastric pressure. The LES pressure is also affected by hormones; however, at present the physiologic role of hormones needs clarification. Muscle strips from the LES have a different length tension curve than the surrounding musculature. This curve is to the left of the curve of the strips of the body of the esophagus, indicating a "stiffness" of the LES. This stiffness allows the sphincter to respond more quickly to stretch reflex and augments its ability to maintain a resting tone. Muscle strips in the LES also have a different membrane potential than either the body of the esophagus or the stomach.[11] These features are important to the normal function of the esophagus. It is therefore important for any surgical procedure to restore to as near to normal as possible these unique features of the LES which are the first line of defense against reflux.

Gastroesophageal Valve ■ Measurement of the lower esophageal sphincter pressure focused attention on the LES almost to the exclusion of other important factors. The role of the diaphragm was downplayed and the GE valve created by the acute angle of His as part of the antireflux barrier has been almost overlooked.[12,13] The valve when viewed through a gastrostomy in a living patient is a flat, lateral leaf approximating against the mucosa of the lesser curve (Fig. 9–1). This arrangement suggests that an increase in intragastric pressure simply pushes the valve medially, thus occluding the lumen and preventing reflux. However, few studies on the human GE valve in situ have been done to clarify the role of the valve, although one study in cadavers suggests that the effect of different antireflux procedures is to increase the flap valve mechanism.[14]

We have recently shown[15] in cadavers without hiatal hernia or esophageal disease that there is a measurable pressure gradient across the GE junction which requires from 7 to 15 cm of water pressure in the stomach before reflux occurs. By simply

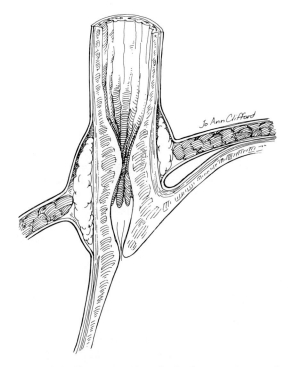

Figure 9–1. The gastroesophageal valve is a musculomucosal valve created by the angle of His. The valve is an important adjunct to the sphincter in preventing reflux. The valve closes against the lesser curve with increased intragastric pressure maintaining a gradient against reflux. The lower esophageal sphincter is normally closed, maintaining a resting pressure greater than intragastric pressure.

depressing the fundus of the stomach to approximately 45 degrees, the angle of His becomes more obtuse, the valve is eliminated, and the osteum of the esophagus is converted into a funnel allowing free reflux and elimination of the gradient. Since there is no sphincter function in the cadaver, the presence of a gradient across the GE junction and the maneuver of depressing the cardia eliminating the valve indicate that the flap valve contributes to the competence of the GE junction in an in situ preparation. This gradient can also be eliminated by dividing the posterior attachment of the GE junction to allow the junction to slide into the chest, thereby creating a hiatal hernia which allows reflux to occur. These observations have been confirmed by Nelems and coworkers at the University of British Columbia and by Mercer and coworkers at the Queens University in Kingston, Ontario, Canada. These studies indicate that the valve created by the angle of His plays a key role in preventing reflux which was previously observed by Allison, Barrett, and others. A gradient can be demonstrated across the valve (see the discussion of GE valve in Chapter 2 on anatomy) in the patient during surgery.

Esophageal Clearance ■ A number of workers, including our group, demonstrated as early as 1959[10] that reflux often occurs in normal subjects, particularly after meals. In the normal individual reflux produces an instantaneous and powerful peristaltic wave that rapidly cleanses the lower esophagus of refluxed material. There is a direct correlation between the duration of exposure to acid reflux and the severity of objective esophagitis.[16] Russell et al.[17] indicated that 41 per cent of patients with GE reflux have delayed esophageal emptying which persists, even after correction of reflux and relief of symptoms. Thus, there appears to be a primary motility defect in many patients with GE reflux. Motility studies on patients with large hiatal hernias and esophagitis have demonstrated a different severe dysmotility, apparently due to the esophagus being accordioned on itself in the chest without its normal anchoring (Fig. 9–2). Normally the GE junction is anchored within the abdomen securely so that it is tethered, usually on a level just above the median arcuate ligament. When anchored at this point, the esophagus has a fulcrum from which it can generate powerful peristaltic waves. With the loss of this tethering or anchoring, the esophagus loses its ability to generate forceful peristaltic waves. In patients with large hiatal hernia and esophagitis, this problem can be corrected by hiatal hernia repair to secure the GE junction at its normal location. The motility returns to normal after proper posterior fixation of the GE junction (Fig. 9–3).

Posterior Fixation ■ The entire GI tract, including the hollow as well as solid viscera in humans and most vertebrate animals, is suspended by the *dorsal* mesentery to the posterior body wall. The esophagus is no exception to this rule. Extensive cadaver dissections demonstrate that the esophagus is primarily fixed posteriorly by a dense plate of fibroareolar tissue extending from the median arcuate ligament all the way above the aortic arch. All other structures, including the anterior and lateral portions of the diaphragm and the anterior and lateral portions of the phrenoesophageal membrane, the liver tunnel, and the left gastric pedicle can be removed and still the esophagus cannot be moved appreciably out of its bed. When this posterior attachment becomes lengthened or attenuated, the GE junction then slides cephalad into the posterior mediastinum with the consequent development of a hiatal hernia.

The posterior attachment of the GE junction by the dorsal mesentery to the preaortic fascia is key to the integrity of the entire barrier to reflux. It has been demonstrated in the cadaver that with division of the posterior attachment, the GE junction slides into the chest and the effect of the GE valve is lost. It has been shown in the living human with hiatal hernia without the normal posterior attachment, the esophagus loses its ability to generate the swallow waves needed to propel a bolus of food into the stomach. Nonpropulsive waves with grossly deranged motility are often seen. When the esophagus is replaced to its normal length by attachment of the GE junction posteriorly to the preaortic fascia, the deranged motility reverts to normal. Dysphagia resulting from the abnormal motility is corrected.

Much attention has been focused on the so-called intra-abdominal esophagus. According to Laplace, when pressure is exerted equally on a small and a large tube, the small tube collapses first. It is therefore assumed that intra-abdominal pressure aids the antireflux barrier by compressing the esophagus and materially assisting the sphincter in maintaining competence. To date, in the living human there has been no documentation of the role of the intra-abdominal esophagus, and in fact, when viewed in patients, the segment is short. Because the sphincter straddles the diaphragm, it is difficult to measure the intra-abdominal esophagus. Further documentation of the role of this segment of the esophagus is necessary before it can be assigned a specific role in the prevention of reflux.

■ Hiatal Hernia

In a patient with hiatal hernia or GE reflux, the components of the antireflux barrier are usually

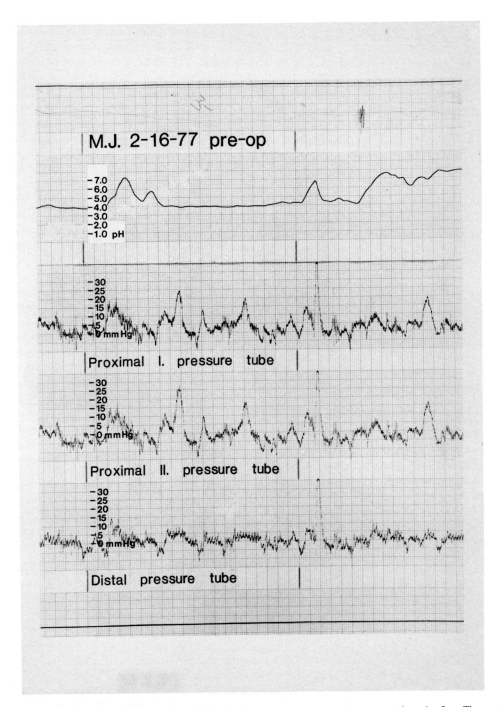

Figure 9–2. Preoperative pH and pressure tracing on a patient with a hiatal hernia with gastroesophageal reflux. The motility is grossly deranged with nonpropulsive waves involving the entire esophagus. This patient had severe dysphagia with inability to swallow food. These phenomena were consistent when reflux was not present.

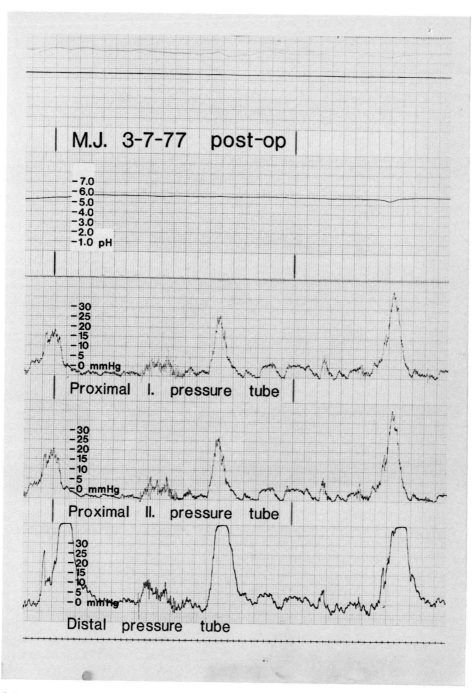

Figure 9–3. Postoperative pH and pressure tracing on patient shown in Figure 9–2 following Hill repair. The swallow waves are orderly and propulsive throughout the esophagus. The dysphagia subsided and the patient was able to resume a normal diet.

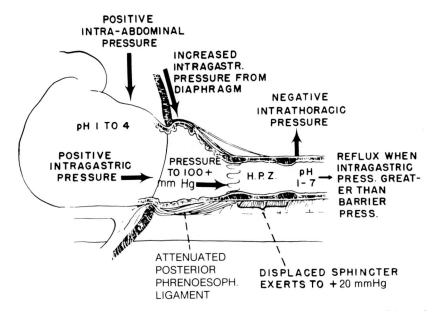

Figure 9–4. With loss of the posterior attachment of the gastroesophageal junction, the sphincter slides up into the posterior mediastinum. The forces that normally assist the sphincter are lost, including the gastroesophageal valve. With the loss of these aids, the sphincter is generally overcome and reflux occurs.

lost. The GE junction loses its posterior attachment and slides into the posterior mediastinum, thereby converting the GE valve to a funnel, which eliminates the gradient created by the valve. In addition, the sphincter may be distracted by the phrenoesophageal membrane (Fig. 9–4). The diaphragm, instead of supporting the GE junction, now actually impinges on the stomach and increases intragastric pressure which further serves to overcome the LES. The net result of all these forces is reflux. Only in those individuals with a competent esophageal sphincter, or in those who have developed a paraesophageal component with maintenance of the gastric "cardial" flap valve, is the antireflux barrier maintained and reflux prevented. In addition to the loss of the valve, esophageal clearance is impaired because the esophagus is accordioned on itself; without a fulcrum or attachment from which to operate, the esophageal peristalsis loses its force in propelling a bolus into the stomach.

■ GE Reflux Without Hiatal Hernia

In the past, hiatal hernia was considered a synonym for GE reflux. This mechanistic and simplistic belief misled clinicians into attaching a multitude of symptoms to a common radiologic finding. Hiebert and Belsey[18] and others have shown that reflux may occur without a hiatal hernia. The cause for failure of the GE junction in these cases is not yet known. The loss of the angle of His and the GE valve may well be an important factor in these patients.

From the preceding discussion, it becomes clear that the aim of an antireflux surgical procedure should be to restore the posterior attachment of the esophagus to aid in the restoration of the valve, esophageal clearance, and sphincter function. Restoration of the valve is also aided by traction on the collar-sling musculature, which accentuates the angle of His and automatically recreates and emphasizes the esophageal valve. Closure of the diaphragm is essential to prevent prolapse of the cardia into the posterior mediastinum and also helps in holding the GE junction in its normal position.

The restoration of the gastroesophageal barrier is aided materially by intraoperative manometrics. We use a number of sophisticated tests before and after surgery to determine the results that are achieved. It is reasonable therefore that we should assess what is being achieved during surgery itself. Unless barrier function is restored during surgery, all the pre- and postoperative tests are useless. If an adequate antireflux barrier is not established, the operation is a total failure. Calibration of the cardia aided by intraoperative measurements of the GEBP is a direct and purposeful effort to preserve and enhance the antireflux barrier.

■ Mature View of the Antireflux Barrier

In summary, the important features of the GE junction that need restoration by antireflux surgery are (1) the lower esophageal sphincter (LES), which maintains a resting tone and remains closed, relaxing and opening with swallowing; (2) esophageal clearance, which clears the esophagus of gastric contents following episodes of reflux; (3) the GE valve, which materially aids the sphincter in preventing reflux; and (4) the posterior fixation, which is important in maintaining the integrity of all the components of the antireflux barrier. The mature view is one recognizing the importance of each of these features.

Confusion and controversy surrounding the antireflux barrier have been compounded by illustrations depicting the GE junction as an open conduit without a sphincter closing mechanism or a valve. Careful survey of the literature shows that the GE junction is invariably shown in the open position which has no relevance to the normal living human (Fig. 9–5).

The normal GE valve closes so efficiently against the lesser curve that it appears when visualized through a gastrostomy as a slit in the mucosa (Fig. 9–6). Studies show that the valve is important in the antireflux barrier and should be depicted in the closed position (see Fig. 9–1). Measurement of the lower esophageal sphincter pressure led most workers to overemphasize the role of the sphincter while ignoring the valve (Fig. 9–7).

The mature view is depicted in Figure 9–8, which includes the sphincter and valve in the *closed* position, fixed posteriorly in the normal location. Loss of any of the key components of the barrier leads to GE reflux.

In addition to restoring the anatomy and function to as near normal as possible, an operative procedure should have durability and should be reproducible in other hands without serious complications.

■ Evaluation and Indications

Because the symptoms of esophagitis, including heartburn and dysphagia, are so common, it is important that the indications for surgery remain strict. The evaluation of the patient must be accurate, otherwise inappropriate operations may be done for the wrong diagnosis. In our GE laboratory, over 15,000 patients have been evaluated by pH and pressure studies with special attention to motility in cases that are not clearly defined by the history and physical examination.

It can be argued that the patient with intractable heartburn, with reflux and dysphagia, does not need sophisticated tests to determine that surgery is indicated. Even with these patients, it is important to know the status of LES, the presence of reflux, the level of gastric acid, and if the patient

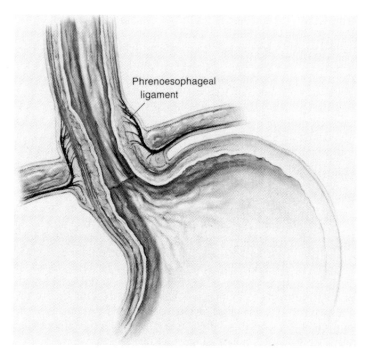

Phrenoesophageal ligament

Figure 9–5. This drawing shows the manner in which the gastroesophageal junction is invariably depicted in the literature. This is no sphincter, no valve, and the gastroesophageal junction is open. The normal gastroesophageal junction is closed except during swallowing, and the gastroesophageal valve represents a strong barrier to reflux. (From Postelwaite RW: Surgery of the Esophagus, 2nd ed. East Norwalk, Conn., Appleton-Century-Crofts, 1986, p. 218.)

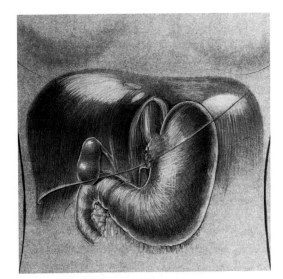

Figure 9–6. The gastroesophageal valve is viewed through a gastrostomy. It closes so effectively against the lesser curve that it can be seen only as a slit in the mucosa. It may be difficult to demonstrate. It represents a musculomucosal leaf that closes against the lesser curve. (See Color Plate I*D*.)

has esophagitis or Barrett's esophagus. It is mandatory to rule out cancer. Only by measuring these baselines will the surgeon know over the long-term whether there has been improvement in the patient's problems. In our experience, motility disorders can often mimic heartburn. A number of patients referred for antireflux surgery have been found after study to have a motility disorder instead of reflux. The important indications for surgery are the following:

Intractability—The most common indication for operation is failure to respond to medical management, or intractability. Medical management is clearly outlined in Chapter 8. If the patient fails this program under guidance of a physician inter-

ested in GI disease, the patient is a candidate for surgery.

Esophagitis—The second most common indication for operation is esophagitis. In the chapter on complications of GE reflux, Dr. Pope outlines the findings in esophagitis. This may vary from edema, and erythema of the mucosa acompanied by spasm, to severe forms of ulcerative esophagitis with stricture. ''Pope's criteria'' for the diagnosis of esophagitis have become well established.

Stricture and ulceration—Approximately 14 per cent of patients in our series were operated for stricture; 2.5 per cent have had *discrete* ulceration with or without stricture. The presence of a stricture usually indicates that refractory esophagitis has

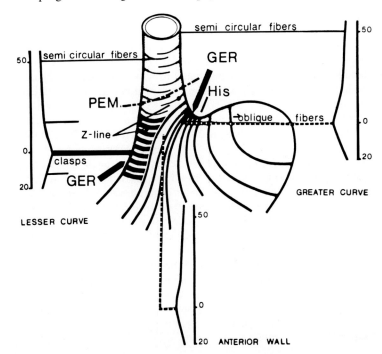

Figure 9–7. This drawing, by Meffert et al., is an excellent depiction of the sphincter and the musculature at the gastroesophageal junction but does not include the gastroesophageal valve.

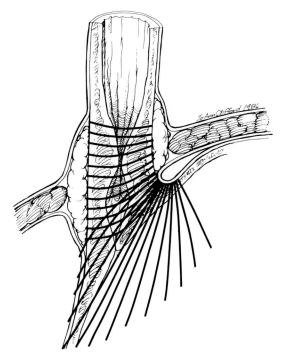

Figure 9–8. The mature view of the gastroesophageal junction is one that brings together the features of the musculature, including the sphincter, the collar sling, and the gastroesophageal valve. These components are fixed posteriorly and in combination make up the gastroesophageal barrier.

been allowed to proceed too long. Peptic ulceration occurs in the stomach in approximately 4 per cent of large hiatal hernias. Bleeding from these ulcers is usually slow and produces a chronic anemia. Perforation has been reported in many series. Perforation of the liver, lung, aorta, and even into the coronary arteries has occurred. These complications are rare but indicate that large hiatal hernias are subject to a variety of problems. In addition to peptic ulceration, large hernias may produce pressure on the heart and lungs and create chest discomfort as well as limitation of cardiorespiratory reserve.

Bleeding—Bleeding from the esophagus is usually chronic and low grade, producing persistent anemia. Rarely, a tear in the esophagus from severe reflux or penetrating ulceration with submucosal bleeding will lead to acute serious bleeding. Approximately 10 per cent of patients operated on in our series had chronic anemia.

Respiratory complications—In the discussion by Dr. Augusto Larrain in Chapter 7, the pulmonary complications of GE reflux are clearly outlined. These complications are often overlooked by physicians. We have operated on a number of patients under long-term treatment for asthma in whom the history indicated that the so-called "asthma" oc-

curred when the patient was lying down or following episodes of reflux. In these individuals, surgery is rewarding because it not only clears the symptoms of reflux, but it eliminates the symptoms related to aspiration or overflow into the tracheobronchial tree.

Large Hernias—In a small group of patients with sliding hiatal hernia, operation is required because the hernia is large enough to produce pressure symptoms in the chest with cardiorespiratory embarrassment. In these individuals, episodes of incarceration may cause pain so severe that it is misinterpreted as a myocardial infarction. In patients with these large hernias, in addition to pressure symptoms, trauma occurs at the point where the diaphragm impinges on the displaced viscus and can lead to what is termed a callous ulceration which may bleed either chronically or acutely.

Finally, there is a group of patients in whom, at both biopsy and endoscopy, *inflammation* of the esophageal mucosa can be seen, although other standard tests fail to show reflux. The patient who presents the paradox of a good sphincter pressure and no reflux during the single pull-through examination on pH and pressure study may be found on more intensive study to have transient relaxation or to have reflux mainly in the upright position. The introduction of 24-hour pH monitoring served to point out those patients who do not reflux in the recumbent position but have severe reflux in the upright position.

■ COEXISTING PROBLEMS

Of 1860 patients operated on in our series, 11 per cent underwent operation because of coexisting problems associated with hiatal hernia. Gallbladder disease was the most common coexisting problem. In these individuals, it is very important that a hiatal hernia be diagnosed and assessed before operation. It is unwise to add a hiatal hernia repair to a routine cholecystectomy or ulcer operation if the patient does not have GE reflux severe enough to warrant the operation. Hiatal hernia is so common that a surgeon may find it in a number of patients with other upper abdominal disease. In many of these cases, the hiatal hernia is asymptomatic. To subject a patient to formal repair of an asymptomatic hiatal hernia invites the complications of the procedure with no benefit to the patient. If a hiatal hernia is suspected in a patient with gallbladder or upper abdominal disease, evaluation of the hiatal hernia before operation should be done so that the surgeon can judge preoperatively whether repair is indicated.

■ *Technique*

■ HILL REPAIR

GE restoration (Hill operation) is accomplished through an upper midline abdominal incision. The abdomen is explored. The pylorus in particular is examined carefully for any evidence of pyloric stenosis which might impede gastric emptying. The triangular ligament of the left lobe of the liver is divided so that the left lobe can be retracted to the patient's right. This exposes the esophageal hiatus with its covering phrenoesophageal membrane. The upper hand retractor is placed. This facilitates exposure. The phrenoesophageal membrane is divided on the diaphragm (Fig. 9–9), keeping as much of the fibroareolar tissue that makes up the phrenoesophageal bundles as possible with the GE junction. It is these bundles that will be used in the repair. The lesser omentum is divided, and the esophageal hiatus is exposed (Fig. 9–10). The esophagus is gently diverted to the patient's right and attachment of the cardia to the diaphragm is divided. As few short gastric arteries as possible are divided (Fig. 9–11). This dissection must be done with care so as not to tear the spleen. Capsular tears of the spleen may be repaired by cautery, suturing, and applying Avitene. Division of the phrenogastric and superior portion of the gastrosplenic ligament mobilizes the upper part of the gasric fundus. The fundus can then be rotated so that the posterior part of the stomach can be visualized (Fig. 9–12). This allows the GE junction

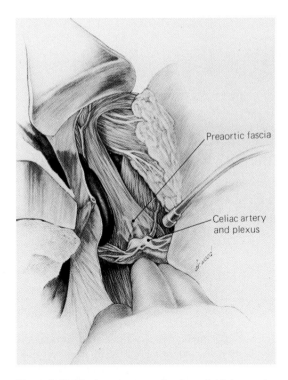

Figure 9–10. The lesser omentum has been divided, exposing the preaortic fascia in the area of the median arcuate ligament and the celiac artery. The phrenoesophageal bundles have been dissected away from the diaphragm.

to be retracted down and the hernia is reduced. The bundles of tissue that constitute the anterior and posterior attachments of the GE junction to the diaphragm, the anterior and posterior phrenoesophageal bundles, then can be displayed. By retracting these caudally, an intra-abdominal segment of esophagus becomes visible. The anterior and posterior vagus nerves are visualized and kept in view so as not to be damaged.

Attention is again turned to the pylorus. If the pylorus is scarred, if the patient has had a duodenal ulcer, or if there is a pyloric diaphragm obstructing the outlet of the stomach, a pryloromyotomy or a pyloroplasty is planned. These findings should be interpreted in the light of the patient's history. If the patient has a history of duodenal ulcer not only should a pylroplasty or pylorotomy be planned, but a vagotomy to decrease the gastric acid should be added. This finding should be anticipated by careful workup preoperatively. Only if the duodenum is markedly scarred or if there is active ulceration should pyloroplasty and vagotomy be performed. We generally employ a highly selective vagotomy and Jaboulay pyloroplasty. If the pylorus is simply scarred and there is no active ulceration, the pylorus may be dilated and a pyloromytomy per-

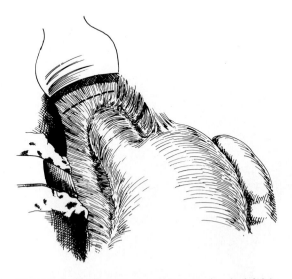

Figure 9–9. The hiatus is exposed by retracting the left lobe of the liver to the patient's right. The dotted line is the line at which the dissection of the fibroareolar tissue from the diaphragm is begun in order to obtain as much fibroareolar tissue of the phrenoesophageal bundles as possible. These bundles are used in fixing the gastroesophageal junction to the preaortic fascia.

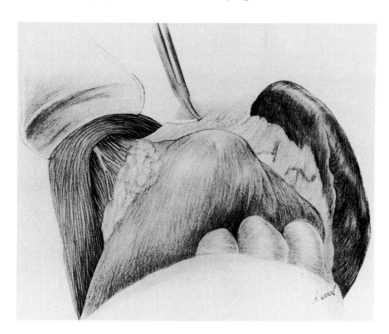

Figure 9–11. The esophagus has been retracted downward and to the patient's right, and the gastrophrenic and gastrosplenic ligaments are divided, dividing as few short gastrics as possible in order to avoid tearing the spleen.

formed. It is imperative to relieve any gastric outlet obstruction to obtain a good result from an antireflux procedure. On the other hand, to add a vagotomy to a routine hiatal hernia repair is unwise. In our experience this has led to complications of vagotomy without benefit to the patient. Retracting the stomach to the patient's left exposes the preaortic fascia. The aorta and the celiac axis are easily felt. The median arcuate ligament (MAL) lies immediately above the celiac trunk (Fig. 9–13). It can be exposed by careful blunt dissection at this point over the midpoint of the aorta. The celiac artery usually arises cephalad to the MAL. When

the free edge of the MAL has been located, the celiac artery can be compressed into the aorta, and the fibroareolar tissue overlying the artery can be carefully divided. An instrument such as a Goodell cervical dilator is then passed beneath the median arcuate ligament. If it is in the correct plane it should simply float beneath the preaortic fascia. If the instrument meets an obstruction, there may be a branch of the celiac in the midline. The branch might be damaged if force is used on insertion.

Dissection of the celiac axis has been the deterrent to performing this operation in many hands. If it is difficult to locate the MAL, if the surgeon

Figure 9–12. The esophagus is rotated clockwise in order to visualize both phrenoesophageal bundles. The vagus nerves are visualized and carefully avoided throughout the repair.

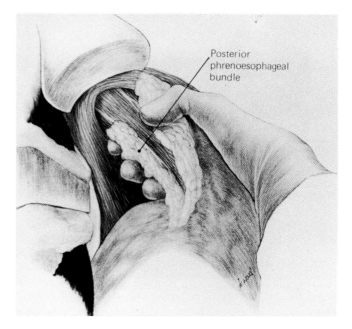

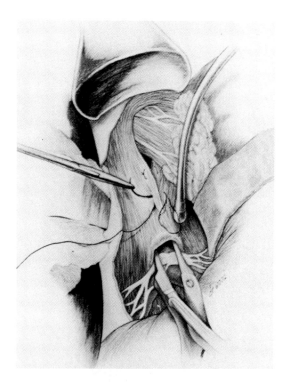

Figure 9–13. The stomach is retracted to the patient's left, exposing the preaortic fascia and the median arcuate ligament. The ligament has been dissected free from the celiac artery, and a Goodell dilator has been placed beneath it. The hiatus is closed loosely about the esophagus with interrupted, heavy silk sutures.

is not familiar with vascular surgery and is uncomfortable in dissecting out the celiac axis, a safer alternative procedure is recommended. By retracting the esophagus to the patient's left, the surgeon can expose the esophageal hiatus. The fibroareolar tissue overlying the aorta and esophageal hiatus can be simply divided by sharp dissection, thereby exposing the aorta. A finger is then passed gently beneath the preaortic fascia down to the celiac artery, and the preaortic fascia is lifted off the aorta. This can then be grasped with a Babcock clamp and the sutures simply placed through the preaortic fascia. This is a much simpler and safer approach than dissecting out the celiac artery. This technique was described by Vansant (Fig. 9–14) and is used by us quite frequently. In passing the finger behind the preaortic fascia, care must be taken not to damage short branches that pass from the aorta to the crura. By staying in the midline, these branches are avoided. If a branch of the celiac or the aorta is avulsed, brisk bleeding may occur. This may be dealt with simply by gentle pressure with a finger, exposure of the branch, and ligation with a vascular suture.

The crura of the esophageal hiatus are loosely approximated behind the esophagus with nonabsorbable sutures. The crura are closed so that a finger can be placed alongside the esophagus, making certain that the closure is not too tight.

The stomach is then rotated in a clockwise direction to expose the posterior part of the stomach, thereby clearly displaying the anterior and posterior bundles of tissue that previously held the GE junction in the diaphragm. The bundles now clearly demonstrated are grasped with special Babcock clamps well above the left gastric artery, taking care not to traumatize the vagal nerves. Strong, nonabsorbable sutures, either O silk or O synthetic material, are used for the repair. Usually five sutures are placed in the anterior and posterior phrenoesophageal bundles and carried through the preaortic fascia (Fig. 9–15). These sutures are placed with the vagus nerve in full view in order not to damage the vagus nerve. A single knot is then placed in the top three sutures which are then clamped with long hemostats. A measurement of the barrier pressure is then obtained by passing the side hole of the modified nasogastric tube through the GE junction (Fig. 9–16). If the pressure is above 55 mm Hg, the sutures are loosened. If it is below 30 mm Hg, the sutures are tightened, depending on the problem at hand. After the proper pressure is obtained, all five sutures are tied and a final pressure measurement is taken. The barrier is about 3 to 4 cm long. Figure 9–17 shows the final appearance of the repair. In addition to restoring the sphincter, the valve of His is accentuated by this procedure and can be readily palpated through the wall of the stomach. The valve measures from 1.5 to 4 cm and is important in prevention of reflux. The valve is readily demonstrated by postoperative upper gastrointestinal x-ray series (Fig. 9–18). In patients who have had previous operations with scarring and destruction of the GE junction, the valve may be destroyed or inadequate. In these cases, a gastrotomy is performed and the valve is secured with sutures in the anterior and posterior edges of the valve, thereby lengthening the valve to 3 to 4 cm.[19]

Attempts to calibrate the cardia with a bougie are unsatisfactory. It is difficult to determine whether the wrap around the bougie is tight or loose.

■ *Intraoperative Manometry*

In 1977 our group first reported the use of a simplified method of measuring the pressure in the GE junction during operation to yield an objective determination of whether an adequate barrier had

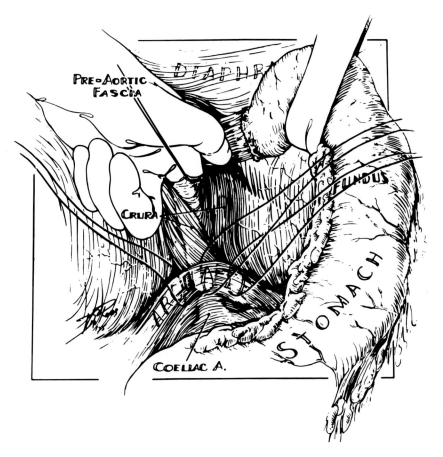

Figure 9–14. A safe approach to the preaortic fascia includes exposure of the esophageal hiatus, division of the fibroareolar tissue over the aorta and the passage of a finger down behind the preaortic fascia. By lifting the fascia off the aorta, sutures simply can be placed in the preaortic fascia or the ligament without dissecting out the median arcuate ligament.

been created.[20] This measurement is obtained by simply modifying the nasogastric tube which is routinely used in these patients. The tip of the smaller Silastic sump portion of the tube is sealed at the end and a 1 mm side hole is cut 12 cm from the tip of the tube (Fig. 9–19). This small Silastic tube (ID 1.2 mm) is attached to a strain gauge and to a manometer that produces a digital reading (Fig. 9–20) as well as tracing that can be viewed by the surgeon. The tube is constantly perfused at a slow rate (0.7 ml/min). This apparatus is identical to the one that has been used in the gastric laboratory for over a decade and has been thoroughly standardized and used on over 15,000 patients at our institution. The side hole is passed across the GE junction at operation, and a baseline pressure is obtained prior to repair. Often there is no pressure whatever in the GE junction. As the side hole passes through the junction, both a tracing and a digital readout are otained. If the pressure is over 55 mm Hg, the sutures which have been placed are loosened. If the pressure is less than 30 mm

Hg, the sutures are tightened. This process is continued until a pressure somewhere between 35 and 45 mm Hg is obtained. The one variable that renders the procedure somewhat difficult is the rate at which the side hole is passed through the GE junction. If it is pulled through too rapidly, a peak pressure may be missed. It should be drawn continuously and slowly through the GE junction to give a valid pressure measurement. With the demonstration of a pressure gradient across the GE valve it is apparent that the measurement obtained at the GE junction is a composite pressure including the sphincter and the valve.

The nasogastric tube which has been used to obtain intraoperative pressures is left in place. On the third or fourth postoperative day, the nasogastric tube is removed. As it is pulled out, the Silastic tube is again attached to the manometer, and a pullout pressure is obtained. This is usually a little less than half of the intraoperative pressure. A barrier pressure of 45 mm Hg at operation generally produces a pressure of 18 to 22 mm Hg postop-

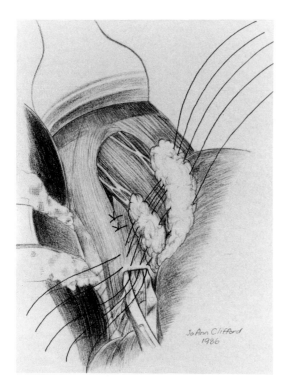

Figure 9–15. The anterior and posterior phrenoesophageal bundles have been demonstrated, and heavy, nonabsorbable sutures are passed through the bundles and the preaortic fascia and median arcuate ligament.

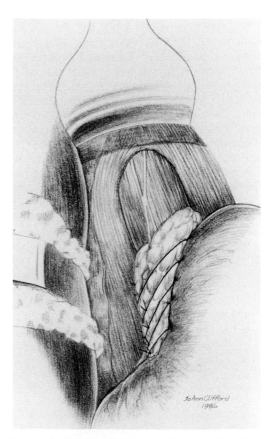

Figure 9–17. The final appearance of the repair. The phrenoesophageal bundles are anchored securely to the preaortic fascia and the median arcuate ligament. The gastroesophageal valve has been accentuated with tension on the collar sling musculature. The vagus nerves have been preserved.

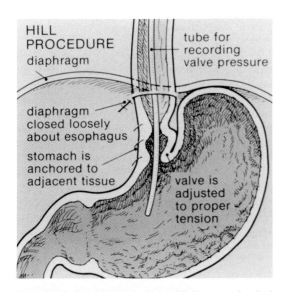

HILL PROCEDURE
diaphragm
tube for recording valve pressure
diaphragm closed loosely about esophagus
stomach is anchored to adjacent tissue
valve is adjusted to proper tension

Figure 9–16. The side hole in the modified nasogastric tube is 12 cm from the tip. The side hole is passed through the sphincter to obtain a sphincter pressure at the time of surgery. The sphincter and the valve are adjusted according to the sphincter pressure obtained until the right level of the LESP is achieved.

eratively. The concept of intraoperative manometry has been debated, but the need for an objective intraoperative method of quality control is obvious. It is worth emphasizing that the preservation of the GE sphincter and restoration of the valve not only produces a barrier to reflux but preserves the unique qualities of the GE junction that have been enumerated in this chapter.

As we will discuss in a subsequent chapter on repair of recurrent hernias, there is no doubt that intraoperative pressure measurement could avoid some of the disastrous complications of the Nissen procedure occurring when the wrap is either too loose to too tight. Further efforts to simplify intraoperative manometrics and to make the technique more readily available are under way. The present technique is safe and simple and requires only a few minutes to obtain valuable information. It is our opinion that in a major antireflux operation so dependent on construction of an adequate barrier, intraoperative assessment of the barrier should become a standard part of any technique that is used.

It is important to point out that the posterior gastropexy is not a fundoplication. The phrenoesophageal bundles are imbricated together and there is actually no wrap of stomach around the lower esophagus. Very often this operation is erroneously described as partial fundoplication or wrap. There is no intention on the part of the authors of this procedure to do a blind wraparound of stomach but rather a careful calibration of the antireflux barrier, restoration of the GE valve, and posterior fixation of the gastroesophageal junction. The basic differences between the gastroesophageal restoration repair and the Nissen repair are as follows:

1. The Hill procedure depends on augmentation of the intrinsic sphincter and its special features. By placing tension on the collar-sling musculature,

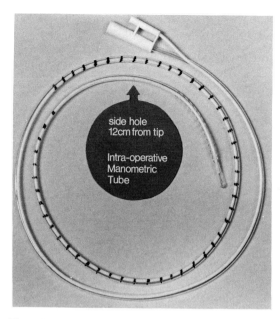

Figure 9–19. The nasogastric tube used for intraoperative manometrics is altered by sealing the tip and punching a side hole through the sump portion of the tube 12 cm from the tip. The tube is then identical to that used in the gastric laboratory in over 15,000 patients.

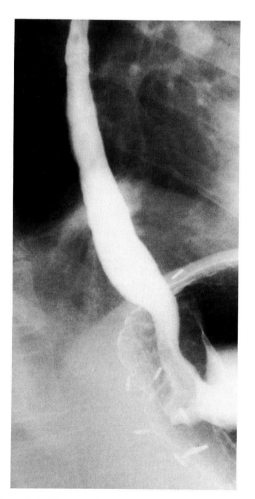

Figure 9–18. Postoperative upper gastrointestinal series shows the appearance of the repair. An intra-abdominal segment of esophagus can be seen, and the gastroesophageal valve has been lengthened and accentuated. The valve closes against the lesser curvature and assists the sphincter in preventing reflux.

the repair automatically accentuates the valve of His, which has now been shown to be important in the prevention of reflux. The Nissen repair, on the other hand, depends on extrinsic pressure of a wrap of stomach around the lower esophagus with indirect pressure on the lower esophagus.

2. The Hill procedure anchors the gastroesophageal junction posteriorly to its normal primary attachment—the preaortic fascia. The Nissen repair is allowed to float freely, and the gastroesophageal junction is not anchored. The unanchored esophagus has no fulcrum from which to operate and very frequently develops a dysmotility.

3. In the Hill procedure no sutures into the esophagus are used because the esophagus has no serosa and no strength. The Nissen procedure employs esophageal sutures to hold the wrap in place. The weakness of these sutures accounts for the frequency of the slipped Nissen. If these sutures are taken deeply, there is a risk of fistula formation.

4. In the Hill procedure intraoperative manometry is used to calibrate the barrier created at operation, giving an objective assessment of the competence of the reflux barrier. In the Nissen procedure the surgeon either relies on a finger or on a bougie and there is no way to tell how tight or how loose the wrap is around these objects.

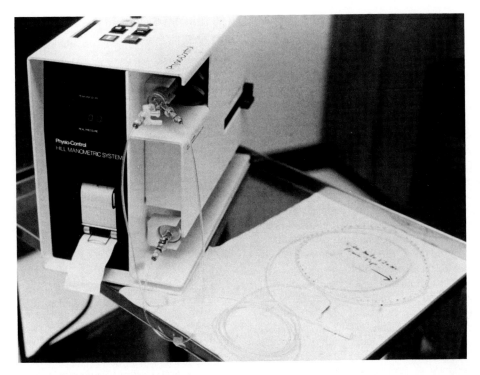

Figure 9–20. The intraoperative pressure tube is attached to a transducer, which in turn is attached to a monitor that displays both a digital readout as well as a tracing to the surgeon during operation.

■ Results of Surgical Therapy

■ PERSONAL EXPERIENCE

The most important criterion of success is patient satisfaction. If a patient is free of heartburn, can eat a full meal, and can resume normal activity including bending over in the garden and indulging in strenuous exercise without reflux or heartburn, then the operation should be considered a success. On the other hand, we have been particularly meticulous in our follow-up using pH and pressure studies two to three months after surgery whenever possible. In those patients who refuse pH and pressure studies we obtain a GI tract x-ray or scintiscan to test the effectiveness of the operation designed to curtail reflux.

Three major retrospective studies of the long-term effect of surgical treatment with the Hill repair have been performed by us in more than 1500 patients out of 1860 patients operated upon over a 24-year period. The results are summarized as follows: excellent or good results have been obtained in over 95 per cent with a failure and recurrence rate of 1.5 to 5 per cent. The complication and mortality rates have been very low, 0.2 per cent, with one death in the last 500 operations for primary repairs. In 299 operations for failed antireflux procedure, the mortality rate has been 1.7 per cent,

and for strictures it was 0.5 per cent. A complication of the Hill repair has been dysphagia, usually transient and present in 5 to 20 per cent of patients. Less than 5 per cent of patients have required dilatation. In one of our series, 48 per cent had dysphagia before surgery, compared to about 20 per cent postoperatively. It should be emphasized that the majority of those patients had no reflux and tolerated this new situation without dilatation. Whether postoperative dysphagia is due to persistent motility disorders encountered preoperatively in 41 per cent of patients has not yet been evaluated. In over 1800 operations we have had brisk bleeding from branches from the aorta or celiac artery in only eight instances. Ligation of these vessels has produced no discernible complications. In one series 28 per cent of our patients had pulmonary symptoms before surgery, and 6 per cent had symptoms postoperatively. There have been four fistulas from the esophagus. Two of these were treated with drainage and expired. These treated early in our experience before Celestin tubes were available. Two were treated with insertion of Celestin tube and survived. Only one fistula occurred in a primary repair. We have not encountered the devastating gastrobronchial, gastroaortic, gastropericardial, and gastrocutaneous fistulas that we have seen with the Nissen procedure.

■ REPRODUCIBILITY

Evaluation of the median arcuate repair by others than the author is important. For an operation to be of value, it should be reproducible in other hands. The median arcuate repair has been performed and reported by a number of surgeons, including Hermreck and Coates,[21] Csendes and Larrain,[22] Thomas et al.,[23] Vansant et al.,[24] and more recently by Warshaw and Ottinger[25,26] of Massachusetts General Hospital. The report by Thomas et al. is important in that the 79 patients operated on were poor risk patients and included a number of chronic alcoholics. Early in their experience, they found persistent herniation in eight patients who were improved symptomatically. With further experience with the technique, Thomas and coworkers had no recurrent herniation in 79 patients over two and one-half years. Howard and Wertheimer reported an experience with 12 patients followed up to three and one-half years with no recurrence. Vansant, et al., have reported treating up to 400 patients with excellent results. Warshaw states that the posterior gastropexy has become the preferred method of surgically treating GE reflux and hiatal hernia at Massachusetts General Hospital. Csendes and Larrain in Santiago, Chile likewise state that the results at their institution have been good with the posterior gastropexy. With extensive preoperative and postoperative testing with pH and pressure studies, Csendes and Larrain achieved a 93 per cent good result and no radiologic recurrence of hiatal hernia in 29 patients followed up to 16 months. The complications of slippage, fistula, and other serious problems that are seen with the Nissen operation have not been reported in any series using the Hill repair.

■ *Summary*

In summary, posterior fixation and barrier restoration (Hill operation) restores the normal posterior fixation of the GE junction. This restores the esophagus to its normal point of attachment or fulcrum, allowing it to generate forceful peristaltic waves to propel food aborally into the stomach. The sphincter is calibrated and the pressure measured so that a range of pressures is created that is high enough to prevent reflux, but not so high as to create dysphagia. The acute angle of His is accentuated by stress on the collar-sling musculature which restores the GE valve. In addition, the diaphragm is closed loosely about the esophagus which prevents herniation of the fundus into the mediastinum and also supports the GE junction.

The mortality and morbidity rates are low, and the operation is reproducible in other hands with good results.

■ REFERENCES

1. Bright K: Account of a remarkable misplacement of the stomach. Guys Hosp Rep, *1*:598, 1836.
2. Bowditch HI: Treatise on Diaphragmatic Hernia. Buffalo, T. Jewett & Co., 1853.
3. Scudder CL: A case of nontraumatic diaphragmatic hernia operation and recovery. Trans Am Surg Assn, 428–439, 1912.
4. Allison PR: Reflux esophagitis, sliding hiatal hernia, and the anatomy of repair. Surg Gynecol Obstet, *92*:419, 1951.
5. Nissen R: Gastropexy as the lone procedure in the surgical repair of hiatus hernia. Am J Surg, *92*:389–392, 1956.
6. Skinner DB, Belsey RHR: Surgical management of esophageal reflux and hiatus hernia. J Thorac Cardiovasc Surg, *53*:33–54, 1967.
7. Toupet A: Technique d'eosophago-gastroplastie avec phreno gastropexie appliquee dans la cure radicale des hernies hiatales et comme complement de l'operation de Heller dans les cardiospasmes. Acad Chir, 394–399, 1963.
8. Hill D: An effective operation for hiatal hernia: An eight year appraisal. Ann Surg, *166*:681–692, 1957.
9. Fyke RE, Code CF, Schlegel JF: The GE sphincter in healthy human beings. Gastroenterologia, *86*:135–150, 1956.
10. Hill LD, Chapman KW, Morgan EH: Objective evaluation of surgery for hiatus hernia and esophagitis. J Thorac Cardiovasc Surg, *41*:60, 1961.
11. Christensen J, Conklin JL: Studies of the origin of the distinctive mechanics of smooth muscle at the esophago-gastric junction. Proceedings of the Fourth International Symposium on Gastrointestinal Motility, Banff, Alberta, September 6–8, 1973, pp 63–71.
12. Barrett NR: Hiatus hernia—a review of some controversial points. Br J Surg, *42*:231, 1954.
13. Collis JL, Kelly TS, Wiley AM: Anatomy of the crura of the diaphragm and the surgery of hiatus hernia. Thorax, *9*:175, 1954.
14. Butterfield WC: Current hiatal hernia repairs: Similarities, mechanisms, and extended indications: An autopsy study. Surgery, *69*:91, 1971.
15. Thor K, Hill LD, Mercer CD, Kozarek RA: Reappraisal of the flap valve mechanism: A study of a new valvuloplasty procedure in cadavers. Acta Chir Scand, *153*:25–28, 1987.
16. Pope CE: Pathophysiology and diagnosis of reflux esophagitis. Gastroenterology, *70*:445–454, 1976.
17. Russell COH, Hill LD, Holmes ER, et al: Radionuclide transit: A sensitive screening test for esophageal dysfunction. Gastroenterology, *80*:887–892, 1981.
18. Hiebert C, Belsey R: Incompetency of the gastric cardia without radiologic evidence of hiatus hernia. J Thorac Cardiovasc Surg, *42*:352, 1961.
19. Thor K, Kozarek RA, Mercer CD, Hill LD: Valvuloplasty: A new surgical procedure. Gastroenterology, *90*:5, 1986.
20. Hill LD: Intraoperative management of lower esophageal sphincter pressure. J Thorac Cardiovasc Surg, *75*:378–381, 1978.
21. Hermreck AS, Coates NR: Results of the Hill antireflux operation. Am J Surg, *140*:764–767, 1980.
22. Csendes A, Larrain A: Effect of posterior gastropexy on GE sphincter pressure and symptomatic reflux in patients with hiatal hernia. Gastroenterology, *63*:19–24, 1972.
23. Thomas AN, Hall AD, Haddad JK: Posterior gastropexy:

Selection and management in patients with symptomatic hiatal hernia. Am J Surg, *126*:148–156, 1973.

24. Vansant JH, Baker JW, Ross DG: Modification of the Hill technique for repair of hiatal hernia. Surg Gynecol Obstet, *143*:637–642, 1976.

25. Warshaw AL: Simplified isolation of the median arcuate ligament for posterior gastropexy. Surg Gynecol Obstet, *154*:733, 1982.

26. Ottinger LW: Transabdominal hiatal herniorrhaphy with median arcuate ligament repair. *In* Malt RA (Ed): Surgical Techniques Illustrated. Boston, Little, Brown & Co., 1976.

MARK IV ANTIREFLUX PROCEDURE

The designation Mark IV was coined to indicate that the final technique emerged as the result of a series of clinical trials of various techniques intended to restore a competent valvular mechanism to the cardia. The fourth and final variant was applied initially in 1952 and has been employed routinely since that time.

■ Specific Preoperative Preparation

When the esophagitis is confined to grades I and II, and when the patient has been on routine medical treatment, in the absence of pulmonary complications, surgical correction can proceed without delay. In cases complicated by more severe esophagitis grades III and IV with dysphagia, an intensive preoperative course of medical therapy may influence significantly the operative program. A history of aspiration pneumonitis or signs indicative of resulting lung damage call for an intensive course of thoracic physiotherapy to reduce the risk of postoperative complications.

A reflux-induced stricture consists of three components: (1) transmural fibrosis from collagen deposition, (2) chronic inflammatory edema and hyperemia associated with the more superficial mucosal ulceration (extensive nonspecific periesophageal lymphadenitis may also be present), (3) muscle spasm in response to the acute inflammatory element. The second and third factors may contribute significantly to the radiologic and endoscopic appearances of a "stricture" and can be reversible.

An intensive course of preoperative medical therapy may reduce the edema and spasm and convert a case in which resection and reconstruction appear inevitable to a simpler therapeutic problem where an antireflux procedure, augmented by dilatation, will prove adequate.

■ Principle of the Mark IV Antireflux Procedure

The basic principle of the Mark IV repair is the restoration of 4 to 5 cm of the lower sphincter zone of the esophagus to the high-pressure region below the diaphragm (Fig. 9–21). The 4 to 5 cm length emerged from three considerations. First, the extent of the sphincter zone cannot be determined with accuracy. Second, the lower esophageal sphincter may play a significant role in the prevention of reflux in the normal subject but once divorced from its relationship to the hiatus, and contending with the negative intrathoracic pressure, it frequently fails to resist the pressure gradient between the stomach and intrathoracic esophagus. Third, this principle emerged during the clinical trials of various techniques and their postoperative assessment.

■ Technique of the Mark IV Repair

Anesthesia ■ Double lumen tracheal intubation is not necessary. A completely atelectatic lung on the side of the thoracotomy is mobile and flaccid and difficult to displace with retractors. A partially inflated lung is easier to control.

Position on the Table ■ The Mark IV antireflux procedure is performed through a left sixth interspace thoracotomy with the patient in the full right lateral position. The patient's spine is maintained in a true horizontal position. The use of a mechanical bridge to open up the thoracotomy incision may cause persistent postoperative back pain and should be avoided.

Mobilization of the Esophagus ■ The mediastinal pleura is incised vertically from diaphragm to aorta. The esophagus is mobilized from the mediastinum in the plane adjacent to the surrounding

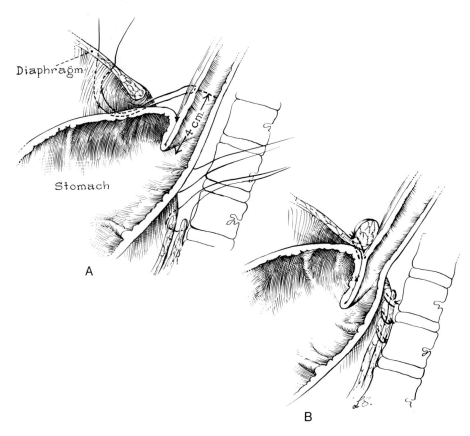

Figure 9–21. *A,* Principle of the Mark IV procedure. *B,* Following reduction. Note the intra-abdominal segment and posterior buttress.

anatomic structures. This technique will minimize the risk of damage to the vagus nerves during the mobilization. Great care is taken to avoid opening the right pleura in order to avoid the unseen accumulation of blood in the right cavity.

Mobilization will involve division of the "middle esophageal artery," a constant vessel running from the descending aorta to the midpoint of the infra-aortic segment of the esophagus. Failure to divide this vessel will result in inadequate mobilization, which is a cause of failure of the Mark IV technique in the hands of the less experienced surgeon. Care is taken to avoid trauma to the vagi. The left vagus is clearly visible during the mobilization; contact with the right vagus can be maintained by palpation on the deeper surface of the organ during the mobilization. Division of the inferior bronchial artery may also be necessary.

Adequate mobilization of the esophagus and cardia is the single most important step in the Mark IV technique and can be achieved only by the thoracic route.

After the proximal mobilization to the aortic arch is complete, the dissection is carried caudally. The

vagus nerves are left in place on the esophagus. Posteriorly, the dissection is carried down to the right crus of the diaphragm.

Mobilization of the Cardia ■ The mobilization of the cardia is commenced anteriorly by the transverse division of the pleural reflection as it passes from the muscular ring of the hiatus to the mediastinum. Upward traction on the esophagus by the encircling tape places tension on the phreno-esophageal membrane to reveal its insertion into the muscular wall of the esophagus. The membrane is divided transversely at right angles to the long axis of the esophagus. The next plane to be entered, the extraperitoneal plane, is identified by the appearance of extraperitoneal fat. The transverse incision of this fatty layer, and further upward traction, will enable the peritoneum to be divided transversely around the anterior aspect of the cardia.

The division of the peritoneal reflection and endoabdominal fascia is continued laterally until the short gastric vessels appear. Division of the upper one or two vessels may be necessary. To the medial side the division is continued until the left lobe of

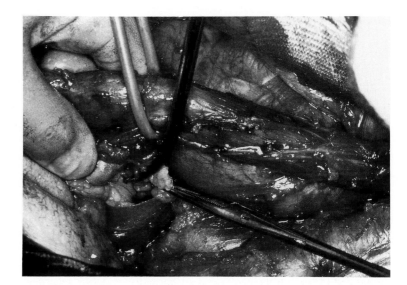

Figure 9–22. Mobilization of the esophagus. The upper gastrohepatic omental band, containing Belsey's artery, is doubly clamped.

the liver appears. The cardia is firmly bound to the posterior abdominal wall and crura by a thick band of tissue, a condensation of the upper limit of the gastrohepatic omentum. This band contains an important vessel known as ''Belsey's artery.''

Accidental division of the band will result in troublesome hemorrhage. To identify this vessel, an index finger is passed downward and medially into the greater sac of the peritoneal cavity to identify the gastrohepatic omentum. The finger then curves posteriorly through the gastrohepatic omentum, which offers little resistance, at a point between the palpable left gastric artery and Belsey's artery in the upper thickened band of the omentum, into the lesser sac, and then upward and laterally behind the cardia. The peritoneum of the lesser sac can be divided onto the exploring finger in the space

between the two halves of the right crus (Fig. 9–22). The band can now be divided between clamps, and a double ligature is placed round the proximal end for greater security. Division of the band and contained vessel results in a dramatic improvement in the mobilization of the cardia (Fig. 9–23).

Another common error is to attempt to identify ''Balsey's artery'' from above. Downward dissection along the posterior aspect of the cardia will enter the plane deep to the visceral peritoneum on the posterior aspect of the stomach and may result in perforation of that organ.

Removal of the Fat Pad ■ The mobilization of the cardia having been completed, the fundus of the stomach is now drawn up into the thorax through the hiatus. The next step is the removal of

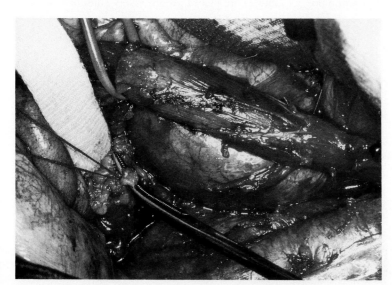

Figure 9–23. Belsey's artery divided. Proximal end doubly ligated. Note improved mobilization of the cardia.

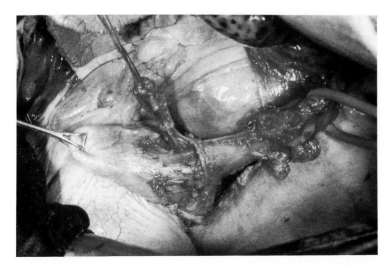

Figure 9–24. Removal of the fat pad. Note lymphenitis due to reflux esophagitis.

the fat pad in front of the cardia and all fibrofatty tissue from the anterior aspect of the esophagus (Fig. 9–24). During the clearing of the anterior aspect of the esophagus, the two vagus nerves are mobilized from the muscle layer in continuity and allowed to drop back posteriorly behind the esophagus. Inadvertent damage to both vagus nerves during the mobilization, which can occur when the local anatomy has been disorganized by previous surgical attempts to control the reflux, will render advisable the extension of the thoracotomy anteriorly, separation of the diaphragm from its origin to the chest wall, and a pyloromyotomy to prevent gastric stasis (Fig. 9–25).

Preparation of the Posterior Buttress ■ Once the mobilization of the esophagus and the cardia has been completed, the posterior buttress can be prepared. The posterior buttress is created by the approximation of the two halves of the right crus. Failure to maintain this buttress will permit a pos-

terior recurrence. Narrowing the hiatus as such plays no significant role in the control of reflux in the context of this technique.

With forward traction on the central tendon of the diaphragm near its medial margin applied by a powerful tissue forceps, the tendinous core of the inner limb of the right crus is tensed into greater prominence as an easily palpable dense band of tissue. The tension on the central tendon will also elevate the inner limb of the right crus off the inferior vena cava. Starting posteriorly near the aorta, strong interrupted sutures of 0 linen thread or silk, preferably on atraumatic needles, are passed through the tensed tendinous core of the inner limb and through the superficial margin of the outer limb, including the firmly adherent overlying pleura. A common mistake is to pass this stitch through the weak intercrural muscle fibers which will not hold sutures. Two or three additional sutures are placed progressively anteriorly at 1 cm

Figure 9–25. Fat pad excised. Mobilization of the vagi for posterior displacement.

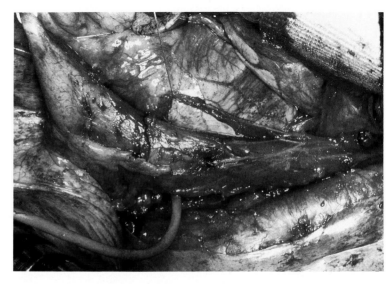

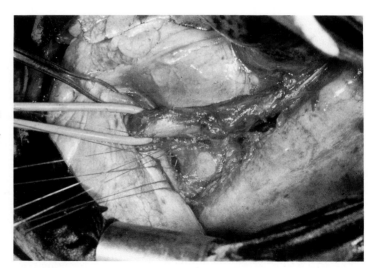

Figure 9–26. Posterior buttressing sutures inserted into the two limbs of the right crus. Note tension applied to the central tendon of the diaphragm.

intervals. An average Mark IV repair requires three such sutures (Fig. 9–26). These sutures are left in place and tied later when the fundoplication has been completed and restored to the abdomen.

The 240-Degree Fundoplication ▪ With the fundus drawn up into the thorax through the hiatus, the 240-degree fundoplication is now created. A 2-0 linen or silk suture on a fine curved atraumatic needle is passed vertically through the seromuscular layer of the stomach about 2 cm below the esophagogastric junction, at the level of the original peritoneal reflection now divided, then vertically through the muscle layer of the esophagus 2 cm above the junction well lateral to the midline of the esophagus. The suture is then reversed and passed down through the muscle layer of the esophagus in the opposite direction 3 to 4 mm nearer the midline of the esophagus and then through the seromuscular layer of the stomach 1 cm medial to the

original point of entry of the stitch (Fig. 9–27). This stitch must not perforate either the gastric or esophageal mucosa.

When the wall is thickened by fibrosis resulting from chronic esophagitis, a deeper bite and more secure grip on the wall of the esophagus can be taken. Protection of the mucosa is enhanced by upward displacement of the esophagogastric junction manually, thus shortening the organ and bunching up the muscle layer off the underlying mucosa. Three mattress sutures are placed in the first row of the fundoplication. The second suture is placed in the midline, and the third is placed medially, nearer the right vagus. The ends of these sutures are shortened independently to prevent a loop of the suture from sawing through the brittle esophageal muscle, and tied very gently to achieve tissue apposition without tissue strangulation. The placement of these sutures is such that when tied

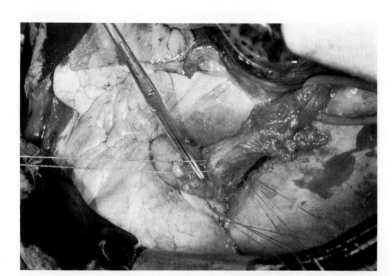

Figure 9–27. Insertion of first row of fundoplicating mattress sutures.

they achieve a 240-degree fundic wrap around the lower 2 cm of esophagus (Fig. 9–28).

The second row of three mattress sutures is first passed through the diaphragm at the point where the central tendon fuses with the muscular ring of the hiatus. With the help of a spoon retractor inserted through the hiatus to protect the abdominal viscera, the suture is passed from above downward through the diaphragm into the bowl of the spoon, then up and out through the hiatus (Fig. 9–29). The further passage of this suture through the wall of the stomach and the muscle layer of the esophagus follows the same pattern as in the first row but is placed 2 cm lower in the stomach and 2 cm higher on the esophagus. Again, with the help of the spoon retractor, the suture is finally passed down through the hiatus and up through the edge of the central tendon 1 cm medial to the original point of the entry. Three sutures are placed in the second row in corresponding locations to those in the first row, to embrace 240 degrees of the circumference of the hiatus and esophagus (Fig. 9–30). They are not tied until after reduction of the hernia. Larger rather than smaller bites of the muscle will ensure a more lasting hold on this layer and discourage any recurrence. The correct placement of these fundoplicating sutures is critical to the success of the operative technique.

Reduction of the Reconstructed Cardia ■ The reconstructed cardia is returned to the abdomen through the hiatus and tucked forward below the diaphragm manually and not by traction on the second row of the fundoplication sutures. With adequate mobilization of the esophagus and cardia, the fundoplication should lie below the hiatus without tension and with no tendency to retract back into the thorax. Once the hernia has been reduced, the ends of the second fundoplicating row are now

shortened independently, again to avoid damage to the esophageal muscle, and to "snuggle" the reconstructed cardia up against the undersurface of the diaphragm. The second row of sutures is again tied very gently. When the technique is correctly performed, there should now be 4 cm of the sphincter zone of the lower esophagus, partially embraced by the fundic wrap, in the high pressure region below the diaphragm and a further 1 cm surrounded by the muscle ring of the hiatus and the two limbs of the right crus when approximated.

Creating the Posterior Buttress ■ The posterior buttressing sutures passed earlier through the two limbs of the right crus are now tied from behind forward to approximate the two limbs. The first throw of the final suture knot is tied and the resulting size of the hiatus assessed for adequacy by digital exploration (Fig. 9–31). If there is no constriction of the esophagus, the knot is completed. When the buttress has been completed, it should be possible easily to pass an index finger through the triangular hiatus posterior to the esophagus (Fig. 9–32). If the finger cannot be passed easily, the final approximating suture should be cut out. It is better to leave the hiatus too loose rather than too tight as mechanical constriction of the lower esophagus plays no part in the control of reflux in this procedure (Fig. 9–33).

Closure ■ The mediastinal pleura is not repaired as residual collections of blood or serum are easier to drain from the pleural cavity than from the mediastinum. A single intercostal catheter is entered in the midaxillary line and positioned with the tip high in the pleural cavity in the paravertebral gutter. No nasogastric tube has been used routinely as the 240-degree fundoplication does not cause the gas bloat syndrome. Should intubation be necessary

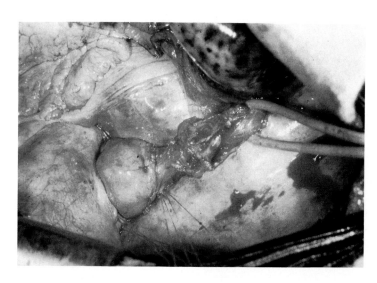

Figure 9–28. First row of three fundoplicating sutures completed. Buttress sutures remain untied.

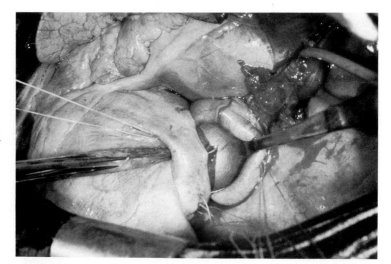

Figure 9–29. Commencement of second fundoplicating layer. First suture passed through diaphragm with help of spoon retractor.

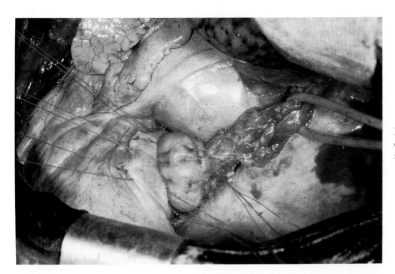

Figure 9–30. Second row of fundoplicating mattress sutures completed. Note spacing of sutures.

Figure 9–31. Hernia reduced manually. Fundoplicating sutures tied. Size of hiatus being checked before last buttressing suture is tied.

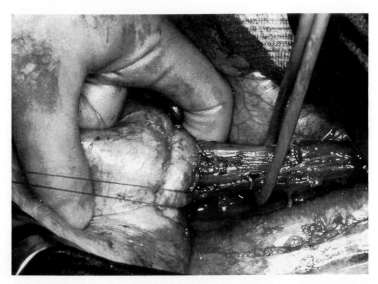

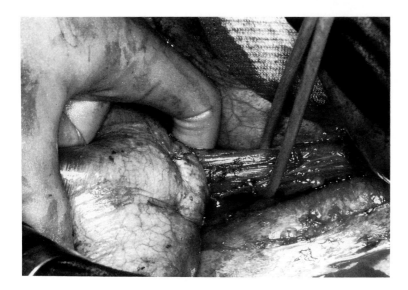

Figure 9–32. Hiatus again checked for excessive constriction after final buttress suture is tied.

later for a specific indication, it can be passed easily through the reconstructed cardia without risk.

The thoracotomy incision is closed with due attention to those steps in the technique designed to minimize post-thoracotomy pain. To recapitulate, the steps in thoracotomy technique designed to minimize postoperative discomfort are as follows:

1. A high thoracotomy, never lower than the sixth interspace.

2. If the posterior end of the seventh rib is divided and 1 cm resected, the seventh neurovascular bundle must be ligated and divided before insertion of the rib spreaders to prevent traction injury to the posterior nerve roots.

3. Aggressive separation of the ribs must be avoided; manual separation of the ribs sufficient only to permit the entry of one hand is maintained by simple spreaders incorporating no mechanical assistance.

4. During closure the sixth and seventh ribs are restored to their original relationship with pericostal sutures to prevent subsequent lung herniation; close approximation of the ribs is a common cause of postoperative pain.

5. Avoidance of sutures in the sensitive intercostal tissues; with correct placement of the drainage catheter no chest wall emphysema will occur.

6. A catheter inserted in the midaxillary line will cause less discomfort than one placed posteriorly.

The intercostal catheter is attached to an underwater seal in the operating room to encourage rapid re-expansion of the lung.

■ Postoperative Care

A chest x-ray is taken in the recovery room to ascertain that the intercostal catheter is correctly

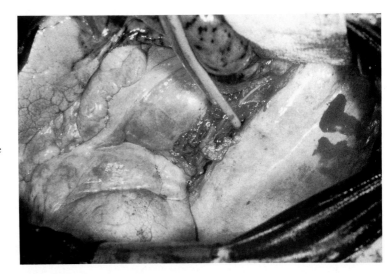

Figure 9–33. The antireflux procedure completed.

positioned, that the lung is re-expanding, and that there is no fluid accumulation in either pleural cavity. Thoracic physiotherapy is commenced as soon as the patient regains consciousness. It is important to explain to the patient that although it will hurt to cough for the first few postoperative days, it will not do any harm. Patients frequently suppress the cough mechanism voluntarily from fear of bursting sutures or promoting complications. Sedation is kept to a minimum to avoid depression of the cough reflex.

Broad-spectrum antibiotic therapy is maintained for the first five postoperative days. The intercostal catheter may be removed at the end of 48 hours or when the drainage of serum falls below 200 ml in the 24-hour period. Sips of clear fluid are permitted on the first postoperative day. The patient is rapidly restored to a semisolid diet. Ice cream is readily accepted by the patient following esophageal surgery. A significant advantage of the thoracic route for antireflux surgery is the avoidance of any trauma to the small intestine and the rapid return of normal peristalsis.

Ambulation is commenced on the evening of the operation or the following morning. While in bed, the patient is nursed with the legs raised to maintain venous drainage. If ulcerative esophagitis was present prior to the operation, antacids are prescribed for the first postoperative month. A postoperative barium swallow study is undertaken to determine that the procedure was correctly performed, to exclude any suture problems in the repair, and to form a basis for comparison with subsequent barium studies.

▪ Postoperative Complications

The general complications are those that may follow any major thoracic surgical procedure, such as wound infection due to operative contamination, cardiovascular accidents, cerebral vascular accidents, deep vein thrombosis, pulmonary embolism, temporary urinary obstruction, various problems arising from the drips, and canulations.

Postoperative Morbidity and Mortality ▪ In an earlier report on a consecutive series of 632 Mark IV procedures, there were eight hospital deaths (1.3 per cent), but only three (0.5 per cent) fatalities were attributable to the operative procedure. Nonfatal complications such as may follow any major surgical procedure were recorded in 5 per cent of the cases. Less than 1 per cent of the complications, including the three directly responsible for the death of the patient, were related to the type of operative procedure. There has been only one fatality in the last 1000 cases, in a patient operated upon in the Middle East.

Pulmonary Atelectasis ▪ Atelectasis of the right lower lobe is frequently observed in the early postoperative chest films. It may cause mild pyrexia but is rarely associated with any pulmonary embarrassment or symptoms. The explanation probably lies in the frequency with which patients with reflux demonstrate minor degrees of aspiration pneumonitis.

A full course of preoperative physiotherapy and a further postoperative course commencing in the recovery room immediately after the patient regains consciousness will reduce the incidence of this relatively minor complication or lead to rapid re-expansion of the atelectatic lobe.

Dysphagia ▪ When the Mark IV procedure has been correctly performed, the patient may experience mild dysphagia for the first postoperative week, resulting from tissue edema in the region of the reconstructed cardia. No treatment is necessary, as the dysphagia will resolve spontaneously. Dysphagia persisting for longer than a week indicates a technical error, the commonest being too aggressive narrowing of the hiatus during the creation of the posterior buttress.

Gas Bloat Syndrome ▪ In contrast to the complications following the 360-degree fundoplication, the ''gas bloat syndrome'' occurs rarely and only temporarily. Attempts to induce the syndrome by administering effervescent drinks have failed. The less aggressive 240-degree fundoplication permits voluntary belching and evacuation of gastric gas, an advantage appreciated by the patient. Any interference with voluntary evacuation indicates a too tight buttress and is avoidable.

Mucosal Perforation during the Fundoplication ▪ As a mucosal perforation due to too deep placement of the fundoplicating sutures in the wall of the esophagus is automatically repaired and supported by the fundic wrap, as in the Thal patch procedure, clinical evidence of a perforation is rarely encountered. Assuming due attention has been paid to dental toilet in the preoperative period, suppurative complications are exceptional. In the event of an operative breach of the esophageal mucosa during the performance of the procedure, this is likely to occur only during the mobilization of the esophagus in a case of recurrent reflux. The mucosa is closed with interrupted sutures of fine monofilament stainless steel wire. The operation is then continued and the suture line buttressed with the fundic wrap as in the standard Mark IV technique.

Intraperitoneal Complications ▪ Failure to secure the proximal end of Belsey's artery with a double ligature during the mobilization of the cardia can lead to intraperitoneal hemorrhage, which may require a laparotomy for its control. Prevention is the correct management.

Any tendency to acute dilatation of the stomach can be corrected by the gentle passage of a nasogastric tube.

Paralytic ileus is mentioned merely to stress its rarity. During an antireflux procedure performed by the thoracic route, the small bowel is rarely seen and is protected throughout from the trauma that precipitates paralysis.

Post-Thoracotomy Pain ■ The occurrence of post-thoracotomy pain persisting beyond the immediate postoperative period could be documented as a disadvantage of the thoracic approach. The incidence of this complication in the 632 patients subjected to a Mark IV repair[3] was 4 per cent. This incidence suggests that pain is preventable in the majority of cases.

■ Modifications of the Mark IV Technique

Application to Cases of Grade III and Grade IV Esophagitis ■ No modifications are introduced into the principle of the procedure. The more chronic and advanced stages of peptic esophagitis are complicated by acquired shortenings of the organ. Even with extensive mobilization of the esophagus up to the aortic arch, difficulty may be encountered in achieving the basic objective of restoring 4 to 5 cm of the sphincter zone to the infradiaphragmatic position. On the credit side, the thickening of the wall of the esophagus, in particular of the muscle layer, enables deeper, more secure bites to be obtained in this layer by the fundoplicating sutures, and some degree of tension on the repair is permissible. Patients with grade III or grade IV esophagitis are prepared for a colon interposition procedure with full bowel prep before being subjected to thoracotomy. The final decision may be made at thoracotomy.

Application to the Management of Type II or Paraesophageal Hernias ■ The large type II hernia has frequently been present since birth, and as a result the esophagus may be congenitally underdeveloped and shortened. An anatomic repair may leave the lower sphincter zone in the low pressure region above the diaphragm and will frequently result in the conversion of a type II hernia into a type I hernia with the immediate creation of reflux and its inherent complications. A formal antireflux procedure is therefore indicated routinely in this situation in addition to restoration of the gastric pouch to the abdomen.

Although most of the herniated stomach may have prolapsed into the right side of the chest, a formal left posterolateral sixth interspace thoracotomy is indicated. The vagus nerves may be displaced some distance away from the lower esophagus by the gastric pouch and are correspondingly more vulnerable to trauma. As much of the hernial sac as possible is resected. The Mark IV procedure is then continued as for the type I hernia. Some degree of tension may be apparent on completing the repair, but every effort should be made to restore an adequate length of the lower sphincter zone below the diaphragm. When the degree of developmental shortening is sufficiently marked to render a satisfactory repair without excessive tension technically impossible, a further alternative is a Collis gastroplasty combined with a Pearson modification of the Mark IV procedure. In the type II hernia the hiatus is frequently abnormally dilated. Up to six or more sutures may be necessary to create the posterior buttress.

Application to Infants and Children with Reflux ■ Infants and children with reflux, usually with complications, may be desperately ill from starvation and anemia and in urgent need of lifesaving surgical treatment. The Mark IV procedure performed through a left thoracotomy is applicable to this age group with no modification in basic technique. The choice of the thoracic approach, and preoperative preparation for a colon interposition procedure enables the final decision regarding the surgical program to be made at operation in the presence of grade III or grade IV peptic esophagitis.

Application to Cases of Recurrent Reflux ■ A transthoracic approach to the problem of recurrent hiatal herniation with reflux affords better exposure, enables the lower esophagus and cardia to be dissected free of the mediastinal adhesions with less risk of trauma to the esophagus, and also permits alternative procedures if a further antireflux operation is contraindicated by the extent of the fibrous adhesions and trauma caused by previous surgery or by acquired shortening of the esophagus secondary to chronic esophagitis.

The approach is the same as for the standard Mark IV procedure. Assuming that only one previous antireflux procedure has been attempted, it may be possible to mobilize the cardia through the hiatus as in the standard operation. Following multiple previous attempts, more extensive adhesions may be encountered. Mobilization may then be achieved with greater safety by extending the exposure to include the upper abdomen. The diaphragm is detached from its costal origin anteriorly and retracted upward. This will permit the mobilization of the cardia and gastric fundus from the diaphragm, liver, and spleen under direct vision and with greater safety. There should be no hesitation in extending the exposure to include the upper abdomen if difficulty is being encountered in the mobilization.

Preservation of the vagus nerves will call for special attention. If doubt arises concerning the integrity of the nerves, the diaphgram is opened in the manner described and a pyloromyotomy performed to prevent gastric stasis. Where the recurrence follows a previous attempt at a Mark IV repair, the partial fundoplication may have prolapsed up into the mediastinum intact. The middle esophageal artery may be found intact, indicating that the cause of the recurrence was inadequate mobilization at the previous operation. After complete mobilization it may be possible to preserve what remains of the wrap and then proceed with a second row of fundoplicating sutures and complete the repair. The recurrence may result from failure of the posterior buttress. The segment of lower esophagus restored to the subdiaphragmatic location may have rotated back up into the mediastinum posteriorly. It may then be necessary only to restore this segment to the intra-abdominal position and reconstruct the posterior buttress.

If the cause of the recurrence is obscure and the anatomy of the cardia confused by the previous surgery, the previous wrap is dismantled after full mobilization and the standard Mark IV technique proceeded with.

Recurrent reflux following multiple failed previous surgical attempts to control the reflux presents the surgeon with a formidable technical challenge.

The ultimate procedure will be resection of the scarred and disorganized cardia and replacement with an interposed isoperistaltic segment of the left colon or jejunum. The interposition, when correctly performed with an 8- to 10-cm segment of the transplant maintained in the high-pressure subdiaphragmatic region, has proved to be an effective reflux controlling mechanism. Patients undergoing further surgery for recurrent reflux should be fully prepared routinely prior to surgery for a colon transplant.

■ REFERENCES

1. Argov S, Goldstein I, Barzilai A: Is routine use of the nasogastric tube justified in upper abdominal surgery? Am J Surg, *139*:849, 1980.
2. Baue A: The Belsey Mark V antireflux procedure. Ann Thorac Surg, *29*:265, 1980.
3. Skinner D, Belsey R: Surgical management of esophageal reflux and hiatus hernia. Long term results with 1030 patients. J Thorac Cardiovasc Surg, *53*:33, 1967.
4. Skinner D, Belsey R, Hendrix T, et al: Gastroesophageal Reflux and Hiatal Hernia. Boston, Little, Brown and Co., 1972.
5. Skinner D, Belsey R: The Surgical Management of Gastroesophageal Reflux. Vol. 2. Surgical Communications, Inc.
6. Stipa S, Belsey R: La Chirurgia Dell'Esophago. Indicazioni e Techniche. Padova, Piccin Editore, 1980.
7. Hiatal Herniorrhaphy. Surgical Treatment Illustrated. Vol. 1. Boston, Little, Brown and Co., 1976.

NISSEN FUNDOPLICATION
Lucius D. Hill

The Nissen fundoplication was initially utilized by Rudolph Nissen in 1936 to protect his closure following the resection of a benign lesion of the cardia. When he reviewed this patient 16 years following the original procedure, Nissen was impressed with the lack of any evidence of esophagitis. He first used the procedure for the primary indication of reflux control in 1955, and published his initial results the following year.[1] Owing to widespread dissatisfaction with Allison repair, which was demonstrating recurrence rates as high as 50 per cent, the procedure was quickly adopted by a large number of surgeons.

■ *Technique*

The original procedure called for the mobilization of the lower 5 to 8 cm of esophagus through an upper midline incision. This includes taking down the gastrohepatic omentum including the hepatic branch of the vagus nerve. With the esophagus on tension with an encircling band, the gastrohepatic ligament is taken down. A large stomach tube is then passed down the esophagus with an accompanying Levine tube to prevent subsequent stenosis. The anterior and posterior walls of the fundus are then wrapped with the right hand to encircle the newly reduced portion of intra-abdominal esophagus. The posterior wall is grasped and stabilized with a Babcock clamp. The posterior wall of the fundus is brought to lie beside its anterior wall counterpart at approximately the level of the GE junction. These two serosal surfaces are then sutured together, starting as high on the esophagus as possible and including the esophagus in the first two stitches. Sutures are then placed 1 to 1.5 cm apart for a distance ranging from 3 to 4 cm. If the patient had previously been identified as an acid hypersecretor, a left truncal vagotomy was also added (Fig. 9–34).

Since its first description the procedure has undergone multiple modifications, both anatomic and technical, predominantly due to dissatisfaction with recurrence rates and complications. It is likely that many of the Nissen fundoplications done today have little in common with their 1956 predecessor.

■ Modifications

Many surgeons complement the fundoplication with a posterior plication of the diaphragmatic crura.[2-6] This is usually accomplished utilizing nonabsorbable sutures to narrow the hiatus to the point where one fingertip can still be inserted easily through the residual orifice, alongside the esophagus. The degree of gastric mobilization can vary from Nissen's original description, in which no

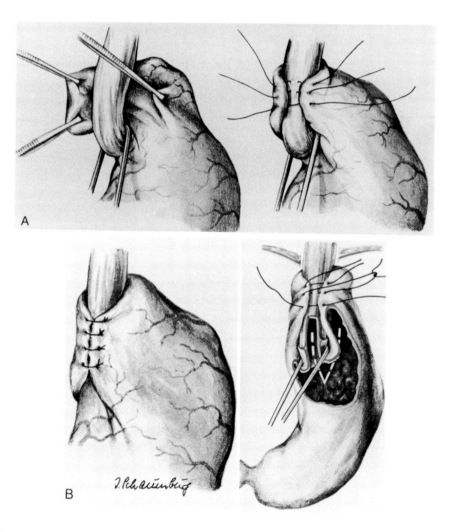

Figure 9–34. *A*, Diagram showing the basic technique of fundoplication. After freeing the peritoneal attachments, the cardia is drawn down in a caudal direction. The posterior wall is then drawn forward medially to the esophagus, thus effecting invagination of the terminal esophagus. *B*, Sutures are then placed 1 to 1.5 cm apart to close the wrap. It can be seen that the upper two sutures include bites of terminal esophagus as well as gastric serosa of the anterior and posterior walls of the cardia. (From Nissen R, Rosetti M: Surgery of the Cardia Ventriculi. Basel, CIBA Ltd., 1963, p 212.)

short gastric vessels are ligated, to the taking down of a portion,[7] or complete mobilization[8,9] of the vasa brevia. The recommendations for stenting the esophagus can vary anywhere from an 18 French nasogastric tube,[5] to a No. 50 mercury-filled bougie.[8]

Predominantly in response to recurrences and the postoperative problems of gas bloat, the fundoplication wrap itself has seen multiple suggested modifications. Nissen suggested a method of tightening the wrap in the very obese patient by using the anterior (rather than the posterior) fundic wall to wrap the intra-abdominal esophagus. This is now known as the Rosetti modification of the Nissen fundoplication[5,10] (Fig. 9–35). Other suggested revisions have included a double plication,[11] an incomplete wrap,[4,12,13] and a loose wrap,[8] or "floppy Nissen."[11] The length of the fundoplication has varied significantly from 6 cm[14] to studies in cadavers which suggested that 4 cm was required to avoid reflux.[15] More recently, animal laboratory studies have shown 2 to 3 cm to be adequate[16] in addition to DeMeester's recommendation of a 1.5 cm or "single stitch" Nissen.[17]

In attempts to ensure the stability of the repair,

thereby avoiding migration of the fundoplication, various authors have suggested fixation of the wrap to the right pillar of the diaphragm,[18] the gastroesophageal junction,[19] and the median arcuate ligament.[4,9] Both Kaminsky[9] and Cordiano[18] noted improvement in esophageal function as determined by pH and manometry with anchoring of the gastroesophageal junction to the preaortic fascia. Other reported modifications include the addition of vagotomy and pyloroplasty[10] and parietal cell vagotomy in selected patients.[20,21]

With this multitude of operative innovations to choose from, this may indicate a potential drawback in critically assessing the success of the procedure. With no gold standard, or essentially classic method of Nissen fundoplication, then each clinical trial must be measured not only by its stated procedure but also by its descriptive account of actual technique.

■ Background

Patients with symptomatic reflux or low-grade esophagitis should be given a trial of nonsurgical

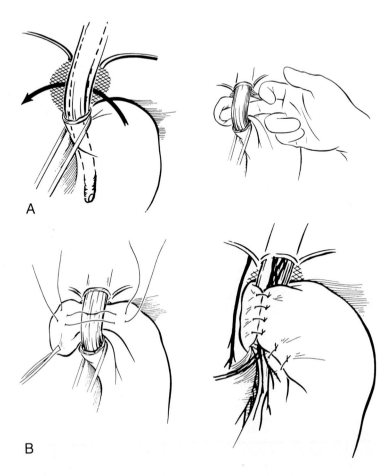

Figure 9–35. *A,* Technique of fundoplication. The peritoneum overlying the cardia is incised, the phrenoesophageal membrane is stripped off, and a 4 to 5 cm segment of distal esophagus is isolated and surrounded with a rubber tube for downward traction. A large bore esophageal probe, inserted by the anesthetist, facilitates identification of the cardia and prevents creating too tight a fundoplication. The anterior fundic wall is gently brought around the esophagus and grasped with an atraumatic clamp. *B,* Seromuscular nonabsorbable interrupted sutures are placed across the esophagus from fundic wall to fundic wall. The wall of the esophagus is not included in the sutures. The sutures are tied to unite the gastric wall in front of the esophagus. The cuff of stomach should be loose, easily admitting one finger. (From Rosetti M, Hell K: Fundoplication for the treatment of gastroesophageal reflux in hiatal hernia. World J Surg, *1*:440, 1977.)

management. Although paradoxically, it has been suggested that even those patients appropriate for initial medical management have increased benefit from surgery.[24]

Absolute indications for surgical intervention include failure to relieve symptoms with medical treatment, severe cases of stricture and ulcerative esophagitis, hemorrhage, or pulmonary aspiration of gastric contents.

Studies in both experimental[25,26] and clinical forums[22,27–29] have suggested that the Nissen fundoplication has potential for good reflux control. Cadaver studies have shown the Nissen is equal to the Hill and better than the Belsey and Thal repairs in controlling GE reflux.[25] The re-establishment of ''normal LES pressure'' is the most often cited mechanism for the Nissen's success at reflux control.[16,22,30,31] However, there is evidence to suggest that there is often little correlation between measurements of pre- and postoperative LES length or amplitude and the presence or absence of reflux.[20,29,32,34] Low LES pressure is not required for reflux to be present, nor does high LES pressure seem to prevent it absolutely. The importance of the angle of His[12] and intra-abdominal esophagus[25] have also been challenged.

Many investigators are coming to accept the theory of the presence of a flap valve mechanism.[2,3,30,32,35] The re-establishment of this flap valve is likely a component of the mechanism whereby GE reflux is brought under control, contradicting the hypothesis of a simple tightening effect.

The presence of a more complicated flap valve mechanism is suggested by the success of various techniques of constructing the fundoplication itself. Most surgeons utilize the 360-degree wrap with various sized intraesophageal stents in place. This technique is supported by experiments in cats using the repair with various degrees of plication follow-ing a lower esophageal circular myotomy. With pre- and postoperative comparison of LES manometry and pH testing, it was shown that a 2 to 3 cm 360-degree wrap was most effective at objectively controlling reflux.[16] Subsequent concern over the postoperative problems of gas bloat and inability to burp and vomit, led investigators to attempt repair with lesser degrees of fundoplication[4,12] (Fig. 9–36). These procedures were not only associated with a decrease in gas bloat but showed maintenance of a good level of reflux control. The simple tightening hypothesis is also undermined by the success of the relatively new ''floppy Nissen'' fundoplication. This technique of purposely constructing a loose wrap, with relatively insignificant increases in LES pressure, effectively controls reflux while limiting postoperative symptoms. This wrap is constructed not only with a 50 French dilator within the esophagus, but also with a No. 15 Hegar dilator external to the esophagus but within the plication (Fig. 9–37). Donahue's series demonstrates good reflux control with one to eight years' follow-up and low complication rate, and provides support for the control of reflux on a physiologic rather than a purely mechanical basis.[8]

More recently, concern has been raised regarding the long-term results of the Nissen repair.[5,34] In one study in which patients were followed for four to seven years postoperatively, there was a documented decrease in manometric LES pressure, and a coincident increase in abnormal esophageal biopsies and asymptomatic reflux demonstrated with acid reflux testing. Although this well-designed trial is noteworthy, the same incidence of recurrence was not seen in other clinical trials with prolonged follow-up[31,36] (Table 9–1).

■ *Complications*

Frequency of postoperative complications has been one area of recent concern with respect to the

Table 9–1. RESULTS OF NISSEN FUNDOPLICATION

Author	Number of Patients	Symptomatic and Anatomic Recurrence	Complications
Bushkin[36]	165	8%	
DeMeester[22]	15		13%
Dilling[27]	37	12.5%	34%
Donahue[8]	77	3%	3%
Ellis[31]	82	10%	19%
Matikainen[3]	20	0%	15%
Menguy-Nissen, modified[4]	61	11%	NR
	54	2%	NR
Negre[5]	94	19%	NR
Nicholson[28]	141	2.9%	NR
Randolph[33]	72	8%	NR
Rossetti[20]	590	12.5%	NR

NR = Not reported.

general usage of the Nissen fundoplication.[37,38,41] The importance of proper patient selection and close attention to operative technique should result in minimizing postoperative symptoms and recurrence.[5,38,39]

The list of potential operative and postoperative complications (Table 9–2) includes slippage of the wrap and significant esophageal and gastric fistulas, which seem to be specific to the Nissen procedure when compared to the other commonly utilized antireflux procedures.

The most common postoperative complication is the gas bloat syndrome with the associated inability to belch or vomit. Reported instances range from 0 to 50 per cent[9,36] with some reporting its presence to some degree in 50 per cent of patients, even after 10 years' follow-up.[5] The associated symptoms with this syndrome are abdominal distention, subdiaphragmatic pressure sensation, and hiccups in 25 per cent.[14] Although the incidence of gas bloat tends to improve with time,[12,36] the initial incidence can be decreased by constructing the wrap with a minimum of tension.[38] This may require ligation of additional short gastric arteries; however, the impressive absence of gas bloat in the floppy

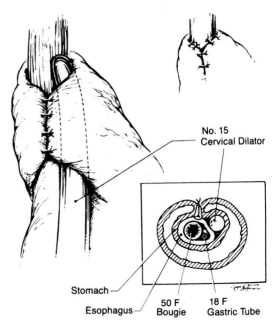

No. 15 Cervical Dilator

Stomach
Esophagus
50 F Bougie
18 F Gastric Tube

Figure 9–37. Floppy Nissen fundoplication is constructed to maximize looseness of wrap by using both anterior and posterior wall of the stomach. Taking care to maintain orientation of greater curvature vessels with respect to left side of gastroesophageal junction, anterior and posterior gastric walls are slipped around esophagus, which is distended by bougie and nasogastric tube. Cervical dilator is positioned prior to placement of sutures to prevent misplacement of sutures and is removed after 4–0 silk sutures have been placed. At right, collar stitches have been placed between top of stomach and esophagus to tether wrap and prevent slipping.

Nissen[8] would seem to justify this additional dissection.

Ellis[31] cites dysphagia as the most common reason for reoperation; in many cases, this is secondary to an unidentified motility disorder, i.e., diffuse spasm, achalasia, or scleroderma (Table 9–3). Postoperative obstruction or dysphagia can be put in either the immediate or late category. Immediate dysphagia can occur in up to 50 per cent of cases

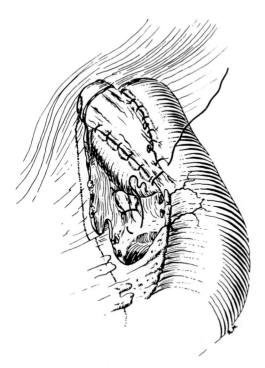

Figure 9–36. Shows the completed partial wraparound. The placement of the first of three anchoring sutures in the median arcuate ligament is shown. Menguy recommends that an Ewald tube or Maloney dilator should be in the esophageal lumen when constructing the wrap. (From Menguy R: A modified fundoplication which preserves the ability to belch. Surgery, 84:304, 1978.)

Table 9–2. OPERATIVE AND POSTOPERATIVE COMPLICATIONS ASSOCIATED WITH NISSEN FUNDOPLICATION*

Gas bloat
Dysphagia, early
    Late
Obstruction
"Slipped Nissen"
Incidental splenectomy
Fundoplication disruption
Paraesophageal hernia
Gastric ulceration
Perforation
Fistula formation
Diarrhea
Increased flatus

*Listed in order of frequency.

Table 9–3. COMPLICATIONS OF NISSEN
FUNDOPLICATION REQUIRING REOPERATION

Complication	Number of Cases
Dysphagia	24
Aperistalsis (10)	
Achalasia (7)	
Diffuse esophageal spasm (2)	
Scleroderma (1)	
"Slipped Nissen" (4)	
Stricture (3)	
Idiopathic (7)	
Recurrent reflux	9
Gas bloat syndrome	2
Paraesophageal hernia	3
Total	38

Source: Leonardi HK, Ellis FH: Complications of the Nissen
fundoplication. Surg Clin North Am, *63*:1162, 1983.

and is usually transient. The majority will resolve
or improve as postoperative edema subsides. A
subpopulation is the group of patients whose dysphagia continues due to a wrap which has been
constructed too tightly. This problem can be improved by stenting the esophagus with at least a
size 50 mercury-filled bougie. It can be avoided
by using intraoperative pressure measurements.
Furthermore, as the evidence increases that fundoplication control of reflux is accomplished on
physiologic rather then mechanical grounds, the
construction of a loose but anchored wrap[8] should
become more generally accepted. The remainder
of the patients in the late dysphagia group result
from either the presence of an unrecognized motility disorder or the development of a paraesophageal hernia or "slipped Nissen." The portion of
patients with motility disorders should be recognized preoperatively. The incidence of paraesophageal hernia can be significantly reduced by routinely adding a posterior crural plication to the
repair. The so-called "slipped Nissen" occurs
when the stomach below the wrap prolapses or
migrates up through the fundoplication, causing
secondary obstruction. By anchoring the wrap to
the crus, preaortic fascia, or median arcuate ligament or inserting several additional sutures from
the lower aspect of the plication to the stomach
just distal to the GE junction, displacement of the
wrap will be avoided.[19]

In reoperative cases of obesity or so called
"shortening of the esophagus," some surgeons
have advocated a transthoracic approach for the
Nissen fundoplication. Some have suggested leaving the wrap itself in the chest.[40] In fact, none of
the circumstances listed above require a thoracic
approach, and a Nissen constructed and left in the
chest has an increased risk for recurrence and serious complications.[41,42]

Incidental splenectomy may be incidental but is
not inconsequential. It occurs in between 2 and 20
per cent of cases and leads to increased morbidity
and mortality rates.[43] Much of the damage is due
to traction tears in the splenic capsule, which cannot subsequently be controlled with topical hemostatic agents of splenorrhaphy. Iatrogenic
splenic trauma can be partially prevented by inserting a sponge posterior to the spleen to take the
tension off the fine gastrosplenic peritoneal attachments and by early ligation of one to two short
gastric vessels when required.

Ulceration in the gastric wrap with subsequent
fistula formation can lead to significantly increased
morbidity and mortality rates (see Chapter 13). It
likely occurs secondary to incomplete emptying
and stasis in the fundoplication. The Nissen procedure comprises a blind wrap of the parietal cell
mass (the most potent producer of hydrochloric
acid). Poor drainage or ischemia of this area causes
gastric ulceration with disastrous results of fistulas,
hemorrhage, and perforation.[37,38,41,42,44] Constructing a "short" or "loose" wrap facilitates emptying
of the pouch formed by the wrap and will decrease
or minimize the occurrence of these potentially disastrous complications.

Gastric ulceration following Nissen fundoplication has motivated several authors to recommend
combining an antireflux procedure with highly selective vagotomy.[20,21] They found that the dissection required for the vagotomy facilitated the construction of the Nissen fundoplication itself. In
addition, separation of the vagus nerves from the
esophagus and placement of the wrap inside the
nerves decreases the potential for damage to the
hepatic branch of the vagus. They also noted that
patients who subsequently developed reflux did not
develop esophagitis.

Although the presence of coexistent refractory
peptic ulcer disease requires the addition of an acid
control procedure, the routine addition of this procedure in all patients is not justified. Most people
with reflux esophagitis are not hypersecretors.
Therefore, it would seem more sensible to refine
one's operative technique to avoid recurrences,
rather than adding the increased risk of lesser curve
necrosis, gastric fistula, and the increased morbidity of a prolonged operation in case recurrence appears.

■ *Summary*

The operation first performed by Rudolph Nissen
in 1936 can be effective in preventing gastroesophageal reflux. Over the last 30 years, the large num-

ber of modifications of the original technique attest to the dissatisfaction with the procedure. Despite these modifications, increasing numbers of reports of complications and failures of the procedure have appeared. The basic problems with the technique are dependence on sutures in the esophagus to prevent slippage of the wrap. Esophageal sutures have little strength and may disrupt, leading to slippage and to fistula formation. Further, the blind wrapping of the parietal cell mass leads to gastric ulcers with the attendant complications of perforation and fistula formation. These complications are detailed in Chapter 13 and appear to be more common with the Nissen procedure than with any other technique.

The most comprehensive review of the total Nissen experience was that of Rosetti and Hell.[10] These authors reviewed the 1400 patients treated by the original Nissen group over a 20-year period. Long-term follow-up was obtained on only 590 patients who underwent fundoplication for simple reflux esophagitis. Eighty-seven per cent of these patients were said to be symptom-free. In 44 patients with complicated gastroesophageal reflux disease, fundoplication produced clinical healing in 84.1 per cent. It is unfortunate in this series that the only documentation of results was by questionnaire and by upper GI tract x-ray series. We have found that the upper GI series is often inadequate in determining effectiveness of an antireflux procedure in terms of correction of reflux. We believe that it is essential to do pH and manometry studies or scintiscanning in as many patients as possible in order to assess the true effect of antireflux therapy.

■ REFERENCES

1. Nissen R: Eine einfache Operation zur Beeinflussung der Refluxoesophagitis. Schweiz Med Wschr, 86:590, 1956.
2. Matikainen M, Kaukinen L: The mechanism of Nissen fundoplication. Acta Chir Scand, 150:653–655, 1984.
3. Matikainen M: Nissen-Rosetti fundoplication for the treatment of gastro-oesophageal reflux. Acta Chir Scand, 148:173–177, 1982.
4. Menguy R: A modified fundoplication which preserves the ability to belch. Surgery, 84:301–306, 1978.
5. Negre JB, Markkula HT, Keyrilainen O, Matikainen M: Nissen fundoplication: Results at 10 year follow-up. Am J Surg, 146:635–637, 1983.
6. Allison PR: Reflux esophagitis, sliding hiatal hernia and anatomy of repair. Surg Gynecol Obstet, 92:419–431, 1951.
7. Ellis FH: Technique of fundoplication. In Stipa S, Belsey RHR, Moraldi A (Eds): Medical and Surgical Problems of the Esophagus. New York, Academic Press, 1981, pp 61–65.
8. Donahue PE, Samelson S, Nyhus LM, Bombeck T: The floppy Nissen fundoplication. Arch Surg, 120:663–668, 1985.
9. Kaminski DL, Codd JE, Sigmund CJ: Evaluation of the use of the median arcuate ligament in fundoplication for reflux esophagitis. Am J Surg, 134:724–729, 1977.
10. Rosetti M, Hell K: Fundoplication for the treatment of gastroesophageal reflux in hiatal hernia. W J Surg, 1:439–444, 1977.
11. Bremner CG, Rabin MR: The Nissen fundoplication operation: Improved technique to prevent complications. In Stipa S, Belsey RHR, Moraldi A (Eds): Medical and Surgical Problems of the Esophagus. New York, Academic Press, 1981, pp 71–74.
12. Alday ES, Goldsmith HS: Efficacy of fundoplication in preventing gastric reflux. Am J Surg, 126:322–324, 1973.
13. Guarner V, Martinez N, Gavino JF: Ten year evaluation of posterior fundoplasty in the treatment of gastroesophageal reflux. Long-term and comparative study of 135 patients. Am J Surg, 139:200–203, 1980.
14. Polk HC, Zeppa R: Hiatal hernia and esophagitis: A survey of indications for operation and technic and results of fundoplication. Ann Surg, 173:775–781, 1971.
15. Lortat-Jacob JL, Maillard JN, Fekete F: A procedure to prevent reflux after esophagogastric resection: Experience with 17 patients. Survey, 50:600–611, 1961.
16. Leonardi HK, Ellis FH: Experimental fundoplication: comparison of results of different techniques. Surgery, 82:514–520, 1977.
17. DeMeester TR (Discussion of Ellis FH, Crozier RE): Reflux control by fundoplication: A clinical and manometric assessment of the Nissen operation. Ann Thorac Surg, 38:387–392, 1984.
18. Cordiano C, Rovere GQD, Agugiaro S, Mazzilli G: Technical modification of the Nissen fundoplication procedure. Surg Gynecol Obstet, 143:977–978, 1976.
19. Hoffman TH, McDaniel A, Polk HC: Slipped Nissen's fundoplication: A stitch in time (letter). Arch Surg, 116:1239, 1981.
20. Bahadorzadeh K, Jordan PH: Evaluation of the Nissen fundoplication for treatment of hiatal hernia. Ann Surg, 181:402–408, 1975.
21. Jordan PH: Parietal cell vagotomy facilitates fundoplication in the treatment of reflux esophagitis. Surg Gynecol Obstet, 147:593–595, 1978.
22. DeMeester TR, Johnson LF, Kent AH: Evaluation of current operations for the prevention of gastroesophageal reflux. Ann Surg, 180:511–525, 1974.
23. Pope CE: Pathophysiology and diagnosis of reflux esophagitis. Gastroenterology, 70:445–454, 1976.
24. Behar J, Sheahan DG, Biancani P, Spiro HM, Storer EH: Medical and surgical management of reflux esophagitis. A 38-month report on a prospective clinical trial. N Engl J Med, 293:263–268, 1975.
25. Butterfield WC: Current hiatal hernia repairs: Similarities, mechanisms, and extended indications—an autopsy study. Surgery, 69:910–916, 1971.
26. Leonardi HK, Lee ME, El-Kurd MF, Ellis FH: An experimental study of the effectiveness of various antireflux operations. Ann Thorac Surg, 24:215–222, 1977.
27. Dilling EW, Peyton MD, Cannon JP, Kanaly PJ, Elkins RC: Comparison of Nissen fundoplication and Belsey Mark IV in the management of gastroesophageal reflux. 134:730–733, 1977.
28. Nicholson DA, Nohl-Oser JC: Hiatus hernia: A comparison between two methods of fundoplication by evaluation of the long-term results. J Thorac Cardiovasc Surg, 72:938–943, 1976.
29. Sillin LF, Condon RE, Wilson SD, Worman LW: Effective surgical therapy for esophagitis. Arch Surg, 114:536–541, 1979.
30. Goodall RJR, Temple JG: Effect of Nissen fundoplication

on competence of the gastro-oesophageal junction. Gut, 21:607–613, 1980.

31. Ellis FH, Crozier RE: Reflux control by fundoplication: A clinical and manometric assessment of the Nissen operation. Ann Thorac Surg, 38:387–392, 1984.
32. Fisher RS, Malmud LS, Lobis IF, Maier WP: Antireflux surgery for symptomatic gastroesophageal reflux: mechanism of action. Dig Dis, 23:152–160, 1978.
33. Randolph J: Experience with the Nissen fundoplication for correction of gastroesophageal reflux in infants. Ann Surg, 198:579–584, 1983.
34. Brand DL, Eastwood IR, Martin D, Carter WB, Pope CE: Esophageal symptoms, manometry, and histology before and after antireflux surgery. A long-term follow-up study. Gastroenterology, 76:1393–1401, 1979.
35. Thor KBA, Hill LD, Mercer CD, Kozarek RA: Reappraisal of the flap valve mechanism: A study of a new valvuloplasty procedure in cadavers. Acta Chir Scand, 153:25–28, 1987.
36. Bushkin FL, Neustein CL, Parker TH, Woodward ER: Nissen fundoplication for reflux peptic esophagitis. Ann Surg, 185:672–677, 1977.
37. Hill LD, Ilves R, Stevenson JK, Pearson JM: Reoperation for disruption and recurrence after Nissen fundoplication. Arch Surg, 114:542–548, 1979.
38. Leonardi HK, Ellis, FH: Complications of the Nissen fundoplication. Surg Clin North Am, 63:1155–1165, 1983.
39. Henderson RD: Nissen hiatal hernia repair: Problems of recurrence and continued symptoms. Ann Thorac Surg, 28:587–593, 1979.
40. Nicholson DA, Nohl-Oser HC: Hiatus hernia: A comparison between two methods of fundoplication by evaluation and long-term results. J Thorac Cardiovasc Surg, 72:938–943, 1976.
41. Mansour KA, Burton HG, Miller JI, Hatcher CR: Complications of intrathoracic Nissen fundoplication. Ann Thorac Surg, 32:173–178, 1981.
42. Balison JR, MacGregor AMC, Woodward ER: Postoperative diaphragmatic herniation following transthoracic fundoplication. Arch Surg, 106:164–166, 1973.
43. Rogers DM, Herrington JL, Morton C: Incidental splenectomy associated with Nissen fundoplication. Ann Surg, 191:153–156, 1980.
44. Hatton PD, Selinkoff PM, Harford FJ: Surgical management of the failed Nissen fundoplication. Am J Surg, 148:760–763, 1984.
45. Nissen R, Rosetti M: In Surgery of the Cardia Ventriculi. Ciba Symposiums, Vol. 11, No. 5/6. Ciba, Ltd., 1963–1964, pp 195–223.

THE NILL PROCEDURE

C. Cordiano ■ G. Inaspettato
L. Rodella

With the advent of improved medical management of patients with reflux esophagitis, the number of patients who require antireflux surgery has declined at the same time that the complexity of the condition of individual patients has increased. The Nissen fundoplication was introduced in 1956 by Rudolph Nissen[1] and was quickly adopted by a large number of surgeons owing to initial reports of good results and its relative ease of construction.

A large experience with the Nissen procedure was gained and many reports appeared, testifying to its efficacy at restoring "normal" lower esophageal sphincter (LES) function.[2–11] However, these reports also began to demonstrate significant problems associated with the Nissen procedure in terms of postoperative dysphagia and gas bloat syndrome (GBS). In response to these problems, many surgeons began experimenting with modifications of the procedure to decrease the incidence of these complications.[12–20]

The Nissen fundoplication has influenced many of the subsequent surgical procedures which appeared in the years following its own introduction (e.g., Toupet, Dor, Vayre-Hureau, Guarner). The only truly new technique, other than the Nissen fundoplication, to emerge since the 1950s is the Hill posterior gastropexy.[21]

■ Mechanism of Action of the Nissen Fundoplication

The actual mechanism of action of the Nissen fundoplication is not known. The relaxation of the fundoplication after swallowing may reach 100 per cent[6,22] owing to the fact that response to vagal stimulus is the same for the gastric fundus and the LES.[23] The competence of the fundoplication is also influenced by the sensitivity of the muscular fibers of the gastric fundus to hormonal stimulation in much the same way as the LES.[7,20,24,25] Furthermore, esophageal motility and the response of the LES to gastrin improves when reflux is controlled and esophagitis eliminated.[6,20] However, the restoration of normal LES function after fundoplication is not achieved solely through neural hormonal mechanisms. Using perioperative manometry, several experimental[8,25] and clinical studies[2,26–30] have shown that LES pressure at rest varies with the degree of wrapping (360, 180, or 90 degrees), the length of the cuff, and the length of the intra-abdominal esophagus.[8,27]

All these elements have influenced the evolution of the present-day Nissen fundoplication, which contains components encompassing both the re-positioning of an esophageal segment fixed pos-teriorly in the abdomen (Hill procedure) and the creation of a short, floppy, or incomplete fundo-plication. For these reasons, the new Nissen pro-cedures, which are influenced both by the original Nissen fundoplication and the Hill operation, we define as "Nill procedures."

■ *Complications of the Nissen Fundoplication*

Peri- and postoperative complications with the Nissen fundoplication can usually be associated with problems in patient selection or operative technique. A typical complication of the Nissen fundoplication is GBS, which can often be asso-ciated with dysphagia. The incidence of GBS is reported to be between 3.6 and 54 per cent.[2-4,9,19,31-35] The pathogenesis of this syndrome is believed to involve the presence of a unidirec-tional flap valve mechanism (between the esoph-agus and the stomach), which produces a trapping of swallowed air without allowing expulsion.[36,37]

Incidence of GBS is increased when the wrap is more than 4 cm[38,39] or constructed too tightly.[38-42] In these cases esophageal peristalsis can overcome the obstacle, but it is impossible to vomit or belch.[38,40-43] A tight wrap creates a relative obstacle to deglutition, requiring more frequent acts of swal-lowing, resulting in increased swallowing of air, thereby augmenting the gas bloat.[9] In many cases, GBS tends to spontaneously resolve in the weeks following surgery.[9,44] However, a portion of pa-tients will have a continuing disability secondary to this complication.

Dumping syndrome[45-47] and postprandial hypoglycemia[47] have been reported in patients fol-lowing Nissen fundoplication. An incidental va-gotomy is the most likely cause of the disturbance, although an alteration in intestinal hormones of unknown origin has also been suggested.[47] Alter-natively, vagal lesions can also give rise to GBS in addition to gastric retention.[48]

Other rare complications include incidental splenectomy[34,49-51] as well as esophagogastric and esophageal fistulas.[52] Gastric ulceration of the ab-dominal and thoracic wrap has a reported incidence of 2 to 3 per cent.[53-60] Most hiatal hernia recur-rences and postoperative deformities of the gastric wrap are related to total or partial dehiscence of the wrap. In some cases, there may be a deformity of the fundoplication without recurrence[43] or slip-ping of the stomach through the fundic cuff (slipped

Nissen or "Teleskop-*phanomen*")[34,40-42,61,62] owing to lack of fixation of the stomach to the cardia or esophagus.

Paraesophageal hernia after fundoplication[38,63] has been reported more frequently in children.[64,65] Migration of the fundoplication into the thorax[66-68] and intussusception of the gastric mucosa cephalad to the fundoplication[21] have also been reported. Many of the above-mentioned complications are the result of improper technique when constructing the fundoplication,[69] of suture reaction,[70] or sec-ondary to early GBS.[9]

■ *The Nill Procedure*

The Nill procedure describes the attempts to re-duce the complications and sequelae associated with the Nissen fundoplication while maintaining its efficacy for reflux control. The basic surgical details of the Nill procedure entail the repositioning of an esophageal segment in the abdomen and maintaining its position with a fixed fundoplica-tion. The fundoplication, which uses the anterior and posterior fundic walls, should not be more than 3 to 4 cm in length, and care should be taken to avoid constructing the wrap too tightly.

These principles are finding greater acceptance in the surgical community and are now widely de-scribed in the literature.[12-15,17-20] Sifers[20] makes a fundoplication in the proximity of the esophago-gastric junction and then fixes the wrap to the gas-trohepatic ligament. Kaminski[17] constructs a typi-cal fundoplication that is fixed to the median arcuate ligament with two of his four fundoplica-tion sutures. Kim[18] and Menguy[19] describe con-structing an incomplete wrap (240 and 270 degrees, respectively), which is fixed to the esophagogastric junction and then anchored to the median arcuate ligament. Csendes[15] also utilizes the median ar-cuate ligament as a fixation point but includes a highly selective vagotomy with his repair. In cases of recurrent hernia, Bremner[12] fixes the fundopli-cation to the right crus of the diaphragm.

Our procedure entails liberating the last 4 cm of the abdominal esophagus following division of the Laimer-Bertelli membrane, and digital dissection of the mesoesophagus. Special care is taken to avoid trauma to the vagus nerves during this dis-section. The posterior wall of the gastric fundus near the cardia is then freed from its attachments for several centimeters, and the wrap is constructed (Fig. 9–38). This involves including the anterior gastric wall, the esophagus, and the posterior gas-tric wall with each suture (Fig. 9–39). We have classically used three sutures; however, the most

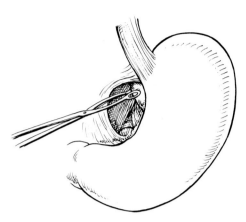

Figure 9–38. Dissection of the small epiploon, freeing the terminal esophagus and cardia and a few centimeters of the posterior gastric wall.

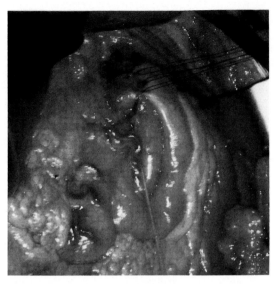

Figure 9–40. Fundoplication is performed with three adsorbable synthetic monofilament sutures; the lowest one should never be placed over the junction between cardia and stomach.

inferior one must never go over the junction of the cardia and the stomach (Fig. 9–40).

If the hiatal ring is strong, we fix the wrap to the right crus of the diaphragm (Fig. 9–41). If the hiatal ring is patulous, we routinely do a hiatoplasty. Alternatively, if the diaphragmatic crus is atrophic and does not offer a strong point for gastropexy, we free the lesser curve for an additional 2 to 3 cm as we would normally do with a highly selective vagotomy. We can then dissect out the median arcuate ligament to which we can fix the wrap (Fig. 9–42). At completion we ensure that the wrap is quite loose, and we find it has deviated posteriorly compared to the esophageal axis.

Until 1980, we used longer wraps (4 to 5 cm) and we constructed the wrap with a nasogastric

tube in the esophageal lumen to avoid making it too tight. Subsequent to 1980 we constructed the "minifundoplication" described above, and calibrated the wrap with digital exploration.

■ ANALYSIS OF CASES

From 1969 to 1985 we have examined 1117 patients with reflux esophagitis. Of these, 385 (34 per cent) have undergone surgical antireflux procedures. In our initial 15 patients we utilized the Vayre-Hureau procedure. We soon abandoned this technique due to dissatisfaction with our early recurrence rate.

Subsequently, from 1970 to 1975, we began our experience with the Nissen fundoplication in 125 patients (group 1). In this group we noted an incidence of recurrent reflux in 6 per cent of cases. The incidence of GBS was 13 per cent in the first six months after the operation; however, in the three years following surgery, with medical therapy and/or endoscopic dilatations, this decreased to 2 per cent.

Starting in 1975, we began to use the "floppy Nissen" with anchoring of the wrap to the right crus. From 1975 to 1979 we treated 208 patients with this technique (group 2).[13,14] The incidence of initial gas bloat syndrome was reduced to 4 per cent during the first six months and to 1 per cent after three years, without a significant increase in

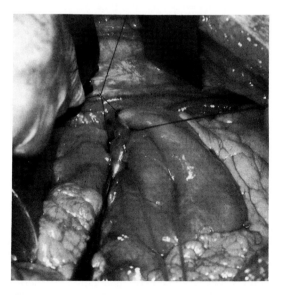

Figure 9–39. The wrap is made, including with every stitch the anterior gastric wall, the abdominal esophagus, and the posterior gastric wall.

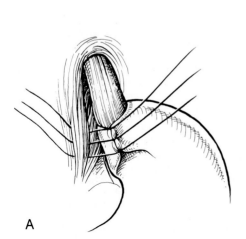
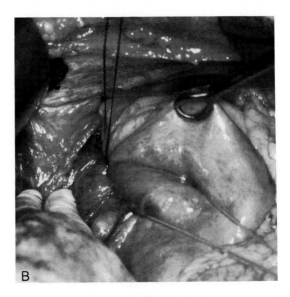

Figure 9–41. *A,* If the hiatal ring is strong enough, the wrap is fixed to the right crus of the diaphragm. *B,* The fixation of the stomach and cardia to the right diaphragmatic crus has been performed.

the incidence of recurrent reflux. These results encouraged us to construct even smaller fundoplications located nearer the gastroesophageal junction.

We have noted that with the widespread acceptance of the newer H$_2$-receptor blockers for reflux, and the improvement in endoscopic dilatation for stricture management, the volume of patients requiring surgical reflux control has declined. As a result, from 1980 to 1985 we have operated on only 37 patients. In three of these cases, there was

a recurrent hiatal hernia, one of which was associated with complete dishiscence of the wrap and delayed gastric emptying. In our simple recurrent cases, we have utilized the "Nill procedure," whereas for the dehiscence we performed an antrectomy with truncal vagotomy and Roux-en-Y gastrojejunostomy.

In one patient who was found to have achalasia (stage 1) associated with hiatal hernia, we utilized a Heller myotomy and Nill procedure with good results. Comparison of results between this group

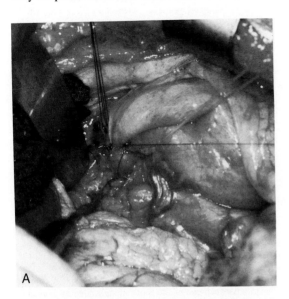
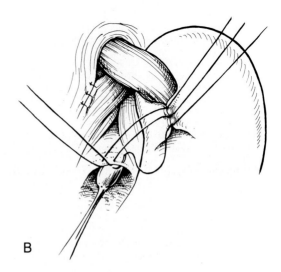

Figure 9–42. *A,* If the hiatus is very large with atrophic crura, we perform a hiatoplasty with interrupted sutures and then research the median arcuate ligament. A Kocher guiding probe is put under the median arcuate ligament. (See Color Plate II*B.*) *B,* The same sutures are used for the fixation to the median arcuate ligament.

and our previous experience is not possible because only 16 of these patients have been followed for a minimum of three years.

■ Conclusions

Our experience demonstrates a continuous evolution of surgical technique in the treatment of hiatal hernia and esophageal reflux and describes an alternative measure for restoring the normal physiologic functions of the terminal esophagus. In this regard, the Hill and Nill techniques are significant steps.

Owing to the significant reduction in the number of patients requiring surgical treatment, resulting largely from improvement in medical therapy, we believe it may be necessary in the future to coordinate follow-up in cooperation with several groups of surgeons utilizing similar methods of surgical reflux control.

■ REFERENCES

1. Nissen R: Eine einfache operation zur beeinflussung der refluxoesophagitis. Schweiz Med Wochenschr, 86:590, 1956.
2. Bushkin FL, Neustein CL, Parker TH, Woodward ER: Nissen fundoplication for reflux peptic esophagitis. Ann Surg, 185:672–677, 1977.
3. DeMeester TR, Johnson LF: Evaluation of the Nissen antireflux procedure by esophageal manometry and twenty-four hour pH monitoring. Am J Surg, 129:94–100, 1975.
4. Dilling EW, Peyton MD, Cannon JP, Kanaly PJ, Elkins RC: Comparison of Nissen fundoplication and Belsey Mark IV in the management of gastroesophageal reflux. Am J Surg, 134:730–733, 1977.
5. Ellis FH, El-Kurd MFA, Gibb SP: The effect of fundoplication on the lower esophageal sphincter. Surg Gynecol Obstet, 143:1–5, 1976.
6. Higgs RH, Castell DO, Farrell RL: Evaluation of the effect of fundoplication on the incompetent lower esophageal sphincter. Surg Gynecol Obstet, 141:571–575, 1975.
7. Leonardi HK, Lee ME, El-Kurd MF, Ellis FH: An experimental study of the effectiveness of various antireflux operations. Ann Thorac Surg, 24:215, 1977.
8. Leonardi HK, Ellis FH: Experimental fundoplication; comparison of results of different techniques. Surgery, 82:514, 1977.
9. Negre JB, Markkula HT, Keyrilainen D, Matikainen M: Nissen fundoplication. Results at 10 year follow-up. Am J Surg, 146:635–638, 1983.
10. Randolph J: Experience with the Nissen fundoplication for correction of gastroesophageal reflux in infants. Ann Surg, 198:579–585, 1983.
11. Sillin LF, Condon RE, Wilson SD, Worman LW: Effective surgical therapy of esophagitis. Arch Surg, 114:536–541, 1979.
12. Bremner CG, Rabin MR: The Nissen fundoplication operation: Improved technique to prevent complications. In Stipa S, Belsey RHR, Moraldi A (Eds): Medical and Sur-

gical Problems of the Esophagus. New York, Academic Press, 1981, p 71.
13. Cordiano C, Agugiaro S, Querci della Rovere G, Motton G, Mazzilli G, Farello GA: Problemi tecnici della fundusplicatio. Acta Chir It, 31:367, 1975.
14. Cordiano C, Querci della Rovere G, Agugiaro S: Technical modification of the Nissen fundoplication procedure. Surg Gynecol Obstet, 143:977, 1976.
15. Csendes A: A modified posterior cardiogastropexy for surgical treatment of GER with the adding of highly selective vagotomy and bougie calibration. In Stipa S, Besey RHR, Moraldi A (Eds): Medical and Surgical Problems of the Esophagus. New York, Academic Press, 1981, p 91.
16. Guarner V, Martinez N, Gavino JF: Ten year evaluation of posterior fundoplasty in the treatment of gastroesophageal reflux. Am J Surg, 139:200–203, 1980.
17. Kaminski DL, Codd JE, Sigmund CJ: Evaluation of the use of the median arcuate ligament in fundoplication for reflux esophagitis. Am J Surg, 134:724–729, 1977.
18. Kim SH, Hendren WH, Donahoe PK: Gastroesophageal reflux and hiatus hernia in children: Experience with 70 cases. J Pediatr Surg, 15:443–453, 1980.
19. Menguy R: A modified fundoplication which preserves the ability to belch. Surgery, 84:301–307, 1978.
20. Sifers EC, Taylor TL, Rick GG, Hartman CR, Tretgar LL: The role of gastrin in the treatment of sliding hiatal hernia with reflux using the refeeding method of fundoplication. Surg Gynecol Obstet, 143:376–380, 1976.
21. Hill LD, Ilves R, Stevenson JK, Pearson JM: Reoperation for disruption and recurrence after Nissen fundoplication. Arch Surg, 114:542–548, 1979.
22. Lipshutz WH, Eckert RH, Gaskins RD: Normal lower esophageal sphincter function after surgical treatment of GER. N Engl J Med, 291:1107, 1974.
23. DeMeester TR: Surgical management of GER. In Castell DO, Wu WC, Ott DJ: Gastroesophageal Reflux Disease: Pathogenesis, Diagnosis, Therapy. Mount Kisko, New York, Futura Publishing Co. 1985, p 243.
24. Duranceau A, LaFontaine ER, Vallieres B: Effects of total fundoplication on function of the esophagus after myotomy for achalasia. Am J Surg, 143:22–28, 1982.
25. Siewert R, Jennewein HM, Waldeck F, Weiser HF: Mechanism of action of fundoplication. J Abdom Surg, 18:131–135, 1976.
26. Behar J: Surgical treatment of reflux esophagitis: How well does it work? Gastroenterology, 77:183–184, 1979.
27. DeMeester TR, Wernly JA, Bryant GH, Little AG, Skinner DB: Clinical and in vitro analysis of determinants of gastroesophageal competence. A study of the principles of antireflux surgery. Am J Surg, 137:39–46, 1979.
28. Lind JF, Crispin JS, McIver DR: The effect of atropine on the GE sphincter. Can J Physiol Pharmacol, 46:233, 1968.
29. Mokka REM, Punto L, Kairaluoma MI, Laitinen S, Larmi TKI: Surgical treatment of axial hiatal hernia reflux complex by Nissen fundoplication. Acta Chir Scand, 143:265–269, 1977.
30. Safaie-Shrazi S, Zike WL, Anvras S, Condon RE, DenBesten L: Nissen fundoplication without crural repair. Arch Surg, 108:424–427, 1974.
31. DeLaet M, Spitz L: A comparison of Nissen fundoplication and Boerema gastropexy in the surgical treatment of gastroesophageal reflux in children. Br J Surg, 70:125–127, 1983.
32. Nicholson DA, Nohl-Oser HC: Hiatus hernia: A comparison between two methods of fundoplication by evaluation of the long-term results. J Thorac Cardiovasc Surg, 72:938–943, 1976.
33. Parola PL, Fortis PA: Il trattamento chirurgico del reflusso

gastro-esofageo. Casistica clinica ed esperienza personale. Min Chir, *39*:165–168, 1984.

34. Polk HC: Fundoplication for reflux esophagitis: Misadventures with the operation of choice. Ann Surg, *6*:645–652, 1976.
35. Woodward ER, Thomas HF, McAlmany JC: Comparison of crural repair and Nissen fundoplication in the treatment of esophageal hiatus hernia with peptic esophagitis. Ann Surg, *173*:782–792, 1971.
36. Butterfield WC: Current hiatal hernia repairs: Similarities, mechanisms, and extended indications: An autopsy study. Ann Surg, *69*:910, 1971.
37. Morgan AG: The place of fundoplication in the treatment of hiatal hernia. Aust NZ J Surg, *40*:329, 1971.
38. Leonardi HK, Crozier RE, Ellis H: Reoperation for complications of the Nissen fundoplication. J Thorac Cardiovasc Surg, *81*:50–56, 1981.
39. Skinner DB: Complications of surgery for gastroesophageal reflux. World J Surg, *1*:485–492, 1977.
40. Henderson RD: Nissen hiatal hernia repair: Problems of recurrence and continued symptoms. Ann Thorac Cardiovasc Surg, 1979; *28*:587–593, 1979.
41. Leonardi HK, Ellis H: Complications of the Nissen fundoplication. Surg Clin North Am, *63*:1155, 1983.
42. Rossmann F, Brantigan CO, Sawyer RB. Obstructive complication of the Nissen fundoplication. Am J Surg, *138*:860–868, 1979.
43. Saik RP, Greenburg AG, Peskin GW: A study of fundoplication disruption and deformity. Am J Surg, *134*:19–24, 1977.
44. Orringer MB, Sloan H: Complications and failings of the combined Collis-Belsey operation. J Thorac Cardiovasc Surg, *74*:726, 1977.
45. Meyer S, Deckelbaum RJ, Lax E, Schiller M: Infant dumping syndrome after gastroesophageal reflux surgery. J Pediatr, *99*:235–237, 1981.
46. Villet R, Boureau M, Hayat P, Weisgerber G: Une complication grave de l'operation de Nissen: le dumping syndrome. A propos de 4 observation. Chir Pediatr, *19*:269, 1978.
47. Zaloga GP, Chernow B: Postprandial hypoglycemia after Nissen fundoplication for reflux esophagitis. Gastroenterology, *84*:840–842, 1983.
48. Siewert JR, Blum AL: Postsurgical syndromes: The esophagus. Clin Gastroenterol, *8*:271, 1979.
49. Danforth DN, Thorbjarnarson B: Incidental splenectomy: A review of the literature and the New York Hospital experience. Ann Surg, *183*:124–129, 1976.
50. Morgenstern L: The avoidable complications of splenectomy. Surg Gynecol Obstet, *145*:525–528, 1977.
51. Rogers DM, Herrington JL, Morton C: Incidental sple-

nectomy associated with Nissen fundoplication. Ann Surg, *191*:153–156, 1980.
52. Mullen JT, Burke EL, Diamond AB: Esophagogastric fistula. A complication of combined operation for esophageal disease. Arch Surg, *110*:826–828, 1975.
53. Bremner CG: Gastric ulcer after the Nissen fundoplication. S Afr Med J, *51*:791, 1977.
54. Bremner CG: Gastric ulceration after a fundoplication operation for gastroesophageal reflux. Surg Gynecol Obstet, *148*:62–64, 1979.
55. DeMeester TR, LaFontaine E, Joelsson BE: The relationship of hiatal hernia to the function of the body of the esophagus and the GE junction. J Thorac Cardiovasc Surg, *82*:547, 1981.
56. Herrington JL, Meacham PW, Hunter RM: Gastric ulceration after fundic wrapping. Vagal nerve entrapment, a possible causative factor. Ann Surg, *195*:574–581, 1982.
57. Maher JW, Cerda JJ: The role of gastric stasis in the genesis of gastric ulceration following fundoplication. World J Surg, *6*:794–799, 1982.
58. Polk HC: Personal communication, 1981.
59. Richardson JD, Larson GM, Polk HC: Intrathoracic fundoplication for shortened esophagus. Treacherous solution to a challenging problem. Am J Surg, *143*:29–35, 1982.
60. Scobie BA: High gastric ulcer after Nissen fundoplication. Med J Aust, *1*:409, 1979.
61. Olson RC, Lasser RB, Ansel H: The slipped Nissen (abstract). Gastroenterology, *70*:924, 1976.
62. Siewert R, Lepsien G, Weiser HF, Schattenmann G, Peiper HJ: Das teleskop-*phanomen*. Eine komplikationsmoglichkeit nach fundoplicatio. Chirurgia, *48*:640–645, 1977.
63. Balison JR, MacGregor AM, Woodward ER: Postoperative diaphragmatic herniation following transthoracic fundoplication. A note of warning. Arch Surg, *106*:164, 1973.
64. Festen C: Paraesophageal hernia: A major complication of Nissen's fundoplication. J Pediatr Surg, *16*:496–499, 1981.
65. Kuffer F, Bettex M: Der hiatushernie des kleinkinder. Fruh und spetkomplikationen nach fundoplication. Z Kinderkir, *14*:153, 1974.
66. Bombeck CT: Gastroesophageal reflux. *In* Nyhus LM, Condon RE (Eds): Hernia. 2nd Ed. Philadelphia, J.B. Lippincott, Co., 1978, p 643.
67. Mansour KA, Burton HG, Miller JI, Hatcher CR: Complications of intrathoracic Nissen fundoplication. Ann Thorac Surg, *32*:173, 1981.
68. Naef AP, Savary M: Conservative operation for peptic esophagitis with stenosis in columnar-lined lower esophagus. Ann Thorac Surg, *13*:543, 1972.
69. Ellis FH: Controversies regarding the management of hiatus hernia. Am J Surg, *139*:782–788, 1980.
70. Henderson RD: Dysphagia complicating hiatal hernia repair. J Thorac Cardiovasc Surg, *88*:922–928, 1984.

HIGHLY SELECTIVE VAGOTOMY, POSTERIOR GASTROPEXY, AND CALIBRATION OF THE CARDIA FOR REFLUX ESOPHAGITIS

Attila Csendes ▪ Italo Braghetto

Posterior gastropexy used as a definitive antireflux operation in patients with reflux esophagitis was introduced by Hill in 1967.[1] The basic principle of this procedure is anchoring the anterior and posterior phrenoesophageal fascial bundles to the preaortic fascia and the median arcuate ligament, thus creating a long, permanent intra-abdominal segment of the esophagus. Larrain modified this operation by adding the concept of calibration of the cardia[2] because several surgical observations indicated that the distal portion of the esophagus and the esophagogastric junction were both dilated in patients with reflux esophagitis.[3-6] The aim of this surgical maneuver is to decrease the diameter of the muscular esophagogastric junction or "cardia" to a normal or smaller than normal diameter. This was first controlled by invaginating the stomach with a finger against the distal end of the esophagus. This maneuver was accepted earlier by Hill and others.[5-8] We have employed this procedure for many years,[3,9,10] but surgical experience and some complications seen during and after surgery led to the introduction of some modifications of the technique.[13-15]

■ Principles of the Antireflux Procedure

We now utilize the following steps in the performance of a definitive antireflux operation:
1. Highly selective vagotomy
2. Calibration of the cardia with three to four stitches using the Hurst No. 32 F bougie as a guide for calibration
3. Closure and approximation of the right crus of the diaphragm behind the esophagus
4. Posterior gastropexy with two stitches to the median arcuate ligament
5. Anterior gastropexy with two stitches in order to avoid a late anterior paraesophageal hernia

Highly Selective Vagotomy. ■ This is done to avoid several problems that can occur during and after antireflux surgery. We perform this for several reasons: The main reason for highly selective vagotomy (HSV) is *technical facility.* Anyone who has performed HSV for duodenal ulcer will understand this point clearly. In patients with reflux esophagitis and in patients with hiatal hernia, there is extensive periesophageal fibrolipomatous tissue with a lymph node reaction that makes it difficult to identify the exact location of the distal esophagus and esophagogastric junction. In these patients with longstanding, severe esophagitis, the distal esophagus suffers "gastrification" with the appearance of Barrett's esophagus. The transmural inflammation alters the surface of the esophageal wall, which looks like gastric serosa. The adipose tissue increases and the esophagus and cardia become dilated. After performing several hundred cases of HSV for duodenal ulcer, we realized that the surgical exposure of the abdominal esophagus, the esophagogastric junction or cardia and lesser curvature, and the angle of His is excellent, allowing us to perform more precise antireflux surgery.

In a majority of antireflux procedures reported by several authors[1-3,6-8,16-19] it has been necessary to divide the lesser omentum or gastrohepatic ligament in order to obtain good exposure of the gastroesophageal (GE) junction. Therefore, the anterior hepatic branch of the vagus nerve is sectioned. A prospective controlled study comparing control cases and patients with reflux esophagitis undergoing HSV with section of the lesser omentum, showed gallstone development in 42 per cent of patients after observation for five years compared to 8 per cent in control subjects observed over this same period ($p < 0.001$). All subjects had normal cholecystograms at the beginning of this study.[20] This finding has not been reported elsewhere.

During the classical Hill-Larrain or Nissen procedures, unless the surgeon is careful, vagal trunks may not be clearly visualized and dissected. Therefore, when calibrating the cardia, it is possible that on occasion these vagal trunks may be cut or perhaps more frequently may be included in the sutures applied for calibration or fundoplication. This unintentional partial or complete vagotomy could be responsible for postoperative symptoms such as gastric distention, diarrhea, and halitosis. This complication can be responsible for the appearance of gastric ulcer secondary to Nissen procedure in 5 per cent of cases.[19,21,22] In our patients undergoing posterior gastropexy with calibration of the cardia, we documented gastric ulcer two to four years following surgery in 5 per cent of patients who previously had normal gastric mucosa on endoscopy. This complication is easily avoided with careful identification of the vagi.

This same complication can result from inappropriate handling of the Latarjet nerves, which has not previously been mentioned in the literature concerning antireflux surgery. These nerves are responsible for gastric emptying of solids and if they are not handled with extreme care (they measure less than 2 mm) during the antireflux repair, nerve damage can also produce symptoms secondary to gastric stasis. During HSV both vagal trunks and the anterior and posterior Latarjet nerves are handled with care to prevent damage.

The addition of HSV to antireflux surgery allows *exact* and very precise calibration of the cardia as all external fatty and inflammatory tissue is removed; thus, any error in proper suture placement can be avoided.

Gastric acid secretion plays an important role in the pathogenesis of reflux esophagitis.[23] There is no increase of basal or maximal acid output in these patients, except in those associated with duodenal ulcer[24] which occurs, in our experience, in

25 per cent of patients.[14] However, reflux of HCl into the esophagus, along with other factors, is responsible for the development of esophagitis and its complications. Medical treatment with H_2-receptor blockers decreases gastric acid secretion, producing symptomatic relief and healing of macroscopic esophagitis.[25,26] Furthermore, we observed in patients with duodenal ulcer who had also had heartburn prior to surgery that following HSV a dramatic and significant decrease in symptoms was noted[27,28] owing to diminution of acid secretion similar to the effect observed with the H_2-receptor blockers. Therefore, HSV has a favorable effect as a permanent "acid secretion blocker." A direct correlation between the duration of esophageal pH below 4 and the number of reflux episodes in one hand and the volume of basal acid secretion on the other hand was demonstrated by Boesby.[29] For these reasons, HSV is advocated in patients with reflux esophagitis.

Delayed gastric emptying is observed in 40 to 50 per cent of patients with reflux esophagitis.[30,31] A lateral beneficial effect of HSV is a slight increase of gastric emptying of fluids after surgery.[32]

Finally, and most important, the extrinsic denervation of the distal esophagus and esophagogastric junction does not alter the dynamics of GE sphincter pressure, both the basal tone and its response to stimulation. We have performed several investigations and the following conclusions have been reached:

1. Resting gastroesophageal sphincter pressure is not changed after extensive isolation of the distal 6 to 7 cm of the esophagus.[26,33–35]

2. The length and location of the gastroesophageal sphincter is not changed.[34,36,37]

3. Gastroesophageal reflux does not increase after HSV alone in duodenal ulcer patients.[28]

4. No significant change occurs in lower esophageal sphincter pressure in spite of an increase in basal serum gastrin.[33,34]

5. Response of GE sphincter pressure to cholinergic stimulation one week following surgery is not changed compared to preoperative response.[34] Even if a decreased response is seen, it returns to normal 12 weeks after surgery, indicating that dysphagia is not due to an "achalasia-like" response.

6. Sphincter relaxation is not altered after HSV nor is amplitude of the peristaltic waves of the distal esophagus.[34]

7. Increase in gastroesophageal sphincter pressure after step-by-step increase in gastric pressure (10, 20, and 30 mm Hg) is not altered after HSV.[35]

Calibration of the Cardia. ■ This essential step in the antireflux procedure is done in order to decrease the dilated distal esophagus and esophagogastric junction or cardia. In a prospective study, we measured at surgery the precise external perimeter of the gastroesophageal junction in 20 control subjects and in 40 patients with reflux esophagitis.[38] This perimeter measured 9 cm in contrast to normal subjects who had a mean perimeter of 6.3 cm ($p < 0.001$). These values correspond to 2.84 and 2 cm in diameter, respectively. In 85 per cent of the 40 reflux esophagitis patients this perimeter measured more than 7.5 cm, while in 95 per cent of the control subjects it measured less than 7.5 cm. There is a direct correlation between severity of esophagitis and a greater perimeter of the cardia. In addition, intraoperative manometry demonstrated that the gastroesophageal sphincter began at the same point as the external landmark of the cardia, that is, at the limit between the gastric serosa and the esophageal longitudinal muscle fibers.

In the beginning, calibration of the cardia was performed with the surgeon's finger against the distal end of the esophagus, but this was variable, depending on the diameter of the surgeon's finger, and it was not possible to determine precisely the actual size of the esophageal lumen. In some cases this resulted in severe constriction of the cardia (two patients) or conversely in a dilated cardia with recurrence of symptoms. Therefore, we adopted the use of a Hurst bougie No. 32, which produces a decrease of the cardia to 10 to 11 mm less than the normal diameter of 2 cm.

Closure of the Hiatus. ■ In approximately 30 per cent of our patients we find a dilated hiatus, and in the remainder it is normal. However, in order to avoid a small postoperative hiatal hernia due to extensive periesophageal and perihiatal dissection, we routinely close the hiatus with two stitches.

Posterior Gastropexy. ■ This procedure is essentially similar to the Hill technique done in order to create a long and permanent segment of intra-abdominal esophagus. However, we do not feel that it is necessary to carefully dissect and visualize the median arcuate ligament. We take the median arcuate ligament along with the crus of the diaphragm, with a Babcock clamp.

Anterior Gastropexy. ■ In order to avoid an anterior paraesophageal hernia (which has occurred in 4 per cent of our late control cases)[14] we put two stitches in the anterior surface of the stomach and tie them to the diaphragm. This paraesophageal type of hernia occurred as a result of the periesophageal dissection and mobilization of the greater curvature necessary for proper antireflux surgery.

■ STEPS IN SURGICAL TECHNIQUE

The patient is positioned with semielevated chest (Grassi's position). A median supraumbilical laparotomy is performed. A rib-lifting retractor is always used (double hand retractor), giving us excellent surgical exposure of the supramesocolic space. Highly selective vagotomy is performed as previously described.[39,40] The dissection is begun at the angle of His, then continues by cutting the proximal branch of the crow's foot of the anterior and posterior Latarjet nerves. The dissection continues proximally at the lesser curvature (which is sutured with interrupted stitches), including isolation of 6 to 7 cm of distal esophagus, to the hiatus, carefully displacing the vagal trunks and the Latarjet nerves with the lesser omentum to the patient's right. The esophagus is mobilized anteriorly and to the left by a pediatric Deaver retractor. This procedure permits visualization of the right and left portion of the right crus of the diaphragm, which is approximated by two nonabsorbable stitches (Fig. 9–43). When the patient has a large hiatal hernia (which is the case in 20 per cent of our patients) the hiatus is also closed anteriorly.

Two seromuscular nonabsorbable sutures are placed in the anterior and posterior surfaces of the stomach, near the lesser curvature, below the cardia. These will be used for posterior gastropexy. These sutures are initially used for traction, facilitating the inspection of both the front and back of the cardia. In order to calibrate the cardia, strong nonabsorbable suture is introduced into the anterior surface of the stomach 1 to 2 cm distal to the limit

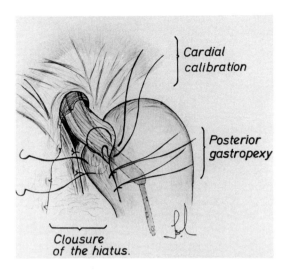

Figure 9–44. Schematic drawing showing the completed closure of the hiatus posteriorly. In addition, the initial two sutures of the repair are seen running from the anterior and posterior phrenoesophageal bundles back to the preaortic fascia. The repair is done over an indwelling No. 32 Hurst's bougie.

between the serosa of the stomach and the muscular wall of the esophagus, perpendicular to the midpoint of the cardia, appearing just at the anatomic border of the cardia, without including the esophagus. This stitch must be seromuscular and should not include the mucosa because it could cause perforation at this level or an ulcer caused by erosion produced by the stitch. Therefore, this suture must include the GE muscular junction and some portion of sling gastric fibers.

The stomach is now very easily rotated to the patient's left for inspection of the posterior wall, and the stitch is placed so that the course of the suture becomes exactly symmetric to that on the front, thus entering at the posterior muscular GE junction and appearing 2 cm distally at the posterior surface of the stomach. This suture is then repeated two to three times toward the left of the cardia and to the angle of His in such a way that we ultimately have three or four stitches for calibration. The sutures are then crossed and calibration of the cardia is evaluated by pushing the No. 32 Hurst bougie into the stomach and pulling it back into the esophagus (Fig. 9–44).

The surgeon invaginates the stomach with a finger, following the tip of the bougie, and a muscular ring should now be felt at the cardia. By pulling the bougie, the diminution of the cardial diameter can be evaluated. The bougie should pass easily, but the cardia should be felt to contract completely when the tip of the bougie is pulled into the esophagus, feeling this ring of muscular tissue. Thus, the opening of the cardia and distal esophagus is converted into a channel.

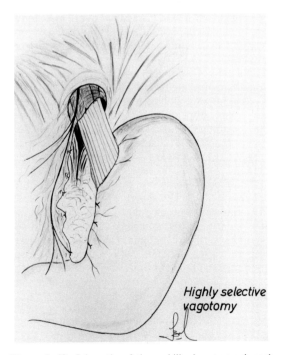

Figure 9–43. Schematic of the mobilized gastroesophageal junction showing the open hiatus posteriorly and the mobilized anterior and posterior vagal branches.

If the result is still not satisfactory, another stitch can be placed to the left. These stitches are tied leaving the bougie in the stomach. Then, the posterior gastropexy is performed using the previous sutures put in place in the lesser curvature. These are tied with the needles intact. The median arcuate ligament is identified in front of the aorta, just proximal to the celiac axis and below the junction of both crura of the diaphragmatic hiatus. The second and third fingers of the surgeon's left hand retract the celiac trunk distally, and a large Babcock clamp is used to firmly grasp the preaortic fascia, including the median arcuate ligament. Without further dissection, each of the two stitches is then passed through this fibrous tissue, by lifting the clamp upward, permitting the sutures to pass easily without damage to the aorta.

After this, two stitches from the gastric fundus to the phrenoesophageal membrane are placed in order to perform the anterior gastropexy (Fig. 9–45).

Calibration is again verified with the bougie which has remained in the stomach during these maneuvers, and it is then withdrawn. A soft nasogastric (NG) tube No. 14 is left in the appropriate position and no abdominal drainage is used. Transfusion of blood is never required, and the entire operation is completed in 60 to 70 min. The NG tube is withdrawn 24 hours after surgery and the patient can drink fluids 48 hours after surgery. Domperidone (10 mg every six hours) is used during the two weeks following surgery. The usual hospital stay is five days. A soft diet is recommended for one to two months following surgery because the patients complain of dysphagia with a regular or bland diet. Clinical evaluation is performed at two months and then again at one year following operation.

■ COMMENTS

Posterior gastropexy with calibration of the cardia (Hill-Larrain procedure) is a well-known surgical technique for patients with reflux esophagitis. We postulate that the addition of HSV greatly facilitates this operation, makes it more reproducible in the hands of other surgeons, and gives more latitude to the surgeon who is performing antireflux procedures.

It is very important to stress that HSV is different from truncal vagotomy and pyloroplasty since we have noted when presenting this technique that others have the two procedures confused. Truncal vagotomy with pyloroplasty was advocated some years ago as a "balanced operation" for patients with reflux esophagitis.[10,41,42] It was mainly used in patients with associated duodenal ulcer, either inactive or active, and also in patients with peptic strictures or severe esophagitis.[9,43] The addition of HSV is not a balanced operation and produces no significant changes at the gastroesophageal sphincter nor increases morbidity or mortality as we have shown in our results. On the contrary, this technique has been shown to have risks similar to other antireflux procedures with a mortality rate of 0.5 per cent. In the Arhus Surgical Group the mortality rate was 0.9 per cent and in the Santiago Group it has been 0.8 per cent. Two patients have died following this operation. In one case the calibration stitches included all layers of the esophagus and a fistula was produced.[44] The other patient who died following this procedure was a 72-year-old male patient with an esophageal stricture and Barrett's syndrome who had necrosis of the lesser curvature. At that time (1979) we did not suture and close the

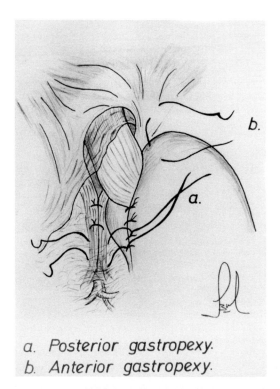

a. *Posterior gastropexy.*
b. *Anterior gastropexy.*

Figure 9–45. Schematic drawing showing the sutures inserted for both the anterior and posterior gastropexies

Table 9–4. REFLUX ESOPHAGITIS IN 240 OPERATED CASES*

Reflux alone	54
Reflux + gallstones	58
Reflux + gastric or duodenal ulcer	67
Reflux + hiatal hernia	61

*Of 240 patients, 115 were males and 125 were females.

Table 9–5. INCIDENCE OF MORBIDITY AND MORTALITY IN REFLUX ESOPHAGITIS

Splenectomy	2	
Intestinal obstruction	2	
Myocardial infarct	1	
Pulmonary embolism	1	
Acute pancreatitis	1	Operative Mortality: 2 cases (0.8%)
Hemoperitoneum	1	
Iatrogenic stricture	2	
Wound infection	3	
Esophagogastric fistula	1	
Lesser curvature necrosis	1	

lesser curvature following HSV. Since this experience we have routinely sutured the lesser curvature, and in 623 cases submitting to HSV we have had no deaths and no lesser curve necrosis.

The addition of HSV to an antireflux procedure has been slowly gaining acceptance by other authors. Sankar et al. proposed its use in 1976 in 27 cases with reflux esophagitis.[45] He showed that antireflux repair was easier with this technique, and reflux after surgery was nil. Bahadorzadek and Jordan in 1975 proposed performance of HSV with Nissen fundoplication.[46] They recognized that the Nissen procedure was greatly facilitated by HSV and was not associated with increased morbidity and mortality without the adverse effects of truncal vagotomy.

Therefore, we postulate that any antireflux procedure that is performed via the abdominal route is greatly facilitated by the addition of HSV, making possible better antireflux surgery without any increased mortality rate and without undesirable side effects observed after truncal or selective vagotomy. In Tables 9–4 and 9–5 we summarized our experience with this technique.

■ REFERENCES

1. Hill LD: An effective operation for hiatal hernia: An eight year appraisal. Ann Surg, *166*:681–692, 1967.
2. Larrain A: Technical consideration in posterior gastropexy. Surg Gynecol Obstet, *122*:299–300, 1971.
3. Csendes A, Larrain A: Effect of posterior gastropexy on gastroesophageal sphincter pressure and symptomatic reflux in patients with hiatal hernia. Gastroenterology, *63*:19–24, 1972.
4. Hill LD: Editorial: Surgery and gastroesophageal reflux. Gastroenterology, *63*:183–185, 1972.
5. Hill LD: Progress in the surgical management of hiatal hernia. World J Surg, *1*:425–438, 1977.
6. Vansant JH, Baker JW, Ross DG: Modification of the Hill technique for repair of hiatal hernia. Surg Gynecol Obstet, *143*:637–642, 1976.
7. Hermreck AS, Coates NR: Results of the Hill antireflux operation. Am J Surg, *140*:764–767, 1980.
8. Thomas AN, Hael AD, Haddad JK: Posterior gastropexy. Am J Surg, *126*:148–156, 1973.
9. Casten DF: Peptic esophagitis, hiatus hernia and duodenal ulcer: a unified concept. Am J Surg, *113*:638–641, 1967.
10. Clarke ID, Gordon HE, Winner RB: Treatment of the hiatus hernia by hiatus herniorrhaphy, vagotomy, and drainage procedure. Am J Surg, *107*:253–257, 1964.
11. Larrain A, Csendes A, Pope CE: Surgical correction of reflux as effective therapy for benign esophageal strictures. Gastroenterology, *69*:578–583, 1975.
12. Uribe P, Csendes A, Larrain A: Evaluation of surgery for gastroesophageal reflux. Rev Med Chile, *101*:125–128, 1973.
13. Csendes A: A modified posterior cardio-gastropexy for surgical treatment of gastroesophageal reflux with the adding of highly selective vagotomy and bougie calibration. *In* Stipa S, Belsey RHR, Misaldi A (Eds): Medical and Surgical Problems of the Esophagus. Symposium No. 43. London, Academic Press, 1981, pp 91–95.
14. Csendes A, Braghetto I, Velasco N: A comparison of three surgical techniques for the treatment of reflux esophagitis: A prospective study. *In* DeMeester T, Skinner D (Eds): Esophageal Disorders; Pathophysiology and Therapy. New York, Raven Press, 1985, pp 177–181.
15. Oster MI, Csendes A, Funch-Jensen P, et al: PCV and modified Hill procedure as surgical treatment of reflux esophagitis: Results in 108 patients. World J Surg, *6*:412–417, 1982.
16. Collis JL: Surgical control of reflux in hiatus hernia. Am J Surg, *115*:465–471, 1968.
17. Cordiano C, Della Rovere GA, Agugiaro S, Mazielli G: Technical modification of the Nissen fundoplication procedure. Surg Gynecol Obstet, *143*:977–978, 1976.
18. Pearson FG, Langer B, Henderson RD: Gastroplasty and Belsey hiatus hernia repair. J Thorac Cardiovasc Surg, *61*:50–63, 1971.
19. Sifers EC, Taylor TL, Rich GG, et al: The role of gastrin in the treatment of sliding hiatal hernia with reflux using the reefing method of fundoplication. Surg Gynecol Obstet, *143*:376–380, 1976.
20. Csendes A, Larach J, Godoy J: Incidence of gallstone development after selective hepatic vagotomy. Acta Chir Scand, *144*:289–291, 1978.
21. Bremner CG: Gastric ulceration after a fundoplication operation for gastroesophageal reflux. Surg Gynecol Obstet, *148*:62–64, 1979.
22. Bushkin FL, Woodward ER, O'Leary JP: Occurrence of gastric ulcer after Nissen fundoplication. Am Surg, *42*:821–826, 1976.
23. Dodds WI, Hogan WI, Helin JI: Pathogenesis of reflux esophagitis. Gastroenterology, *81*:376–394, 1981.
24. Csendes A, Larrain A, Uribe P: Gastric acid secretion in

patients with symptomatic gastroesophageal reflux and patients with esophageal strictures. Ann Surg, *179*:119–121, 1974.

25. Behar I, Brand DL, Brown FC, Castell DO, et al: Cimetidine in the treatment of symptomatic gastroesophageal reflux. Gastroenterology, *74*:441–448, 1978.
26. Wesdorf ICE, Bartelsman J, Schipper MEI, Tytgat GN: Effect of long-term treatment with cimetidine and antacids in Barrett's esophagus. Gut, *22*:724–727, 1981.
27. Braghetto I, Csendes A, Velasco N: Gastroesophageal reflux in gastric and duodenal ulcer patients before and after definitive surgical treatment. A prospective study in esophageal disorders. *In* DeMeester T, Skinner D (Eds): Esophageal Disorders: Pathophysiology and Therapy. New York, Raven Press, 1985, pp 155–163.
28. Csendes A, Oster MI, Moller IT, Flynn I, et al: Gastroesophageal reflux in duodenal ulcer patients before and after vagotomy. Ann Surg, *188*:804–808, 1978.
29. Boesby S: Relationship between gastroesophageal acid reflux, basal gastroesophageal sphincter pressure and gastric acid reaction. Scand J Gastroenterol, *12*:547–553, 1977.
30. Maddern OJ, Chatterton BE, Collins PJ: Solid and liquid gastric emptying in patients with gastroesophageal reflux. Br J Surg, *72*:344–347, 1985.
31. Velasco N, Hill LD, Gannan RM: Gastric emptying and GER. Am J Surg, *144*:58–62, 1982.
32. Wilbur BG, Kelly KA: Effects of proximal gastric and truncal vagotomy on canine gastric activity, motility, and emptying. Ann Surg, *178*:295–299, 1973.
33. Csendes A, Oster M, Brandsborg O: Gastroesophageal sphincter pressure and serum gastrin in relation to food intake before and after vagotomy. Scand J Gastroenterol, *13*:437–441, 1978.
34. Csendes A, Oster M, Moller IT, Brandsborg M, et al: Effect of extrinsic denervation of the lower end of the esophagus on study and cholinergic stimulated gastroesophageal sphincter in man. Surg Gynecol Obstet, *148*:375–378, 1979.

35. Csendes A, Oster M, Brandsborg O, Moller IT, et al: Effect of vagotomy on human gastroesophageal sphincter pressure in the resting state and following increases in intraabdominal pressure. Surgery, *85*:419–424, 1979.
36. Braasch IW, Sala LE, Ellis EH, et al: Parietal cell vagotomy. Its effect on lower esophageal sphincter function. Arch Surg, *115*:699, 1980.
37. Oowen JPC, Wittebal P, Geverts WJC, et al: Lower esophageal sphincter function after highly selective vagotomy. Arch Surg, *114*:908–910, 1979.
38. Csendes A, Miranda M, Espinoza M, et al: Perimeter and location of the muscular gastroesophageal junction or cardia in control subjects and in patients with reflux esophagitis or achalasia. Scand J Gastroenterol, *16*:951–956, 1981.
39. Amdrup E: Parietal cell (highly selective) vagotomy for duodenal ulcer. *In* Dudley H, Robb C, Smith R (Eds): Operative Surgery: Abdomen. 3rd Ed. London, Butterworths, 1977, pp 137–141.
40. Csendes A, Velasco N, Amat J, et al: Highly selective vagotomy: Preoperative studies and mortality. Rev Chil Cir, *31*:165–170, 1979.
41. Herrington JL: Treatment of esophageal hiatal hernia. Arch Surg, *84*:379–389, 1962.
42. Pearson FG, Store RM, Parrish RM: Role of vagotomy and pyloroplasty in the therapy of symptomatic hiatus hernia. Am J Surg, *117*:130–137, 1969.
43. Mustard RA: A survey of techniques and results of hiatus hernia repair. Surg Gynecol Obstet, 1970; *130*:131–136, 1970.
44. Csendes A, Braghetto I: Reflux esophagitis. Acad Cir, *28*:307–318, 1984.
45. Sankar MY, Old JM, Trinder P, Base AAK, et al: The advantages of combining posterior gastropexy with proximal gastric vagotomy. Clin Gastroenterol, *10*:389–392, 1976.
46. Bahadorzadek K, Jordan PH: Evaluation of the Nissen fundoplication for treatment of hiatal hernia: Use of parietal cell vagotomy without drainage as an adjunctive procedure. Ann Surg, *181*:402–408, 1975.

THE MODIFIED TOUPET PROCEDURE
Kjell Thor

The Toupet procedure was first described in 1963 and is a partial fundoplication usually performed transabdominally behind the esophagus.[1] This procedure was developed to be used in conjunction with the Heller myotomy in order to prevent reflux, but also to avoid ''gas bloat'' syndrome or ''l'incapacité d'éructation'' so commonly described after total fundoplication. This procedure is presented here with slight modifications, but without change of the original principle.

■ Indications

The most obvious indication for operation is failure to respond to full medical therapy, including diet and postural measures under the guidance of a gastroentrologist or physician with a special interest in this field. It is also important to verify that the patient's symptoms have arisen from the esophagus and not from any other sources. This includes careful preoperative investigation: endoscopy with biopsy, x-ray, 24-hour pH measurement, and motility studies.

Another common indication for antireflux surgery is reflux esophagitis. At endoscopy this is seen as either erosion, edema, erythema, ulceration, or a stricture representing the end result of the chronic, persistent inflammation causing fibrosis and narrowing of the lumen. Ulcerations may cause hemorrhage, either as chronic blood loss or less frequently as major upper gastrointestinal hemorrhage.

The appearance of aspiration of reflux material into the lung producing chronic respiratory problems such as asthma, pneumonia, chronic bronchitis, bronchiectasis, or lung abscess further strengthens the indication for surgery.

Finally, there is a group of patients in whom both at endoscopy and at biopsy no inflammation can be seen and in whom the other tests will not show any significant increased reflux. In this small group of patients with a sliding hiatal hernia, operation may be required because the hernia produces pressure symptoms in the chest, causing compression of the surrounding organs with conjoint respiratory embarrassment as well as episodes of incarceration of the stomach with obstructive symptoms and severe chest pain.

■ *Technique*

An incision is made through the upper abdominal midline; the left triangular ligament is divided; and the left lobe of the liver is retracted to the right. The upper hand or the Riesler retractor is used to elevate the thoracic wall or to facilitate exposure. In order to avoid tension in the gastrosplenic vessels during the operation, a wet compress is placed behind the spleen if the spleen is not attached to the abdominal wall by adhesions. The phrenoesophageal membrane is divided just as it leaves the diaphragm. Care should be taken at this stage not to damage the vagus nerves or the ascending branch of the left gastric artery.

The diaphragm surrounding the esophagus with the right and left crus is dissected completely free, and the distal esophagus is mobilized to a minimum of 5 cm. Both vagus nerves are identified, and the right vagus nerve is dissected completely free from the esophagus. A rubber band is then placed behind the esophagus which allows constant distal traction during the subsequent operative maneuvers. By division of the phrenogastric and superior portion of the gastrosplenic ligament along with two or three short gastric vessels, the upper part of the gastric fundus is mobilized. The mobilization of the fundus and the dorsal upper part of the stomach can often be done without sharp dissection and division of the small vessels. At this point, the median arcuate ligament is identified by placing the index finger between the preaortic fascia and the aorta through the hiatus of the diaphragm. The median arcuate ligament is grasped with a Babcock forceps and left in place to be used later in the procedure.

Two or three O nonabsorbable sutures are placed

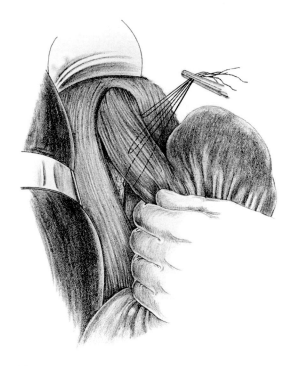

Figure 9–46. Two to three nonabsorbable sutures placed in the left crus. These are left untied with needles on so they can later be used for fixation of the fundus to the left crus.

in the left crus, leaving them untied with their needles on (Fig. 9–46). They will later be used for the fixation of the fundus to the left crus. The top of the fundus together with the anterior part of the fundus is thereafter passed from the left side, behind the esophagus, to the right side, where it is picked up by two Babcock forceps. The fundus portion should actually stay in place behind the esophagus without tension in order to avoid excessive external pressure on the esophageal wall or strain on the gastrosplenic vessels. Nonabsorbable sutures are used for all procedures. A suture is placed which includes the upper part of the right crus, the fundus, and the esophageal wall (Fig. 9–47). Care should be taken to avoid penetration of the sutures into the esophageal lumen or the gastric cavity, or to damage the vagi. Three to four sutures are then placed between the fundoplication and the right border of the esophagus. Thereafter, a second row is made which fixes the fundoplication to the right diaphragmatic crus. The distal or the two distal sutures include the median arcuate ligament which earlier has been identified. A similar procedure is then done on the left side by the use of the sutures placed in the left diaphragmatic crus before placing the fundus of the stomach behind the esophagus. The final row of sutures between fundus and esophagus should be placed so that the fundus of the stomach encircles the esoph-

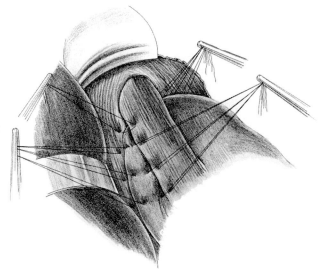

Figure 9–47. Placement of suture including upper part of the right crus, fundus, and esophageal wall.

agus for about 250 degrees (Fig. 9–48). No attempt is made to narrow the hiatal orifice by separate sutures except for very large hernias. When there is a large hiatus, sutures are placed in front of the esophagus to close the hiatus anterior to the esophagus. The rationale to close the diaphragm in front is to allow it to act as a pinchcock around the esophagus.

The original procedure can also be done transthoracically through a thoracotomy through the seventh or eighth left intercostal space. After division of the inferior pulmonary ligament up to the inferior pulmonary vein, the mediastinal pleura is

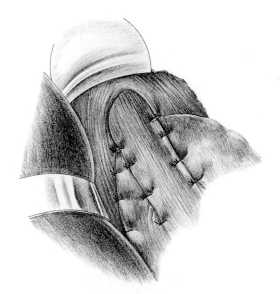

Figure 9–48. Final row of sutures between the fundus and the esophagus placed in such a way that the fundus of the stomach encircles the esophagus about 250 degrees.

opened, and the distal third of the esophagus is dissected free circumferentially. An incision is made in the muscular part of the diaphragm to avoid interference with the hiatal region. After mobilization of the esophagus, the procedure is carried out as described through the intra-abdominal incision.

■ Results

It is difficult to assess the results of different antireflux procedures since the outcome of an operation obviously depends on patient selection, indications for surgery, and the objective criteria for assessment, both pre- and postoperatively. Furthermore, there is no uniform standard of what we mean by ''recurrence.'' Many studies do not include objective criteria such as pH and pressure measurements, whereas others do. Is an operation to be considered successful if the patient no longer has heartburn but has a hiatal hernia on x-ray and esophagitis at endoscopy? Or has the patient a recurrence if symptoms, though less severe, persist without objective signs of recurrence? These questions will undoubtedly be answered differently by different investigators.

One hundred patients operated upon according to the modified Toupet procedure recently have been investigated, with a minimum of three years follow-up. All patients have been followed both pre- and postoperatively with x-ray, pressure manometry, Bernstein tests, pH measurement, and endoscopy with biopsy. Good or excellent results have been obtained in over 90 per cent with a recurrence rate of 7 per cent, no operative deaths, and one splenectomy.[2] Previous good results with a recurrence rate under 10 per cent have previously been published without the presence of the gas bloat syndrome found in patients after Nissen fundoplication.[3,4]

This operation accentuates the angle of His or the flap valve mechanism, which can be clearly seen when viewed from an endoscope postoperatively. The flap valve mechanism may be an important factor in preventing gastroesophageal reflux (see chapters on Surgery and Motility). Furthermore, this procedure increases the LES pressure to a third or half of that of total Nissen fundoplication.[3] This might explain why patients having had a Toupet procedure will not present with a gas bloat syndrome or inability to vomit.

■ REFERENCES

1. Toupet A: Technique d'oesophago-gastroplastie avec phrénogastropexie appliquée dans la cure radicale des hernies hiatales et comme complément de l'opération de Heller dans les cardiospasmes. Acad Chir, *89*:394, 1963.
2. Thor K, Silander T: Long-term results after the modified Toupet procedure for gastroesophageal reflux. Acta Chir Scand, 1987, in press.
3. Boutelier P: Résultats d'une série homogène de reflux gastrooesophagiens traités par valve tuberositaire rétro-oesophagienne fixée. Actual Chir, *1*:77, 1978.
4. Jonsell G, Boutelier P: Gastroesophageal reflux. Evaluation of two fundoplication methods by intraoperative esophageal manometry. Acta Chir Scand, *493*:(suppl) 47, 1979.

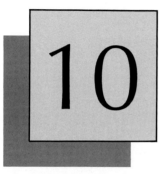

Surgery for
Peptic Esophageal Stricture

Lucius D. Hill ▪ *C. D. Mercer*

Rokitanski[1] first recognized peptic ulceration and stricture of the esophagus a century ago. Over the century few problems of the gastrointestinal tract have created more controversy regarding etiology and management than reflux stricture of the esophagus. The consensus and conflict about surgical management of peptic esophageal stricture presently favors conservative antireflux procedures with dilatation rather than resection.

Much of the controversy regarding strictures arose from a very unfortunate statement made by Norman Barrett in 1950.[2] He said, ''Any portion of the gullet lined by columnar epithelium must be stomach.'' He presented the hypothesis that columnar epithelium above the diaphragm represented ''congenital shortening of the esophagus with an attenuated intrathoracic stomach.'' A short time later Allison and Johnstone[3] described the columnar epithelium–lined esophagus and stated that the tubular portion of the gullet, even though lined with columnar epithelium above the diaphragm, was indeed esophagus. Despite Allison and Johnstone's clear and careful description, the term ''Barrett's esophagus,'' connoting a short esophagus with intrathoracic stomach, has become accepted in the surgical literature and has led to many unfortunate interpretations and erroneous modes of therapy.

Some idea of the prevalence of columnar-lined esophagus in gastroesophageal reflux emerged from a study by Naef et al.[4] They reviewed the results of 6000 endoscopies and found changes suggestive of reflux esophagitis in 1225 cases. One hundred forty (10 per cent of those patients with esophagitis) were noted to have columnar or Barrett's epithelium.

The evidence for acquired columnar-lining of the esophagus based on observations by Mossberg[5] and others show conversion of squamous epithelium to columnar epithelium as a process of creeping substitution, as the squamous mucosa is eroded by esophagitis and replaced by columnar epithelium that may or may not contain parietal cells. From these and countless other studies, it becomes evident that Allison and Johnstone's description was the correct one in that the lower esophagus, and in fact all the esophagus, may be lined with columnar epithelium and indeed is not, as Barrett described, ''stomach above the diaphragm.'' This is an important observation since the decision to resect the esophagus rather than do a simple antireflux procedure is often based on the misinterpretation that the columnar-lined esophagus is stomach.

The term ''short esophagus'' continues to reappear in the literature despite the fact that there has yet to be a study that has given any scientific determination of the length of a so-called ''short esophagus.'' In a series of patients undergoing antireflux operation and dilatation for peptic esophageal stricture, we have yet to encounter a so-called short esophagus, except in a small number of patients who have had perforation or repeated bougienage with complete destruction of the esophagus. We have reserved resection for this type of patient only. Other incorrect notions regarding strictures are that lower esophageal sphincter is destroyed in these patients and patients with stricture have an ulcer diathesis with hypersecretion of gastric acid. Many peptic strictures are termed undilatable and yet with careful bougienage can be dilated, especially intraoperatively, with the esophagus on the stretch to eliminate tortuosity.

The unfortunate term "short esophagus" with an attenuated intrathoracic stomach and an undilatable stricture has led to surgical treatment of these strictures by complex and formidable operations, which frequently include gastric resection or esophageal resection with a variety of reconstructions and plastic operations on the stricture. The mortality and morbidity rates in these operations range from as high as 10 to 15 per cent. In addition, few of these procedures corrected the underlying problem of reflux of gastric contents, which is the sine qua non for the development of a peptic or alkaline esophageal stricture.

In 1970 we reported our experience with 37 patients with advanced strictures treated with a simplified antireflux procedure.[6] Following successful antireflux procedures, these strictures and ulcers opened up with surprising rapidity. Dilatation was done during surgery and was required in less than half of the patients postoperatively. There was one fatality from a myocardial infarction and the five-year follow-up indicated an excellent result in 85 per cent of patients.

A representative patient in the reported series had a stricture of the midesophagus with a deep penetrating ulcer shown in Figure 10–1. She had been unable to swallow solid food for three years and had been told that she had an undilatable stricture with a short esophagus. At operation, however, with the esophagus straightened and tortuosity eliminated, bougies could be passed and the stricture was dilated. An antireflux procedure was done and three weeks postoperatively a repeat upper gastointestinal x-ray showed the stricture to be opened. This patient was done in 1970 and remains well, swallowing all solid food, and now has a normal upper GI series. Figure 10–2 shows a type of composite study that was done in 10 patients. All 10 studies showed that the peptic stricture occurred at the squamocolumnar junction. There was ulceration at this point and the esophagus from the level of the stricture down was lined with glandular epithelium, with or without parietal cells. In Figure 10–2 it can be seen that reflux was corrected and a high-pressure zone indicating a competent barrier to reflux was located below the diaphragm. Figure 10–3 shows a stricture high in the esophagus. This patient was also treated by surgery and dilatation, and three months later (Fig. 10–4) the upper GI series showed almost complete disappearance of the stricture, and the pH and pressure study showed

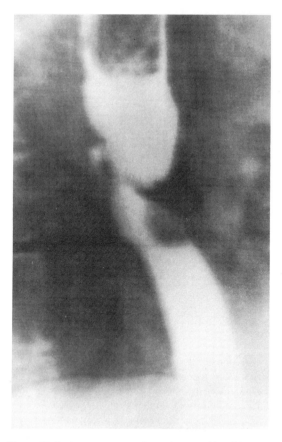

Figure 10–1. A very narrow stricture is seen with a deep penetrating ulcer in a patient considered to have an undilatable stricture and short esophagus. This patient was treated with a simplified antireflux procedure.

complete correction of reflux with a good high-pressure zone below the diaphragm. This patient remains well 18 years following operation.

The close association between barrier pressure and correction of reflux is shown in a 14-year-old patient who was operated upon for severe stricture (Fig. 10–5). The postoperative LESP was only 9 mm Hg, and reflux was not corrected. The stricture persisted. The patient was reoperated and the only parameter which was changed was that the barrier pressure was raised to 25 mm Hg and reflux was corrected. The stricture healed within two months, and the patient remains well 13 years after operation (Fig. 10–6). This patient clearly illustrates the point that unless the antireflux procedure is effective, the stricture indeed will not heal. It is this failure to correct reflux that has led many surgeons to the conclusion that only a resection will answer the problem in the patient with a peptic stricture. It is obvious that a technique that does

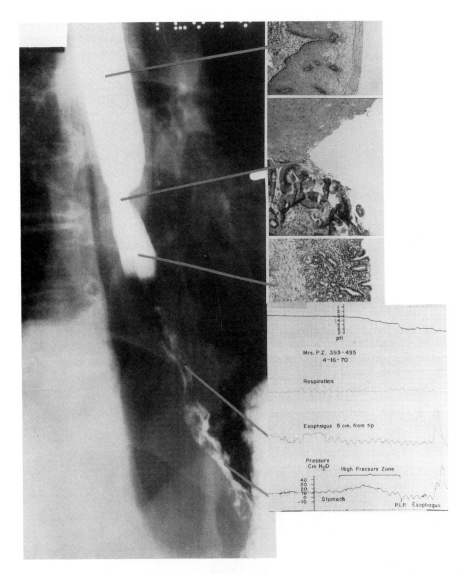

Figure 10–2. A composite postoperative study done in the patient shown in Figure 10–1 three weeks following surgery. The previous stricture has been dilated and an antireflux procedure done. Reflux has been corrected as evidenced by the pH and pressure study and the stricture has opened up. The patient remains well 16 years following surgery. In all the composite studies done on patients with reflux strictures, the stricture is shown to occur at the squamocolumnar junction with columnar lining of the lower esophagus.

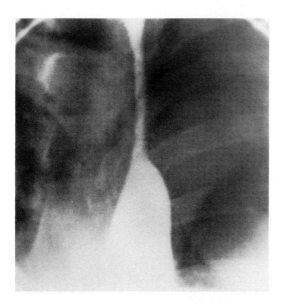

Figure 10–3. A very dense stricture high above the aortic arch treated by simplified antireflux procedure.

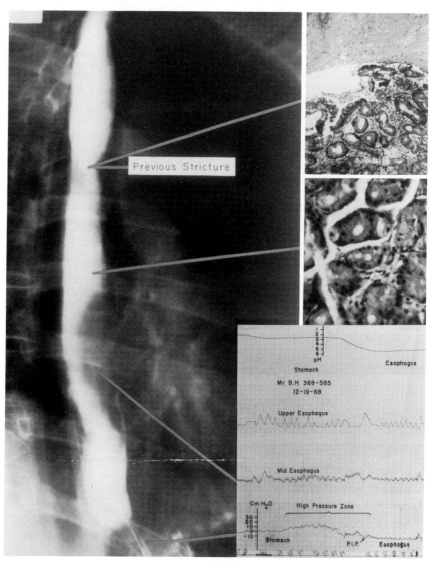

Figure 10–4. Composite study done one month postoperatively on patient shown in Figure 10–3. The previous stricture above the aortic arch has healed and reflux has been corrected as shown on the pH tracing.

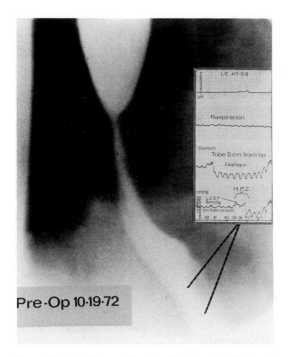

Figure 10–5. A 16-year-old male who had a simplified anti-reflux procedure for a very tight midesophageal stricture. The sphincter pressure was raised to only 9 mm Hg, which is inadequate, and reflux was not corrected. The stricture persisted.

not correct reflux will indeed fail to heal the stricture.

The findings of our original study have been confirmed by an experience now of 231 patients in whom antireflux procedures have been done. Based on these findings and supported by additional composite studies, our concepts of esophageal stricture is illustrated in Figure 10–7. This diagram shows that a stricture occurs at the squamocolumnar junction with the tubular esophagus below the stricture having all the manometric characteristics of the esophagus, even though lined with gastric epithelium. A small hiatal hernia is almost always present. The sphincter is at the GE junction just above the diaphragm and can be brought below the diaphragm without undue tension on the esophagus. The GE junction can be anchored to the preaortic fascia, and the GE barrier pressure can be increased to the point where reflux can be corrected. This experience clearly shows that when a surgeon is faced with a reflux stricture of the esophagus, rather than subject the patient to a formidable resection, a simplified approach should be considered. The simplified approach has a lower mortality and morbidity rate and a high rate of satisfaction.

This original report created a great deal of controversy and misunderstanding, but since the report, the majority of surgeons have abandoned re-

section of the stricture with its increased risk for a simplified antireflux procedure and dilatation.

Our own experience has expanded, and we recently reported[7] 170 patients undergoing antireflux operations with dilatation for stricture. We analyzed 160 of these patients with a mean follow-up of 47 months (range, 6 to 240 months), and we indicated that the consensus in the conflict about surgical management of peptic esophageal stricture presently favors conservative antireflux procedure with dilatation rather than resection. However, emphasis is now shifting to the controversy of conservative surgical treatment versus medical management with dilatation alone. An analysis of the effect of the timing of surgery on outcome was done. The patients were divided into three groups. Group 1 underwent antireflux surgery following at most one preoperative dilatation and no previous esophageal surgery. Group 2 had at least one previous esophageal operation prior to remedial surgery. Group 3 had more than one preoperative dilatation but no previous esophageal surgery.

The results (good, fair, or poor) were evaluated by one investigator blinded to pH and manometric measurements. Patients with good results were asymptomatic or had frequent minimal dysphagia not requiring postoperative treatment or at most a single dilatation. Fair results occurred in patients with slight symptomatic improvement but still requiring frequent dilatation or antireflux therapy. Poor results were obtained in patients with no improvement or worsening or symptoms requiring frequent dilatation or reoperation. Fair and poor results were combined as poor for analysis or variables when the number of patients in this group of patients was small.

The timing of esophageal surgery significantly affected the result. There were 107 patients in group 1. There were 90 per cent good, 9 per cent fair, and 1 per cent poor results. In the 31 patients in group 2 there were 52 per cent good, 23 per cent fair, and 25 per cent poor results. Twenty-two group 3 patients[7] showed 45 per cent good, 23 per cent fair, and 32 per cent poor results.

This study suggests that patients undergoing primary repair without multiple previous dilatations have a much better long-term result than patients who have had multiple dilatations or who had previous surgery. It is interesting that the patients with multiple dilatations fared worse than the patients who had had previous surgery. There is no doubt that multiple dilatations traumatize the esophagus, leading to periesophagitis and compromise of the esophageal motility.

The introduction of intraoperative manometry had a beneficial effect on results. Prior to intraoperative manometry, 71 per cent of 69 patients

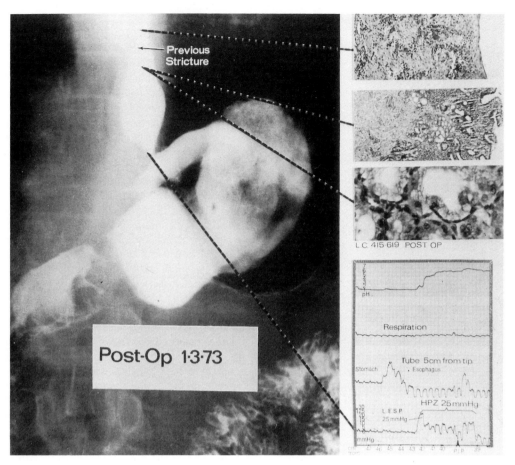

Figure 10–6. The patient shown in Figure 10–5 has been reoperated upon and the sphincter pressure was raised to 25 mm Hg; reflux has been corrected as demonstrated on the pH tracing, with the previous stricture healed. The patient remains well 13 years after surgery.

had good results. After intraoperative manometry, 85 per cent of 91 patients had good results (p <0.05). The presence of postoperative reflux evaluated in 63 patients had a detrimental effect on results.

The presence of Barrett's esophagus had no effect on clinical outcome. Thirty-seven patients had histologic proof of Barrett's mucosa lining the esophagus. The results in these patients were 76 per cent good and 24 per cent poor. This result was the same as is in those patients without columnar epithelium. Age and sex of the patient had no effect on the results.

Operative complications included dysphagia in 19 per cent of patients. Nine per cent had minimal dysphagia requiring either single dilatation or no treatment. Ten per cent had moderate dysphagia requiring more than one dilatation. The splenectomy rate was 10 per cent, half of these occurring in group 2 patients with previous operations and extensive abdominal adhesions. Pulmonary complications occurred in 3 per cent, gastroesophageal

fistula in 1 per cent, bolus obstruction in 1 patient, subdiaphragmatic abscess in 1 per cent, and miscellaneous complications in 3 per cent. The operative mortality rate was 1.7 per cent. One patient died of an intracranial hemorrhage, one had a myocardial infarction, a third patient had organ failure secondary to intra-abdominal sepsis, and a fourth patient had a gastroesophageal leak. This patient had had two previous failed Nissen fundoplications.

Resection has been reserved for patients, as seen in Figure 10–8. This patient had had multiple dilatations and had been undergoing self-dilatation for 18 years, finally perforating the esophagus, which was entirely destroyed. She required an esophagogastric anastomosis and has done well. Another patient is shown in Figure 10–9. This patient was done as an emergency for perforation of a giant ulcer into the posterior portion of the pericardial sac. This patient also had an esophagogastric anastomosis to the upper third of the esophagus and represents the only survivor of an

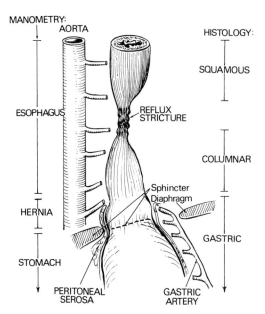

Figure 10–7. A synthesis of the current concept of peptic strictures is shown. A small hiatal hernia results in an incompetent gastroesophageal junction, which allows reflux to damage the esophagus. The squamous mucosa is replaced by creeping substitution by columnar epithelium so that the stricture may rise all the way to the aortic arch. The esophagus is not shortened and the tubular portion of the gullet from the stricture to the stomach has all the manometric characteristics of the esophagus.

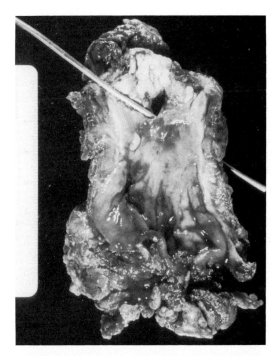

Figure 10–8. Postoperative resected specimen from a 71-year-old patient who had been undergoing self-dilatation as well as dilatations in a number of medical centers for 18 years. The esophagus was perforated during self-dilatation and emergency esophagogastric resection was done. Note that the stricture is at the squamocolumnar junction and the large perforation is at the area of narrowing. This patient remains well five years after operation.

esophagopericardial fistula of whom we are aware. Only in these patients with destroyed esophagus have we employed resection. We have used colon in those with high perforation but prefer the stomach for esophageal replacement. We employ a right thoracotomy incision and do an extensive inkwelling or invagination of the esophagus into the stomach to prevent reflux or anastomose the stomach to the esophagus in the neck.

Dilatation combined with an antireflux procedure is now employed by a number of surgeons throughout the world, including Hayward,[8] Herrington et al.,[9] Moghissi,[10] and many others. It should certainly be considered by any surgeon encountering a peptic stricture before undertaking a large resectional procedure.

■ *Investigations*

Prior to any form of therapy, adequate investigations must include an upper GI x-ray to define the anatomy of the stricture and the presence or absence of a hiatal hernia. A pH and pressure study is necessary to document sphincter pressure and the presence of GE reflux as well as the presence or absence of secondary or primary motility dis-

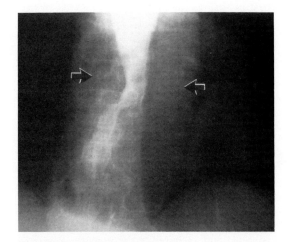

Figure 10–9. Barium roentgenogram of a patient with a giant gastric ulcer having eroded into the posterior wall of the pericardium. Emergency esophageal resection followed by esophagogastrostomy has resulted in the only survivor of an esophagopericardial fistula of which we are aware.

orders, which would not benefit from an antireflux procedure. It is imperative that carcinoma be ruled out in any patient with presumed benign peptic stricture of the esophagus by endoscopy with brush cytologic examination and multiple biopsies, which must be repeated if the tissue is not diagnostic.

■ Principles of Surgical Management

The most important concept in this simplified approach is that the GE junction can be reduced into the abdomen without tension in virtually all patients and that the esophagus is, in fact, not shortened. In the past, the stricture was often assumed to be present at the GE junction, and this resulted in endless arguments about where the esophagus ends and the stomach begins. However, it is now well documented that the stricture occurs at the squamocolumnar junction. The lower esophageal sphincter is the landmark between the stomach and the esophagus, just as the pyloric sphincter separates the stomach and the duodenum.

■ Technique

Once the diagnosis of benign esophageal stricture is established, dilatation is performed with one of the many presently available esophageal dilators, usually prior to surgery. At surgery the left chest as well as the abdomen is prepared in case the stomach is fixed by adhesions in the thorax. An upper abdominal incision is made and the upper hand retractor is placed. At the time of surgery dilatation is repeated if necessary, either antegrade or retrograde. If the stricture is difficult to dilate from above, a high gastrostomy is done, which allows for added information from direct inspection and palpation of the stricture as well as dilatation.

Following dilatation the esophagus is further freed by blunt and sharp dissection in the posterior mediastinum. The GE junction is brought down into the abdomen. The hiatus is closed snugly about the esophagus. Since correction of reflux now becomes the principal aim of surgery, meticulous care is taken to achieve this end. The GE junction is calibrated and anchored to the preaortic fascia by the technique described in the chapter on surgery for GE reflux. Calibration is aided by intraoperative manometrics, which assures the surgeon that an adequate barrier to reflux is achieved. The GE junc-

tion is fixed permanently to the preaortic fascia without tension.

In those patients with low-lying strictures or patients who have had multiple dilatations in whom the GE junction is grossly compromised, we have recently added the valve restoration technique.[11,12] The technique consists of viewing the musculomucosal valve at the angle of His through a gastrostomy, which has already been done to enable the retrograde dilatation. The valve is grasped and extended caudally, and sutures are placed in the anterior and posterior edges of this valve to fix it in a lengthened position in order to give further protection to reflux and strengthen the antireflux barrier. This technique is described in detail in the chapter on surgery for reflux esophagitis and Chapter 13 on Failed Antireflux Procedures.

Postoperatively, if the patient is unable to swallow solids with ease, dilatations are performed and an additional biopsy can be obtained to correlate the level of the stricture with the histologic lining of the esophagus. Pullout pressures of the LES are determined when the nasogastric tube with the attached manometric catheter is removed. Postoperative pH and pressure studies are performed on all patients approximately three months later to assess for reflux and to measure the pressure in the lower esophageal sphincter.

■ Results

In the past 20 years 231 patients have been treated with this simplified technique of esophageal dilatation and posterior fixation with cardial calibration. The treatment of the last 78 patients was aided by intraoperative manometry.[13–15] Our follow-up of these patients is by personal and telephone interview, along with pH and pressure or upper GI x-rays whenever possible, and averages three and one-half years. Patients in this series were previously reported.[6] In those patients who have had a primary repair without multiple previous dilatations good results have been obtained in 90 per cent of patients.

We feel that our results indicate that the primary surgical procedure for a reflux stricture offers the best hope for preventing further reflux and allows the stricture to heal. Intraoperative manometry provides a useful method for intraoperative objective assessment of the efficacy of the surgery.

■ Conclusion

Our clinicopathologic analysis clearly demonstrates that peptic strictures are located at the squamocolumnar junction superior to the lower esophageal sphincter. The esophagus in these patients is not shortened. The lower esophageal sphincter had not been destroyed. Once the LES is returned to its normal location below the diaphragm and calibrated, it functions efficiently with a normal pressure. Once the sliding hiatus hernia has been corrected and the antireflux barrier has been restored, reflux will cease and the esophagitis and ulcerations will heal. The stricture following adequate dilatation will not recur if the insult (i.e., GE reflux) causing it to form can be stopped.

For the past 20 years we have used this simplified technique in our patients with good results. There seems to be little need for a high-risk procedure such as esophageal resection with gastrointestinal reconstruction in any patient with a benign peptic esophageal stricture except for those unfortunate patients with the most severe and recurrent stricture following multiple dilatations and failed antireflux surgery.

■ REFERENCES

1. Barrett NR: Chronic peptic ulcer of the oesophagus lined with gastric mucous membrane. Thorax, 8:87, 1953.
2. Barrett NR: Chronic peptic ulcer of the esophagus and esophagitis. Br J Surg, 38:175, 1950.
3. Allison PR, Johnstone AS: The esophagus lined with gastric mucous membrane. Thorax, 8:87, 1953.
4. Naef A, Savary M, Ozzello L: Columnar-lined lower esophagus, an acquired lesion with malignant predisposition. J Thorac Cardiovasc Surg, 70:826–835, 1975.
5. Mossberg SM: The columnar lined esophagus (Barrett's syndrome): An acquired condition. Gastroenterology, 50:671, 1966.
6. Hill LD, Gelfand M, Bauermeister D: Simplified management of reflux esophagitis with stricture. Ann Surg, 172:638–651, 1970.
7. Mercer CD, Hill LD: Surgical management of peptic esophageal stricture: Twenty-year experience. J Thorac Cardiovasc Surg, 91:371–378, 1986.
8. Hayward J: The treatment of fibrous stricture of the esophagus associated with hiatal hernia. Thorax, 16:45, 1961.
9. Herrington JL Jr, Wright RS, Edwards WH, Sawyers JL: Conservative surgical treatment of reflux esophagitis and esophageal stricture. Ann Surg, 181:552, 1975.
10. Moghissi K: Conservative surgery in reflux strictures of the oesophagus associated with hiatal hernia. Br J Surg, 66:221–225, 1979.
11. Thor K, Kozarek RA, Mercer CD, Hill LD: Valvuloplasty, a new surgical antireflux procedure (abstract). Gastroenterology, 90, 1986.
12. Thor K, Hill LD, Mercer CD, Kozarek RA: Reappraisal of the flap valve mechanism: A study of a new valvuloplasty procedure in cadavers. Ann Surg, 1986 (submitted for publication).
13. Hill LD: Intraoperative measurement of lower esophageal sphincter pressure. In Stipa S, Belsey RHR, Moraldi A (Eds): Medical and Surgical Problems of the Esophagus. Serona Symposium No. 43. London, Academic Press, Inc., 1981, pp 106–109.
14. Hill LD, Velasco N, Russell COH, Ilves R: Results of Hill antireflux operation before and after intraoperative manometry. Abstr Gastroenterol 80(5):1174, May 1981.
15. Hill LD: Intraoperative measurement of lower esophageal sphincter pressure. J Thorac Cardiovasc Surg, 75:378–382, 1978.

11

Paraesophageal Hernia

C. Dale Mercer ▪ *N. Velasco*
Lucius D. Hill

Paraesophageal hiatus hernia is a rare condition which can result in life-threatening complications. This form of hernia occurs in approximately 2 per cent of patients for whom surgery is required for diaphragmatic hernias and in less than 1 per cent of all patients having a hiatus hernia. In this condition, stomach and at times other viscera herniate alongside the esophagus through the esophageal hiatus. However, the lower esophageal sphincter lies in its normal intra-abdominal position, fixed firmly by the posterior phrenoesophageal fascial complex. The location of the gastroesophageal (GE) junction below the diaphragm separates the true paraesophageal hernia from the two other types of hernias through the esophageal hiatus. In the other two types, the sliding hernia and the combined sliding and paraeosphageal hernia, the GE junction slides into the posterior mediastinum above the diaphragm. In these patients reflux is usually present.

Paraesophageal hernias, being similar in all respects to hernias in general, produce symptoms as a consequence of their size. They may contain viscera which can incarcerate or strangulate. As well, this form of hernia is repaired by reducing the contents of the hernia, excising the hernia sac, and closing the neck of the hernia. Occasional confusion occurs with the definition of the term paraesophageal hernia. A parahiatal hernia has been reported by a few authors. This type of hernia occurs through a hole in the diaphragm separated from the esophageal hiatus by a segment of diaphragm. This hernia is even rarer than the parae-

sophageal type.[1,2] We have questioned the occurrence of such congenital herniation of the stomach through a separate opening in the diaphragm and have been unable to find any actual operative photographs delineating any segment of the diaphragm lying between the hernia and the esophagus.[3] In addition, in all of our operative experience repairing diaphragmatic hernias as well as examining many cadaver dissections, at no time have we been able to identify this form of hernia.

In paraesophageal hernia the esophagus lies in its normal position, fixed intra-abdominally by the firm posterior phrenoesophageal ligament, a structure consisting of fibroelastic tissue extending from the esophageal wall onto the hiatal rim of the diaphragm. Anteriorly and laterally the components of the phrenoesophageal complex are very attenuated and along with the peritoneum form the sac of the herniation. In this form of hernia the stomach rolls up into the posterior mediastinum anterior to the esophagus such that the greater curve lies superiorly. However, the gastroesophageal junction lies in its normal intra-abdominal position. This anatomic arrangement (Fig. 11–1) allows for competency of the cardia as documented by normal pH and pressure studies and therefore the absence of gastroesophagel reflux symptoms in these patients. As these hernias enlarge, greater amounts of gastrointestinal tract may become incarcerated in the chest. At times the entire first portion of the duodenum may ascend into the thorax (Fig. 11–2). As more viscera becomes incarcerated in the chest, the esophageal hiatus widens considerably and at this

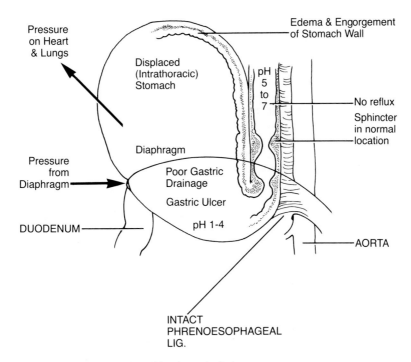

Figure 11–1. Abnormal function in paraesophageal hernia, sagittal view.

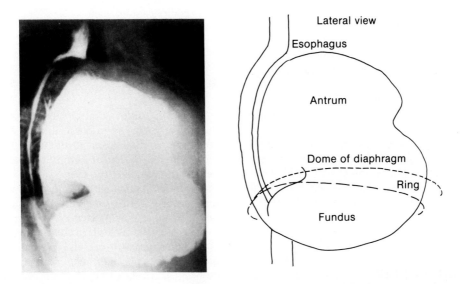

Figure 11–2. Lateral view of massive paraesophageal hernia showing the esophagus in its normal location with the gastroesophageal junction below the diaphragm fixed posteriorly. The stomach has rolled up through a large ring adjacent to the esophagus. The first portion of the duodenum is in the thorax.

point with incarceration in the chest the posterior phrenoesophageal component may become lax, allowing the gastroesophageal junction to slide up into the chest and resulting in a combined paraesophageal and sliding hiatus hernia. Pearson et al. have identified, in 53 cases of massive hiatal hernia with incarceration, that this situation is always present and implies the need for an adequate antireflux operation.[4] It is imperative to define preoperatively whether there is a pure paraesophageal hernia or a combined sliding and paraesophageal hernia. Measurement of pH and pressure may be difficult to perform because of the acute angulation of the GE junction at the diaphragm. If reflux is present, the hernia must be corrected as a sliding hernia. The repair must include an antireflux procedure.

■ *Natural History*

Paraesophageal hernias present a benign course until the patient reaches middle age, at which time symptoms of postprandial distress, retching, and a sensation of nausea after eating become common. Patients may also experience substernal pressure after eating, presumably related to a dilated intrathoracic gastric segment. This pressure is often relieved with belching or vomiting. Patients do not complain of gastroesophageal reflux. Symptoms are often well tolerated until one of the following complications occurs: ulceration in the herniated portion of the stomach, hemorrhage, volvulus and obstruction, or pulmonary complications such as aspiration.

In our reported series there has been a 30 per cent incidence of chronic bleeding secondary to gastric ulceration within the intrathoracic segment of stomach.[5] The ulceration is caused by poor gastric emptying and by trauma from torsion of the gastric wall and pressure from the diaphragm. Management of this ulceration mandates surgical correction of the problem because the underlying pathophysiologic defect is mechanical. Antacid therapy will not allow healing of the ulcer because the underlying problem is interference with gastric drainage and continued trauma to the gastric wall, interfering with the blood and lymphatic supply of the stomach.

■ *Complications*

The most feared complication is volvulus and strangulation with infarction of the contained vis-

cus and possible perforation into the mediastinum, resulting in mediastinitis. These complications often result in symptoms diagnosed initially as myocardial infarction or some other major intrathoracic catastrophe.

Other complications include pulmonary conditions varying from dyspnea to pneumonia. Dyspnea may be particularly evident following ingestion of a heavy meal, whereas complications of pneumonitis, basilar bronchiectasis, and lung abscess occur because of repeated episodes of aspiration. Aspiration occurs because of the obstruction of the distal esophagus as well as the fact that the pressure effects of the large hernia in the chest make effective coughing difficult.

It is of interest that most of the patients seen by us with massive paraesophageal hiatus hernias were known to have had the hernia for many years prior to surgery. As is generally the case, only a few had symptoms to suggest complications. However, both the physicians and surgeons caring for these patients felt that the condition was harmless as long as it was asymptomatic despite the frequent reports of morbidity and even death with associated complications.

It would appear that the very striking radiologic changes usually present in frail and elderly patients deter many surgeons from operating. Unfortunately, this converts a technically easy, elective procedure with low morbidity and minimal mortality rates to a very complicated emergency operation with great risks once complications develop. Skinner et al. documented a series of 21 patients who were treated medically because of minimal symptoms. In this series six patients died with complications such as strangulation, perforation, or hemorrhage.[6]

■ *Diagnosis*

The diagnosis of paraesophageal hernia is frequently suspected from plain films of the chest in which an air-fluid level posterior to the heart is seen (Fig. 11–3). Upper gastrointestinal series are helpful in evaluating the extent of the stomach involved in the hernia and also provide some information about gastric emptying. Infrequently, barium enema examination may show part of the transverse colon making up the herniated viscus. One should perform pH and pressure studies to determine whether one is dealing with a true paraesophageal hernia in which there is a competent cardia and no reflux or with a combined or sliding hernia in which gastroesophageal reflux may be present. The operation in this latter case would be

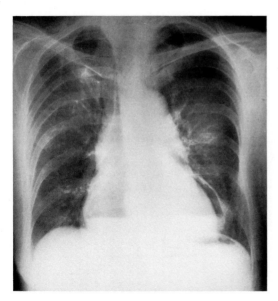

Figure 11–3. Chest x-ray showing a paraesophageal hernia behind the heart with a large air-fluid level.

an antireflux repair rather than simple reduction of the hernia, as is the case for paraesophageal hernia.

■ Treatment

The presence of a paraesophageal hiatus hernia alone is a sufficient indication for surgery provided that the risks of elective transabdominal or transthoracic surgery are not prohibitive. Episodes of incarceration, bleeding, or obstruction are obvious indications for immediate surgery. There has been a reluctance to operate on these patients, presumably because of previous poor results in patients who have had sliding hiatal hernias. This lack of a clear understanding of the natural history of this condition by physicians who do not routinely deal with these patients has deterred clinicians from recommending surgery for paraesophageal hernia. However, in contrast to the results of surgical intervention in sliding hiatus hernia, repair of paraesophageal hiatus hernia has met with almost complete success in the elective case. If the condition is accurately diagnosed and the operation is performed properly, there should be few, if any, recurrences.

■ Surgical Technique

Once the surgeon understands the pathologic anatomy of patients with paraesophageal hernia,

the surgeon will realize that it is a technical mistake to free the esophagus circumferentially from the posterior part of the hiatus. As described above, the posterior phrenoesophageal ligament is intact and functioning properly, maintaining the lower esophageal sphincter in its normal location within the abdominal cavity. Any dissection posterior to the esophagus will disrupt this ligament, allowing the terminal sphincter to migrate into the chest, creating an iatrogenic sliding hiatus hernia.

The paraesophageal hernia may be approached either transthoracically or transabdominally. The technique is essentially the same for both routes. Using the transabdominal approach, the surgeon may be surprised to find that no portion of the stomach is present within the abdomen (Fig. 11–4), but a transthoracic approach would reveal the inverted stomach visible in the posterior mediastinum. The hernial contents are carefully and usually easily reduced by slow manual traction. Once all the abdominal contents have been replaced intra-abdominally, the sac of the hernia is excised from the posterior mediastinum by a combination of blunt and sharp dissection. Re-expansion of the lungs with reduction of the hernia will cause the hernial sac to collapse down into the abdomen, making the dissection easier. The dissection of this sac may be difficult if it has been there for a long time and is firmly adherent to mediastinal tissue. In this situation excision of the majority of the sac and closure of the hernial orifice should be performed, but dissection of the entire sac is not necessary.

Once the hernia is reduced, it is advisable for the surgeon to reassess the problem. Figure 11–5 shows the arrangement in a true paraesophageal hernia. The esophagus lies posteriorly, fixed in its normal position. If an intraoperative pressure study is done, it will show the sphincter lying in its usual location, functioning normally. It has been interesting to us that the sphincter, which is not in contact with the preaortic fascia, functions normally, especially because there is a sharp angle at the gastroesophageal junction representing an accentuated valve mechanism so that in true paraesophageal hernia, both the sphincter and the valve mechanism are preserved. If manometric studies show that the sphincter lies in the thorax, the surgeon then is dealing with a sliding hernia, and the usual antireflux procedure should be done. If, however, the sphincter is in its normal location, it is a technical mistake to tear down the posterior attachments.

The diaphragmatic opening is then closed with interrupted heavy nonabsorbable sutures with Teflon pledgets. It has been our experience that the diaphragmatic tissues are strong enough to hold

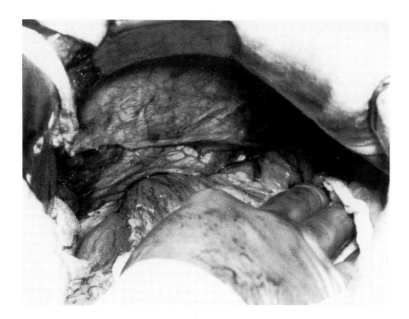

Figure 11–4. At surgery, the entire stomach is up in the thorax. Only the first portion of the duodenum can be seen protruding from the enlarged esophageal hiatus.

sutures well, even in the elderly patient in whom there is a huge hernial orifice. We have not utilized Marlex or other foreign material to close the opening because the diaphragmatic rim is lax enough to come together well. The crural muscles are reapproximated. This should be done anterior to the esophagus so as not to disrupt any of the posterior attachments. This closure should be snug enough to allow a surgeon's index finger to be inserted alongside the esophagus in which a Levine tube is present. These sutures in the crura and in the anterior portion of the phrenoesophageal membrane should be placed in such a way that the lower esophageal sphincter is not under any distracting pressures that would prevent closure and promote gastroesophageal reflux.

Fixation sutures should be placed along the lesser curvature down to the preaortic fascia to prevent a sliding hernia from developing later. In Figure 11–6 the completed repair shows the large opening in the diaphragm closed anterior to the esophagus. Several fixation sutures are placed along the lesser curve to the preaortic fascia. With a mixed type paraesophageal and sliding hernia a formal antireflux repair and sphincter calibration are necessary. Gastrointestinal hemorrhage from bleeding ulcer can be repaired easily by simple suturing of the ulcer. An antireflux operation utilizing vagotomy and pyloroplasty is not necessary in these patients because the ulceration is not on the basis of an acid pepsin mechanism. There have

Figure 11–5. After the paraesophageal hernia is reduced, the esophagus can be seen posteriorly fixed in its normal location, functioning normally. The gastroesophageal angle and flap valve are also intact.

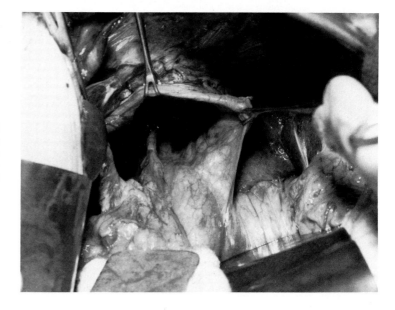

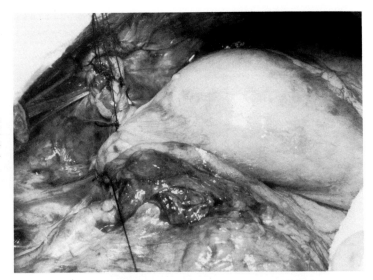

Figure 11–6. The completed operation showing the large esophageal hiatus closed anterior to the esophagus. Fixation sutures are placed from the lesser curve to the preaortic fascia to prevent a subsequent herniation.

been no recurrences in the uncomplicated cases of paraesophageal hernia or in those with ulceration and hemorrhage in the incarcerated stomach.

■ Incarcerated Paraesophageal Hernia

In a previous report[7] we indicated that around 30 per cent of the patients with paraesophageal hernia seen in our experience develop incarceration. Incarceration represents a surgical emergency

that often is not appreciated. Review of the history of patients with incarcerated paraesophageal hernia shows that they have had the hernia for many years. During this time the patient may develop substernal pain and pressure or a gastric ulcer from the poorly drained stomach. It appears that as long as the entire stomach is in the chest, incarceration does not occur.

The first step in the development of an incarcerated hernia is the prolapse of the distended fundus into the abdomen (Fig. 11–7). With further distention of the antrum and the fundus, the patient develops obstruction at multiple points. The mid-

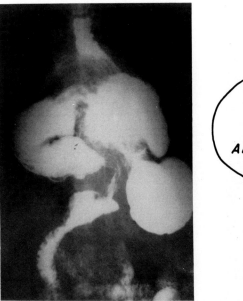

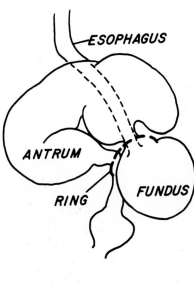

Figure 11–7. The first step in incarceration of a paraesophageal hernia is prolapse of the fundus into the abdomen through the diaphragmatic opening.

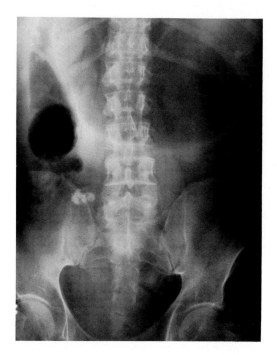

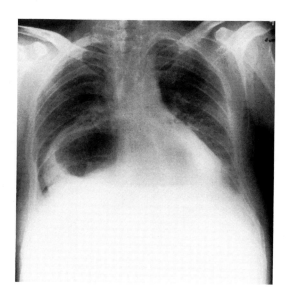

Figure 11–9. Plain film of the chest and abdomen showing a large incarcerated paraesophageal hernia with the antrum grossly distended in the thorax. The patient is in shock.

Figure 11–8. The same patient as shown in Figure 11–7 with a flat plate of the abdomen showing the grossly distended fundus in the abdomen. This could not be decompressed with a nasogastric tube and required emergent surgery.

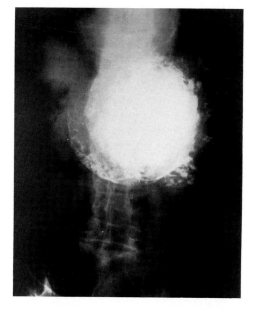

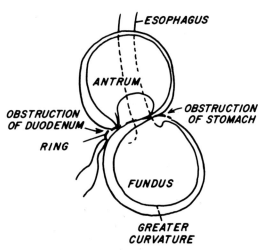

Figure 11–10. The fundus prolapsed into the abdomen becomes distended as does the antrum, producing a dumbbell-shaped shadow with incarceration of both the antrum and the fundus of the stomach, with the fundus being in the abdomen and the antrum in the thorax.

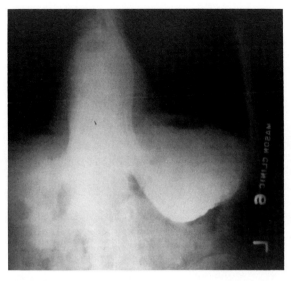

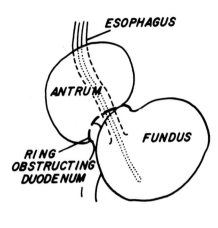

Figure 11–11. Further distention of the fundus and antrum leads to incarceration and obstruction of the distal esophagus, the midportion of the stomach, and the first portion of the duodenum by the enlarged esophageal hiatus.

portion of the stomach, the terminal esophagus, and the first portion of the duodenum are all obstructed by the ring of the diaphragm. A flat plate of the abdomen will show the enormously dilated fundus filling the entire upper abdomen (Fig. 11–8). A concomitant chest x-ray will show the enormously dilated antrum behind the heart, displacing the thoracic viscera (Fig. 11–9). Barium swallow will clearly show the dumbbell-shaped appearance of the stomach in both the chest and the abdomen (Fig. 11–10).

The pathophysiology of an incarcerated hernia is shown in Figure 11–11. In essence, there are two closed-loop obstructions as well as obstruction of the esophagus and the duodenum. At this point, the patient is in serious distress and represents a surgical emergency. If this goes unrecognized, both the antrum and the fundus are subject to gangrene and perforation. If a nasogastric tube can be inserted past the GE junction into the fundus, the stomach can be decompressed. Following the rush of gas and gastric juice, the patient will improve

rapidly and can be prepared for an elective operation that carries very low morbidity and mortality rates. If a nasogastric tube cannot be passed beyond the gastroesophageal junction because of the severe compression, then the patient should be taken to surgery immediately.

At operation the enormously dilated and nearly gangrenous fundus will be seen in the abdomen, or if the thoracic approach is used, the dilated antrum is seen in the chest. It may be necessary to divide the rim of the diaphragm and to do a gastrostomy in order to decompress the markedly distended stomach. Following reduction of the hernia it is again important to determine whether the surgeon is dealing with a pure paraesophageal hernia, in which case repair that is described for elective repair of paraesophageal hernia is indicated. If the gastroesophageal junction is in the thorax and the surgeon is dealing with a sliding hernia, an antireflux procedure is then indicated, along with closure of the large opening in the diaphragm.

Table 11–1 shows the analysis of 23 patients

Table 11–1. RESULTS OF TREATMENT IN COMPLICATED AND UNCOMPLICATED PARAESOPHAGEAL HERNIAS

Type of Hernia	Number of Patients (%)	Treatment Results
Uncomplicated	13 (40%)	Excellent; no deaths, no recurrences
Complicated	10 (30%)	Excellent; no deaths, no recurrences, all ulcers healed
Volvulus, incarceration, obstruction, decompression	6 (18%)	Good; no deaths, 15% morbidity rate, no recurrences
Not decompressed	4 (12%)	Two preoperative deaths (mortality rate, 50%), two survivors
Total	23 (100%)	

treated for paraesophageal hernia and dramatically shows the difference in outcome in patients who are diagnosed early and have an elective repair with no complications or recurrence, as opposed to those patients who are diagnosed late and develop serious complications. In the four patients in whom decompression was not possible, two died before reaching the operating room with cardiac arrest and two were salvaged by removal of the near gangrenous stomach. This experience clearly underscores the fact that incarcerated paraesophageal hernia has a high mortality rate. It follows that paraesophageal hernia is subject to serious complications, and if the patient is a reasonable risk for surgery, elective repair of the paraesophageal hernia is clearly indicated.

■ *Summary*

True paraesophageal hernia is a rare condition and must be clearly differentiated from sliding hernia and the combined paraesophageal and sliding hernia. A large paraesophageal hernia presents the threat of incarceration and strangulation, which has considerable mortality and morbidity rates. In the good risk patient repair should result in very low risk and a very low long-term recurrence rate of less than 1 per cent. Therefore, a paraesophageal hernia in a patient who is a reasonable risk for surgery should be repaired.

■ REFERENCES

1. MacDougall JT, Abbott AC, Goodhard TK: Herniation through congenital diaphragmatic defects in adults. Can J Surg, 6:302, 1963.
2. Sweet RH: Thoracic Surgery. 2nd ed. Philadelphia, W.B. Saunders, 1954.
3. Hill LD, Tobias JA: Paraesophageal hernia. Arch Surg, 96:735, 1968.
4. Pearson FG, Cooper JD, Ilves R, Todd TRJ, Jamieson WRE: Massive hiatal hernia with incarceration: A report of 53 cases. Ann Thorac Surg, 35:45–51, 1983.
5. Hill LD, Mercer CD: Paraesophageal hernia. *In* JL Cameron (Ed): Current Surgical Therapy. Burlington, Ontario, B.C. Decker, Inc., 1984, pp 22–24.
6. Skinner DB, Belsey RHR, Russell PS: Surgical management of esophageal reflux and hiatus hernia—long term results with 1030 patients. J Thorac Cardiovasc Surg, 53:33, 1967.
7. Hill LD: Incarcerated paraesophageal hernia. A surgical emergency. Am J Surg, 126:286–291, 1973.

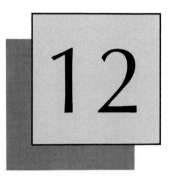

12

Barrett's Esophagus and Esophageal Adenocarcinoma

Brian J. Reid ∎ *Rodger C. Haggitt*
Cyrus E. Rubin

Barrett's esophagus is a condition in which the stratified squamous mucosa of the esophagus is replaced by a metaplastic columnar mucosa.[1-5] Barrett's esophagus develops as a complication in 10 to 12 per cent of patients with chronic gastroesophageal reflux and predisposes to the development of adenocarcinoma.[5-11] Although Barrett's esophagus can be associated with several clinical complications of gastroesophageal reflux, including benign peptic stricture,[1,8,12,13] esophageal ulceration,[1,8,14-16] nocturnal aspiration, and chronic obstructive pulmonary disease (COPD),[17] the predisposition to develop adenocarcinoma is responsible for the present intense clinical and research interest in this condition. In this chapter we will concentrate on the association of Barrett's esophagus with esophageal adenocarcinoma. Readers interested in more general information on Barrett's esophagus are referred to comprehensive reviews of the subject.[18-22]

∎ Definitions

Barrett's esophagus is usually defined by the presence of columnar mucosa proximal to the lower esophageal sphincter.[18,23] The length of columnar lining necessary to qualify as Barrett's esophagus has usually been set at 2 or 3 cm. This definition has several intrinsic difficulties. First, the exact relationship between the squamocolumnar junction and the lower esophageal sphincter is difficult to

determine; second, there may be short lengths of columnar mucosa within the esophagus in some normal individuals[24]; and third, such a definition based on a manometric landmark does not help the practicing gastroenterologist who relies on endoscopy to identify Barrett's esophagus. As will be explained later, we propose an alternate definition of Barrett's esophagus.

Although the normal esophagus may contain islands of gastric mucosa, these are most often located in the cervical region. These islands are usually attributed to embryonic rests of normal gastric epithelium and differ from Barrett's esophagus because they are separated from the stomach by a substantial length of squamous epithelium.[25] Although adenocarcinoma has rarely been reported in association with such islands, there is no evidence that they are associated with an increased risk of carcinoma.[10,25]

The literature on Barrett's esophagus has been confused by the multiplicity of names and definitions given to the three types of columnar mucosa said to be associated with it. This confusion is largely a semantic problem in the definition of metaplasia. This is especially important because it appears that only the metaplastic mucosa has a malignant potential in Barrett's esophagus, and its presence should therefore be the sine qua non for the diagnosis of Barrett's esophagus. One definition of metaplasia is the abnormal transformation of one fully differentiated mucosa into another type of fully differentiated mucosa normally seen lining another organ. By this definition normal gastric mucosa lining the tubular esophagus would be considered metaplastic. For example, fundic mucosa normally found in the proximal stomach might be considered metaplastic if found lining the tubular esophagus. Yet, careful study has shown that fundic mucosa occurred in only 16 of 287 biopsies of Barrett's tubular esophagus and that it was then confined to the distal 3 cm of tubular esophagus[26] where it may also be found in normal individuals without Barrett's esophagus. Most gastric fundic mucosa found in biopsies taken above the diaphragm originates in a hiatal hernia, whether or not the endoscopist has recognized the presence of the hernia. Hiatal hernia is stomach which has been displaced above the diaphragm; fundic mucosa is its normal lining and is therefore not metaplastic. Gastric cardiac mucosa is found frequently in the distal 3 cm of both normal and Barrett's tubular esophagus[24,26,27]; therefore, it, too, is not metaplastic in this location.

What about the columnar mucosa in tubular Barrett's esophagus proximal to the distal 3 cm? In our experience, most of this mucosa is completely different because it represents a special type of columnar mucosa, which contains a broad spectrum of mucus-secreting columnar cells that may be confused with intestinal mucosa. For this reason some observers consider this special epithelium to be ''intestinalized'' or to have undergone ''intestinal metaplasia.'' Electron microscopic studies of biopsies of this Barrett's specialized metaplasia suggest that it may be gastric in origin.[28] Presumably, it originates from multipotent gastric cells that grow proximally to replace the squamous mucosa that has been destroyed by acid peptic digestion during gastroesophageal reflux disease. *These displaced columnar cells meet a second definition of metaplasia, i.e., the transformation of normally differentiated epithelium to an abnormally differentiated one.*

Barrett's specialized metaplastic epithelium contains a spectrum of mucus-secreting cells with different morphologic features (Fig. 12–1). Goblet cells contain mucus that stains intensely with Alcian blue at pH 2.5. Other cells retain the configuration of gastric surface cells; some of these secrete a mucus that is Alcian blue positive, while others secrete clear mucus. Some cells have a partially developed brush border, but these cells are not fully intestinalized because they also contain mucous granules. Other cells resemble the cells of the mucous neck region and may represent mucous neck cells that migrated to the surface without differentiating. The common denominator is that all these epithelial cells contain secretory granules of mucus. Morphologically, there are all gradations

of change between the various cell types.[28] Proximal to the distal 3 cm of tubular Barrett's esophagus over 90 per cent of biopsies from columnar mucosa show Barrett's specialized metaplasia.[26,27] Fundic gland mucosa is almost never seen in such proximal biopsies, and pure cardiac gland mucosa is rare, although patches of cardiac gland mucosa can be found in areas of Barrett's specialized metaplastic epithelium.[26,27] Barrett's specialized metaplasia almost always involves the surface and foveoli or pits of the superficial or luminal portion of the mucosa. The specialized metaplasia can occupy the full thickness of the mucosa; alternatively, the basal half of the mucosa might be occupied by cardiac glands.[26,27] We reserve the diagnosis of Barrett's esophagus for patients whose biopsies show Barrett's specialized metaplastic epithelium in the tubular esophagus. Available data indicate that it is this epithelium that is associated with an increased risk of adenocarcinoma.[10,29–32]

■ *Clinical Features*

The usual clinical manifestations of Barrett's esophagus are those of gastroesophageal reflux or its complications. Thus, heartburn, regurgitation, dysphagia, and gastrointestinal bleeding are frequently reported in association with Barrett's esophagus.[18–21] Nocturnal aspiration of refluxed gastric contents and even COPD are less frequently recognized complications. Although reflux as measured by objective tests tends to be more severe in patients with Barrett's esophagus, heartburn may not be severe in such patients. In the largest study reported, 11 per cent of 1225 patients with chronic peptic esophagitis were found to have Barrett's esophagus on endoscopy.[6] In another preliminary report, 13 per cent of patients with uncomplicated gastroesophageal reflux were reported to have Barrett's esophagus.[33] Obviously the patients in both these series were selected on the basis of having sufficiently severe disease to require an endoscopy. The true prevalence of Barrett's esophagus in the population of patients with gastroesophageal reflux disease remains to be established.

Dysphagia in patients with Barrett's esophagus may be caused by benign peptic stricture, by carcinoma, or by an underlying motility disorder such as scleroderma.[34] Many benign peptic strictures of the esophagus occur in patients who have Barrett's esophagus—in one series, 44 per cent of peptic strictures were associated with Barrett's epithelium.[12] Peptic strictures in Barrett's esophagus usually develop at the proximally relocated squamocolumnar junction; distal to the stricture one finds

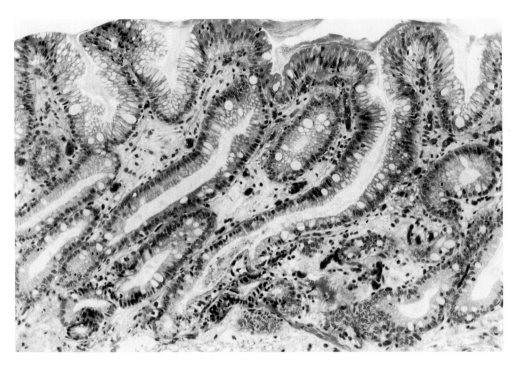

Figure 12–1. Barrett's specialized metaplastic epithelium. Goblet cells resembling those found in the intestine are interspersed among columnar cells, some of which closely resemble gastric surface cells, while others resemble absorptive cells. The small, evenly spaced, basally located nuclei indicate that this biopsy is negative for dysplasia. (H & E, ×260)

Barrett's specialized metaplastic epithelium. In cases in which the stricture occurs near the junction of the tubular esophagus and hiatal hernia, cardio-fundal or fundic mucosa may be found. If no Barrett's specialized metaplasia is seen this is not considered Barrett's esophagus. On the other hand, a short segment of such specialized epithelium may be present and this probably represents an early form of Barrett's esophagus.

Gastrointestinal blood loss results from erosions or ulcerations in either the squamous or metaplastic lining of the tubular esophagus. Such bleeding can vary from chronic, occult blood loss to acute massive gastrointestinal hemorrhage.[16,35]

Esophageal adenocarcinoma is the most feared complication of Barrett's esophagus. The clinical characteristics of 121 patients with Barrett's adenocarcinomas reported in the literature have been summarized.[20] The average age at diagnosis of adenocarcinoma was 57 years (range, 23 to 88 years). Esophageal adenocarcinoma has a predilection for men with a male:female ratio of 3 to 5.5:1[9,10,20] and appears to be more common in Caucasians. Dysphagia is the most common presenting complaint. As many as one-third of reported cases of Barrett's adenocarcinoma have minimal or no antecedent symptoms of gastroesophageal reflux.[20] This paradoxic finding may reflect inadequate historical information, or the fact that once Barrett's esophagus

develops, the patient may become asymptomatic because reflux onto columnar epithelium may not be associated with the symptoms caused by reflux onto squamous epithelium. Some patients, when carefully questioned, may recall symptoms that underwent spontaneous remission several years previously. Some series,[10] but not all,[30] suggest that a heavy smoking history is a risk factor for developing Barrett's esophageal adenocarcinoma.

Malignancies arising in sites other than the esophagus have been said to occur with increased frequency in patients with Barrett's esophagus.[36–38] In one series, 25 of 115 (22 per cent) patients with Barrett's esophagus had extraesophageal malignancies.[38] The head, neck, and lung were the most common sites reported and the high prevalence of cigarette smoking and alcohol abuse was postulated to play a role in the development of these cancers.

Sontag and colleagues found an apparently high prevalence of adenomatous polyps and adenocarcinoma of the colon in patients with Barrett's esophagus.[37] Unfortunately, because asymptomatic, age- and sex-matched control subjects were not studied, more data will be required to assess the frequency of colonic neoplasia in patients with Barrett's esophagus.

Therapy in patients with Barrett's esophagus is directed toward the control of gastroesophageal reflux symptoms.[18] Antireflux therapy is described in more detail elsewhere in this book, but initial therapy usually consists of histamine-2 receptor blockers (H_2-blockers) and antacids as needed. Metoclopramide or bethanechol may be added to H_2-inhibitors for patients whose symptoms are not controlled by life-style changes and initial medical therapy. We reserve antireflux surgery for patients with symptoms refractory to medical therapy or with severe complications such as recurring strictures, repeated pulmonary aspiration, or bleeding ulcers that do not heal. There is no clear evidence that antireflux surgery causes regression or disappearance of metaplastic epithelium or that it prevents the development of adenocarcinoma. Partial regression of metaplastic epithelium has been reported in a few cases after antireflux surgery,[7,10,39] but others have not found such regression and have even observed progression to adenocarcinoma despite antireflux surgery.[6,40] For this reason we do not recommend prophylactic antireflux surgery to prevent development of adenocarcinoma in uncomplicated Barrett's esophagus if the patient's symptoms can be controlled by medical therapy.

■ Endoscopic Appearance

The normal stratified squamous mucosa of the tubular esophagus has a pink-white color. The junction between the whiter squamous mucosa of the esophagus and more salmon-pink columnar mucosa of the stomach lies in the region of the lower esophageal sphincter. The squamocolumnar junction is also referred to as the ora serrata or Z-line because the junction of the two epithelial types often occurs as a wavy interface extending over 1 or 2 cm. In Barrett's esophagus the ora serrata is proximally displaced and represents the junction between the proximal squamous mucosa and the more distal specialized metaplastic columnar mucosa.[41] The proximally relocated ora serrata in Barrett's esophagus is often asymmetric and may extend over a greater length than normal.

Long segments of esophageal mucosa lined by Barrett's specialized metaplastic epithelium are usually obvious at endoscopy, but there are potential sources of error in detecting and estimating the length of the columnar-lined segment by endoscopy. Some very long segments of Barrett's specialized metaplasia may be missed if the endoscope is passed "blindly" beyond a proximally relocated ora serrata in the upper esophagus. This error can be avoided by searching for the ora serrata if it is not discovered in its usual position in the distal esophagus. The distance of the ora serrata from the teeth should be recorded. Occasionally, the bright red appearance of marked squamous esophagitis may cause confusion by obscuring the junction with the gastric mucosa. In such cases biopsy will establish the correct diagnosis.

Patients with gastroesophageal reflux and Barrett's esophagus almost always have hiatal hernias.[42] In fact, we have never seen a patient with Barrett's esophagus who did not have a hiatal hernia. It is important for the endoscopist to recognize hiatal hernias so that biopsies taken from them are not mistakenly classified as "Barrett's esophagus" with its associated implications for the development of malignancy. Typically the hernial pouch has gastric folds that run from the stomach through the diaphragmatic hiatus and disappear just distal to the lower esophageal sphincter.[42] The region of the lower esophageal sphincter can usually be recognized endoscopically in the normal individual at the distal end of the tubular esophagus by the presence of a circumferential mucosal rosette that can be opened by gentle insufflation of air.[42] In Barrett's esophagus the lower esophageal sphincter region is usually more patulous, but it is still recognizable as the distal end of the tubular esophagus. Hiatal hernias can be recognized as pouches, lined with a reddish orange columnar mucosa typical of stomach extending between the lower esophageal sphincter region and the diaphragmatic pinchcock or hiatus. The diaphragmatic pinchcock or hiatus can be recognized as a concentric narrowing of the lumen that closes intermittently with respiration or sniffing.[42]

■ Histology of the Columnar Epithelial Esophagus

Paull and colleagues[41] described three different patterns of epithelium in Barrett's esophagus: gastric fundic, junctional epithelium resembling that of the gastric cardia, and specialized columnar epithelium. In studies utilizing a standardized biopsy protocol at the University of Washington and UCLA, gastric fundic type mucosa in its normal form has not been identified above the distal 3 cm of the tubular esophagus, i.e., above the lower esophageal sphincter zone.[26,27] However, studies that include children suggest that fundic epithelium may be present in columnar-lined esophagus above the lower esophageal sphincter zone.[43,44] Our working classification of esophageal columnar epithelium is shown in Table 12–1.

The cardiac type of mucosa has been the most variable in our experience. In adult patients with only short (<3 cm) segments of columnar-lined

Table 12–1. HISTOLOGIC FEATURES OF COLUMNAR-LINED ESOPHAGUS

Type of Epithelium	Surface/Pits	Glands
Gastric fundic*	AB negative mucous cells	Fundic
Cardiac	AB negative mucous cells	Mucous
Specialized metaplastic†	Flat or villiform configuration, AB positive goblet cells, AB positive or negative mucous cells	Mucous or metaplastic

*Gastric fundic epithelium rarely, if ever, occurs in the adult with a true columnar-lined esophagus; most such biopsies were inadvertently taken from a hiatal hernia.

†The diagnosis of Barrett's esophagus is limited to patients with specialized metaplastic epithelium.

AB = Alcian blue pH 2.5.

esophagus, it may be the only type of mucosa present; in others, patches of cardiac mucosa are interspersed with specialized metaplastic epithelium.

As mentioned above, specialized metaplastic epithelium is highly distinctive and has therefore been considered diagnostic of Barrett's esophagus when seen in a biopsy from the tubular esophagus. This specialized columnar epithelium may be found in mucosa with a villiform surface, but it is most frequently seen in mucosa that has a flat or only faintly villiform configuration. The epithelium covering the flat surface and pits or the villiform projections has two types of cells: goblet cells and columnar cells (see Fig. 12–1). The goblet cells contain mucin that stains positively with Alcian blue at pH 2.5. Histochemical studies show that this goblet cell mucin most often contains a mixture of sialomucin and sulfated mucins. In general, the sialomucins predominate.

The columnar cells between the goblet cells may resemble normal gastric foveolar cells or intestinal absorptive cells but do not have all the typical features of either. The brush border, if present, is only partially developed, in contrast to the fully developed, refractile brush border of the mature intestinal absorptive cell. The columnar cells are also unlike normal gastric surface cells, for they frequently contain Alcian blue positive mucin in variable quantities. Histochemical studies to differentiate sialomucins from sulfomucins in columnar cells disclose that sialomucins are more often present.

Several studies have claimed an increased risk of adenocarcinoma in patients with sulfated mucins in the *columnar* cells of specialized metaplasia, but this claim has been based on circumstantial evidence and not on prospective follow-up data.[45,46] We have found that the sensitivity and specificity of sulfated mucins for predicting the presence of dysplasia or cancer are too low to be of clinical value in managing patients. By electron microscopy, granules within the columnar cells more closely resemble cells of the mucous neck region of the stomach, suggesting that this cell might be the precursor of the metaplastic epithelium in Barrett's esophagus.[28]

In clinical practice, we use the term "Barrett's metaplasia" for patients in whom the columnar-lined esophagus contains specialized metaplastic epithelium as defined by the combination of Alcian blue positive goblet cells and columnar cells described above. Because such patients appear to be the ones at risk for developing adenocarcinoma, our surveillance activities have focused on them.

Dysplasia is defined as unequivocally neoplastic epithelium confined within the basement membrane of the glands within which it arose. Rarely, when dysplastic epithelium proliferates to form a mass, it becomes an adenoma. Dysplasia in Barrett's esophagus can be recognized histologically by a combination of architectural and cytologic abnormalities (Fig. 12–2). Dysplastic glands may retain their normal configuration, but more often have irregular or even grossly distorted architecture. The glands are lined by cells with crowded, stratified, hyperchromatic nuclei. In other examples, the nuclei are large, are hyperchromatic, contain large nucleoli and show a loss of nuclear polarity, but lack the crowding and stratification mentioned above. Dysplasia in Barrett's esophagus has been subdivided into low-grade and high-grade forms in a manner analogous to that for dysplasia complicating ulcerative colitis. The category high-grade dysplasia encompasses carcinoma in situ. The diagnosis of intramucosal carcinoma is made when malignant cells invade into the lamina propria but do not extend below the muscularis mucosae. Until invasion of the lamina propria is present, the lesion does not have the capacity to metastasize. The diagnostic criteria for differentiating reactive or regenerative hyperplasia due to inflammation from low-grade dysplasia are not sharply defined, resulting in the category of "indefinite" for dysplasia. In practice, we have lumped indefinite with low-grade dysplasia as interobserver variability in separating them is high and because they have similar management implications.[47]

We have employed DNA analysis by flow cy-

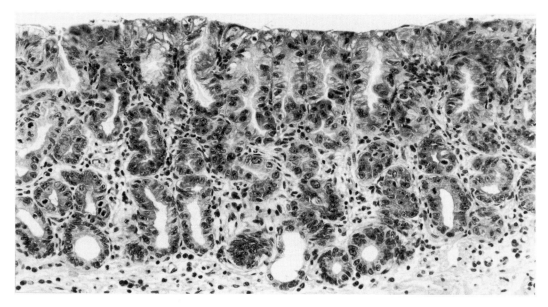

Figure 12–2. Barrett's esophagus with high grade dysplasia. In this example of high grade dysplasia, there is less distortion of the glandular architecture than usually seen. The epithelium is no longer recognizable as Barrett's specialized metaplastic epithelium because there is a marked diminution in mucus secretion. The nuclei are enlarged and hyperchromatic and vary markedly in size and shape. The nuclei are no longer evenly spaced and basally oriented but tend to be piled up on one another and have no consistent relationship to the base of the cell (loss of polarity). These dysplastic cells are still confined within the basement membrane of the glands within which they arose. (H & E, ×210)

tometry to more fully characterize the biologic nature of the alterations in Barrett's esophagus. Our preliminary data suggest that abnormal DNA content and cell cycle abnormalities correlate well with the histologic diagnosis of dysplasia. Further study may prove that flow cytometry is a valuable adjunct to histologic diagnosis in identifying patients who merit intensive endoscopic biopsy surveillance.[48]

■ *Incidence and Prevalence of Barrett's Adenocarcinoma*

Shortly after Barrett's original description of the columnar-lined esophagus, several reports appeared that linked it to primary esophageal adenocarcinoma.[49,50] Barrett's associated esophageal adenocarcinomas are now being reported with increasing frequency, as are adenocarcinomas of the gastric cardia.[51-54] These two tumors are now the most common adenocarcinomas of the upper gastrointestinal tract.[54] Anatomic, epidemiologic, and pathologic similarities between Barrett's and cardiac adenocarcinomas have led to speculation that some cardiac carcinomas may have arisen in short segments of Barrett's metaplasia.[52]

Although there is no doubt that Barrett's esophagus is a premalignant condition with an increased

risk of adenocarcinoma, the magnitude of the risk is difficult to ascertain. Accurate data to define the incidence of adenocarcinoma in Barrett's esophagus will require prospective serial endoscopic biopsy evaluation of large numbers of patients who have been characterized by uniform definitions of Barrett's esophagus and who have been shown to be free of adenocarcinoma at entry into a surveillance program. Such data are not available at the present time. Retrospective analyses have estimated a 30- to 40-fold increase in the risk of esophageal adenocarcinoma compared to the expected rate.[38,40] These retrospective analyses have estimated one case of adenocarcinoma in 81 to 411 "patient years" of follow-up.[38,40,55]

Several studies have estimated the prevalence of adenocarcinoma in Barrett's esophagus.[30] In Naef's classic study of 1225 patients who had endoscopy for peptic esophagitis, 140 had Barrett's esophagus and 12 had esophageal adenocarcinoma. Thus, the prevalence of Barrett's esophagus among patients with peptic esophagitis who underwent endoscopy was 11.4 per cent and the prevalence of adenocarcinoma was 8.6 per cent of those who had Barrett's esophagus.[6] These data are comparable to the results of several other large series in which the overall prevalence of adenocarcinoma at the time of diagnosis of Barrett's esophagus was 7.8 per cent, with a range of 0 to 14.8 per cent.[8,38,40,56-59] Two surgical series found a much higher prevalence of esophageal adenocarcinoma, but these figures probably reflect the selection bias of patients referred for surgery.[7,10]

Several factors may lead to over- or underestimation of the prevalence of adenocarcinoma in Barrett's esophagus, and the published estimates should be interpreted with caution. An example of the impact of the histologic definition of Barrett's esophagus is illustrated in a retrospective study that reported a 7 per cent (8 of 115) prevalence of adenocarcinoma in patients with Barrett's esophagus.[38] Only 77 of the 115 patients with ''Barrett's'' esophagus in this series had Barrett's specialized metaplastic epithelium. All 8 patients with cancer had specialized metaplastic epithelium. No patients without specialized metaplastic epithelium had cancer. Thus, a revised prevalence of 10.4 per cent (8 of 77) might be more appropriate for this group of patients. Two patients in this series developed cancer in follow-up; both had specialized metaplastic epithelium. None of 38 patients without specialized metaplastic epithelium developed cancer on follow-up.[38] Barrett's adenocarcinomas could also be underestimated if cancers occurring in the distal esophagus were classified as gastric in origin. In some series, all adenocarcinomas involving the distal 10 cm of esophagus have been uncritically dismissed as gastric carcinomas.[60]

The prevalence of esophageal adenocarcinoma can also be overestimated because patients with cancer are more likely to be symptomatic and therefore to have endoscopy. One preliminary study prospectively estimated the prevalence of adenocarcinoma in patients with Barrett's esophagus who did not have symptoms of cancer, but only those directly related to gastroesophageal reflux (heartburn, regurgitation, or frequent antacid use). Of 54 such patients, two had adenocarcinoma, a prevalence of 3.7 per cent.[33]

■ Dysplasia and Adenocarcinoma

Because the great majority of patients with Barrett's esophagus will never develop adenocarcinoma of the esophagus, there is a need for indicators of increased cancer risk to select patients in whom more frequent endoscopic biopsy surveillance would justify its costs. One such indicator is dysplasia, especially high-grade dysplasia. Dysplasia in Barrett's esophagus refers to an unequivocally neoplastic transformation in the epithelium. Several lines of evidence suggest that high-grade dysplasia is a premalignant lesion in Barrett's

esophagus. First, retrospective studies of resected Barrett's adenocarcinomas have demonstrated high-grade dysplasia in the mucosa adjacent to the carcinoma in approximately 90 per cent of the cases in which it was sought.[10,29,30,31,61,62] Second, some patients who have undergone esophagectomy for high-grade dysplasia had previously unrecognized adenocarcinomas in their resected specimens.[10,63] Finally, evaluation of the DNA content of dysplastic epithelium in some patients with Barrett's esophagus has shown aneuploidy, like that observed in carcinoma.[48]

The natural history of high-grade dysplasia in Barrett's esophagus remains unknown. Most of the available data implicating high-grade dysplasia as a precursor of adenocarcinoma in Barrett's esophagus have been derived by studying the mucosa surrounding adenocarcinomas that had been surgically resected.[10,29,30,31,61-63] Although such studies can be used to establish an association between high-grade dysplasia and adenocarcinoma, they cannot be used to determine if dysplasia is an obligatory precursor of carcinoma or to determine the time course for the development of carcinoma from high-grade dysplasia. Such retrospective studies also cannot determine the risks of a coexisting, but inapparent adenocarcinoma when endoscopic biopsies of Barrett's esophagus show only high-grade dysplasia.

A few patients have undergone esophagectomy because endoscopic biopsies showed high-grade dysplasia; some of these patients have had unsuspected adenocarcinoma discovered in the surgical specimen.[10,62,63] In most of these reported cases, however, the endoscopic appearance of the mucosa and the number and site of endoscopic biopsies were not specified. One recent study reported seven patients with high-grade dysplasia in mucosa that was endoscopically unremarkable.[64] All seven patients were evaluated by a methodical and extensive biopsy protocol prior to esophageal resection. The preoperative diagnosis was compared to the final diagnosis as established by extensive evaluation of the excised surgical specimen and was found to correctly predict high-grade dysplasia without adenocarcinoma in four patients and adenocarcinoma in the remaining three. All three adenocarcinomas were early; two were intramucosal and one extended into the submucosa without involvement of the muscularis propria or the adventitial lymph nodes. These data clearly indicate that a systematic endoscopic biopsy protocol can detect high-grade dysplasia and early adenocarcinoma at a stage in which they are treatable and potentially curable. The data also suggest that a systematic endoscopic biopsy evaluation may be able to minimize the possibility of an unsuspected coexisting adenocarcinoma. Accurate preoperative diagnosis is especially helpful in deciding on surgery for patients who are poor surgical risks.

Only anecdotal data are available about the natural history of high-grade dysplasia in patients who do not already have an adenocarcinoma. One patient has been reported who progressed from Barrett's metaplasia negative for dysplasia through high-grade dysplasia to adenocarcinoma in 38 months.[65] A second patient in whom high-grade dysplasia persisted for 42 months prior to surgery has also been reported; this patient had only high-grade dysplasia in the resected specimen.[64] Many more patients with high-grade dysplasia will need to be evaluated before definitive statements can be made concerning its natural history. It is possible that the natural history of high-grade dysplasia in the individual patient with Barrett's esophagus will prove unpredictable because of wide variation in the time course of developing adenocarcinoma in different patients.

Even less is known concerning the natural history of low-grade dysplasia, mostly because of the difficulty in recognizing it reproducibly.[48] Although some studies report reversal of low-grade dysplasia with medical or surgical therapy for gastroesophageal reflux,[10,63,66] the available data do not rule out the possibilities that either the endoscopic sampling was inadequate to detect persisting low-grade dysplasia or that the low-grade dysplasia really represented regenerative or reparative changes rather than true dysplasia. Although it seems quite likely, it is not known for certain that low-grade dysplasia is a precursor of high-grade dysplasia; nor is it known whether adenocarcinoma can arise directly from low-grade dysplasia.

■ Endoscopic Biopsy Surveillance

We believe that all patients with longstanding symptoms of gastroesophageal reflux should be evaluated endoscopically, even if their symptoms are easily controlled with medical therapy because endoscopy would allow identification of the subset who have Barrett's esophagus. Furthermore, those patients with unsuspected Barrett's esophagus may already have an adenocarcinoma that will produce symptoms only after it has become unresectable.[20] When the diagnosis of Barrett's esophagus is first made, we recommend four quadrant biopsies at 2-cm intervals throughout the columnar-lined tubular esophagus, as well as biopsies of target lesions such as ulcers, erosions, or strictures, no

matter how insignificant they may appear endoscopically. Direct-vision brush cytologic examination at the time of biopsy may be complementary, but requires special interest and expertise by the cytopathologist for accurate interpretation. If the capability for flow cytometry is available, we recommend that at least one biopsy of each 2-cm level of the columnar-lined esophagus and any target lesion be evaluated for DNA content.

If the systematically taken biopsies are negative for dysplasia histologically, if they show no evidence of aneuploidy or abnormalities of proliferation by flow cytometry, and if the brush cytologic finding is benign, how often should patients be reevaluated? Several long-term prospective studies are in progress to answer this question, but the data generated thus far are insufficient to make conclusive recommendations. Until such data are available, we believe that repeat endoscopic evaluation at two- or three-year intervals is appropriate, provided that a complete evaluation has been performed initially. Before antireflux surgery is performed in a Barrett's patient, we carry out a systematic preoperative biopsy evaluation to seek unsuspected high-grade dysplasia or early adenocarcinoma, as these findings would modify the surgical approach.

Pessimism has been expressed concerning the value of endoscopic surveillance because many of the tumors that have been discovered were unresectable for cure. This has not been borne out in centers that have expertise in proper biopsy sampling, processing, and interpretation.[64]

If high-grade dysplasia is detected in a biopsy from mucosa that showed no gross abnormality endoscopically, we recommend early re-endoscopy with multiple biopsies of the area of dysplasia to determine its extent and to search for a coexisting adenocarcinoma.[64] No general recommendations for management can be made if at re-endoscopy only high-grade dysplasia is found. Some of these patients probably merit surgery, but the available data are not adequate to determine which ones. Each patient with high-grade dysplasia must be evaluated individually weighing the usual clinical factors when considering surgery. For patients with high-grade dysplasia who are not deemed surgical candidates, but who would be if adenocarcinoma were documented, we repeat biopsies in three months and at six-month intervals thereafter. If such a course of endoscopic surveillance is undertaken, it should be recognized by both the physician and the patient that large areas of dysplasia are more difficult to sample adequately than smaller ones.

At least four general cautions should be made concerning high-grade dysplasia in Barrett's esophagus. First, because high-grade dysplasia in Barrett's esophagus is relatively rare in unselected patients, most pathologists do not have the opportunity to see many cases and therefore have not gained experience in its evaluation. For this reason, most general pathologists would be wise to seek an expert second opinion before surgical resection is considered. Second, our discussion applies to the patient in whom high-grade dysplasia is detected in mucosa that appears endoscopically unremarkable. If the high-grade dysplasia is associated with gross findings suggesting adenocarcinoma such as a malignant-appearing narrowing, a deep ulceration, or a mass, repeat biopsies at the first opportunity are indicated. Third, some adenocarcinomas are so well differentiated that they can be distinguished from high-grade dysplasia only by demonstrating invasion below the muscularis mucosae. This may be difficult because endoscopic biopsies usually do not obtain significant amounts of submucosal tissue and because recurring ulceration associated with Barrett's esophagus may obliterate the muscularis mucosae, the landmark which must be traversed to prove submucosal invasion. Fourth, it should be obvious that the evaluation intervals we have recommended are of necessity arbitrary because of our lack of knowledge concerning the natural history of high-grade dysplasia.

Theoretically, patients with low-grade dysplasia merit more frequent biopsy surveillance than patients without dysplasia. However, as we discussed above, there is considerable interobserver disagreement concerning the diagnosis of low-grade dysplasia.[47] For patients in whom several experienced gastrointestinal pathologists diagnose low-grade dysplasia or in whom there is an objective abnormality by flow cytometry, repeat endoscopic biopsy at six-month intervals may be justified.

Once early esophageal adenocarcinoma is documented, the treatment is surgical resection if the patient is considered an acceptable surgical candidate. Because adenocarcinoma or high-grade dysplasia may be multicentric or involve large areas of esophageal mucosa, and because specialized metaplasia may become dysplasia, the entire columnar-lined segment should be completely removed if the patient undergoes surgery.

■ ACKNOWLEDGMENTS

Supported by NIDDK Program Project Grant #PO1 AM32971 and American Cancer Society Grant PDT-316.

■ REFERENCES

1. Barrett NR: The lower esophagus lined by columnar epithelium. Surgery, *41*:6, 1957.
2. Barrett NR: Chronic peptic ulcer of the oesophagus and "oesophagitis." Br J Surg, *38*:175–182, 1950.
3. Allison PR, Johnstone AS: Oesophagus lined with gastric mucous membrane. Thorax, *8*:87, 1953.
4. Mossberg SN: The columnar-lined esophagus (Barrett syndrome)—an acquired condition? Gastroenterology, *50*:671–676, 1966.
5. Hamilton SR: Pathogenesis of columnar cell-lined (Barrett's) esophagus. *In* Spechler SJ, Goyal RK (Eds): Barrett's Esophagus. Pathophysiology, Diagnosis, and Management. New York, Elsevier, 1985, pp 29–37.
6. Naef AP, et al: Columnar-lined lower esophagus: An acquired lesion with malignant predisposition. J Thorac Cardiovasc Surg, *70*:826–835, 1975.
7. Radigan LR, et al: Barrett esophagus. Arch Surg, *112*:486–491, 1977.
8. Messian RA, et al: Barrett's esophagus. Am J Gastroenterol, *69*:458–466, 1978.
9. Harle IA, et al: Management of adenocarcinoma in columnar-lined esophagus. Ann Thorac Surg, *40*:330–336, 1985.
10. Skinner DB, et al: Barrett's esophagus. Comparison of benign and malignant cases. Ann Surg, *198*:554–566, 1983.
11. Witt TR, et al: Adenocarcinoma in Barrett's esophagus. J Thorac Cardiovas Surg, *85*:337–345, 1983.
12. Spechler SJ, et al: The prevalence of Barrett's esophagus in patients with chronic peptic esophageal strictures. Dig Dis Sci, *28*:769–774, 1983.
13. Lackey C, et al: Stricture location in Barrett's esophagus. Gastrointest Endosc, *30*:331–333, 1984.
14. Wesdorp I, et al: Treatment of reflux oesophagitis with ranitidine. Gut, *24*:921–924, 1983.
15. Thompson WG, Barr R: Pharmacotherapy of an ulcer in Barrett's esophagus: Carbenoxylone and cimetidine. Gastroenterology, *73*:808–810, 1977.
16. Kothari T, et al: Barrett's ulcer and treatment with cimetidine. Arch Intern Med, *140*:475–477, 1980.
17. Davidson JS: High pectic stricture of the oesophagus. Thorax, *31*:1–14, 1976.
18. Spechler SJ, Goyal RK: Barrett's esophagus. N Engl J Med, *315*:362–371, 1986.
19. Bozymski EM, et al: Barrett's esophagus. Ann Intern Med, *97*:103–107, 1982.
20. Sjogren RW, Johnson LF: Barrett's esophagus: A review. Am J Med, *74*:313–321, 1983.
21. Trier JS, Curtis RL: Barrett's esophagus. Progr Gastroenterol, *4*:231–251, 1983.
22. Spechler SJ, Goyal RK (Eds): Barrett's Esophagus. Pathophysiology, Diagnosis, and Management. New York, Elsevier, 1985.
23. Goyal RK: Columnar cell-lined (Barrett's) esophagus. A historical perspective. *In* Spechler SJ, Goyal RK (Eds): Barrett's Esophagus. Pathophysiology, Diagnosis, and Management. New York, Elsevier, 1985, pp 1–17.
24. Hayward J: The lower end of the esophagus. Thorax, *16*:36–41, 1961.
25. De La Pava S, Pickren JW, Adler RH: Ectopic gastric mucosa of the esophagus, a study on histogenesis. NY State J Med, *64*:1831–1835, 1964.
26. Reid BJ, Rubin CE: When is the columnar-lined esophagus premalignant? Gastroenterology, *88*:1552, 1985.
27. Weinstein W, et al: A histologic evaluation of Barrett's esophagus using a standardized endoscopic biopsy protocol (abstract). Gastroenterology, *86*:1296, 1984.
28. Levine DS, Rubin CE: Electron microscopic evidence for

the gastric origin of Barrett's metaplasia and dysplasia (abstract). Gastroenterology, *90*:1519, 1986.

29. Smith RRL, et al: The spectrum of carcinoma arising in Barrett's esophagus: A clinicopathologic study of 26 patients. Am J Surg Pathol, *8*:563–573, 1984.

30. Haggitt RC, Dean PJ: Adenocarcinoma in Barrett's epithelium. *In* Spechler SJ, Goyal RK (Eds): Barrett's Esophagus. Pathophysiology, Diagnosis, and Management. New York, Elsevier, 1985, pp 153–166.

31. Thompson JJ, et al: Barrett's metaplasia and adenocarcinoma of the esophagus and gastroesophageal junction. Hum Pathol, *14*:42–61, 1983.

32. Appleman HD, et al: Distinguishing features of adenocarcinoma in Barrett's esophagus and in the gastric cardia. *In* Spechler SJ, Goyal RK (Eds): Barrett's Esophagus. Pathophysiology, Diagnosis, and Management. New York, Elsevier, 1985, pp 167–187.

33. Schnell T, et al: Endoscopic screening for Barrett's esophagus (BE), esophageal adenocarcinoma (AdCa) and other mucosal changes in ambulatory subjects with symptomatic gastroesophageal reflux (GER) (abstract). Gastroenterology, *88*:1576, 1985.

34. Halpert RD, et al: Adenocarcinoma of the esophagus in patients with scleroderma. AJR, *140*:927–930, 1983.

35. Borrie J, Goldwater L: Columnar cell-lined esophagus: Assessment of etiology and treatment. J Thorac Cardiovasc Surg, *71*:825–834, 1976.

36. Sheahan DG, Berman MA: Barrett's mucosa with multiple carcinomas of the esophagus and oral cavity. J Clin Gastroenterol, *8*:103–107, 1986.

37. Sontag SJ, et al: Barrett's oesophagus and colonic tumours. Lancet, *1*:946–948, 1985.

38. Spechler SJ, et al: Adenocarcinoma and Barrett's esophagus: An overrated risk? Gastroenterology, *87*:927–933, 1984.

39. Brand DL: Regression of columnar esophageal (Barrett's) epithelium after anti-reflux surgery. N Engl J Med, *302*:844–848, 1980.

40. Cameron AJ, et al: The incidence of adenocarcinoma in columnar-lined (Barrett's) esophagus. N Engl J Med, *313*:857–859, 1985.

41. Paull A, et al: The histologic spectrum of Barrett's esophagus. N Engl J Med, *295*:476–480, 1976.

42. Boyce WH: The esophagogastric junction: 25 years looking and learning. ASGE Distinguished Lectureship, May, 1984.

43. Dahms BB, Rothstein FC: Barrett's esophagus in children: A consequence of chronic gastroesophageal reflux. Gastroenterology, *86*:318–323, 1984.

44. Hassall E, Weinstein W, Ament M: Barrett's esophagus in childhood. Gastroenterology, *89*:1331–1337, 1985.

45. Jass JA: Mucin histochemistry of the columnar epithelium of the oesophagus: A retrospective study. J Clin Pathol, *34*:866–870, 1981.

46. Peuchmaur M, Potet F, Goldfain D: Mucin histochemistry of the columnar epithelium of the oesophagus (Barrett's oesophagus): A prospective biopsy study. J Clin Pathol, *37*:607–610, 1984.

47. Reid BJ, et al: Criteria for dysplasia in Barrett's esophagus: A cooperative consensus study. Gastroenterology, *88*:1552, 1985.

48. Reid BJ, Haggitt RC, Rubin CE, Rabinovitch PS: Flow cytometry complements histology in detecting patients at risk for Barrett's adenocarcinoma. Gastroenterology, *93*:1–11, 1987.

49. Morson BC, Belcher JR: Adenocarcinoma of the oesophagus and ectopic gastric mucosa. Br J Cancer, *6*:127–132, 1952.

50. Armstrong RA, Blalock JB, Carrera GM: Adenocarcinoma of the middle third of the esophagus arising from ectopic gastric mucosa. J Thor Surg, *37*:398–403, 1958.

51. MacDonald WC: Clinical and pathologic features of adenocarcinoma of the gastric cardia. Cancer, *29*:724–732, 1972.

52. Wang HH, et al: Comparative features of esophageal and gastric adenocarcinomas: Recent changes in type and frequency. Hum Pathol, *17*:482–487, 1986.

53. Levine MS, et al: Adenocarcinoma of the esophagus: Relationship to Barrett mucosa. Radiology, *150*:305–309, 1984.

54. Kalish RJ, et al: Clinical, epidemiologic, and morphologic comparison between adenocarcinomas arising in Barrett's esophageal mucosa and in the gastric cardia. Gastroenterology, *86*:461–467, 1984.

55. Sprung DJ, et al: Incidence of adenocarcinoma in Barrett's esophagus. Am J Gastroenterol, *79*:817, 1984.

56. Bremner CG: Benign strictures of the esophagus. Curr Probl Surg, *19*:401–489, 1982.

57. Menguy R: On the malignant potential of acquired short esophagus. Arch Surg, *114*:260–263, 1979.

58. Hawe A, Payne WS, Weiland LH, Fontana RS: Adenocarcinoma in the columnar epithelial lined lower (Barrett) oesophagus. Thorax, *28*:511–514, 1973.

59. Ransom JM, Patel GK, Clift SA, Womble NE, Read RC: Extended and limited types of Barrett's esophagus in the adult. Ann Thorac Surg, *33*:19–27, 1982.

60. American Joint Committee for Cancer Staging and End Results Reporting: Clinical Staging System for Carcinoma of the Esophagus. CA, *25*:50–57, 1975.

61. Haggitt RC, et al: Adenocarcinoma complicating columnar epithelium-lined (Barrett's) esophagus. Am J Clin Pathol, *70*:1–5, 1978.

62. Schmidt HG, et al: Dysplasia in Barrett's esophagus. J Cancer Res Clin Oncol, *110*:145–152, 1985.

63. Lee RG: Dysplasia in Barrett's esophagus. Am J Surg Pathol, *9*(12):845–852, 1985.

64. Reid BJ, et al: Barrett's esophagus: High grade dysplasia and intramucosal carcinoma detected by endoscopic biopsy surveillance. Gastroenterology, *90*:1601, 1986.

65. Skinner DB, et al: Surgical treatment of Barrett's esophagus. *In* Spechler SJ, Goyal RK (Eds): Barrett's Esophagus. Pathophysiology, Diagnosis, and Management. New York, Elsevier, 1985, pp 211–221.

66. Riddell RH: Dysplasia and regression in Barrett's epithelium. *In* Spechler SJ, Goyal RK (Eds): Barrett's Esophagus. Pathophysiology, Diagnosis, and Management. New York, Elsevier, 1985, pp 143–152.

13

Failed Antireflux Procedures

Lucius D. Hill

The worth of any surgical operation can be measured in part by the incidence of failure or recurrence of the problem for which the operation was performed. The persistence of reflux and recurrence of herniation after antireflux surgery has been significant in many reports over the last 20 years. It is only recently, however, that reports dealing specifically with this problem have appeared in any numbers.

Present-day antireflux procedures are successful in the majority of cases. However, a significant number of patients have persistent or recurrent symptoms following repair and at times have severe, life-threatening complications. These failures of antireflux procedures have been a deterrent to surgery and have compromised the confidence of gastroenterologists and other physicians in surgery for reflux.

An antireflux operation is, with few exceptions, an elective procedure, and the surgeon has ample time to do a complete and satisfactory repair that should offer the patient long-lasting relief of the symptom complex.

Our experience with failed antireflux procedures includes 303 patients who were referred for reoperation after having had 380 previous repairs. The types of procedures and numbers of operations are shown in Table 13–1.

Over the last 15 years we have compiled three reports of our experience with failed antireflux procedures. The findings and trends seen in these reports are reviewed in this chapter.

One of the first reports from the United States dealing with failed antireflux procedures was compiled by our group in 1971.[1] The report included 63 patients, who had 71 antireflux operations. The Allison repair was the most common procedure, being used in 56 of the previous operations. Only 3 patients had had Nissen repairs.

An analysis was done in each of our reports to determine the cause of failure of the previous operation, and an effort was made to determine whether failure was the fault of the surgeon or was due to an inherent defect in the operation.

In our first report it was found that the most common cause for recurrent reflux was failure to construct an adequate barrier to reflux at the gastroesophageal (GE) junction. At reoperation the GE junction was grossly patulous in these individuals. This finding has been persistent in subsequent reports and appears to be the most common cause of failure of all antireflux operations. Figure 13–1 depicts the patulous cardia resulting from failure to calibrate the gastroesophageal junction at surgery. Many of these patients reported that reflux was noted immediately after surgery, indicating that the surgeon had failed to calibrate the cardia sufficiently to prevent reflux. This type of failure occurred in all operations, including the Allison, the Nissen, and the Belsey repairs as well as those reported to have had the posterior gastropexy or Hill operation.

In Table 13–1 a large group of patients with indeterminate repairs is shown. There were 75 patients who had 100 previous operations. In these patients we were unable to determine, either from

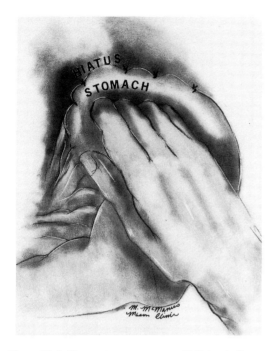
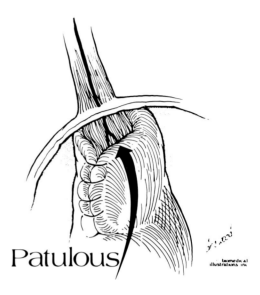

Figure 13–1. The most common cause of failed antireflux procedures is the patulous gastroesophageal junction created at surgery resulting from failure to construct an adequate barrier to reflux.

the previous operative note or at the time of surgery, the kind of repair that had been done. Some of these had modifications of standard procedures. Others had unidentifiable operations that appeared to have no relationship to an antireflux operation.

In the Allison and Belsey repairs shown in Table 13–1 the second most common cause for failure was inadequate fixation sutures that allowed the stomach to again herniate back into the mediastinum. In the crural repairs there were no fixation sutures, the operation consisting solely of bringing the crura together. Five patients with crural repairs recurred while in the hospital, as evidenced by postoperative upper GI x-rays showing the stomach back in the chest. Unfortunately, we continue to see procedures of this kind done, even today.

An important observation that appeared in our original review was that ancillary procedures such as gastric resection, vagotomy, and drainage procedures failed to prevent esophagitis if reflux was not corrected. A number of patients in our early reports had severe esophagitis despite the fact that vagotomy had rendered them hypochlorhydric. Gastric contents, containing enzymes and small amounts of hydrochloric acid, are clearly irritating to the esophageal mucosa and will produce alkaline esophagitis, which may be as severe as the esophagitis that occurs in patients with normal gastric acid.

Table 13–1. FAILED ANTIREFLUX OPERATIONS*

Type of Operation	Number of Operations	Number of Patients
Nissen	148	120
Allison	65	52
Belsey	32	25
Hill	15	13
Heller	2	2
Crural	10	9
Thal	2	1
Paraesophageal	2	2
Angelchik	4	4
Indeterminate		
Transthoracic	14	8
Abdominal	86	67
Total	380	303

*A total of 380 operations in 303 patients.

Another important observation gained from our earlier experience that is pertinent at the present time is that patients with severe respiratory symptoms are not relieved by ancillary procedures such as gastrectomy, vagotomy, and pyloroplasty, or drainage procedures. If reflux continues, respiratory symptoms will persist. This important aspect of the patient's disease is in no way alleviated by acid-reducing procedures. Gastric juice, regardless of its pH, is highly irritating to the tracheobronchial tree.

The ratio of operations for failed antireflux procedures in relation to primary repairs is unfortunately increasing dramatically at our institution. In the 1960s 12 per cent of 351 antireflux operations were done for recurrent hernias. In the 1970s, 20 per cent of 744 operations were remedial procedures. Between 1980 and 1984, 25 per cent of 450 cases were reoperations for failed antireflux procedures. Seventy per cent of the most recent 180 operations were done for failed Nissen fundoplications. These unfortunate surgical results are the prime reason for the reluctance on the part of physicians to refer patients for antireflux surgery. The increasing number of reports of reoperation for failed antireflux procedures with a preponderance of Nissen operations is significant across the country.

Over the years the Nissen procedure has become much more common in this country and our second report in 1979 dealt with reoperation for disruption and recurrence after Nissen fundoplication.[2] We reported 25 patients with failed Nissen operations and again noted that the most common cause for failure was the patulous or incompetent repair in which there had been a failure to construct an adequate barrier to reflux at the original procedure. This type of failure is shown in Figure 13–2. This photograph, taken at operation, shows the surgeon's fingers being invaginated into the incompetent or patulous GE junction. Many of these patients indicated that reflux was noted immediately after surgery, showing the surgeon had failed to calibrate the cardia sufficiently to prevent reflux.

The second most common failure of the Nissen procedure is the so-called ''slipped Nissen.'' This is shown in Figure 13–3 and occurs when the wrap, which should be placed around the gastroesophageal junction, slips down to the junction of the upper and middle third of the stomach. This not only fails to control reflux but partially obstructs the stomach and actually promotes reflux and causes severe dysphagia. In addition, we have found that a number of these patients have a serious dysmotility of the esophagus, apparently caused by a combination of esophagitis and the esophagus being accordioned on itself and unable to generate

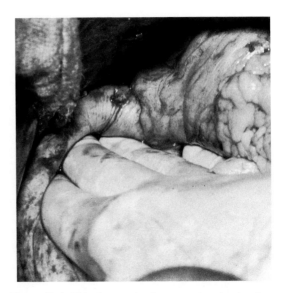

Figure 13–2. This photograph taken at surgery showing four of the surgeon's fingers invaginated through the patulous gastroesophageal junction.

propulsive peristalsis. A slipped Nissen, in the author's opinion, occurs because the sutures that are taken in the esophagus to anchor the wrap have very little strength. The esophagus has no serosal coat, is the weakest portion of the entire GI tract, and sutures placed in the esophagus pull out readily. If the sutures are taken too deeply, the risk of fistula formation is considerable. It is for these reasons that the Hill repair avoids sutures in the esophagus.

The Nissen fundoplication may disrupt completely, again because the esophageal sutures are weak, as shown in Figure 13–4. The fundoplication may disrupt partially, as seen in Figure 13–5. This partial disruption resembles the slipped Nissen when seen on upper GI x-rays. If the surgeon makes the wrap too tight, the Nissen may obstruct as seen in Figure 13–6. The wrap may be so tight that obstruction is complete and reoperation is imperative.

In addition to these common causes of failure of the Nissen procedure, a wide variety of life-threatening complications were seen in our series. These have been reported in our most recent review of 118 failed Nissen operations.[3] In one patient, the gastric mucosa intussuscepted cephalad to the wrap, completely obstructing the patient and requiring reoperation (Fig. 13–7). Figure 13–8 shows a patient who had a Nissen repair which became obstructed. The surgeon reoperated and noted that there was loss of continuity between the lower esophagus and stomach. He placed in a gastrostomy for feeding purposes, and a GI series showed complete loss of continuity between the end of the esophagus and the stomach.

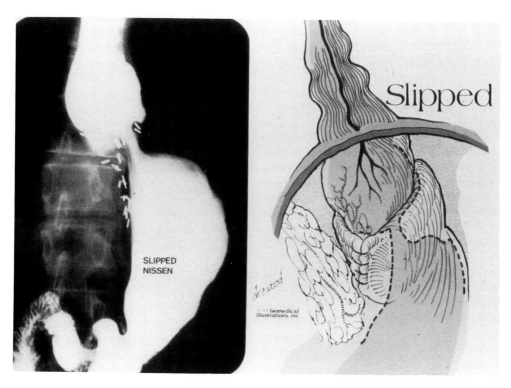

Figure 13–3. Second most common cause for failure of an antireflux procedure is the so-called "slipped Nissen."

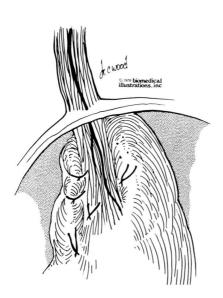

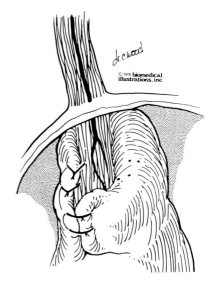

Figure 13–4. The sutures placed in the esophagus and the serosa of the stomach pull out, allowing the wrap to disrupt completely.

Figure 13–5. Partial disruption of a Nissen fundoplication occurs when part of the sutures pull out of the weak muscularis of the esophagus and the serosa of the stomach, producing a clinical picture similar to the slipped Nissen.

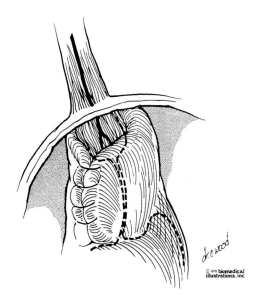

Figure 13–6. Failure to calibrate the cardia allows the wrap to be too tight, producing complete obstruction of the gastroesophageal junction.

A variety of life-theatening fistulas have been seen in our series. Predominantly these were limited almost exclusively to the Nissen procedure. Figure 13–9 shows a patient who had a Nissen fundoplication which slipped, causing a large gastric ulcer in the obstructed pouch to perforate on the seventh postoperative day. Following drainage of a subphrenic abscess, the patient developed a gastrocutaneous fistula, requiring intensive care for two months before the fistula could be brought under control and rerepair was accomplished. Figure 13–10 shows a fistula occurring following a transthoracic Nissen repair in which a gastric ulcer perforated into the left lung, forming a gastrobronchial fistula. Figure 13–11 shows a patient who developed a slipped Nissen followed by a large gastric ulcer which penetrated through the stomach, through the diaphragm, and into the right lung to form a gastrobronchial fistula into the right lung.

Figure 13–12 shows a patient who developed a slipped Nissen followed by formation of a large posterior gastric ulcer in the obstructed pouch. This posterior gastric ulcer penetrated through the stomach and into the aorta. An alert surgeon, Edwin James, was able to control the aorta, evacuate an enormous clot from the stomach, and close the opening in the aorta before the patient exsanguinated. This patient represents the only survivor of a gastroaortic fistula of which we are aware.

In Figure 13–13 a challenging complication is demonstrated. This patient was admitted to the Coronary Care Unit with a tentative diagnosis of myocardial infarction. The ECG showed changes indicating inferior myocardial injury. Dr. William Traverso recognized that the patient had a Nissen repair that had slipped and a large gastric ulcer had formed. On barium swallow and CT scan a connection between the stomach and the pericardium was demonstrated. At operation a huge gastric ulcer in the gastric pouch above the slipped repair had penetrated through the stomach, the diaphragm, and the pericardium. The base of the ulcer was the myocardium. The ulcer was taken down and closed and the gastroesophageal junction was anchored to the preaortic fascia. This patient represents the only recovery of a gastropericardial fistula of which we are aware. The gastric wrap was left in place. The patient then developed a recurrent ulcer in the gastric wrap, which perforated into the liver. This required a total gastrectomy. This case supports the observation that the gastric wrap is subject to gastric ulcers with lethal complications. The wrap should be taken down during operations for failed Nissen repairs.

One patient with postoperative empyema was found at reoperation to have multiple gastric perforations in a fundoplication that had migrated and incarcerated in the thorax.

This array of challenging problems required careful preoperative assessment and intraoperative and postoperative management.

■ *Preoperative Assessment*

Preoperative assessment of patients who have had previous antireflux surgery must include a careful history to determine if the patient is suffering with symptoms that are disabling enough to warrant reoperation. All the patients in our series had had medical management under the guidance of a gastroenterologist and had failed medical management. All had disabling symptoms or life-threatening complications. Following a careful history and assessment of the patient's condition, diagnostic tests include upper GI barium x-ray, endoscopy with biopsy when necessary, esophageal radionuclide scintigraphy, and esophageal manometric and pH testing.

In a survey of 93 patients who had preoperative manometry the test was normal in 50. Thirty-seven patients had nonspecific manometric abnormalities characterized by frequent tertiary contractions with occasional high-amplitude, prolonged duration of peristaltic waves. Four patients had manometric evidence of collagen vascular disease and two had achalasia. Gastroesophageal reflux as measured by pH probe preoperatively was present in 73 of these patients and absent in 20. The lower esophageal

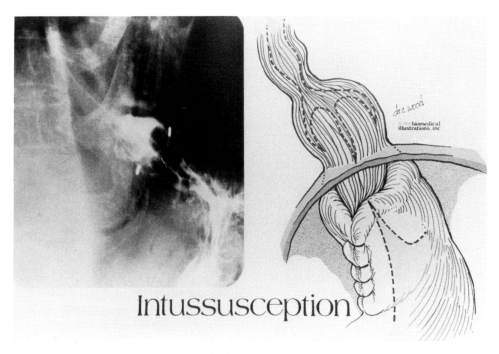

Figure 13–7. Mucosal intussusception cephalad through the wrap produced nearly complete obstruction in this patient who was suffering from severe dysphagia.

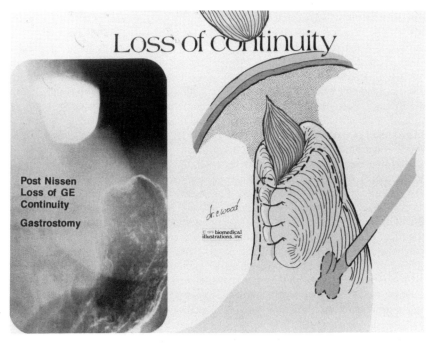

Figure 13–8. Following two failed antireflux procedures, continuity between the esophagus and stomach was lost, requiring jejunal interposition.

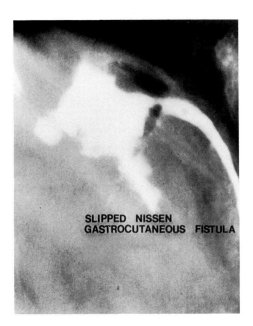

Figure 13–9. Gastrocutaneous fistula following Nissen fundoplication resulting from perforated gastric ulcer, which had formed in the obstructed pouch.

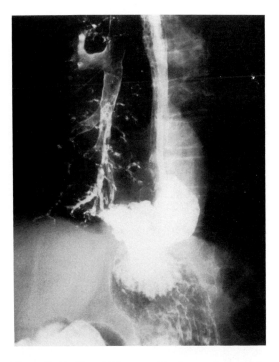

Figure 13–11. Slipped Nissen resulting in gastrobronchial fistula into the right lung.

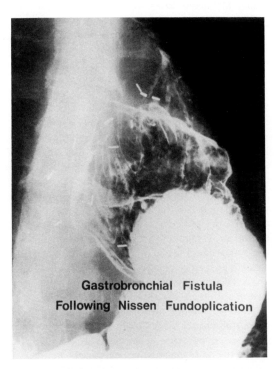

Figure 13–10. Gastric ulcer resulting from a slipped Nissen penetrated through the stomach, the diaphragm, and into the right lung producing a gastrobronchial fistula.

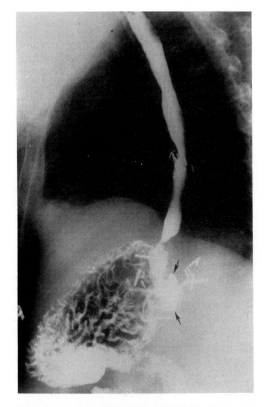

Figure 13–12. Slipped Nissen producing a large posterior ulcer, which perforated into the aorta. Operative correction resulted in the only known survivor of a gastroaortic fistula.

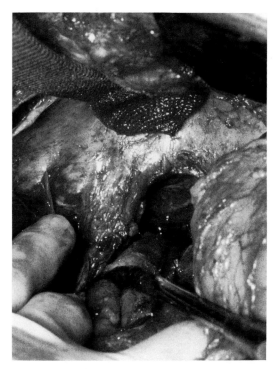

Figure 13–13. Surgical picture of the challenging complication of a gastropericardial fistula. This represents a case of true heartburn.

sphincter pressure was measured pre-, intra-, and postoperatively in nearly all patients. The mean lower esophageal sphincter pressure preoperatively was 11.1 ± 0.8 mm Hg (range of 0 to 32 mm Hg). Mean intraoperative pressure was 48.4 ± 0.8 mm Hg (range of 38 to 58 mm Hg). Postoperative pressures were 18.5 ± 0.9 mm Hg (range of 10 to 27 mm Hg).

In addition to preoperative diagnostic considerations, the patient's risks should be considered. Since these are technically difficult operations, they may require tedious dissection. The patient's pulmonary and cardiovascular status need to be thoroughly appraised. If the patient has been bleeding chronically or even acutely, hypovolemia should be corrected with preoperative blood transfusions. If the patient has been operated upon multiple times and the gastroesophageal junction has been destroyed as assessed by endoscopy, motility studies, and barium x-rays, consideration for resection rather than attempting to restore a destroyed esophagus should be made.

In our series of 303 patients, resection has been utilized in six patients with destroyed GE junctions. It is also important to determine preoperatively if the patient has had a transthoracic repair, which might indicate that the stomach is adherent to contiguous structures in the chest. In these cases, the appropriate hemithorax is prepared because a counterincision may be required in these patients in order to free the GE junction and bring it below the diaphragm.

■ Surgical Technique

The surgical approach to this diverse group of failed fundoplications was individualized, depending on the nature of the failure. In an analysis of the last 118 patients, 104 had the fundoplication taken down followed by reconstruction of the gastroesophageal junction (Hill repair). Seven patients had Hill repairs with the addition of vagotomy and pyloroplasty, either because the vagus nerve had been unknowingly cut previously or damaged during takedown of the fundoplication. The patient with multiple gastric perforations required takedown of the fundoplication with fundectomy and drainage of an empyema. The various fistulas were dealt with on an individual basis. The gastrocutaneous fistula was oversewn and a Hill procedure was performed after takedown of the fundoplication. The abdominal gastrobronchial fistula was identified at surgery and transected with a stapling device. After transecting the fistula, the fundoplication was taken down with meticulous dissection and a reconstruction of the gastroesophageal junction (Hill repair) was performed. The patient with loss of gastrointestinal continuity required resection of the fibrous cord and a jejunal interposition.

A previously unreported problem is shown in Figure 13–14. This patient has a Nissen repair which unfortunately was placed below the left gastric artery. This automatically creates a serious obstruction of the midportion of the stomach. Following this procedure the patient was unable to swallow solids, had serious gas bloat, and had continuous regurgitation. At a second surgery, another surgeon placed an Angelchik prosthesis around the wrap, again below the left gastric artery. This compounded the problem and the obstruction became complete. At reoperation, the Angelchik prosthesis was removed. A dense fibrous reaction to the prosthesis had formed around the stomach. This was dissected free, the wrap was taken down, and the gastroesophageal junction was reconstructed.

The GE junction in many of these patients is grossly abnormal and a simple antireflux procedure may not be enough. In an effort to improve the results in the management of recurrent hernias, a valvuloplasty technique has been employed in surgery for failed antireflux procedures. This adjunct has been a significant contribution to the management of the difficult antireflux operation. After the

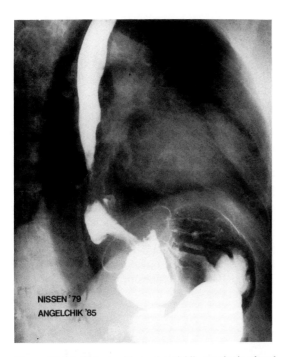

Figure 13–14. Patient with an Angelchik prosthesis placed below the left gastric artery for failed Nissen repair, also placed below the left gastric artery, resulting in complete obstruction. A dense fibrous reaction was noted to have formed around the stomach.

repair is taken down, the GE valve is palpated. If it has been destroyed, a gastrostomy is performed and the valvuloplasty technique that is described in the chapter on surgery for gastroesophageal reflux is employed.

It is worth repeating here that this procedure is based on cadaver dissections, as reported in the Chapter 2 on anatomy, and consists first of grasping the lateral edge of the esophageal introitus viewed through the gastrostomy with Babcock clamps. With a finger in the esophageal introitus the gastroesophageal valve is lengthened by placing sutures in the anterior and posterior edges of this valve, carrying the suture line cephalad up through the incisura to increase the length of the valve to 2.5 to 4 cm. These sutures are taken through and through the gastroesophageal walls. Intraoperative and postoperative pressure measurements indicate that this technique clearly lengthens the valve and offers an ideal solution in the patient with a damaged esophagus. The valve offers little or no obstruction to the flow of food and fluid into the stomach and yet offers considerable resistance to retrograde flow.

The valve can also be lengthened by placing sutures on the outside. By rotating the esophagus to the patient's right, a row of posterior sutures is placed vertically, from the incisura upward, ex-

tending the valve onto the esophagus 1.5 to 2 cm. After the posterior row is placed, a similar anterior row, starting at the angle of His on the stomach, is placed to approximate the gastric cardia to the esophagus and to lengthen the valve to 1.5 to 2 cm. The valve technique is necessary only if the standard Hill antireflux procedure does not produce a sufficient valve. This can be determined by palpation through the stomach or by visualization through the gastrostomy if one has been done to dilate the esophagus.

If the phrenoesophageal bundles are deficient and the GE junction is scarred, the standard antireflux procedure may not produce a sufficient gastroesophageal valve. In patients in whom a primary repair is done, the standard antireflux procedure produces an excellent 2 to 3 cm valve that is long-lasting, but when the tissues are deficient, this may not be possible. The valve reconstruction has been utilized in 25 patients with excellent results.

Intraoperative measurement of the barrier pressure at the GE junction has been used in all the reoperations we have done.

■ The Angelchik Prosthesis

The Angelchik prosthesis has been used in an estimated 20,000 patients across the United States.[4] An increasing number of reports of migration of the prosthesis into quadrants of the abdomen and into the chest have been noted.[5-7] A more serious problem is erosion of the prosthesis into the stomach and passage per rectum or obstruction at the pylorus.[8-10] A number of these cases are being seen as well.

We have removed six Angelchik prostheses that have either migrated from or obstructed the esophagus or partially eroded into the stomach. A patient with an obstruction resulting from the Angelchik prosthesis is shown in Figure 13–15. In all these patients at surgery a dense fibrous ring has been noted around the prosthesis and the gastroesophageal junction has generally been partially obstructed. Long-term follow-up on the Angelchik prosthesis is needed before it can be recommended as a routine. Temple of England[11,12] has reported problems with the Nissen repair including obstruction, migration, and erosion. Durrans et al.[13] and Wale et al.[14] found dysphagia and recurrent symptoms severe enough to warrant removal of the prosthesis in 10 per cent of cases. These authors, along with Watson,[4] Bombeck,[15] and others, recommend abandonment of the use of the Angelchik prosthesis.

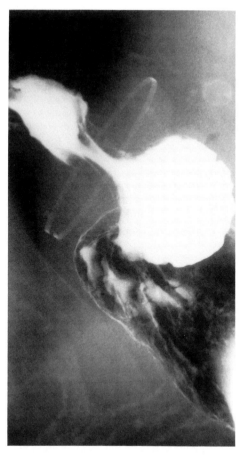

Figure 13–15. Patient with an obstruction resulting from the placement of an Angelchik prosthesis showing the dense fibrous ring noted to form in all these patients around both the prosthesis and the gastroesophageal junction.

■ *Mortality and Morbidity Rates*

The operative mortality rate in our experience of reoperative antireflux surgery has been 1.9 per cent. One patient died from postoperative intra-abdominal sepsis and one from pancreatitis complicated by multisystem organ failure. One late death of related causes occurred 10 weeks postoperatively. A patient died of cardiac arrest during a prolonged hospitalization complicated by gastric perforation and empyema. The remaining three patients died of cardiovascular accidents. Results were excellent to good in 86 per cent of the patients. Fair results occurred in 10 per cent of patients who were improved but required antacid therapy or intermittent dilatation. Poor results occurred in around 5 per cent of patients who were either no better clinically or were actually more symptomatic than preoperatively.

At the present time nearly all the reoperations performed at this institution are for failed Nissen

procedures. Only rarely has a Belsey, Thal, or Allison technique been seen. It is worth emphasizing that we have not seen the devastating fistulas, obstructions, and the life-threatening complications of the Nissen technique with the Belsey or the Allison procedure. In addition, a significant number of patients have had an antireflux operation that is unidentifiable. These variations include simple closure of the hiatus with no other sutures being employed and a variety of gastropexies and valvuloplasties that have no relation to any of the standard operations.

The Collis-Nissen and the Collis-Belsey procedures are employed apparently in large numbers in some centers in the East. These procedures have not been employed in any numbers in the Western United States, and we have seen only two patients with the Collis procedure in whom a reoperation was required.

■ *Summary and Comment*

Patients who require reoperation for failed antireflux procedures represent only a fraction of the patients who have trouble after these operations. The gas bloat syndrome emphasized by Woodward et al.[16] has been commented on by many surgeons. The persistence of reflux and the occurrence of gastric ulcers as well as recurrent herniation have all been documented with recurrence rates up to 13 per cent over four and one-half years as emphasized by Mokka et al.[17] It is only when these become so severe that they become intolerable that patients submit to reoperation. In our most recent analysis of failed antireflux procedures, it is interesting that the mean time interval between the failed fundoplication and remedial surgery was 50 months (range of 1 to 156 months). However, the mean time interval to onset of recurrence of symptoms was only 12 months. This indicated that the patients suffered with severe, disabling symptoms for an average of 38 months before submitting to reoperation. During this interval, the surgeon, the internist, ant the patient together did their utmost to make the best of a failed situation. If the patient had had more than one operation, which was the case in 35 patients with failed Nissen procedures, reluctance to undergo a third or fourth procedure is understandable.

The first report from this country dealing specifically with recurrent hiatal hernia was our report in 1971[1] in which we described 63 patients having had a variety of operations who developed recurrent problems of sufficient severity to warrant reoperation. Although reports of a high rate with antireflux operations had been noted around the world, reports dealing specifically with this problem were slow in appearing. Since the report in 1971, reports of failed antireflux operations have become much more common.

Belsey and Skinner reported on 98 recurrences in 1972.[18] The highest recurrence rates were in children under two years of age and in patients with strictures. Of these, only 45 required reoperation. Thirty-three Belsey-type repairs were successful in 26 patients. Resection was carried out in 11, with good results in 10. In 1977 Bremner reported 60 patients with significant symptomatic recurrence after antireflux procedures.[19] It is interesting that in only 17 of these was there an anatomic recurrence. In 41 patients the sphincter pressure was below normal, being zero in 15 patients. Esophageal spasm was noted in 16 and a normal sphincter pressure was noted in the remainder. These data correlate well with our analysis of 96 patients with failed antireflux procedures in whom the mean lower esophageal sphincter pressure preoperatively was 11 mm Hg $\pm$ 0.8 mm Hg (range of 0 to 32 mm Hg). Seventy-nine of the 96 patients in our group had gastroesophageal reflux, while 20 had no reflux on conventional pH and pressure testing. In the 20 patients with no reflux, obstruction from a slipped Nissen and dysphagia from dysmotility and esophageal spasm were present.

As the Nissen procedure has become more popular, more and more reports dealing with failed antireflux procedures have concentrated primarily on the Nissen procedure. Our report in 1979 of reoperation for disruption and recurrences after Nissen fundoplication was apparently the first report dealing specifically with the Nissen repair.[2] We, like others, found that most of the recurrent hernias being reported during the last decade are related to the Nissen fundoplication. The frequency of failed antireflux operations being performed in this country is impossible to determine without knowing the total number of operations being done.

The report of Ellis and coworkers[20] is important in that of the 25 cases reported 8 were from their own series. Ellis is one of the most experienced esophageal surgeons in the world, and if eight of his own cases needed reoperation, this suggests that the surgeon who infrequently operates on the esophagus will have more failures with the Nissen procedure. Recent review of the literature shows that during the last eight years, 271 cases of Nissen reoperations have been reported in large series. Many smaller series of three to four operations have also appeared. A study by Negre[21] indicates an extremely high incidence of postfundoplication symptoms in 226 patients followed for five and one-half years. Forty-four per cent of these patients had difficulty swallowing, 31 per cent were unable to vomit, 19 per cent were unable to belch, 12 per cent had abdominal pain, and 10 per cent had dyspepsia, findings which clearly restricted the success of the Nissen procedure.

Hatton et al.[22] reported that 20 per cent of all antireflux surgery at their institution stemmed from complications of the Nissen fundoplication, the indications for reoperation being dysphagia (57 per cent), recurrent reflux (36 per cent), and bloating (7 per cent). Of these patients requiring reoperation, 29 per cent required esophageal resection, either at the time of remedial surgery or following a subsequent failed fundoplication. The surgical technique of performing a Nissen fundoplication transthoracically and leaving the wrap within the chest resulted in a 40 per cent complication rate in a series by Mansour, which led them to conclude that this practice should be severely condemned.[23] There are also a number of reports of gastric ulcer forming in the Nissen wrap,[24] and there are reports of life-threatening complications including gastric left ventricular fistula and gastropericardial fistula with pericardial abscess and death.[25,26]

The report of Little et al.[27] is a significant report which represents a large series of 61 patients undergoing repeat antireflux procedures. Twenty-seven of these patients had more than one Nissen repair. Eight had at least three previous attempts at repair. Little recommended a transthoracic repair for multiple operations. We have found the transthoracic approach unnecessary except where the esophagus is virtually destroyed or the stomach is adherent to contiguous structures in the chest. Little stated, ''It is dismaying to note the number of patients in whom either a clearly inappropriate anatomic repair of a hiatal hernia or a crural repair was performed. In these patients failure can be attributed to a lack of understanding of or familiarity with the principles and technique of antireflux surgery.'' We agree emphatically with Little's statement that many antireflux procedures across the country are done by surgeons who rarely operate on the esophagus, and one only needs to read the previous note to realize that the failure can be attributed to a lack of understanding of the principles of antireflux surgery. However, we would add that the increasing number of reports of failure with the Nissen procedure indicate that the operation itself may well be flawed for the reasons we outlined. Many of the patients operated on by us had been previously operated on by board-certified surgeons in large medical centers.

As the incidence of failed Nissen fundoplications has increased, it has accounted for a higher and higher percentage of reoperations. In our most recent analysis of the Nissen fundoplication we have concluded that there are five reasons for failure of the Nissen fundoplication:

First, the wrap is done in a blind fashion around the distal end of the esophagus using a Maloney bougie or other stent in the esophagus. This in no way gives any indication of the sphincter pressure during the procedure. It is impossible to tell how tight the wrap is around the bougie. In addition, there are no attempts to alter the wrap to obtain an adequate sphincter pressure during surgery.

Second, sutures are placed from the seromuscular layer of the stomach through the muscularis of the esophagus. The esophagus has no serosa. The sutures therefore have a tendency to pull out of the muscularis, resulting in either fistula formation or allowance of the wrap to migrate distally. If the sutures pull out of the seromuscular layer of the stomach, the wrap then disrupts.

Third, there is no calibration of the cardia, which we feel is mandatory so that the patient at the time of surgery will have a sphincter pressure adjusted to an adequate level.

Fourth, the fundoplication is not anchored. The gastroesophageal junction is normally anchored, as is the entire GI tract, by the dorsal mesentery to the posterior body wall. By creating a fundoplication, these posterior attachments are destroyed, allowing the wrap to migrate into the chest or slip up and down in the abdomen. Without a fulcrum, the esophagus has difficulty generating peristaltic waves strong enough to propel food aborally. This may well account for much of the dysphagia and gas bloat syndrome associated with the Nissen. Cordiano in Chapter 9C on the Nill procedure points out that his results improved after anchoring the wrap to the preaortic fascia. He showed by manometry that the esophageal motility was better in the anchored esophagus.

Fifth, if the Nissen fundoplication is performed transthoracically and left in the thorax, the wrap represents an iatrogenic, paraesophageal hernia which may suffer all the attendant complications of that type of herniation. Gastric ulcers, incarceration, and rupture have been seen by our group in patients with transthoracic fundoplications.

Intraoperative manometry, in our opinion, could well prevent many of the complications reported in this chapter. The patulous gastroesophageal junction, the most common cause of failure of antireflux procedures, can be prevented by the use of intraoperative manometrics which objectively demonstrates to the surgeon whether an adequate range of barrier pressure has been created. The obstructed antireflux procedure can likewise be prevented by determining at the time of operation that the barrier pressure is not too high.

During reoperation for failed antireflux procedures, intraoperative manometrics is very helpful because anatomy is obscured and adhesions are present, particularly after multiple operations. With the aid of intraoperative pressure measurements, the surgeon not only can locate the barrier but determine if an adequate barrier has been reconstructed. If the barrier pressure cannot be raised adequately, the valvuloplasty procedure is added.

In conclusion, the large number of complications and the failure rate with antireflux surgery that are being reported around the world are alarming. If we are to restore the confidence on the part of the gastroenterologist and other physicians, it is imperative that surgeons pay attention to the details and principles of antireflux surgery. It is obvious from ours and others' experience, that the first operation is the optimal time to do the definitive repair. Antireflux surgery is nearly always elective. The surgeon has ample time to utilize proper techniques aided with modern technology. With modern instrumentation being readily available, the surgeon has the ability to determine precisely what is being done at surgery. With these newer techniques, the mortality, morbidity, and complication rates of reoperations should be preventable.

■ REFERENCES

1. Hill LD: Management of recurrent hiatal hernia. Arch Surg, *102*:296–302, 1971.
2. Hill LD, Ilves R, Stevenson JK, Pearson JM: Reoperation for disruption and recurrence after Nissen fundoplication. Arch Surg, *114*:542–548, 1979.
3. Mercer CD, James EC, Hill LD: Post Nissen syndrome (to be published).
4. Watson A: Angelchik antireflux prosthesis. Br J Surg, 72:935–936, 1985.
5. Starling JR, Reichelderfer MO, Pellet JR, Belzer FO: Treatment of symptomatic GE reflux using the Angelchik prosthesis. Ann Surg, *195*:689–691, 1982.
6. Temple JG, Taylor TV, Williams A: A simple operative prosthetic treatment for GE reflux. J Roy Coll Surg Edinb, 29:16–17, 1984.
7. Pickelman J: Disruption and migration of an Angelchik oesophageal antireflux prosthesis. Surgery, *93*:467–468, 1983.
8. Lackey C, Potts J: Penetration into stomach—a complication of the Angelchik prosthesis. JAMA, *248*:350, 1982.
9. Van der Brandt G, Huibregtsch K, Tyfgat L: Endoscopical removal of an antireflux prosthesis. Acta Endosc, *13*:47–50, 1983.
10. Lilly MP, Slatsky F, Thomson W: Intraabdominal erosion and migration of the Angelchik prosthesis. Arch Surg, *119*:849–853, 1984.
11. Weaver RM, Temple JG: Angelchik prosthesis for gastroesophageal reflux: Symptomatic and objective assessment. Ann R Coll Surg Engl, *567*:299–302, 1985.
12. Temple JG: Personal communication.
13. Durrans S, Armstrong CP, Taylor TV: The Angelchik antireflux prosthesis—some reservations. Br J Surg, *72*:526–527, 1985.

14. Wale RJ, Royston CMS, Bennett JR, Buckton GK: Br J Surg, 72:520–524, 1985.
15. Bombeck CT: The choice of operations for gastrooesophageal reflux. In Watson A, Celestin LR (Eds): Disorders of the Oesophagus. London, Pitman, 1984.
16. Woodward ER, Thomas HF, McAlhany JC: Comparison of crural repair and Nissen fundoplication for the treatment of esophageal hiatal hernia with peptic esophagitis. Ann Surg, 173:782–792, 1971.
17. Mokka REM, Laitinen S, Punto L: Hiatal hernia repair. Ann Chir Gynaecol, 65:369–375, 1976.
18. Belsey RHR, Skinner DB: Management of esophageal strictures. In Skinner DB, Belsey RHR, Hendrix TR, Zuidema GD (Eds): Gastroesophageal Reflux and Hiatal Hernia. Boston, Little, Brown, 1972, Chap 14, pp 173–196.
19. Bremner CG: Gastric ulcer after the Nissen fundoplication: A complication of alkaline reflux. S Afr Med J, 51:791–793, 1977.
20. Leonardi HK, Crozier RE, Ellis FH: Reoperation for complications of the Nissen fundoplication. J Thorac Cardiovasc Surg, 81:50–56, 1981.
21. Negre JB: Post fundoplication symptoms. Do they restrict the success of Nissen fundoplication? Ann Surg, 198:698–700, 1983.
22. Hatton PD, Selenkoft PM, Harford FJ: Surgical management of the failed Nissen fundoplication. Am J Surg, 148:760–763, 1984.
23. Mansour KA, Burton HG, Miller JI, Hatcher CR: Complications of intrathoracic Nissen fundoplication. Ann Thorac Surg, 32:173–178, 1981.
24. Bushkin FL, Woodward ER, O'Leary JP: Occurrence of gastric ulcer after Nissen fundoplication. Am Surgeon, 42:821–826, 1976.
25. Nakhgevana KB, Parra LA: Gastric left ventricular fistula: An ususual complication of Nissen fundoplication. Contemporary Surg, 23:57–60, 1983.
26. Ikard RW, Jacobs JR: Gastropericardial fistula and pericardial abscess: An unusual complication of subphrenic abscess following Nissen fundoplication. S Med J, 67:17–19, 1974.
27. Little AG, Ferguson MK, Skinner DB: Reoperation for failed antireflux operations. Surgery, 91:511–517, 1986.

Motility Disorders

Martin D. Gelfand

Interest in motility disorders of the esophagus as a possible explanation of noncardiac chest pain has been kindled by advances in diagnostic abilities and therapeutic choices. These patients do not have gastroesophageal reflux, for the discomfort is not the typical burning sensation and does not respond to antacids or potent drugs that decrease acid secretion. Moreover, obvious acid reflux is not usually present on studies attempting to confirm this problem. Since reflux is not the cause, these complaints are now being attributed to esophageal dysmotility.[1,2]

Improvements in esophageal manometric technique have uncovered patterns of increased contractility. Although at times present in a patient when free of distress, they more often need to be provoked by pharmacologic or physical agents. Unfortunately, even this occurs in less than half of patients suspected of an esophageal source of pain.[3]

New insights into both medical and surgical treatment of esophageal motor disorders have kept pace with the increased number of patients whose chest symptoms are being identified as esophageal in origin. The role of precise manometric diagnosis is becoming increasingly clear as treatment evolves for each specific motor abnormality.

■ Clinical Presentation

The symptoms of esophageal motility disorders are chest pain and dysphagia. The chest discomfort tends to be central, substernal, and persistent. It may radiate cephalad to neck, jaw, and back, and even down the left arm. Its intensity may vary from a dull ache to a severe, crushing pain that may lead to a trip to a hospital and admission to the coronary care unit. The pain rarely comes on during a meal. Rather, it is spontaneous, perhaps brought on by stress, but not infrequently awakening the patient at night. A residual soreness may last into the next day, and attacks may be multiple, each lasting 5 to 30 min in one day.

The patient may not realize there is difficulty swallowing during pain, for he or she will not feel like ingesting anything. To discover a temporal association between the chest pain and esophageal function may require the patient being told to eat or drink when pain starts as an attempt to elicit dysphagia. Manometric evaluation may be inconclusive when the patient is pain-free and may be impossible to arrange at the time of an attack; thus, this instruction may yield the only information that confirms the diagnosis of esophageal spasm, albeit a subjective judgment. A large glass of liquid rapidly imbibed may produce the sensation of going down slowly, as if over a series of ledges, regurgitation before entering the stomach, or increased pain. However, normal individuals were shown to dilate their esophagus when pain was induced by ingestion of cold liquids.[4] A subgroup of patients will not have dysphagia at the time of their chest pain owing to a similar mechanism. Attacks of pain are usually intermittent and do not produce weight loss. Heartburn, if present, is not severe and does not precede the symptoms of dysmotility.

■ *Differential Diagnosis*

Before ascribing chest discomfort to esophageal motor disease, the diagnosis of angina pectoris must be excluded. Even patients referred specifically to a gastroenterologist must be suspected of possible angina, and the results of a treadmill electrocardiogram should be reviewed. With any hint that the discomfort relates to exertion, angina is especially likely. The pain of coronary insufficiency may seem esophageal because it can be nocturnal, postprandial, and transiently relieved by eructation. Some patients assume strange postures in an attempt to relieve their angina by "reducing" their hiatal hernia. Associated dyspnea, diaphoresis, or dizziness can occur with either source, as can a feeling of doom or radiation of the discomfort into jaw or arm. Identifying dysphagia at the time of chest pain best reassures that the esophagus and not the heart is the culprit. A few patients may have both esophageal and heart disease with indistinguishable complaints. Medical treatment for each fortunately employs the same drugs. Pain refractory to medical management mandates consideration of further cardiac studies so that additional treatment for either heart or esophageal disease will resolve the problem.

Diffuse esophageal spasm had been suspected as often being precipitated by gastroesophageal reflux.[5] This currently does not appear to be true.[6,7] Pain with swallowing can occur from a severely acid-eroded esophagus, but radiologic or manometric abnormalities are localized to the distal esophagus. When heartburn is a prominent symptom, confirmed reflux should be treated, but symptoms from underlying motor disease may well remain. Surgery to correct reflux will similarly not eliminate a patient's dysmotility complaints.

Severe, persistent substernal pain frequently results from a sudden insult to the esophagus from an exogenous substance and not intrinsic spasm. Tetracycline therapy is the commonest setting. This drug lodging in the esophagus will cause an inflammatory reaction with secondary spasm that may take 7 to 14 days to dissipate and requires only reassurance and analgesia.[8] Everyone given this medication should be instructed to remain upright and swallow a large glass of water before and after ingesting the capsule. Other drugs that can do this are potassium, theophylline and indomethacin, as well as cromolyn inhalant. Similar symptoms can also occur in viral diseases, such as hepatitis, mononucleosis, and pericarditis. These either systemically or by local extension can affect the esophagus. Again, no specific treatment is needed. Not only in the compromised host but even in the normal person, *Candida* may be the cause.[9] Usually only inspection for thrush or a barium x-ray to reveal typical findings is required before initiating drug treatment.

Of concern in the patient with chest pain and dysphagia is the possibility of cancer. Symptoms are more likely progressive and produce weight loss. Anorexia or nausea may already be prevalent. Diagnostic studies are done, even if only to exclude a neoplasm.

The thoracic outlet syndrome can mimic esophageal motor disease, but this diagnosis is uncommon or at least rarely recognized. If repetitive use of the upper extremities precipitates the chest discomfort, further investigation is warranted.

Esophageal dysmotility has on occasion followed truncal vagotomy. Temporary dysphagia has been attributed to extrinsic mechanical obstruction caused by intraoperative periesophageal trauma.[10] A number of patients, however, develop persistent dysphagia with an irreversible motility disturbance similar to achalasia.[11]

■ *Classification*

The recognition of different manometric patterns has enabled a classification of esophageal motor disorders. Although the symptoms of dysmotility in each category may be similar, and the etiology, currently unknown, may prove to be the same, the disorders when looked at separately may be more easily characterized. Moreover, optimal treatment may differ and depend on knowledge of the particular form.[12]

■ ACHALASIA

The most distinctive as well as longest recognized and best understood motor disease is achalasia. It is appreciated on barium radiography as a widened, flaccid esophagus with a short, symmetric "bird's beak" narrowing at the cardioesophageal junction. Delayed barium emptying allows a column to form in the esophagus. The increased sphincter tone prevents air from normally appearing in the gastric fundus (Figure 14–1).

The typical symptom complex is slowly progressive, intermittent dysphagia to both liquids and solids. Any degree of chest discomfort may also be experienced. Severe, crushing pain may arise from concomitant spasm, as in "vigorous" achalasia, or a milder pressure sensation from fluid or food distending the esophagus. It may even be described as burning with transient relief by an ant-

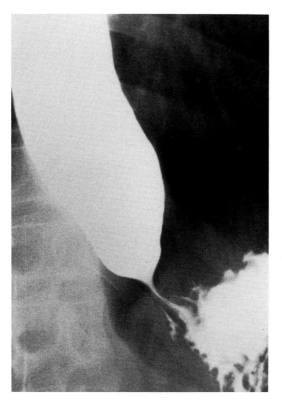

Figure 14–1. Achalasia. Barium x-ray showing dilated esophagus and characteristic narrowing (bird-beak) at gastroesophageal junction. Note absence of gastric air bubble.

acid, but reflux is, by the nature of the disease, always absent. Nocturnal regurgitation of sweet-tasting, undigested material may lead to coughing and aspiration. A more accelerated form of the disease may present with rapidly progressive dysphagia and weight loss. This must be differentiated from "secondary" achalasia caused by a neoplasm at the cardioesophageal junction. The source of this tumor is usually gastric, but lung, pancreas, and lymphomas have been described in this area, even in conjunction with marked esophageal widening. By the cancer invading the myenteric plexus, the sphincter loses its innervation to relax and appears unyielding. Also, inexplicably, aperistalsis affects the body of the esophagus. Resection of the neoplasm results in return of peristalsis.[13]

The manometric criteria for achalasia are (1) absence of peristalsis; (2) elevated lower esophageal sphincter (LES) pressure; and (3) incomplete LES relaxation. In the lower two thirds of the esophagus, the smooth muscle portion, all swallow waves are aperistaltic. Their amplitude can vary from very low in most patients to above normal in those with a "vigorous" form of this disease (Figs. 14–2 and 14–3).[14] Swallow waves may be repetitive and appear spontaneously without deglutition. LES pressure ranges from high-normal to markedly elevated (up to three times normal). Occasionally, not all the usual features are apparent, an entity termed "pseudoachalasia."[15] These patients may not respond as well to the usual treatment.

Although failure of relaxation of the LES is part of the definition of the disease, its demonstration manometrically is not mandatory, for no diagnostic confusion should result with the other features present. In a dilated esophagus the catheter assembly may not pass through the cardioesophageal junction by simple gravity. The LES pressure can then only be obtained by tying a suture to the assembly and held by a biopsy forceps through an endoscope, so that it can be passed into the stomach by direct vision. As the forceps is released and endoscope removed, the assembly remains in the stomach and can be withdrawn through the LES, determining its pressure.

■ DIFFUSE ESOPHAGEAL SPASM

The hypercontractile motility disorder, diffuse esophageal spasm (DES), has classically been believed to be the chief esophageal cause of severe chest pain.[16] Because radiologic and manometric features of DES may also be seen in asymptomatic persons, the diagnosis is a clinical one based on symptoms with typical test findings. Why one patient is symptomatic in this instance and another is not is still a mystery.

Barium study reveals diffuse, powerful contractions, appearing as "curling," that obliterate the normal esophageal peristaltic sequence. Less noticeable waviness or scalloping of the margin of the barium-filled esophagus also may indicate dysmotility. The presence of a pulsion diverticulum, usually epiphrenic, is an important sign of spasm.[17]

Manometrically, nonperistaltic contractions may be repetitive, increased in duration (>6 sec), increased in amplitude (>150 mm Hg), and spontaneous. However, normal peristaltic function is also intermittently present. LES pressure is usually normal, with complete relaxation upon deglutition. DES may over years evolve into achalasia, with "vigorous" achalasia perhaps being in the middle of this spectrum.[18] The esophagus in spasm, moreover, manifests the same supersensitivity of a denervated organ to cholinergic agents such as Mecholyl (no longer available), as earlier noted in achalasia.[19] Patients with DES may have a thickened esophageal wall that can be appreciated by surgical palpation or visualized by computer tomography.

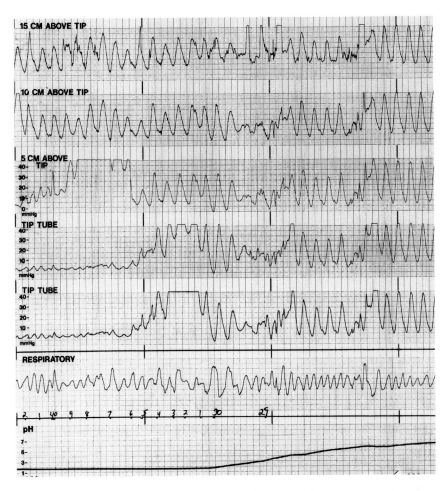

Figure 14–2. Motility study at a speed of 2.5 mm/sec showing repetitive, aperistaltic swallow waves that are normal amplitude with an elevated sphincter pressure compatible with vigorous achalasia.

■ SUPERSQUEEZE ("NUTCRACKER") ESOPHAGUS

As patients with noncardiac chest pain were studied with improved fidelity recording systems, a manometric pattern different from DES was recognized. The very high amplitude, peristaltic swallow waves seen were termed "nutcracker esophagus." This is a poor term because it implies aperistalsis, and should be replaced by the name, "supersqueeze," which is already being used by some. Mean amplitude in the distal esophagus greater than 150 mm Hg with individual waves over 180 mm Hg qualifies for this diagnosis. Increased duration of contraction should also be present, and may be even more specific than amplitude in defining this patient group (Fig. 14–4). Supersqueeze is a far more common finding in the motility lab than DES.[20]

Supersqueeze is not known to evolve into DES or achalasia. Its persistence on follow-up manom-

etry was seen by the author in a patient seven years after his initial manometry showed an identical supersqueeze pattern. Radiologic recognition may be difficult. Clinically, these patients are indistinguishable from ones with DES.

■ HYPERTENSIVE LES

Some patients in the manometry laboratory demonstrate an elevated LES pressure but normal peristalsis in the body of the esophagus, which at times can include features of diffuse spasm. This group of patients, called hypertensive sphincter, may complain more of dysphagia than chest pain.[21] Treatment should be aimed at decreasing LES strength.

■ NONSPECIFIC MOTOR ABNORMALITIES

Other abnormal findings noted at manometry consist of multiple peaked wave forms, decreased

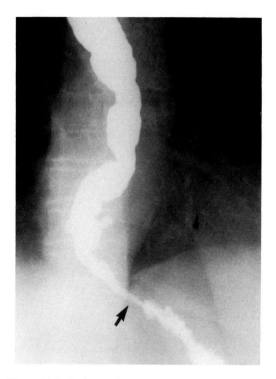

Figure 14–3. Barium study showing asymmetric tertiary contractions of esophagus and typical distal esophageal appearance of achalasia (arrow). This 78-year-old woman with recent onset of rapidly progressive symptoms did very well after a long myotomy for the "vigorous" form of this disease.

amplitude peristaltic waves, increased duration of waves, and isolated simultaneous or spontaneous contractions.[22] These may be similar in importance to abnormal ST-T waves in an electrocardiogram. Perhaps they will evolve into a more specific pattern or become more abnormal with provocative agents. Symptoms relate to these nonspecific findings with less certainty.

■ *Pathophysiology*

The cause of motor abnormalities of the esophagus is unknown. Our understanding is limited by our inability to ascertain what is occurring at the molecular level. Measuring motor activity alone ignores the electrical, neurochemical, and myogenic failures that lead up to the disordered muscle contraction. It is little wonder, then, that the precipitating stimulus of this process has remained elusive.[23]

Dysfunction of the LES or body of the esophagus can be measured manometrically and split into various categories. However, these may be manifestations of the same disease. There are, moreover,

numerous generalized conditions that affect the esophagus, causing disordered motility. These include collagen vascular diseases, neuromuscular disease, and diabetes. Aging alone has been described as a source of a boggy, aperistaltic esophagus. But the term "presbyesophagus" is of less value than the manometric classification of the motor disturbance.[24]

Microscopic study of the esophagus has been limited by the inability to acquire a meaningful number of organs, as motor disorders are not soon fatal. The most consistent lesion in achalasia is ganglion cell degeneration with loss of the myenteric plexus.[25,26] This neurogenic abnormality occurs not only in the esophageal wall but also in the extraesophageal vagus nerve. The intracytoplasmic inclusions characteristically present in the brain stem in Parkinson's disease have been found in the esophageal myenteric plexus in two patients with achalasia, suggesting a relationship between these diseases.[27] The achalasia esophagus has a reduced number of vasoactive intestinal polypeptide (VIP) fibers. VIP has been proposed as an inhibitory neurotransmitter in smooth muscle activity. A decreased level can contribute to the incomplete relaxation and increased pressure of the LES in achalasia.[28] The familial occurrence of achalasia has suggested a genetic component or common environmental pathogen.[29] Smooth muscle hypertrophy is evident at the LES in achalasia, and in the vigorous form and DES may involve the esophagus to the level of the aortic arch.

■ *Diagnostic Studies*

A review of the diagnostic studies available for motility disorders should help establish a logical approach to their use. Assessment of the heart as a source of chest pain is an early essential part of the evaluation. Coexistent heart disease and esophageal dysmotility indicate that the role the gullet plays in causing symptoms cannot be determined until the degree of coronary insufficiency is appreciated.[30]

The importance of the patient's observation of dysphagia at the time of chest pain bears repetition. Since esophageal motor disorders have transient objective changes rarely occurring during a meal or motility testing, their documentation is a vexing problem. Therefore, the patient should note during an attack how a glass of water or piece of bread or apple is swallowed.

The barium swallow is not to be overlooked. Cinefluorography, often stated as indispensable, is frequently not available and is not necessary to the

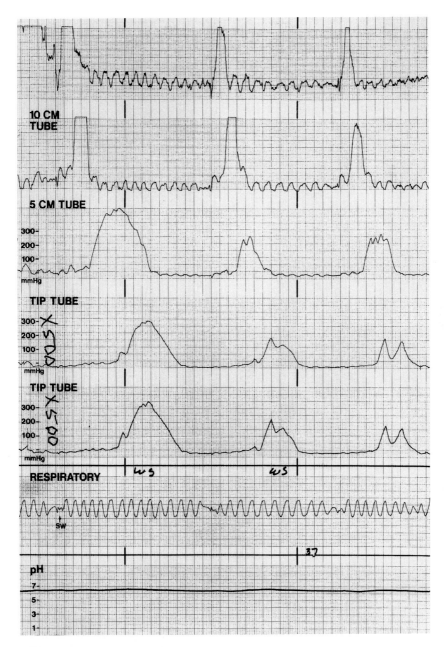

Figure 14–4. Motility study at a speed of 2.5 mm/sec showing increased amplitude contractions that are broad and indicative of a ''supersqueeze'' esophagus.

careful and informed fluoroscopist. Attention to the cardioesophageal junction will focus on its structural integrity and allow interpretation of how easily this area opens with deglutition. Swallow waves can be assessed for peristalsis, noting the occurrence of tertiary waves or obvious incoordination. Identification of the telltale diverticulum may help confirm hypercontractility (Fig. 14–5). Other observations such as air in the stomach, tumefaction in the fundus, widening of the esophagus, or in-

flammatory changes are, of course, also recorded. Usually the evaluation will not stop here, but valuable information may be obtained.

Fiberoptic endoscopy is utilized except when the clinical situation is clear without it, such as drug ulceration in a young person. In suspected achalasia endoscopic inspection passing into the stomach excludes malignancy and benign inflammatory strictures. Muscular resistance of the LES and tertiary contractions are difficult to judge, but nodu-

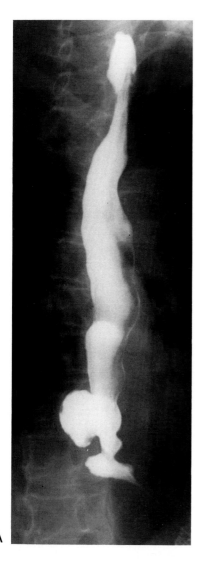

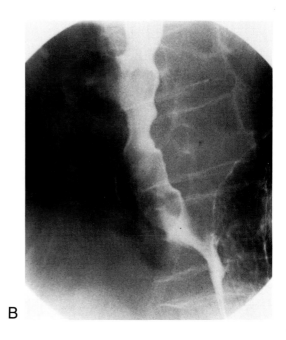

Figure 14–5. *A,* Barium study showing a wide-mouthed diverticulum in a 77-year-old man who had experienced an esophageal diverticulectomy 20 years previously. *B,* His barium study after pneumatic dilation performed for gradual worsening of dysphasia secondary to achalasia with the diverticulum no longer apparent.

larity and rigidity should warn of a structural abnormality rather than primary motor disease. Endoscopy detects mucosal inflammation with more sensitivity than barium study.

Manometric examination of the esophagus is the definitive test for dysmotility. Even with an abnormal barium study, more precise definition of the LES and body of the esophagus may be clinically useful. After LES pressure is recorded, motility in the esophagus is measured using at least three catheters 5 cm apart in response to 10 sips of water each 30 sec apart. Abnormalities may be apparent even when the patient is not having pain, but a normal study in patients strongly suspected of having esophageal spasm is frustratingly common. Confusingly, a few patients, who by chance developed chest pain while undergoing manometry, were found to have no change in their motility from when they were not having pain.[31] In achal-

asia, by contrast, the characteristic abnormalities are present at all times.

Because patients so infrequently have their pain during baseline manometric examination, provocative testing was proposed to produce symptoms while undergoing study that can then be correlated with a change in motility.[3] This is analogous to treadmill testing to elicit ECG changes and chest pain in a patient with suspected angina.

Numerous pharmacologic agents were tried to induce dysmotility with the most effective and safest being edrophonium (Tensilon), 80 μgm/kg, given intravenously. Concomitant provocation of the patient's chest discomfort also could be induced and is necessary for a positive interpretation of the test (Fig. 14–6). Edrophonium increases amplitude height in both patients and normal volunteers, with only the duration of swallow waves becoming significantly longer in patients in whom chest pain

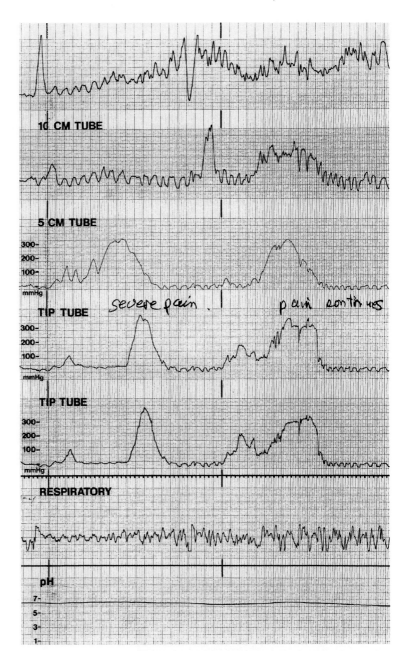

Figure 14–6. Motility study at a speed of 2.5 mm/sec showing a "supersqueeze" pattern in conjunction with the appearance of severe, substernal chest pain after intravenous Tensilon.

was induced.[32] Replication of chest pain, therefore, appears to be the decisive factor in identifying those patients with true esophageal dysfunction, with manometric changes being meaningless. Even abnormal baseline manometric findings did not predict pain with edrophonium, an observation complicating their interpretation. Without a perfect means for diagnosing esophageal chest pain, the value of any test to identify these patients is open to question. Inflation of an esophageal balloon has shown promise as a provocative test (Castell, abstract). Food ingestion in the upright position is another maneuver that may replace edrophonium

administration as a better means of detecting dysmotility in conjunction with eliciting chest pain and dysphagia (Mellow, abstract).

Radionuclide scintigraphy can examine esophageal function. This technique uses a gamma camera to measure the transit of tagged technetium sulfur colloid. Liquid boluses are administered to the patient in the supine position. A computer displays the rate of passage of the bolus through each third of the esophagus. The pattern for each area can delineate achalasia and DES.[33] This test will probably not identify the supersqueeze, but can serve as an alternative if manometry is unavailable or intubation of the catheter assembly cannot be tolerated. Although abnormal scintiscans have been described in patients with presumed noncardiac chest pain and normal manometry, any claim of greater sensitivity is difficult to interpret. No advantage over manometry has been proved.

Solid food scintigraphy with the patient upright is the study closest approximating normal food ingestion. This measure of esophageal emptying is an excellent means of assessing the success of treatment in achalasia.[34] The percentage of food remaining in the esophagus 20 min after ingestion gives an objective comparison after whatever therapy has been used.

Patients with hypercontractility may benefit from being examined for a thickened esophageal wall. Computed tomography (CT) of the chest can accurately measure esophageal wall thickness, with normal being up to 3 mm.[35] Identifying a long segment of muscular hypertrophy indicates that surgery would require a longitudinal myotomy (Fig. 14–7). Excessive wall thickness by itself is a nonspecific finding and may be focal in malignant as well as other benign conditions.

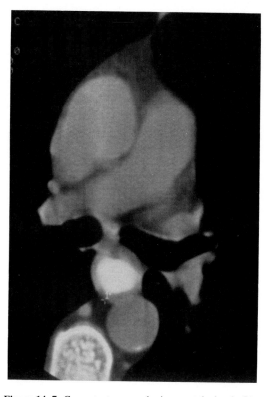

Figure 14–7. Computer tomography image at the level of just below the aortic arch showing a thickened (4.5 cm) esophageal wall in the same patient whose motility is shown in Figure 14–2.

■ Treatment

The aim in achalasia is to destroy partially the unyielding, high-pressure LES. As emptying is improved, esophageal stasis and its consequences are reduced. Even though peristalsis usually does not return, the patient feels as if deglutition is normal. This can be achieved by either pneumatic dilation using an instrument to tear the sphincter muscle or by surgical myotomy.[36,37] Dilatation may be the more accurate term but is less commonly used and may sound affected.

This chapter does not purport to be a syllabus on how to perform a pneumatic dilation.[38] A few observations, though, may be of theoretical and practical benefit. Before the dilation, structural stenosis should be excluded by successful passage of a large mercury dilator. These Maloney or Hurst bougies by themselves never satisfactorily treat achalasia. Esophageal residue should be emptied from a dilated esophagus by aspirating from a large nasogastric or Ewald tube. The dilation is performed with the patient in the supine position. With an uncooperative patient or child, general anesthesia using a cuffed endotracheal tube can be given in the fluoroscopy room without affecting the likelihood of the procedure's success.[39] Preferred balloons include the Browne-McHardy, or if a guidewire is necessary owing to tortuosity of the esophagus, the Mosher bag. This also will work in a patient with a small gastric pouch from a subtotal gastrectomy as its coiled spring tip will bend back on itself, allowing proper positioning of the bag. Other types have assuredly served experienced clinicians well. Preliminary results with the microvasive achalasia balloon system have been excellent, and this may evolve into the instrument of choice (Kozarek, Gelfand and Christie, abstract).

Although the patient would like immediate success from a single dilation, the outcome may not be apparent for a month. A good result produces lifelong benefit without further treatment. If a 30- or 35-mm ballon proves unsuccessful, dilation with the next larger balloon may be attempted. If this, too, fails, surgery should be suggested. Assessment of LES pressure and a solid-food scintiscan one month after treatment gives objective data to help interpret residual symptoms. A post-treatment LES pressure of 7 to 15 mm and a 20-min scintiscan of less than 20 per cent should indicate an excellent result.

The Mason Clinic 10-year (1974–1983) experience is an example of results that should be expected from both forms of treatment and correlates well with data from other institutions.[40] Pneumatic dilation was performed in 57 patients, with 76 per cent of those with an adequate follow-up having an excellent result. Surgery was utilized in 26 patients, 82 per cent of whom were markedly improved at follow-up, even though many had previous unsuccessful treatment elsewhere. Two patients were perforated at dilation and required surgical drainage. Both recovered and swallow well without sequelae. This is similar to the accepted 5 per cent perforation rate that patients should be warned about prior to the procedure. Pneumatic dilation can be employed successfully in patients not helped by surgical myotomy (Fig. 14–8).[39] Immediately after dilation, the patient may be examined for a perforation.[41] After positioning semi-erect, the gag reflex is tested by a sip of water. If that is not aspirated, first a water-soluble contrast medium and then a barium solution is swallowed to look for extravasation, which usually presents above the diaphragm and to the left and posterior of the esophagus. Even if none is apparent, the patient should be kept in the hospital overnight, with hourly temperatures recorded. If a fever develops, the patient should have a chest x-ray and repeat contrast study. A walled-off excrescence indicates a contained perforation that usually can be treated with antibiotics alone. If afebrile, the patient may be given a clear liquid supper and regular meals the next day. Although substernal burning may be an early complaint postdilation, this does not indicate reflux; which is rarely a problem following pneumatic dilation. Peristalsis may inexplicably return in perhaps 20 per cent of patients after pneumatic dilation and after surgery as well (Fig. 14–9).[42] Routine long-term follow-up of patients with achalasia is not necessary. An increased risk of esophageal carcinoma is reported, especially with longstanding, untreated disease, but the incidence is small.[43] Surveillance would be costly and is of no established benefit.

Before discovery of calcium-channel blockers, drug therapy for esophageal motility disorders consisted principally of the antispasm effects of nitrates.[44,45] Studies with the new class of agents, especially nifedipine, however, have demonstrated a reduction of LES pressure and inhibition of contractions in the body of the esophagus.[46] These findings suggested the use of these drugs in achalasia.[47,48] Experience with them has shown partial relief of symptoms, and when the risks associated with dilation or surgery in an ill or aged patient are excessive, they can be tried. Patients with continued difficulty after treatment and especially those with vigorous achalasia may also benefit. Nifedipine, 10 to 20 mg, administered three to four times daily, has the advantage of rapid sublingual absorption when the capsule is punctured.

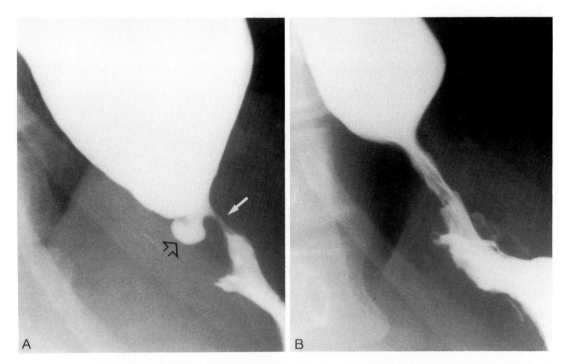

Figure 14–8. *A,* Barium study showing a markedly dilated esophagus with a pseudodiverticulum in the dependent portion and a short area of marked narrowing at the cardioesophageal junction after two prior surgical procedures for achalasia. *B,* After pneumatic dilation in this 12-year-old girl barium rapidly enters the stomach, the pseudodiverticulum is no longer seen, and there is no narrowing at the cardioesophageal junction.

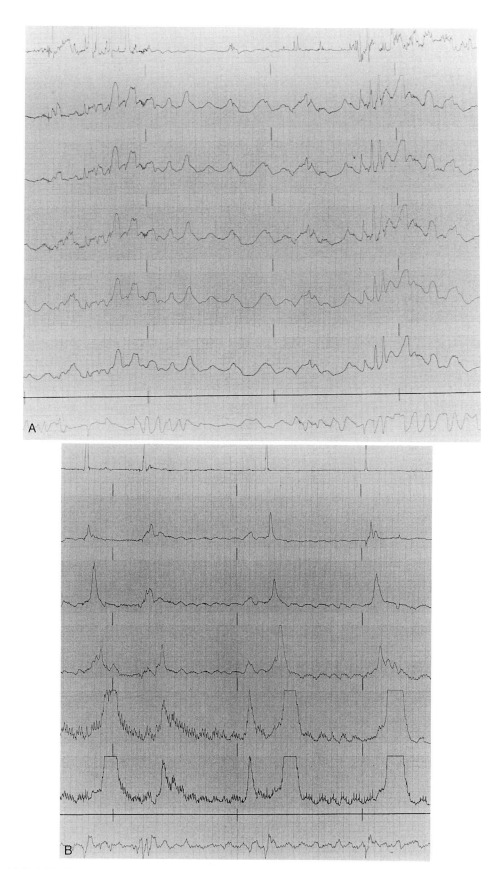

Figure 14–9. *A,* Motility study at the body of the esophagus showing aperistaltic, low-amplitude swallow waves typical of achalasia. *B,* Motility study of the same patient one month after surgical cardiomyotomy appearing normal as peristalsis and improved amplitude are now present.

The calcium-channel blockers may be an important advance in treating the hypercontractile dysmotilities. Contraction amplitude is reduced in both the aperistaltic waves of diffuse spasm and the long duration peristaltic waves of super-squeeze.[49] These drugs may not be more active than nitrates, but they possess different and perhaps less troublesome side effects. If one drug proves intolerable, one from the other group should be tried. The dose of drug chosen should be pushed as high as possible to achieve an optimal response. The calcium-channel blocker, diltiazem, 90 mg, administered up to four times daily, may be better tolerated than nifedipine and perhaps even more effective in decreasing the amplitude of swallow waves in the body of the esophagus.

Before drug treatment for esophageal dysmotility is considered, the patient's symptoms should be assessed for severity and frequency. Any precipitating cause should, of course, be eliminated. Some patients require merely reassurance, as knowing that the cause of the chest discomfort is not cardiac may make it tolerable. Patients who only have occasional severe pain may do best with only sublingual nitroglycerin during an attack. More frequent symptoms suggest daily treatment with perhaps a calcium-channel blocker as first choice. The natural history of spasm or super-squeeze is unknown, except for the rare person who progresses to achalasia. Patients can be told that their symptoms should not get worse. Drugs once started can readily be stopped, although rebound worsening of symptoms may occur. Patients may, however, function well without them. Usually, dysmotility is chronic, with symptoms persisting over years. The final chapter to this frustrating disorder has not been written, for these heterogeneous disorders are providing clues grudgingly. The co-ordinated efforts of talented investigators and observant clinicians are continually amassing data that will eventually solve the riddle of noncardiac chest pain.

■ REFERENCES

1. Brand D, Martin D, Pope C: Esophageal manometrics in patients with angina-like chest pain. Am J Dig Dis, 22:300–304, 1977.
2. Clouse RE, Stenson WF, Avioli LV: Esophageal motility disorders and chest pain. Arch Intern Med, 145:903–906, 1985.
3. Benjamin SB, Richter JE, Cordova CM, et al: Prospective manometric evaluation with pharmacologic provocation of patients with suspected esophageal motility dysfunction. Gastroenterology, 84:893–901, 1983.
4. Meyer W, Castell DO: Human esophageal response during chest pain induced by swallowing cold liquids. JAMA, 246:2057–2059, 1981.
5. Siegel CI, Hendrix TR: Esophageal motility abnormalities induced by acid perfusion in patients with heartburn. J Clin Invest, 42:686–695, 1963.
6. Burns TW, Venturatos SG: Esophageal motor function and response to acid perfusion in patients with symptomatic reflux esophagitis. Dig Dis Sci, 30:529–534, 1985.
7. Richter JE, Johns DN, Wu WC, et al: Are esophageal motility abnormalities produced during the intraesophageal acid perfusion test? JAMA, 253:1914–1917, 1985.
8. Amendola MA, Spera TD: Doxycycline-induced esophagitis. JAMA, 253:1009–1011, 1985.
9. Brown JW, McKee WM: Acute monilial esophagitis occurring without underlying disease in a young male. Am J Dig Dis, 17:85–88, 1972.
10. Carter SL: Resolution of postvagotomy dysphagia. JAMA, 240:2657–2658, 1978.
11. Gelfand MD: Irreversible esophageal motor dysfunction in postvagotomy dysphagia. Am J Gastroenterol, 76:347–350, 1981.
12. Vantrappen G, Janssens H, Hellemans J, et al: Achalasia, diffuse esophageal spasm, and related motility disorders. Gastroenterology, 76:450–457, 1979.
13. Tucker HJ, Snape WJ, Cohen S: Achalasia secondary to carcinoma: Clinical and manometric features. Ann Intern Med, 89:315–318, 1978.
14. Sanderson DR, Ellis FH, Schlegel JF, et al: Syndrome of vigorous achalasia: Clinical and physiologic observations. Dis Chest, 52:508–517, 1967.
15. Hogan W, Caflisch C, Winship D: Unclassified oesophageal motor disorders simulating achalasia. Gut, 10:234–240, 1969.
16. Fleshler B: Diffuse esophageal spasm. Gastroenterology, 52:559–564, 1967.
17. Hodes SE, Korsten MA: Fixed corkscrew pattern of the esophagus. Am J Gastroenterol, 73:249–251, 1980.
18. Kramer P, Harris LD, Donaldson RM: Transition from symptomatic diffuse spasm to cardiospasm. Gut, 8:115–119, 1967.
19. Kramer P, Ingelfinger FJ: Esophageal sensitivity to Mecholyl in cardiospasm. Gastroenterology, 19:242–253, 1951.
20. Benjamin SB, Gerhardt DC, Castell DO: High amplitude, peristaltic esophageal contractions associated with chest pain and/or dysphagia. Gastroenterology, 77:478–483, 1979.
21. Code C, Schlegel J, Kelley M: Hypertensive lower esophageal sphincter. Proc Staff Mayo Clin, 35:391–399, 1960.
22. Herrington PJ, Burns TW, Balart LA: Chest pain and dysphagia in patients with prolonged peristaltic contractile duration in the esophagus. Dig Dis Sci, 29:134–140, 1984.
23. Cohen S: Classification of the esophageal motility disorders. Gastroenterology, 84:1050–1051, 1983.
24. Hollis JB, Castell DO: Esophageal function in elderly men: A new look at "presbyesophagus." Ann Intern Med, 80:371–374, 1974.
25. Casella RR, Brown AL, Sayre GP, et al: Achalasia of the esophagus: Pathologic and etiologic consideration. Ann Surg, 160:474–486, 1964.
26. Csendes A, Smok G, Braghetto I, et al: Gastroesophageal sphincter pressure and histological changes in distal esophagus in patients with achalasia of the esophagus. Dig Dis Sci, 30:941–945, 1985.
27. Qualman SJ, Haupt HM, Yang P, et al: Esophageal Lewy bodies associated with ganglion cell loss in achalasia. Similarity to Parkinson's disease. Gastroenterology, 87:848–856, 1984.
28. Aggestrup S, Uddman R, Sundler F, et al: Lack of vasoactive intestinal polypeptide nerves in esophageal achalasia. Gastroenterology, 84:924–927, 1983.

29. Kilpatrick ZM, Milles SS: Achalasia in mother and daughter. Gastroenterology, 62:1042–1046, 1972.

30. Henderson RD, Wigle ED, Sample K, et al: Atypical chest pain of cardiac and esophageal origin. Chest, 73:24–27, 1978.

31. Clouse RE, Staiano A, Landau DW, et al: Manometric findings during spontaneous chest pain in patients with presumed esophageal "spasms." Gastroenterology, 85:395–402, 1983.

32. Richter JE, Hackshaw BT, Wu WC, et al: Edrophonium: A useful provocative test for esophageal chest pain. Ann Intern Med, 103:14–21, 1985.

33. Blackwell JN, Hannan WJ, Adam RD, et al: Radionuclide transit studies in the detection of oesophageal dysmotility. Gut, 24:421–426, 1983.

34. Holloway RH, Krosin G, Lange RC, et al: Radionuclide esophageal emptying of a solid meal to quantitate results of therapy in achalasia. Gastroenterology, 84:771–776, 1983.

35. Reinis JW, Stanely JH, Schabel SI: CT evaluation of thickened esophageal walls. AJR, 140:931–934, 1983.

36. Csendes A, Velasco N, Braghetto I, et al: A prospective randomized study comparing forceful dilation and esophagomyotomy in patients with achalasia of the esophagus. Gastroenterology, 80:789–795, 1981.

37. Vantrappen G, Hellemans J: Treatment of achalasia and related motor disorders. Gastroenterology, 79:144–154, 1980.

38. Castell DO, Johnson LF: Esophageal Function in Health and Disease. New York, Elsevier, 1983.

39. Gelfand MD, Christie DL: Pneumatic dilation under general anesthesia after unsuccessful cardiomyotomy for achalasia. J Clin Gastroenterol, 1:317–319, 1979.

40. Gelfand MD: Achalasia: importance of early detection and treatment. Bull Mason Clin, 39:1–9, 1985.

41. Stewart ET, Miller WN, Hogan WJ, et al: Desirability of roentgen esophageal examination immediately after pneumatic dilation for achalasia. Radiology, 130:589–591, 1979.

42. Lamet M, Fleshler B, Achkar E: Return of peristalsis in achalasia after pneumatic dilatation. Am J Gastroenterol, 80:602–604, 1985.

43. Chuong JJ, DuBovik S, McCallum RW: Achalasia as a risk factor for esophageal carcinoma. Dig Dis Sci, 29:1105–1108, 1984.

44. Mellow MH: Effect of isosorbide and hydralazine in painful primary esophageal motility disorders. Gastroenterology, 83:334–340, 1982.

45. Swamy N: Esophageal spasm: Clinical and manometric response of nitroglycerin and long-acting nitrites. Gastroenterology, 72:23–27, 1977.

46. Traube M, Hongo M, Magyar L, et al: Effects of nifedipine in achalasia and in patients with high-amplitude peristaltic esophageal contractions. JAMA, 252:1733–1736, 1984.

47. Berger K, McCallum RW: Nifedipine in the treatment of achalasia. Ann Intern Med, 1982; 96:61–62, 1982.

48. Gelfond M, Rozen P, Gilat T: Isorbide dinitrate and nifedipine treatment of achalasia: A clinical, manometric and radionuclide evaluation. Gastroenterology, 83:963–969, 1982.

49. Richter JE, Spurling TJ, Cordova CM, et al: Effects of oral calcium blocker, diltiazem, on esophageal contraction studies in volunteers and patients with "nutcracker" esophagus. Dig Dis Sci, 29:649–656, 1984.

15

Surgery for Motility Disorders of the Esophagus

C. Dale Mercer ▪ *Kjell Thor*
Lucius D. Hill

Surgical therapy for motility disorders of the esophagus requires a clear understanding of both the physiology of normal esophageal function and the pathophysiology of the specific disease process. Because this type of surgery usually alters esophageal function rather than anatomy, the surgeon must know what the surgical endpoint is and how it can be measured. Preoperative investigations are critical to obtain an accurate diagnosis of the disease and an understanding of the esophageal dysfunction. The full value of the modern diagnostic battery of tests is essential when attempting to differentiate motility disorders and their various subtypes. Objective intraoperative assessment of results obtained at surgery allows the surgeon the comfort of identifying what results are being obtained. If necessary, the operation can be altered to provide a better postoperative result. The recent introduction of intraoperative manometry to these patients has been a major technical advance.[1]

A number of primary motility disorders—defects occurring in the absence of systemic disease, including achalasia, vigorous achalasia, diffuse esophageal spasms, nutcracker esophagus, segmental spasm, and hypertensive sphincter—may require surgical treatment following failed medical management. Secondary motility disorders (esophageal dysfunction associated with systemic disease), such as scleroderma, infrequently require surgical therapy, and then only as a last resort following failed maximal medical management. Other secondary disorders, e.g., diabetes mellitus, presbyesophagus, chronic idiopathic intestinal pseudo-obstruction, and Chagas' disease, rarely require surgical treatment.

▪ Achalasia

The main principle in the surgical management of patients with achalasia is division of the lower esophageal sphincter musculature so that a swallowed bolus will pass into the stomach. An important corollary of this principle is to prevent gastroesophageal (GE) reflux from occurring postoperatively, since this complication in a patient with inadequate esophageal peristalsis can be disastrous.

The indications for surgical treatment of achalasia are multiple. These include myotomy as a primary treatment modality, or rescue following failed pneumatic dilation. There are many claims by internists and surgeons that pneumatic dilatation or surgical myotomy is the treatment of choice in the management of achalasia.[2–5] We believe that in early achalasia pneumatic dilatation is a useful treatment modality, but should it fail, or if the disease is longstanding at the time of diagnosis, then surgery is the treatment of choice. Surgical myotomy is safer than pneumatic dilatation in patients with megaesophagus because it may be extremely difficult to properly position the pneumatic bag across the lower esophageal sphincter in the very tortuous and dilated esophagus. Heller myotomy may also be more difficult in advanced cases.[6] Associated conditions such as esophageal diverticula and peptic ulcer disease are more adequately treated with surgery than with pneumatic dilatation. The rarely associated hiatus hernia is a definite surgical indication, since a concomitant hiatus hernia repair can be performed and the lower esophageal sphincter adjusted to an appropriate level to both allow swallowing and prevent reflux. Intraoperative manometry in these rare cases is critically important to identify the length of the myotomy, as well as the sphincter pressure created at the time of the hiatus hernia repair. Another indication for surgery is vigorous achalasia with failed medical management. A standard Heller procedure with proximal extension of the myotomy determined by intraoperative manometric pressure measurements eliminates the high-pressure zone.[7,8]

The surgical procedure of choice for patients with achalasia is the modified Heller esophagomyotomy, initially described by Heller in 1914 and modified by Zaaijer in 1919.[9,10] Heller's operation utilized a myotomy, both on the anterior and posterior surfaces of the esophagus, whereas the most common modification consists of an extramucosal myotomy on the anterior wall of the esophagus.

Even though the Heller myotomy has been accepted as the surgical treatment of choice for achalasia of the esophagus, great debate still exists with regard to the length of the myotomy, both proximally and distally, and the necessity for concomitant antireflux procedures.[11] The length of the myotomy onto the esophagus has variously been described as extending 8 cm,[12] 5 cm,[14] 2.5 cm,[15] and 1 cm[13] onto the fundus of the stomach. Other reports either do not specify the length of the myotomy on the stomach or avoid extending the incision onto the stomach.[7] Likewise, there is a great diversity of opinion with regard to the proximal extension of the myotomy. Some advise carrying the incision proximally for 5 cm, whereas others extend it to the inferior pulmonary vein or up to the level of the aortic arch.[7,15,16]

■ TECHNIQUE

Esophagomyotomy may be done either transthoracically or transabdominally. We have had experience with both approaches and now prefer to use the transabdominal approach because it allows better visualization of the GE junction and a more precise myotomy.

An upper midline incision is made and the upper hand retractors are inserted, allowing full visualization of the upper abdomen. After thorough abdominal exploration, attention is turned to the gastroesophageal junction. The nasogastric tube that has been modified to do intraoperative pressure measurements is palpated and a baseline measurement of the lower esophageal sphincter (LES) is obtained.[1,17] Particular attention is paid to the length of the sphincter that needs to be shortened. After obtaining a baseline measurement of the lower esophageal sphincter (Fig. 15–1), the left triangular ligament of the liver is incised and the liver is retracted laterally. Care is taken to preserve the attachments of the esophagus to the diaphragm, thus preventing the creation of an iatrogenic hiatus hernia. An anterior incision through the phrenoesophageal membrane is done to expose the esophagus. The anterior vagus nerve is identified and carefully preserved. A gastrostomy is done and a finger is then placed into the introitus of the esophagus cephalad through the sphincter to palpate the length of the sphincter and to allow for careful division of the LES under direct vision. Some surgeons use this technique,[18] while others use intraesophageal bougies[19] or Foley catheters.[6] The myotomy is commenced at the cephalad end of the LES and carried distally until approximately 1 cm or less of the sphincter is left. At this point, the finger is removed and a pressure measurement is obtained, showing partial division of the sphincter. If more than 1 cm of sphincter remains, additional muscle is divided under direct vision down to the point where there is less than 1 cm of sphincter remaining. A final measurement of the sphincter is obtained, assessing both the length and the pressure (Fig. 15–2). If the pressure is still very high in the remaining sphincter, the sphincter is dilated digitally, stretching the remaining muscle fibers. A length of 1 cm or less with a pressure of 12 to 20 mm Hg is ideal. The myotomy is extended around 50 per cent of the circumference of the esophagus.

Following the myotomy, the introitus of the esophagus is visualized with attention to the gastroesophageal valve, which is a flat musculomucosal valve created by the angle of His at the greater curvature of the GE junction. The valve closes against the lesser curve. The valve is grasped with Babcock clamps and pulled caudally. Under direct vision, sutures are then placed in the anterior and posterior aspects of this valve (valvuloplasty). The suture lines are carried cephalad through the incisura, lengthening the valve to 4 to 4.5 cm. After the valve has been lengthened, a pressure measurement is again obtained to determine that the length of the valve is adequate, usually 4 cm. The sutures are placed in the anterior and posterior aspects of the valve with a finger through the GE junction to make certain that the lumen is adequate. The valve technique is shown in Figure 15–3.

This valve represents an ideal solution in acha-

PERSISTENT ACHALASIA
LENGTH: 4 cm

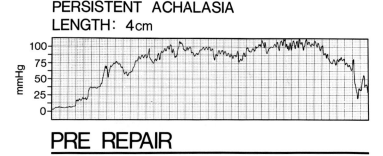

Figure 15–1. A baseline barrier pressure is obtained prior to myotomy, showing a high pressure over a length of 4 cm.

PRE REPAIR

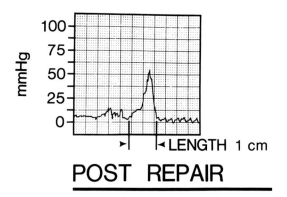

POST REPAIR

Figure 15–2. Following myotomy, there remains only a short length of sphincter 1 cm or less with a markedly lower pressure.

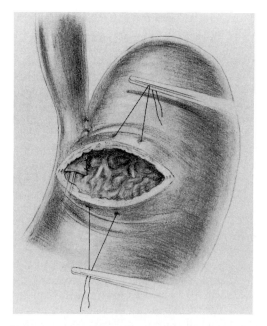

Figure 15–3. Following myotomy the gastroesophageal valve is accentuated by placing sutures in the anterior and posterior edges of the valve and carrying the suture line up through the incisura to lengthen the valve to 3 to 4 cm.

lasia, as it offers no obstruction to the passage of food and fluid into the stomach but offers considerable resistance to retrograde or cephalad flow (see section on flap valve in Chapter 2, on anatomy). This is a new technique developed after extensive experimentation on cadavers and the early results have been very encouraging.[20,21] Postoperatively, the valve can be visualized through the fiberoptic endoscope and appears as an effective one-way flutter valve.

Following careful measurement of both the sphincter and the newly created valve, the gastrostomy is closed in two layers. The wound is irrigated and then closed.

Some authors report using the Nissen or Belsey fundoplication or other antireflux procedures routinely at the time of Heller myotomy.[13,22] This has been advocated because of the concern that in performing an adequate myotomy, the sphincter is rendered incompetent, allowing reflux. Also, too aggressive dissection of the distal esophagus in performing a myotomy creates an iatrogenic hiatus hernia if the attachments are destroyed, because division of the posterior attachments of the GE junction allows the GE junction to slide up into the chest. When the GE junction slides cephalad, the angle of His and the valve are lost, rendering the GE junction incompetent. We feel that it is contraindicated to perform an antireflux procedure following a Heller operation. To perform a Nissen or other antireflux procedure will simply add an obstruction to an esophagus that has poor motility and produce severe dysphagia.

With the technique that we have just described, an antireflux procedure is unnecessary. A fundoplication replaces the functionally obstructed LES with an anatomically obstructing gastric wrap in the distal esophagus. We have had experience with a number of patients having fundoplication following Heller myotomy who have developed serious dysphagia. These patients represent a complex surgical challenge. The sphincter has been destroyed and the esophagus is obstructed. It is in the patients who will require reoperations following myotomy that the new operation (valvuloplasty) with restoration of the gastroesophageal valve has been particularly effective. The use of intraoperative manometry also is important in clearly demonstrating the length of the remaining sphincter. With a length of less than 1 cm and a pressure of 12 to 20 mm Hg at surgery, the postoperative result is excellent.

Infrequently, a lower esophageal diverticulum is found in conjunction with achalasia of the esophagus. Diverticula have been reported in 2 to 4 per cent of patients with achalasia.[3,23] This diverticulum should be excised at the time of the Heller myotomy. (See Chapter 16, on esophageal diverticula, rings, and webs.)

The Heller myotomy was traditionally carried out through a transthoracic approach. Many surgeons prefer this approach, while others use the transabdominal approach.[3,7,24,25] We and others have used both approaches, preferring the transthoracic approach when preoperative manometric studies indicate a diagnosis of vigorous achalasia, or one in which the high-pressure zone extends far into the proximal esophagus.[6,26]

If the Heller myotomy is to be performed through a transthoracic approach, a double lumen endotracheal tube is used so that the left lung can be collapsed at the time of surgery, thereby facilitating exposure through a left anterolateral thoracotomy through the bed of the resected sixth rib. The lung is deflated and the mediastinal pleura overlying the esophagus is incised. The esophagus is identified, taking care not to traumatize the vagus nerve. However, it is not mobilized out of its bed. Next, a counterincision in the left hemidiaphragm is performed, dividing the muscle in a radial fashion so as not to injure any branches of the phrenic nerve. The fundus of the stomach is then identified and a gastrostomy is performed in the fundus so that a finger can be passed into the stomach up through the lower esophageal sphincter. A myotomy is performed similarly to that described for the transabdominal approach using intraoperative manometry to determine the length of the myotomy required. Once an adequate myotomy has been obtained, a valvuloplasty may be added and the gastrostomy closed in two layers. The counterincision in the diaphragm is resutured in a pant-over-vest repair with interrupted No. 1 silk sutures, and the chest is drained with a chest tube and closed in layers.

After surgery, the nasogastric tube is left in place for three days, at which time it is withdrawn through the lower esophageal sphincter, allowing a pressure measurement to be obtained. With the removal of the tube, the patient is begun on clear fluids and advanced to a soft diet over the next two weeks. If the nasogastric tube is inadvertently removed, care must be taken not to perforate the esophagus through the thinned mucosa and submucosa if it is reinserted. If insertion of a nasogastric tube is required following its initial removal, it should be placed using fluoroscopic guidance to assure correct positioning.

The technique of intraoperative manometry has previously been described.[1] In 17 patients with achalasia, the average premyotomy pressure was 42 mm Hg over an average length of 5.5 cm. Following the myotomy, the pressure was reduced to 20 mm Hg over 2.1 cm in length.

■ COMPLICATIONS AND RESULTS

The main intraoperative complication of Heller myotomy is inadvertent perforation of the esophageal mucosa and submucosa. If this does occur, simple suture closure is necessary. A Gastrografin swallow prior to removal of the nasogastric tube will ensure that there is no leak from the distal esophagus.

Other complications that may occur are persistent dysphagia, caused by an inadequate myotomy or proximal esophageal dysmotility. Gastroesophageal reflux secondary to an overzealous myotomy results in progressive dysphagia following development of a peptic esophageal stricture.

The clinical results following Heller myotomy are difficult to assess because of the chronicity of the condition and the fact that the proximal esophagus lacks effective peristalsis, even at the completion of the surgical myotomy. Some studies find equally good results with pneumatic dilatation or myotomy,[27] but most reports show surgical treatment giving better clinical results.[28–30] Csendes et al.[30] have the only prospective randomized study comparing pneumatic dilatation with esophagomyotomy and have reported excellent or good results in 100 per cent of patients undergoing surgery and only 60 per cent of those undergoing dilatation. They also documented reduced sphincter pressure in 75 per cent of the myotomy patients, but in only 49 per cent having dilatation. An interesting finding in this study is that 31 per cent of myotomy patients had a positive provoked acid reflux test, whereas only 7 per cent of those with dilatation have a similar result. Other large series report clinical results following myotomy as excellent or good in from 70 to 90 per cent.[5,7,23] Mortality rates in recent series vary between 0 and 0.4 per cent.[5]

Between 1974 and 1986 we treated 32 patients with Heller myotomy, 11 of whom had previous failed pneumatic dilatation. Twenty-four of 28 patients (85 per cent) had excellent or good results. Four patients had poor results and four had inadequate follow-up. In no patient with follow-up was there any evidence of reflux.* No antireflux repairs or medical management for reflux was required in these patients. Mean follow-up was 64 months. In each instance, intraoperative manometry was utilized to determine the extent of myotomy.

We have also studied an additional 11 patients who had incapacitating dysphagia following a Heller operation done elsewhere for presumed achalasia. Symptoms began an average of nine months following the previous operation. The causes of dysphagia were diverse, including: (1) inadequate myotomy with either persistent or recurrent achalasia in seven; (2) hiatus hernia with reflux esophagitis and either spasm or stricture in two; and (3) incorrect diagnosis and treatment of the primary condition in two patients, each of whom developed a stricture. In these patients, individualized investigation and treatment were necessary and included a repeat Heller operation utilizing intraoperative manometry in five patients, Hill antireflux repair in four patients, and takedown of the concomitant Nissen fundoplication and extension of the myotomy in two patients, one of whom required a Hill antireflux repair. One patient required further surgery, and one required multiple dilatations postoperatively. In each case, the remedial operations were more difficult than the primary repair, owing to extensive adhesions in the upper abdomen with obliteration of the normal anatomy of the distal esophagus. Since the introduction of the valvuloplasty, five patients with multiple previous operations for achalasia have been reoperated upon with good results in all. The follow-up for these patients is from three months to one year. Thus far, the results are encouraging.[21] Intraoperative manometry was a critical adjunct in determining the adequacy of the repeat Heller operation or antireflux repair so as to prevent further postoperative dysphagia.[31]

Ellis in 1984 reported an extensive experience with the Heller procedure in 113 patients. He emphasized that the myotomy should be limited and that an antireflux procedure is unnecessary. Of 103 patients followed for an average of 6.75 years, 94 had a good result. We agree entirely with Ellis' conclusions and would add that the valvuloplasty should improve the results, as it avoids an antireflux procedure.[32]

■ Vigorous Achalasia

This variant of achalasia should be treated with a transthoracic myotomy, since the proximal ex-

tension of the myotomy, as determined by intraoperative manometry, is at a higher level than can be dealt with through a transabdominal approach. The muscularis of the esophagus is thickened over a longer distance than in the usual variation of achalasia. Care must be exercised not to traumatize the vagus nerve, and the muscularis must be dissected from the underlying submucosa about 50 per cent of the circumference of the esophagus. The distal esophagus should not be mobilized out of its bed, since mobilization may result in an iatrogenic hiatus hernia. Frequently, vigorous achalasia is associated with other pathologic entities, e.g., epiphrenic diverticula. These diverticula should be excised at the time of the long myotomy. If diverticula are excised without performing a myotomy, the esophagotomy site may disrupt because of the high-pressure nonperistaltic contractions.

■ Diffuse Esophageal Spasm

This relatively rare primary motility disorder is manifested clinically by chest pain and intermittent dysphagia and manometrically by frequent tertiary waves, some of which are of higher amplitude and long duration. If the diagnosis has been accurately determined with esophageal manometry, treatment with muscle relaxants, i.e., nitroglycerine or calcium channel blockers, is indicated. If chest pain and dysphagia are incapacitating, surgical treatment with a transthoracic long esophagomyotomy is the treatment of choice.* In these cases the approach is transthoracic, since the myotomy extends proximally usually to the level of the aortic arch. The extent of the myotomy has been controversial, with some authors suggesting myotomy to the level of the aortic arch,[33] and others suggesting even higher levels of myotomy.[34,35] The extent of the distal myotomy is also controversial. In this form of esophageal motor disorder, the distal high-pressure zone relaxes normally with swallowing, and therefore, myotomy of this normal muscle is unnecessary and can result in reflux esophagitis. We and other investigators[33] favor preserving the distal esophageal high-pressure zone, utilizing intraoperative manometry to identify both the pressure in the lower esophageal sphincter and the length of the sphincter. However, one study has shown that patients with a myotomy excluding the distal high-pressure zone had intractable postoperative dys-

---

*All four patients with poor results had some dysphagia requiring dilation which has corrected the dysphagia. None require dilation now.

*At surgery the musculature of the esophagus is markedly thickened up to 1.5 cm, extending to or above the aortic arch (Fig. 15–4).

phagia and required distal extension of the my-otomy.[36]

As in achalasia, there are various proponents to the addition of a Nissen fundoplication to prevent reflux.[36] We feel this is unnecessary because the distal high-pressure zone functions normally and can be preserved accurately with the use of intra-operative manometry. If an additional procedure were to be performed, we would advocate the val-vuloplasty, because this offers no resistance to the aboral flow.

The results of surgery in this group are not as consistently good as in those patients with acha-lasia. Six patients prior to myotomy had a mean intraesophageal pressure of 41 mm Hg over a length of some 13 cm. Following myotomy with the use of intraoperative manometry, the high-pres-sure zone was reduced to 22 mm Hg, and this occurred over the distal 2 cm of esophagus. Over a mean follow-up of 29 months, five patients had an excellent result and one patient had a poor result. Gastroesophageal reflux did not develop in any pa-tients. Only one had dysphagia following the pro-cedure. The only poor result occurred in a patient who had had three previous operations on the distal esophagus, causing extensive scar and stricture for-mation.

Four patients with segmental esophageal spasm in which the distal esophagus was spastic and as-sociated with esophageal diverticula have been treated. Hypertrophied muscle distal to the diver-ticulum was incised, eliminating the manometri-cally defined area of high-pressure zone. The di-verticula were excised and the esophagotomy

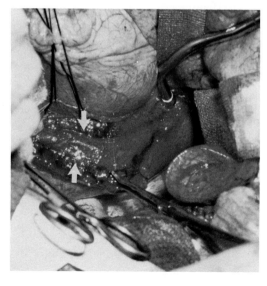

Figure 15–4. Transthoracic long myotomy in a patient with diffuse spasm shows the musculature to be markedly thickened (arrows), up to 1.5 cm all the way up to the aortic arch.

oversewn. Prior to surgery, the mean intraesopha-geal pressure was 60 mm Hg over 5 cm in length. Following the myotomy, these pressures were re-duced to 25 mm Hg over 2 cm in length. Three patients had excellent results, while another patient had an esophageal leak with subsequent empyema which cleared with drainage. Reflux did not occur during the two-year follow-up.

■ *Nutcracker Esophagus*

This is a relatively rare condition, usually well managed by medical therapy with calcium channel blockers or nitroglycerine. We have seen one pa-tient with severe, unrelenting chest pain associated with dysphagia in whom all medical measures had been tried without any symptomatic relief. Pneu-matic dilatation of his distal esophagus was at-tempted, and this actually provoked pain rather than relieving it. Since the relationship between nutcracker esophagus and diffuse esophageal spasm has not been completely defined, we felt that therapy with a long esophagomyotomy might improve the symptoms.

At operation, the entire esophageal musculature from the aortic arch to the lower esophageal sphinc-ter was thickened, and we performed an esoph-agomyotomy down to the level of the distal sphinc-ter, which was preserved. Following surgery and for two years, the patient has remained completely asymptomatic and has had no further episodes of chest pain or dysphagia. The future surgical man-agement of nutcracker esophagus remains to be evaluated, but surgery may play a role in those patients who are refractory to medical manage-ment.

■ *Scleroderma*

Esophageal involvement with scleroderma is one of the manifestations of progressive systemic scle-rosis. These patients complain of heartburn and dysphagia. The dysphagia is usually caused by ab-sent peristalsis or the presence of a reflux-induced peptic esophageal stricture. Surgery for this con-dition should be undertaken only following a pro-longed course of maximum medical therapy that has failed in alleviating the severe dyspeptic symp-toms or during which a peptic esophageal stricture developed. The patient should be evaluated pre-operatively for other evidence of systemic involve-ment, and only if he or she is an acceptable surgical candidate should this operation be undertaken. A variety of repairs have been utilized. In each case, an antireflux repair with dilatation of the sphincter was used. Repairs include the modified Collis-Belsey gastroplasty,[37] the Thal-Nissen procedure,[38] and the Collis-Nissen procedure.[39,40] A number of authors have even recommended esophagus resection and replacement.[41,42] These operations were undertaken in patients who had nondilatable strictures.

Even though all patients survived these operations and were able to eat postoperatively, and the majority were significantly improved, the quality of the result after operation in patients with scleroderma was certainly inferior to the results of similar procedures carried out in patients without this disease.[37]

We have followed eight patients who underwent the Hill posterior fixation and sphincter calibration procedure over a mean period of four years. Two of these patients had previous antireflux surgery, one a Belsey repair and one a Nissen fundoplication, both of which had failed. All eight patients had peptic esophageal strictures and complained of severe dysphagia as well as heartburn. Maximal medical management and dilatation had failed in each patient. All strictures required endoscopy, and the biopsy findings were benign. Esophageal motility studies confirmed the absence of peristalsis in the esophagus. However, each patient had marked spontaneous reflux at the time of pH and pressure studies, with reduced lower esophageal sphincter pressure. Six of our patients have had good results following surgery. One patient with a good result now requires dilatation on an annual basis, rather than every two to three weeks as it was preoperatively. Two patients had poor results with significant postoperative dysphagia persisting. In this disease we also use intraoperative manometry, as it allows us to calibrate the sphincter to an adequate level to prevent reflux, and yet not cause dysphagia in those patients without peristalsis.

Since the introduction of the new valvuloplasty procedure, we have operated on one patient with scleroderma with a previously failed Angelchik prosthesis. In that patient, the valvuloplasty procedure was performed without posterior fixation. At present, 12 months after surgery, no reflux has occurred.

Since the surgical treatment of stricture in patients with scleroderma does not affect their underlying disease, these patients must be aware that the surgical treatment is purely a palliative form of therapy. Because of progressive diminishment of esophageal peristalsis, complete eradication of the dysphagia is often not possible.

■ *Summary and Conclusion*

With new advances in technology, surgery for motility disorders is becoming more accurately controlled. The complexity of motility problems demands accuracy in both diagnosis and surgical technique. With the application of intraoperative manometry, results of surgery for motility disorders have improved.

■ REFERENCES

1. Hill LD, Asplund CM, Roberts PN: Intraoperative manometry; adjunct to surgery for esophageal motility disorders. Am J Surg, *147*:171–174, 1984.
2. Vantrappen G, Hellemans J, Deloof W, Valembois P, Vandenbroucke J: Treatment of achalasia with pneumatic dilatations. Gut, *12*:268, 1971.
3. Ellis FH Jr, Kiser JC, Schlegel JF, Earlman RJ, McVey JL, Olsen AM: Oesophagomyotomy for esophageal achalasia: Experimental, clinical and manometric aspects. Ann Surg, *166*:640, 1967.
4. Payne WS, King RN: Treatment of achalasia of the esophagus. Surg Clin North Am, *63*(4):963–970, 1983.
5. Harley HRS: Achalasia of the Cardia. Bristol, Ed J. Wright & Sons, Limited, 1978.
6. Nanson EM: Treatment of achalasia of the cardia. Gastroenterology, *51*:236, 1966.
7. Sarijamis C, Mullard KS: Oesophagomyotomy of achalasia of the cardia. Thorax, *30*:539, 1975.
8. Gelfand MD, Mercer CD, Hill LD: A Ten Year Experience with Pneumatic Dilatation and Surgery for Achalasia. Presented at American College of Gastroenterology, June 1984.
9. Heller E: Extramukose Kardioplastik beim Chronischen Kardiospasmus mit Dilatation des Oesophagus. Mitt Grenzgeb Med U Chir, *27*:141, 1914.
10. Zaaijer JH: Cardiospasm en andere Slakarmaandoenignen. Zentralbl Chir, *46*:57, 1919.
11. Barrett NR, Franklin RH: Concerning the unfavourable results of certain operations performed in the treatment of cardiospasm. Br J Surg, *37*:194, 1949.
12. Steichen FM, Heller E, Ravitch MM: Achalasia of the esophagus. Surgery, *47*:877, 1960.
13. Belsey R: Functional disease of the oesophagus. J Thorac Cardiovasc Surg, *52*:164, 1966.
14. Havard C: Para-oesophageal hernia of the stomach complicating Heller's operation. Thorax, *18*:139, 1963.
15. Douglas R, Nicholson F: The late results of Heller's operation for cardiospasm. Br J Surg, *47*:250, 1959.
16. LeRoux BT, Wright JT: Cardiospasm. Br J Surg, *48*:619, 1961.
17. Hill LD: Intraoperative measurement of lower esophageal sphincter pressure. J Thorac Cardiovasc Surg, *75*:378–382, 1978.
18. Drake EH: Surgical treatment of cardiospasm. N Engl J Med, *266*:173, 1962.
19. Adams CWM, Brain RHF, Ellis FC, Kauntze R, Trounce JR: Achalasia of the cardia. Guy's Hosp Rep, *110*:191, 1961.
20. Thor K, Hill LD, Mercer CD, Kozarek RA. Reappraisal of the flap valve mechanism: A study of new valvuloplasty procedure in cadavers. Acta Chir Scand, *153*:25–28, 1987.
21. Thor K, Kozarek RA, Mercer CD, Hill LD. Valvuloplasty:

A new surgical procedure. Gastroenterology, 90:1666, 1986.

22. Menguy R: Management of achalasia by transabdominal cardiomyotomy and fundoplication. Surg Gynecol Obstet, 133:482–484, 1971.
23. Payne WS, Ellis FH Jr, Olsen AM: Achalasia of the oesophagus. Arch Surg, 81:411, 1960.
24. Barlow D: Problems of achalasia. Br J Surg, 48:642, 1961.
25. Browse NL, Carter SJ: The late results of Heller's operation in the treatment of achalasia. Br J Surg, 49:59, 1961.
26. Olsen AM, Ellis FH Jr, Creamer B: Achalasia (cardiospasm). Am J Surg, 93:299, 1957.
27. Bennett JR, Hendrix TR: Treatment of achalasia with pneumatic dilatation. In Bayless TM: Management of Esophageal Disease. Modern Treatment, Vol. 7, No. 6. New York, Harper & Row, 1970.
28. Yan J, Christensen J: An uncontrolled comparison of treatments for achalasia. Ann Surg, 182:672–676, 1975.
29. Okike N, Payne WS, Neufield DM, et al: Esophagomyotomy versus forceful dilatation for achalasia of the esophagus; results in 899 patients. Ann Thorac Surg, 28:119–125, 1979.
30. Csendes A, Velasco N, Braghetto I, Henriquez A: A prospective randomized study comparing forceful dilatation and esophagomyotomy in patients with achalasia of the esophagus. Gastroenterology, 80:789–795, 1981.
31. Haqelberg RS, Mercer CD, Hill LD: Diagnosis and Treatment of Dysphagia Following Surgery for Achalasia. Presented at Washington State Chapter of A.C.S., June 1984.
32. Ellis FH, Crozier RE, Watkins EJ: Operation for esophageal achalasia. Results of esophagomyotomy without an antireflux operation. J Thorac Cardiovasc Surg, 88:344, 1984.

33. Leonardi HK, Shea JA, Crozier RE, Ellis FE Jr: Diffuse spasm of the esophagus. Clinical manometric and surgical considerations. J Thorac Cardiovasc Surg, 74:736–743, 1977.
34. Henderson RD, Pearson FC: Reflux control following extended myotomy in primary disordered motor activity (diffuse spasm) of the esophagus. Ann Thorac Surg, 22:278–283, 1976.
35. Henderson RD, Ho CS, Davidson JW: Primary motor activity of the esophagus (diffuse spasm); diagnosis and treatment. Ann Thorac Surg 18:327–366, 1974.
36. Henderson RD: Diffuse esophageal spasm. Surg Clin North Am, 63(4):951–962, 1983.
37. Pearson FC, Henderson RD: Experimental and clinical studies of gastroplasty in the management of acquired short esophagus. Surg Gynecol Obstet, 136:737, 1973.
38. O'Leary JP, Hallenbeck JI, Woodward ER: Surgical treatment of esophageal stricture in patients with scleroderma. Am J Surg, 41:131, 1975.
39. Orringer MB, Orringer JS, Dabish L, et al: Combined Collis-gastroplasty-fundoplication operation for scleroderma reflux esophagitis. Surgery, 90:624, 1981.
40. Orringer MB: Surgical management of scleroderma reflux esophagitis. Surg Clin North Am, 63(4):859–867, 1983.
41. Akiyama H: Esophageal anastomosis. Arch Surg, 107:512, 1973.
42. McLaughlin JS, Raig R, Woodward MF: Surgical treatment of strictures of esophagus in patients with scleroderma. J Thorac Cardiovasc Surg, 61:641, 1971.

16

Rings, Webs, and Diverticula

Lucius D. Hill ▪ C. Dale Mercer

A great deal of controversy is present in the medical literature concerning the nature of esophageal rings and webs. Both terms have been used for the same entity, thereby creating confusion as to the pathologic condition being described. Webs are traditionally described as thin membranes consisting of mucosa and submucosa only, whereas rings are thicker and consist of mucosa, submucosa, and muscularis. However, this description would indicate that the best known ring—Schatzki's ring—is actually a web. Because of this confusion we and others[1] favor an anatomic classification of rings and webs: (1) upper esophageal webs (Paterson-Kelly, Plummer-Vinson syndrome), (2) midesophageal webs, and (3) lower esophageal webs and rings (Schatzki's ring).

Both rings and webs must be differentiated from benign peptic esophageal strictures, malignant annular tumors, and the muscle contractions that occasionally appear on a barium swallow. The margins of rings and webs are usually sharp and thin compared to longer tapered margins of strictures. Malignant strictures are longer than webs with shouldering and axial asymmetry. Webs and rings radiographically do not change over years, whereas muscle contractions are transient, changing from minute to minute, and benign and malignant strictures may be progressive prior to treatment of the disease.

▪ Webs

Esophageal webs are infrequently accomplished by diverticula, usually occurring proximal to the web. We have reported one such case of an upper esophageal web in association with a Zenker's diverticulum[2] (Fig. 16–1). It is very important to exclude the presence of a web when treating patients with diverticula because this could result in

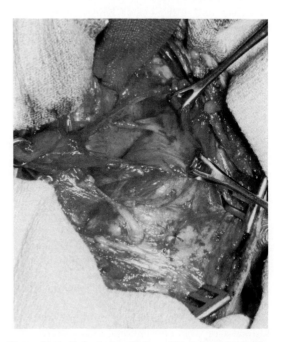

Figure 16–1. Zenker's diverticulum with esophageal web. The diverticulum has been opened and the margins are grasped with Babcock clamps. A web is identified within the lumen of the esophagus at the level of the cricopharyngeus muscle. This was divided, the diverticulum excised, and a cricopharyngeal myotomy performed.

201

early postoperative dysphagia if it were to go unrecognized and untreated.

Webs are often incomplete with an eccentric lumen and therefore usually do not cause total obstruction. Sometimes patients are completely asymptomatic but a web is found incidentally on upper gastrointestinal x-ray done for other reasons. If webs are symptomatic, the most common symptom is dysphagia, usually for solids only.

■ UPPER ESOPHAGEAL WEB

The upper esophageal web located in the postcricoid region occurs in 12 to 15 per cent of selected patients with dysphagia.[3,4] However, because of the difficulty diagnosing these lesions with cineradiography, the true incidence remains a question. The relationship of upper esophageal webs to the Plummer-Vinson syndrome is unclear. In 1919 Brown-Kelly[5] and Paterson[6] separately described upper esophageal dysphagia in anemic females who also had glossitis. Two years later Vinson presented 69 cases from the Mayo Clinic patients with dysphagia who had no esophagoscopic abnormalities.[7] In this report he indicated that Plummer had been the first to recognize this condition. These reports have resulted in the syndrome being referred to in the United States as Plummer-Vinson syndrome and in the United Kingdom as the Paterson-Kelly syndrome. Others[8] identified iron deficiency anemia and the syndrome gradually expanded to include glossitis, cheilosis, koilonychia, brittle fingernails, and splenomegaly.

The pathogenesis of cervical webs is unknown; however, their association with iron deficiency anemia led to the suggestion that iron deficiency anemia caused the web. However, epidemiologic studies have not shown any correlation between iron deficiency and cervical esophageal webs. Indeed, some studies have identified iron deficiency anemia in only 50 per cent of patients with webs.[9] The web causes dysphagia and may lead to a decrease in iron ingestion in a few patients, and because the symptoms occur mostly in women, the monthly menstrual cycle may also contribute to the anemia.[1] Upper esophageal webs are also associated with an increased incidence of carcinoma in the upper esophagus,[10] but this has not been supported by all authors.[11]

The diagnosis is confirmed by upper gastrointestinal x-ray, but conventional radiography is not sufficient. Cineradiography during the swallowing act is the most sensitive method available to show the esophageal web. This method distinguishes webs from other web-like phenomena that are usually due to insignificant mucosal foldings.[4,12]

Cineradiography techniques can distinguish the anterior, thin web from the smooth, posterior indentation of the cricopharyngeus muscle. Endoscopically, webs are identified if the endoscope is passed under direct vision; however, often they are missed because the endoscope has passed through the web and ruptured it before it has been identified. Treatment of webs consists of endoscopic rupture and iron replacement if the patient has iron deficiency anemia. If the web cannot be ruptured endoscopically, then dilatation may be necessary, but this is required infrequently. Results are excellent. Rarely recurrent dysphagia requires repeat dilatation, but surgical removal of the web is not necessary.

An anecdotal report of an atypical upper esophagus web mimicking the Paterson-Kelly, Plummer-Vinson syndrome identified a web formed at the squamocolumnar junction with ectopic gastric mucosa below and squamous epithelium above.[13]

■ MIDESOPHAGEAL WEBS

Webs in the body of the esophagus covered by squamous epithelium may be single or multiple and occur along the entire length of the esophagus.[14,15] The etiology is unclear, but in some patients the web is probably congenital, even though symptoms did not occur until adulthood.[16] These are usually treated with endoscopic dilatation with relief of the dysphagia.

■ LOWER ESOPHAGEAL WEB

Lower esophageal webs are distinct from lower esophageal rings and consist of a diaphragm formed of mucosa and submucosa. Patients with these webs present similarly to those having lower esophageal (Schatzki's) ring. Pathologically the submucosa is mildly inflamed, but the stimulus to produce this inflammation is uncertain. It may be difficult to distinguish radiologically a lower esophageal web from a Schatzki's ring. The diagnosis is suspected in middle-aged people presenting with intermittent dysphagia. The treatment is similar to that for Schatzki's ring, consisting of dilatation.

■ *Lower Esophageal Ring (Schatzki's Ring)*

The lower esophageal ring described by Schatzki[17] occurs at the squamocolumnar junction and may be asymptomatic or present with intermittent dysphagia. Asymptomatic rings are observed in 6 to 14 per cent of patients undergoing routine barium meal examinations.[18] Patients with intermittent dysphagia from a Schatzki's ring are identified in about 0.5 per cent of all upper GI examinations.[19]

The ring as defined by Schatzki was composed of only esophageal mucosa. Others felt the ring was a constant, anatomic structure with muscular thickening, but little is really known about the pathogenesis of these rings.[17,20] Various hypotheses have included plication of the esophageal mucosa, resulting in a transverse mucosal fold—congenital, developmental, or inflammatory in origin. The ring occurs often in patients with a hiatus hernia and is always present at the squamocolumnar junction.[21] The upper surface of the ring is covered by squamous epithelium, but the lower surface is covered by columnar epithelium. At the core of the ring is submucosal connective tissue, which occasionally exhibits a mild degree of chronic inflammation and minimal fibrosis.

These patients have intermittent dysphagia to solid food and are usually over 50 years of age. Chest pain is uncommon, but a few will develop heartburn and reflux symptoms indicating a concomitant hiatus hernia. Occasionally they present as a complete bolus obstruction, usually with impacted meat (the steakhouse syndrome) at the level of the ring. If the esophageal opening is greater than 20 mm in diameter, there is no history of dysphagia, but in those patients with an opening of less than 13 mm intermittent obstruction will occur.[18]

The diagnosis is made by the typical x-ray appearance of the distal esophageal ring (Fig. 16–2). It is important to fully distend the esophagus with barium to delineate this ring. A barium tablet may hang up at the level of the ring. Endoscopy usually shows no evidence of esophagitis, but there may or may not be a concomitant hiatus hernia. Manometric studies have been performed with confusing results. The lower esophageal sphincter pressure has been found to be normal in some studies[22] and low in others.[23]

Treatment of this condition depends on symptoms. Asymptomatic patients with lower esophageal rings do not require treatment. Many symptomatic patients benefit by chewing their food well. A dilatation is occasionally necessary and is usually curative if performed with a dilator up to a 50 French size. There are no long-term studies on the results of treatment of this disease, but most patients will be completely cured with dilatation. Some authors use pneumatic dilatation with equally good results, but again, long-term studies are lacking.[24] Infrequently surgical treatment is necessary.[25] In these situations a gastrotomy with digital dilatation of the ring is effective in treating the dysphagia. Most of these patients should have a concomitant hiatus hernia repair to prevent reflux and any further stricture. We prefer a transabdominal approach to the hiatus with a high lying gastrotomy. Through this gastrotomy the Schatzki's ring can be visually inspected, digitally fractured, and dilated. The gastrotomy is closed and a posterior fixation and sphincter calibration (Hill procedure) is performed such that the sphincter is returned to the abdomen and calibrated to an adequate pressure.

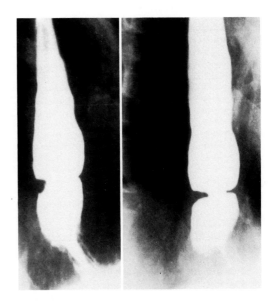

Figure 16–2. Lower esophageal (Schatzki) ring. A lower esophageal ring is identified as well as a small sliding hiatus hernia. Left half shows results after dilatation, and the right half shows the appearance before dilatation.

■ Diverticula of the Esophagus

Esophageal diverticula are blind pouches of one or more layers of the esophageal wall. Diverticula are classified according to (I) anatomy, (II) histology, and (III) pathophysiology (Table 16–1). Anatomically, diverticula occur in the pharyngoesophageal region (Zenker's diverticula), midesophagus, and epiphrenic esophagus. The histologic classification depends on the layers of the esophageal wall. Diverticula are either true, in which all layers of the esophageal wall are present, or false, in which the diverticulum consists of mucosa and submucosa only. The classification relating to pathophysiology divides diverticula into pulsion or traction types. Pulsion diverticula occur at

Table 16–1. CLASSIFICATION OF ESOPHAGEAL DIVERTICULA

Differentiating Features		Type	Description
I.	Anatomy	a. Pharyngoesophageal (Zenker's)	Potential weak area between lower fibers of inferior pharyngeal constrictor and upper fibers of cricopharyngeus
		b. Midesophageal	Midesophagus
		c. Epiphrenic	Distal esophagus
II.	Histology	a. True	All layers of esophageal wall present in diverticulum
		b. False	Wall of diverticulum consists of mucosa and submucosa only
III.	Pathophysiology	a. Pulsion	Secondary to segmental area of elevated intraluminal pressure
		b. Traction	Secondary to tug from surrounding structure, i.e., chronically inflamed carinal lymph nodes

the level of segmental areas of elevated intraluminal pressure, while traction diverticula occur where chronically inflamed lymph nodes tug at the esophageal wall. The anatomic site of the diverticulum helps in defining its pathophysiology in that the proximal and distal diverticula, i.e., pharyngoesophageal and epiphrenic diverticula, are pulsion diverticula, whereas the midesophageal diverticula is usually a traction type of diverticulum.

■ PHARYNGOESOPHAGEAL DIVERTICULUM (ZENKER'S DIVERTICULUM)

Zenker's diverticulum is an acquired, false, pulsion type of herniation of the pharyngeal mucosa penetrating through the potential weak area between the lowermost fibers of the inferior pharyngeal constrictor muscle and the upper fibers of the cricopharyngeus muscle. The condition was first described by Ludlow[26] 100 years prior to Zenker's description.[27] Ludlow was able to correctly identify both the pathophysiology and anatomy of this condition from his autopsy studies of a single case.

Patients presenting with dysphagia have 1.8 per cent incidence of pharyngoesophageal diverticula.[28] These are the most frequent types of diverticula in the esophagus and are usually encountered in patients over 50 years of age.

Zenker's diverticula occur through a weakened area in the midline posteriorly between the oblique fibers of the inferior pharyngeal constrictor muscle and the transverse fibers of the cricopharyngeus muscle.[29] Most investigators believe that the diverticula develop as a result of localized increase in intraluminal pressure, causing the mucosa to push out through this potential weak area. However, the evidence substantiating this fact is contradictory. Some studies show normal relaxation of

the upper esophageal sphincter, but the relaxation occurs at an incorrect time in the swallowing sequence.[30] Others have identified cricopharyngeal spasm,[31,32] presumably as a result of hypertrophy of the cricopharyngeus muscle (Fig. 16–3). This finding has been refuted by others[33] using a special radial arrangement of manometric catheters.

Ellis found that the pressure in the upper esophageal sphincter in patients with Zenker's diverticula is actually lower than in normal patients, but there was an abnormal temporal relationship between the pharyngeal contraction and cricopharyngeal muscle relaxation.[34,35] We, and others,[36] have been unable to identify this premature cricopharyngeal contraction as a cause for Zenker's diverticula because the events occurring at the upper sphincter take place almost simultaneously. Monitoring devices at present are unable to distinguish events with this rapidity. Symptoms related to Zenker's diverticula depend on the stage of development of the diverticulum.[37] Initially when the diverticulum is small, the patient is asymptomatic. However, later in the development the opening of the pouch allows food to accumulate in the diverticulum, causing a foreign body sensation in the throat after meals. Occasionally the patient will have regurgitation and aspiration following eating or drinking. These are particularly prominent at night. In the final stage the diverticulum is large and its orifice lies in the plane of the esophagus, allowing food to preferentially pass into the diverticulum and compress the esophagus (Fig. 16–4). Obstructive esophageal symptoms predominate, and the dysphagia becomes progressively worse. Aspiration pneumonia may become a problem and malnutrition can develop. Halitosis and hoarseness of the voice due to recurrent laryngeal nerve compression are infrequent symptoms.[38] Interesting but rare complications include malabsorption of medications with loss of drug bioavailability,[39] squamous cell car-

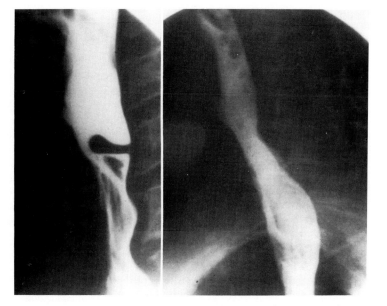

Figure 16–3. Hypertrophy of the cricopharyngeus muscle. A prominent cricopharyngeus muscle causes dysphagia in a patient without a Zenker's diverticulum. Left plate was taken prior to myotomy; right plate was taken after cricopharyngeal myotomy.

cinoma developing in the diverticulum,[40] and esophagotracheal fistulas.[41]

Physical examination is usually unremarkable in patients with Zenker's diverticula. A diagnostic physical finding present in patients with large diverticula is a gurgling sensation with manual compression of the neck (Fig. 16–5). The diverticulum is best demonstrated by a barium swallow in which anterior, lateral, and oblique views are obtained. Occasionally cineradiography is necessary to identify the diverticula if they are small.[42] Endoscopy in these patients may be hazardous; the scope will easily pass into the thin-walled diverticulum and thus potentially could cause rupture. Therefore, we do not recommend this investigation. Patients with asymptomatic diverticula do not require surgical treatment but those in whom early symptoms of dysphagia develop should be treated prior to development of complications, i.e., aspiration pneumonia.

Over the years, surgical management has

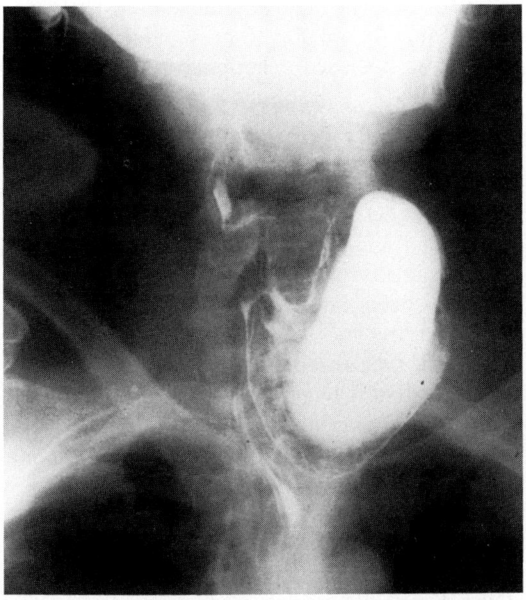

Figure 16–4. Large Zenker's diverticulum. The esophagus lies in the plane of the orifice of the diverticulum causing preferential passage of barium into the diverticulum. The diverticulum compresses the esophagus causing deviation and obstructive symptoms.

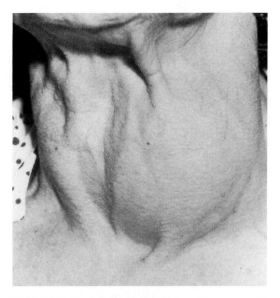

Figure 16–5. Large Zenker's diverticulum. The x-ray of this patient is shown in Figure 16–4. Manual compression of the soft mass on the left side of the neck created a gurgling sensation and reduction in size of the mass.

evolved from early attempts at creating an esophagocutaneous fistula[43] through the two-stage diverticulectomy.[44,45] The two-stage diverticulectomy was performed such that the diverticulum was isolated and sewn under the skin incision allowing the fascial planes of the neck to close prior to the second operation at which time the sac was removed. This was utilized to eliminate the devastating septic complications, such as mediastinitis, that had occurred previously with esophagocutaneous fistula. Presently the one-stage diverticulectomy pioneered by Harrington[46] is the usual treatment method. This has been found to be an effective method of treating esophageal diverticula, and recently stapling techniques have become available for excision of the diverticulum.[47] The newest modification of the one-stage diverticulectomy has been the addition of a cricopharyngeal myotomy, which is used in addition to the diverticulectomy for large diverticula but may be used as a primary procedure for smaller diverticula[48] or as an adjunct to diverticulopexy.[49]

We use the one-stage diverticulectomy with cricopharyngeal myotomy, and since intraoperative manometry is useful in surgery of motor disorders of the esophagus,[50] we use this technique in the management of patients with Zenker's diverticulum. We are at present studying the results of surgery following the introduction of intraoperative manometry to determine its role in operative management of these patients (Fig. 16–6). Preopera-

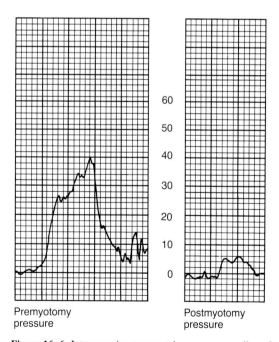

Premyotomy
pressure

Postmyotomy
pressure

Figure 16–6. Intraoperative manometric pressure recording of the cricopharyngeus muscle before and after myotomy. Prior to myotomy the pressure in the sphincter was 40 mm Hg; after myotomy the pressure was reduced to 8 mm Hg.

tively a modified nasogastric sump tube with the second lumen sealed at the tip and a recording orifice 12 cm from the tip is inserted and used as a manometric catheter to determine intraoperatively the pressure measurement in the upper esophageal sphincter. General anesthesia is utilized and a left oblique cervical skin incision is performed along the anterior border of the sternocleidomastoid muscle. This muscle is then retracted laterally exposing the anterior belly of the omohyoid muscle, which is divided. The middle thyroid vein is exposed and ligated if necessary to facilitate the upward retraction of the thyroid gland. Next the carotid sheath is retracted laterally and the inferior thyroid artery may be ligated between ligatures if it interferes with the exposure. The recurrent laryngeal nerve is identified throughout the procedure and is carefully preserved. The esophagus is now identified anterior to the prevertebral fascia, and the diverticulum is mobilized from the surrounding tissues. The sac is completely dissected down to the neck of the diverticulum. The apex is then opened and a finger is inserted to identify the sphincter.

A myotomy is performed through the cricopharyngeus muscle by dividing the longitudinal and circular muscle layers just distal to the diverticulum for a distance of 2 to 3 cm. This muscle is then dissected from approximately one half of the circumference of the mucosal tube of the esophagus, with care being taken not to enter the mucosa. The redundant diverticulum is removed, ensuring that enough mucosa remains to prevent stricture when the mucosa is closed. The mucosa is closed with a running 3–0 chromic suture following which the muscle layer overlying the site is reapproximated with interrupted silk sutures. Following closure, the manometric catheter is again drawn through the sphincter to determine if a high-pressure zone still exists distally in which case a myotomy is carried further caudally until the entire sphincter musculature has been transected (Fig. 16–6). The neck is drained and the wound closed in layers. The nasogastric tube is removed 24 hours after surgery and the patient is begun on liquids by mouth. The drain is removed following the institution of liquids by mouth, and a soft diet may be started at home 1 to 2 weeks later.

Our results have been excellent with this technique. We have had no operative mortalities and no complications of fistula, stenosis, or recurrence of the diverticula since introduction of intraoperative manometry. The role of manometry is still being determined in contrast to hiatus hernia surgery in which it has proved to be effective. We have had one patient who developed transient hoarseness following resection of a giant diverticulum, but this resolved after a few months.

■ MIDESOPHAGEAL DIVERTICULUM

These diverticula are frequently asymptomatic and are traction diverticula associated with lymphadenopathy in the parabronchial region caused by a variety of chronic inflammatory processes. The extrinsic processes in the inflamed lymph nodes lead to traction on the wall of the esophagus and therefore result in a true diverticulum becoming manifest. These diverticula are usually quite small and because of their small size they are frequently asymptomatic. If symptoms do exist, they consist of mild retrosternal chest pain and occasionally dysphagia. This type of diverticulum leads to the same complications as diverticula in the colon, including diverticulitis, perforation, fistula formation, and hemorrhage. The diverticulitis may result in abscess formation of localized mediastinitis.[51] Fistulas can occur between the esophagus and any of a number of mediastinal vessels.[52,53] Midesophageal diverticula resulting in fistula account for approximately 15 per cent of the nonmalignant esophageal fistulas.[54] Chronic bleeding occurs occasionally from these diverticula, and infrequently this bleeding may be massive.

Midesophageal diverticula are diagnosed with a barium swallow. Multiple views may be necessary to identify the diverticula. These are usually widemouthed diverticula and occur in the midportion of the esophagus. Endoscopy adds little to the diagnostic process but may be of benefit in those patients with esophagorespiratory tract fistula to rule out the presence of malignancy.[55]

Surgery is necessary for those patients developing complications of the diverticula. Ulceration occurring in the diverticulum can be a lethal complication because bleeding may be massive. Another patient may present in shock with upper gastrointestinal hemorrhage. The bleeding site may be difficult to identify, and a high index of suspicion for this reason will aid in the diagnosis. The surgery should be performed through a right thoracotomy incision in which the diverticulum and abscess, if present, can be identified. The defect in the esophageal wall is dissected out and closed in two layers, with catgut in the inner layer and another layer of nonabsorbable sutures. Periesophageal abscesses require drainage followed by diverticulectomy. Occasionally the inflamed diverticulum results in a fistulous tract to the bronchus resulting in bronchiectasis. This segment of the lung needs to be excised at the time of excision of the fistula and closure of the diverticulum.

■ EPIPHRENIC DIVERTICULA

Epiphrenic diverticula are uncommon forms of pulsion diverticula accounting for approximately 4 per cent of some 437 patients with esophageal diverticula seen at the Lahey Clinic.[56] They are located between 5 and 10 cm above the cardioesophageal junction and emerge predominantly from the right posterolateral wall of the esophagus. They may vary in size from less than 1 cm to greater than 10 cm in diameter and may be single or multiple. These diverticula usually develop proximal to an organic or functional obstruction of the esophagus and are frequently associated with other conditions as documented by Allan and Clagett in their 160 patients at the Mayo Clinic.[57] These associated conditions include hiatus hernia with reflux esophagitis, diffuse esophageal spasm, segmental spasm[50] (Fig. 16–7), achalasia (Fig. 16–8), eventration of the diaphragm, and even carcinoma of the esophagus. This association led to the hypothesis that these diverticula develop a congenitally weak area in the distal esophagus, which is subjected to prolonged, elevated intraluminal pressure. This results in a progressive outpouching of the mucosa and submucosa similar to the development of a Zenker's diverticulum. However, the vast majority of patients with motility disorders and hiatus

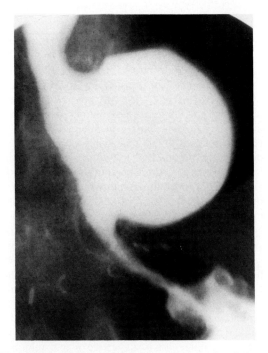

Figure 16–7. Epiphrenic diverticulum. This large diverticulum developed proximal to the site of a failed Heller myotomy in a patient with achalasia. Note the narrow "bird's beak" esophagus distal to the diverticulum. The patient required diverticulectomy and repeat esophagomyotomy.

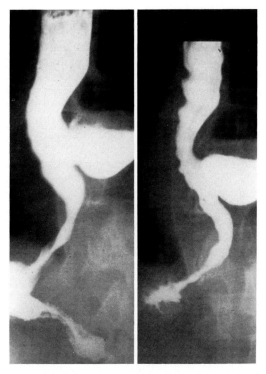

Figure 16–8. Epiphrenic diverticulum in a patient with segmental spasm. Note the barium-air-fluid level in the diverticulum as well as the tertiary contractions in the right x-ray. Esophageal manometry reveals a high pressure zone above and below the diverticulum.

hernias do not develop diverticula, and the presence of a congenital, weakened area in the esophagus has never been proved.

Most patients with epiphrenic diverticula are over 50 years of age, and many are asymptomatic or have vague, ill-defined symptoms that are not diagnostic. A wide variety of symptoms may be present, relating to the underlying esophageal disorder or the presence of a diverticulum in which food and saliva accumulate and become putrified. Dysphagia occurs either because of hangup of food in the diverticulum or because of the concomitant motor disorder of the esophagus. Regurgitation occurs as a result of nocturnal emptying of the diverticular sac. If the diverticulum is very large, the sac, when filled with material, may cause obstruction by extrinsic pressure or angulation of the esophagus. Fever indicates inflammation of the diverticulum, respiratory tract complications such as aspiration, or infrequently perforation of the diverticulum. A chest x-ray with an air-fluid level in the pericardial region is suggestive of an epiphrenic diverticulum.

The diagnosis is confirmed with a barium esophagogram, which also identifies associated lesions such as hiatus hernia, achalasia, or diffuse spasm.

Endoscopy is unnecessary to establish the diagnosis, but it may be helpful in identifying the associated lesion, particularly hiatus hernia with esophagitis. This procedure must be performed very carefully because these diverticula have very thin walls and inadvertent perforation is possible. Esophageal motility studies, cineradiography, and esophageal radionuclide scintigraphy are helpful in determining the associated motility disorders, a necessary part of any anticipated surgical management. Failure to treat associated disease is the most common reason for persisting symptoms following surgical resection of the diverticulum.

The natural history of patients with epiphrenic diverticula is unpredictable. Some slowly progress over years and have symptoms at a late date. Others remain asymptomatic for many years, while still others seek medical attention for the underlying motility problem. Infrequently complications of the diverticulum occur including diverticulitis, abscess, hemorrhage, and perforation. Aspiration occasionally occurs resulting in bronchopulmonary infection.

Treatment is necessary in symptomatic patients, for appearance of symptoms indicates enlargement of the diverticula or progression of the motility disorder. Surgical resection of the diverticulum as well as a surgical approach to the underlying esophageal problem is the treatment of choice. Resection of the diverticulum can best be performed through a right thoracotomy. The diverticular sac is dissected from the surrounding tissue down to the mouth of the diverticulum, at which point the redundant mucosa and submucosa are excised and the diverticular orifice is closed with a running chromic suture. If the patient has achalasia, a Heller myotomy should be performed (see Chapter 14, on surgery for motility disorders). If the manometry studies preoperatively indicate that the patient has vigorous achalasia or diffuse esophageal spasm, a long myotomy is necessary utilizing intraoperative manometry (see Chapter 14). Patients with concomitant hiatus hernia and esophagitis should have a combined thoracoabdominal approach resecting the diverticulum, closing the mouth of the diverticulum, and then repairing the hiatus hernia with posterior fixation and sphincter calibration (Hill procedure) (see Chapter 8, on surgery for gastroesophageal reflux). Experience has shown that patients undergoing diverticulectomy alone have significantly more complications than those patients treated by diverticulectomy and long esophagomyotomy. There are, at present, no long-term results of treatment with diverticulectomy and myotomy in patients with epiphrenic pulsion diverticulum and diffuse esophageal spasm.

■ REFERENCES

1. Rinaldo JA: Esophageal webs and rings. *In* Vantrappen G, Hellemans J (Eds): Diseases of the Esophagus. New York, Springer Verlag, 1974, pp 571–589.
2. Mercer CD, Hill LD: Esophageal web associated with Zenker's diverticulum: A possible cause for postoperative dysphagia. Canad J Surg, 28:375–376, 1985.
3. Elwood PC, Jacobs A, Pitman RG, et al: Epidemiology of the Paterson-Kelly syndrome. Lancet, 2:716–720, 1964.
4. Ekburg O, Nylander G: Webs and web-like formations in the pharynx and cervical esophagus. Diagnostic Imaging, 52:10–18, 1983.
5. Brown-Kelly A: Spasm at the entrance to the oesophagus. J Laryng Otol, 34:285–289, 1919.
6. Paterson DR: A clinical type of dysphagia. J Laryng Rhin Otol, 34:289–291, 1919.
7. Vinson PO: Hysterical dysphagia. Minn Med, 5:107–108, 1922.
8. Waldenström J, Hollen L: Iron and epithelium. Some clinical observations. Acta Med Scand, 90:380–405, 1938.
9. Wynder EL, Fryer JH: Etiologic consideration of Plummer-Vinson (Paterson-Kelly) syndrome. Ann Intern Med, 49:1106–1128, 1958.
10. Shamma MH, Benedict EB: Esophageal webs. N Engl J Med, 259:378–384, 1958.
11. Seaman WB: The significance of webs in the hypopharynx and upper esophagus. Radiology, 89:32–38, 1967.
12. Seaman WB: Pharyngeal and upper esophageal dysphagia. JAMA, 235:2643–2646, 1976.
13. Weaver GA: Upper esophageal web due to a ring formed by a squamocolumnar junction with ectopic gastric mucosa (another explanation of the Paterson-Kelly, Plummer-Vinson syndrome). Dig Dis Sci, 24:959, 1979.
14. Ikard RW, Rosen HE: Midesophageal web in adults. Ann Thorac Surg, 24:355, 1977.
15. Shiflett DW, Gilliam JH, Wu WC, Austin WE, Ott DJ: Multiple esophageal webs. Gastroenterology, 77:556, 1979.
16. Kelley ML Jr, Frazer JP: Symptomatic midesophageal webs. JAMA, 197:143–146, 1966.
17. Schatzki R, Gray JE: Dysphagia due to the diaphragm-like localized narrowing in the lower esophagus (lower esophageal ring). Roentgenology, 70:911–922, 1953.
18. Schatzki R: The lower esophageal ring: Long-term follow-up of symptomatic and asymptomatic rings. Am J Roentgenol, 90:805–810, 1963.
19. Schatzki R, Gray JE: The lower esophageal ring. Am J Roentgenol, 75:246–261, 1956.
20. Ingelfinger FJ, Kramer P: Dysphagia produced by a contractile ring in lower esophagus. Gastroenterology, 23:419–430, 1953.
21. Goyal RK, Glancy JJ, Spiro HM: Lower esophageal ring. N Engl J Med, 282:1298–1305, 1355–1362, 1970.
22. Eckardt VF, Adami B, Hucker H, et al: The esophagogastric junction in patients with asymptomatic lower esophageal rings. Gastroenterology, 79:426–430, 1980.
23. Rinaldo JA, Gahagan T: The narrow lower esophageal ring: Pathogenesis and physiology. Am J Dig Dis, 11:257–265, 1966.
24. Mossberg SM: Lower esophageal ring treated by pneumatic dilatation. Gastroenterology, 48:118–121, 1965.
25. Postlethwait PW, Sealy WC: Experience with the treatment of 59 patients with lower esophageal web. Ann Surg, 165:756–779, 1967.
26. Ludlow A: A case of obstructed deglutition from a preternatural dilatation of, and bag formed in, the pharynx (communicated by Hunter WJ). Med Observ Inquiries, 3:85, 1967.
27. Zenker FA, Ziemssen H: Krankheit des Oesophagus in Handbuch des Speciellen Pathologie und Therapie. Leipzig, F.C. Vogel, 1877.
28. MacMillan AS: Statistical study of diseases of the esophagus. Surg Gynecol Obstet, 60:394, 1935.
29. Killian G: La boudre de l'oesophage. Ann Mal Oreille Larynx, 34:1, 1908; cited by Moersch and Judd, Surg Gynecol Obstet, 58:781, 1934.
30. Negus VE: The etiology of pharyngeal diverticula. Bull Johns Hopkins Hosp, 101:209, 1957.
31. Cross FS, Johnson GF, Gerein AN: Esophageal diverticula associated neuromuscular changes in the esophagus. Arch Surg, 83:525, 1961.
32. Cross FS: Esophageal diverticula related neuromuscular problems. Ann Otol Rhinol Laryngol, 77:914, 1968.
33. Winans CS: The pharyngeal closure mechanism: A manometric study. Gastroenterology, 63:768, 1972.
34. Ellis FH, Schlegel F, Lynch VP, Payne WS: Cricopharyngeal myotomy for pharyngoesophageal diverticulum. Ann Surg, 170:340, 1969.
35. Ellis FH Jr: Pharyngoesophageal diverticula and cricopharyngeal incoordination. Mod Treat, 7:1098, 1970.
36. Knuff TE, Benjamin SB, Castell DO: Pharyngoesophageal (Zenker's) diverticulum: A reappraisal. Gastroenterology, 82:734, 1982.
37. Lahey FH, Warren KW: Esophageal diverticula. Surg Gynecol Obstet, 98:1–28, 1954.
38. Becker H, Ungeheuer E: Zur Klinik und Therapie des Oesophagus Divertikels. Med Klin, 65:589–594, 1970.
39. Baron SH: Zenker's diverticulum as a cause for loss of drug availability. A "new" complication. Am J Gastroenterol, 77:152–153, 1982.
40. Som ML, Deitel M: Carcinoma in a large pharyngoesophageal diverticulum. Arch Surg, 94:35, 1967.
41. Stanford W, Barloon TJ, Lu CC: Esophagotracheal fistula from a pharyngoesophageal diverticulum. Chest, 84:229–231, 1983.
42. Ekberg O, Wylander G: Lateral diverticula from the pharyngoesophageal area. Radiology, 146:117–122, 1983.
43. Micoladoni K: Study of the operative treatment of diverticula of the esophagus. (Ein beitrag zur Operativen Behandlung der Oesophagus Divertikel.) Wien Med Wochenschr, 27:6015–6031, 1877; cited by Saint, Arch Surg, 19:53, 1929.
44. Lahey FH: Esophageal diverticulum. JAMA, 1101:994, 1933.
45. Goldman EE: Die Ziveidentige Operation von Pulsions Divertikeln der Speiserohre. Beitr Klin Chir, 61:741, 1909; cited by Saint, Arch Surg, 19:23, 1929.
46. Harrington SW: Pulsion diverticula hypopharynx: A review of forty-one cases in which operation was performed and a report of two cases. Surg Gynecol Obstet, 69:364–373, 1939.
47. Hoelm JG, Payne WS: Resection of pharyngoesophageal diverticulum using stapling device. Mayo Clin Proc, 44:738–741, 1969.
48. Sutherland HD: Cricopharyngeal achalasia. J Thorac Cardiovasc Surg, 43:114–126, 1962.
49. Belsey R: Functional disease of the esophagus. J Thorac Cardiovasc Surg, 52:164–188, 1966.
50. Hill LD, Asplund CM, Roberts PN: Intraoperative manometry: Adjunct to surgery for esophageal motility disorders. Am J Surg, 147:171–174, 1984.
51. Webster BH: Spontaneous perforation of an oesophageal diverticulum. Report of a case with survival. Dis Chest 31:345–348, 1957.
52. Cheitlin MD, Kamin EJ, Wilkes DJ: Midesophageal diverticulum: Report of a case with fistulous connection with

the superior vena cava. Arch Intern Med, *107*:252–259, 1961.

53. Powell MEA: A case of aortic-esophageal fistula. Br J Surg, *45*:55–57, 1957.

54. Coleman FP, Bunch GH Jr: Acquired nonmalignant esophagotracheobronchial communications. Dis Chest, *18*:31–48, 1950.

55. Naclerio EA: Diverticula of the thoracic esophagus. Am J Surg, *93*:218, 1957.

56. Boyd DP, Adams HD: Esophageal diverticulum. N Engl J Med, *264*:641, 1961.

57. Allen TH, Clagett OT: Changing concepts in the surgical treatment of pulsion diverticula of the lower esophagus. J Thorac Cardiovasc Surg, *50*:455, 1965.

17

Perforation, Rupture, and Injury of the Esophagus

C. D. Mercer ▪ Lucius D. Hill

Perforation, rupture, and injury of the esophagus usually result in severe, acute, life-threatening injuries often requiring prompt surgical management. Unfortunately, the diagnosis is often delayed, causing a change in the therapeutic options and an increase in the mortality rate.

Classification of injuries of the esophagus[1,2] (Table 17–1) divides the injuries into two groups. Extraluminal causes include penetrating wounds, blunt external trauma, and intraoperative injuries, while intraluminal causes of injury include intrinsic forces such as Mallory-Weiss tears or Boerhaave's spontaneous rupture of the esophagus. Intraluminal causes of injury with extrinsic force occur with tears from instrumentation, foreign bodies, ingestion of caustics or acids, and air pressure.

Table 17–1. CLASSIFICATION OF INJURIES AND WOUNDS OF THE ESOPHAGUS

I. Extraluminal causes of injury
  A. Penetrating wounds
  B. Externally applied blunt trauma
  C. Operative accidents
    1. Suture or tear
    2. Trauma to wall or blood supply

II. Intraluminal causes of injury
  A. Intrinsic (from within body)
    1. Mallory-Weiss tear
    2. (Boerhaave) spontaneous esophageal rupture
  B. Extrinsic (force from outside body)
    1. Instrumentation
    2. Foreign body
    3. Ingestion of caustics or acids
    4. Air pressure

■ Perforation and Ruptures of the Esophagus

Esophageal perforation remains a major challenge for the thoracic surgeon and a substantial cause of further complications and death for the patient. For nearly two decades there has been a debate between conservative, nonoperative therapy and prompt operative intervention.[3,4] As well, during that time a variety of surgical approaches have been recommended as the definitive answer to all cases of perforation (Fig. 17–1). This has ultimately led to confusion in the management of these patients.

Extraluminal causes of injury are seen infrequently. However, intraluminal causes are becoming more common, particularly with the increased frequency of a variety of endoscopic therapeutic maneuvers. Esophageal perforation constitutes both a medical and surgical emergency, but with modern improved critical care monitoring and potent intravenous antibiotics, survival is improving. In spite of these advances, mortality rates, depending on the time of diagnosis, site of perforation, and coexisting disease, still range between 15 and 30 per cent.

Intraluminal causes of perforation are the most common form of esophageal injury. Of these types, instrumentation as an extrinsic force remains the most frequent cause of perforated esophagus. In these patients the perforation occurs most commonly through the posterior wall of the cervical esophagus. This occurs in from 0.1 to 1.5 per cent

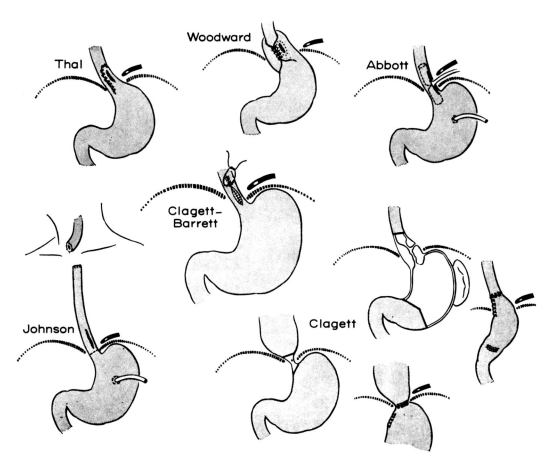

Figure 17–1. A variety of methods of managing distal esophageal perforations, both early and late, includes the Thal fundic patch, complete fundoplication in the Woodward procedure, decompression with a T-tube in the Abbott procedure, full suture and drainage in the Clagett-Barrett procedure, complete defunctionalization of the esophagus, the cervical esophagostomy and gastrostomy in the Johnson procedure, and resection of the lesion with esophagogastrostomy or colon interposition when concomitant disease is present in the Clagett procedure.

of patients, depending on the type of endoscopic procedure performed.[5–7] With increasing skill and use of the fiberoptic endoscope, the incidence of this is declining, even though the frequency of endoscopic procedures is increasing. Other less common sites for endoscopic perforation are the narrowing at the level of the aortic arch and the gastroesophageal junction. The presence of a benign or malignant stricture increases the risk of perforation, especially when dilatation (pneumatic or hydrostatic) of the stricture is performed.[8] A variety of palliative prostheses and tubes is available to be passed across the stricture. These can also perforate the esophagus since they must be placed endoscopically by *blind* pulsion techniques. Accidental or intentional ingestion of sharp foreign bodies, such as fish bones or pieces of metal, occasionally cause esophageal perforation and mediastinitis. These perforations also occur at the anatomic sites of narrowing of the esophagus as

described above. Caustic ingestion occasionally results in perforation of the esophagus, and this will be dealt with at length in Chapter 18. Anecdotal reports of perforation occurring with high-pressure air guns also exist.

Intrinsic intraluminal injury spans a spectrum of disease entities. At one end the Mallory-Weiss syndrome[9] results in mucosal injury and gastrointestinal hemorrhage. This bleeding often stops spontaneously but may be massive and life-threatening. At the other end of the spectrum spontaneous perforation or Boerhaave's syndrome[10] results in transmural rupture of the distal esophagus. This may be particularly lethal because of the delay in diagnosis or the presence of existing and predisposing esophageal conditions.[11]

Extraluminal causes of injury are rare. Penetrating wounds of the esophagus are usually associated with injuries to other structures in the neck, thorax, or abdomen, and it is these associated injuries that are most evident clinically and that often result in a high mortality rate.[12] Such injuries may cause a delay in diagnosis and treatment of the esophageal injury. External blunt trauma is an extremely uncommon cause of esophageal perforation and when present, concomitant injuries predominate. Operative injury to the esophagus, either at the time of thoracotomy or laparotomy, occurs infrequently but has been reported with pulmonary resections,[13] repair of paraesophageal and sliding hiatus hernia,[14] and vagotomy.[15] Interference with the blood supply to the wall of the esophagus uncommonly causes ischemic necrosis and perforation of the esophagus.[16]

The etiology of perforated esophagus in a combined series of 23 cases from the Virginia Mason Medical Center and the University of California San Francisco Hospital over an 8-year period is shown in Table 17–2. This includes seven gunshot wounds, ten iatrogenic disruptions, four Boerhaave's spontaneous ruptures, one foreign body perforation, and one perforation of a peptic esophageal ulcer.

■ CLINICAL PRESENTATION

Clinical presentation of a patient with a perforated esophagus depends on the etiology of the perforation, the length of time from perforation to diagnosis, and the site of the perforation. If the perforation is due to external trauma the nature and extent of associated injuries to blood vessels, other mediastinal organs, or intra-abdominal contents will determine the presentation. Consequently, the clinical manifestations of esophageal injury itself are usually obscured by concomitant injuries. This often results in delay in diagnosis and treatment of the esophageal injury. Delay in diagnosing the esophageal perforation alters the pathogenesis from a chemical injury to a more severe bacterial infection. Initially saliva, gastric acid, and bile create chemical inflammation, usually in the mediastinum and pleura. Bacterial colonization quickly follows

Table 17–2. ETIOLOGY OF ESOPHAGEAL PERFORATION

Trauma (gunshot wounds)	7
Iatrogenic	10
Esophagoscopy (4)	
Dilatation (3)	
Intraoperative (2)	
Nasogastric tube (1)	
Postemetic (Boerhaave)	4
Foreign body	1
Peptic ulceration	1
Total	23

and results in a rapid septic course with signs of shock and sepsis predominating. If a perforated esophagus is not suspected as the etiology of the sepsis, valuable time is lost, making management more difficult.

The site of perforation also determines the clinical presentation. Salivary contamination from a perforated cervical esophagus spreads into the superior mediastinum and into the surrounding tissues of the neck. Perforation of the thoracic esophagus results in direct mediastinal contamination, which develops more rapidly than after cervical perforation. Mediastinal pleural ruptures, resulting in soilage of the intrapleural space with respiration then disseminate the infection within the mediastinum as the negative intrathoracic pressures draw gastric contents into the mediastinum and pleural spaces. This pleural contamination causes significant intravascular fluid volume depletion and signs of hypovolemia, shock, and sepsis prevail.

A patient with a perforation of the abdominal esophagus from surgery or with instrumentation may present with both generalized peritonitis and mediastinitis with transit of the contaminants through the esophageal hiatus into the mediastinum. When two cavities, the thorax and abdomen, are contaminated, a combined thoracoabdominal approach may be necessary to deal adequately with the perforation and drain the mediastinum.

Coexisting disease also influences the clinical presentation of patients with perforation. Peptic esophageal strictures (Fig. 17–2), malignancies, and achalasia produce symptoms specific to each disease in addition to the symptoms of perforation when this occurs during treatment of the underlying condition.

Most patients with esophageal perforation complain of pain, dysphagia, fever, and some degree of respiratory distress. The pain is localized either to the neck, chest, or epigastrium, depending on the site of perforation. The pain on cervical perforation is aggravated by swallowing and neck movement. Upper abdominal pain occurs with both thoracic and abdominal perforations, which may result in diagnostic error. At the time of perforation, the patient may have noticed a tearing or bursting sensation, especially in spontaneous Boerhaave's ruptures. Mediastinal air migrates upward, resulting in palpable subcutaneous emphysema in the neck in approximately one half of the patients with perforated esophagus. The air trapped in the mediastinum causes a crunching sound on auscultation of the chest (Hamman's crunch). This is associated with extensive and long-standing injuries.

The diagnosis of esophageal rupture is established when a suspicious clinical presentation is confirmed by the demonstration of an esophageal

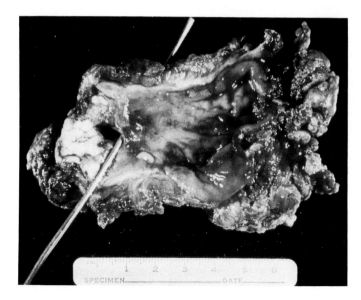

Figure 17–2. Esophageal perforation at the site of a chronic peptic esophageal stricture in a patient who had been dilating herself for many years.

fistula. Plain radiographs of the neck may show air in the prevertebral space (Fig. 17–3). Radiograph of the chest early in the course of disease often shows mediastinal or subcutaneous emphysema. Air in the mediastinum takes on the shape of a V at the cardiophrenic angle (Naclerio's sign)[17]; however, if initial films are negative, repeat films may show the sudden onset of emphysema. Chest x-ray can show other signs of perforated esophagus including pneumothorax or hydropneumothorax.

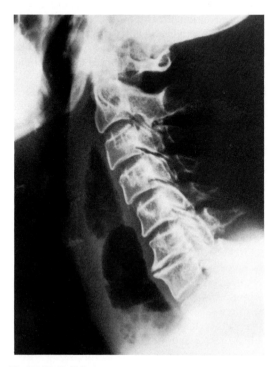

Figure 17–3. Subcutaneous neck emphysema secondary to an esophageal perforation. The air distends the prevertebral space.

Later films show mediastinal widening caused by trapped air and mediastinal fluid.

The site of perforation should be localized using esophagograms with water-soluble contrast medium. If the initial study is negative and clinical findings are suspicious, a repeat examination one hour later is recommended. Radiologic technique, however, does not always give an exact impression of the size of the leak.[18] Esophagoscopy has been utilized in the diagnosis of questionable causes but it is risky in these ill, unstable patients. Upright abdominal x-rays show the intra-abdominal free air when the abdominal esophagus has been perforated.

The frequency of diagnostic error is often as high as 50 per cent, especially in patients with spontaneous perforation of the esophagus.[19] The differential diagnosis is extensive and includes pancreatitis, myocardial infarction, dissecting aortic aneurysm, pneumothorax, mesenteric thrombosis or embolus, pulmonary embolus, perforated peptic ulcer, strangulated diaphragmatic hernia, and acute cholecystitis.

■ TREATMENT OF ESOPHAGEAL PERFORATION

The operative approach to perforation of the esophagus depends on the site of perforation, whether or not there is coexisting disease or injury, and the time from perforation to treatment. Immediately following the diagnosis, all patients with perforated esophagus should be placed on intravenous antibiotics, intravenous fluids, and if possible, nasogastric decompression of the stomach. Obviously no single treatment is applicable to all cases of esophageal perforation. In most instances, the perforation can be identified and repaired early following injury; however, delay in diagnosis may result in a septic course and a fatal outcome.

If the injury occurs as an iatrogenic, intraoperative perforation, sound surgical judgment must be exercised regarding treatment. When appropriate, simple repair of the perforation with two layers of nonabsorbable sutures is effective. Occasionally the underlying disease, for instance peptic stricture, achalasia, or cancer, can be treated simultaneously. Endoscopic injuries following dilatation are usually evident to the endoscopist, and emergency surgery with simple suture repair of the laceration is the treatment of choice. Occasionally a patient may exhibit only minimal signs and symptoms of contamination of the pleural cavity. In these situations, a carefully observed nonoperative course including elimination of oral intake, nasogastric suction, intravenous fluids, and broad-spectrum antibiotics may be followed. Perforations of the neck usually respond well to supportive measures and drainage of the neck.[20] There is rarely any need to perform a direct repair and the perforation is actually seldom seen.

Drainage is of primary importance in all forms of esophageal lacerations. Intrathoracic injuries require adequate drainage of both the mediastinum and pleural cavity. Neck wounds with esophageal injury require drainage of the neck while intraabdominal perforations require mediastinal and peritoneal drainage. If, following closure, a postoperative disruption occurs, antibiotic coverage, nutritional support, and adequate mediastinal drainage will often allow for healing of the fistula. Primary repair of the esophagus should be buttressed with adjacent viable tissue such as mediastinal pleura, gastric fundus, diaphragmatic pedicle flap, intercostal muscle bundle, or pericardium. Operative management of patients with delayed diagnosis of esophageal perforation or spontaneous perforation is more complex, as outlined in the next section.

■ SPONTANEOUS RUPTURE (BOERHAAVE'S SYNDROME)

Spontaneous rupture of the esophagus is an uncommon, life-threatening event. If left untreated, there is a 100 per cent mortality rate and even when prompt treatment is instituted, there is a 15 to 30 per cent operative mortality rate. When this condition is recognized early and treated within 24 hours, primary closure of the esophageal tear is usually successful. However, when the diagnosis is not confirmed within the first 24 hours, other forms of therapy must be utilized.

Many causes of Boerhaave's syndrome have been reported. Vomiting is the usual precipitating cause, but rupture has been reported following other forms of straining such as vigorous coughing or weight lifting. The syndrome has also occurred in the absence of straining, as in those patients with esophagitis or distal esophageal obstruction. We have treated a patient who had no precipitating cause for perforation, even in retrospect.

The tear is linear, approximately 2.5 cm long, occurring on the left side of the distal esophagus. Mediastinal widening and air are seen early. The mediastinal pleura ruptures or is digested, allowing a pleural effusion, with or without pneumothorax, to develop. Crepitus is palpable in the neck. Later in the course of the disease Hamman's sign is positive in 20 per cent of patients. Patients complain of severe substernal or epigastric pain and pleuritic lower chest pain. This is accompanied by fever and prostration. Chest x-ray shows typical signs previously described. Water-soluble esophagograms confirm the diagnosis. The incidence of diagnostic error is as high as 50 per cent in patients with Boerhaave's syndrome.[19] The most frequent misdiagnoses are perforated peptic ulcer and acute myocardial infarction. In one series the correct diagnosis was made within the first 12 hours in only 21 per cent of patients.[21]

Therapy includes drainage of the pleura and mediastinum, elimination of the source of contamination, and provision of adequate nutrition.[22] The first successful surgical repair was performed by Barrett in 1946.[23] Since then, primary closure of the defect with nonabsorbable sutures with drainage of the pleura and mediastinum has been advocated for those cases recognized within the first 24 hours. After 24 hours, there is a high incidence of breakdown of the suture line, and the risk of operative death increases severalfold. Sawyer found that patients treated within the first 24 hours had an operative mortality rate of 13 per cent, and those treated after 24 hours had a 56 per cent mortality rate.[24]

Several alternatives have been proposed for the treatment of esophageal rupture when diagnosed more than 24 hours after the rupture has occurred. Many of these alternative procedures require multiple stage operations. These include early esophagogastrostomy,[25] use of a Thal patch,[26] exclusion and diversion in continuity,[27] insertion of a large silastic T-tube to externalize the perforation and confine the fistula to a manageable tract,[21] use of a pleural patch,[28] and use of an intercostal pedicle graft for reinforcement.[29] Unfortunately these procedures have been associated with operative mortality rates as high as 56 per cent.[24] In addition to the necessity for repeat operation, a long hospital stay, increased expense, and increased morbidity are common to these procedures.

In patients with delayed diagnosis of esophageal perforation we have used a Celestin tube.[30] It is simple, both in concept and execution, has a low operative risk, and is completely reversible, requiring only brief general anesthetic and esophagoscopy for its removal. The tube overcomes the obstruction distal to the tear produced by the lower esophageal sphincter. This physiologic obstruction causes the perforation to be the route of least resistance for egress of esophageal contents. The time-honored dictum for fistulas of the GI tract that a fistula will not close in the presence of a distal obstruction holds equally true for the esophagus. This distal obstruction is relieved by the Celestin tube, which allows easy passage of esophageal contents into the stomach.

The surgical technique is similar to that described in the original article by Celestin.[31] A gastrotomy is performed through the anterior wall of the stomach. The obturator of the Celestin tube is passed down the esophagus into the stomach. The tube is then pulled downward into the esophagus and positioned such that the flange is located above the perforation, which has been previously identified with the esophagoscope. The distal end of the Celestin tube is transected where it will be attached to the anterior abdominal wall and a side opening is cut in the tube. The tube is sutured to the anterior abdominal wall with a prolene suture through the stomach wall so that it will not displace. The suture is taken through the fascia into the subcutaneous tissue. The site of abdominal wall fixation is marked on the skin so that the suture can be cut with a small incision, allowing division of the retained suture and removal of the tube with the esophagoscope without a major secondary operation. The stomach is attached to the abdominal wall around the fixation suture. The anterior gastrotomy is closed in two layers. A feeding jejunostomy is placed, and the abdominal cavity is drained. A minithoracotomy is required to adequately drain the mediastinum and pleural cavity.

The Celestin tube offers a number of advantages. First, the tube stents the gastroesophageal junction in the open position. Second, the operation is simple and does not require extensive dissection of the esophagus. Third, if a stricture is present, the tube provides a stent across the strictures. Fourth, the operation can be done in severely debilitated patients with a minimum of operating time.

An illustrative case is shown in Figure 17–4. This 46-year-old man sustained a Boerhaave's rupture of the distal esophagus which was diagnosed

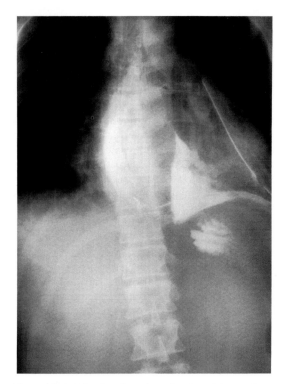

Figure 17–4. A late Boerhaave's perforation of the esophagus demonstrating leak of Gastrografin.

promptly and repaired with chromic catgut sutures. The patient became septic four days after the initial operation, at which time an anastomotic leak was suspected. A Gastrografin swallow showed leakage of contrast material into the left side of the chest and mediastinum producing a V-shaped shadow at the cardiophrenic angle, or Naclerio's sign, indicating a breakdown of the suture line. The patient was taken to the operating room, and a Celestin tube was inserted by the technique previously described (Fig. 17–5).

The patient began swallowing liquids on the third postoperative day. At the end of one week he was eating soft foods and was discharged to commence work two weeks after the Celestin tube was inserted. Six weeks after placement of the Celestin tube, he returned and the Celestin tube was removed by first incising the skin under local anesthetic, dividing the prolene suture, grasping the Celestin tube through the esophagoscope, and retrieving it without surgery. An upper GI series two months after insertion of the Celestin tube showed complete healing of the stricture with a normal-appearing esophagus (Fig. 17–6). To date, six patients have been treated by this method with recovery in all. This patient illustrates several important points. As Barrett pointed out, the perforation should be closed with nonabsorbable suture material since absorbable suture material may be digested quickly by the contaminated pleural contents. Stenting of the esophagus with insertion of a Celestin tube allows food and fluid to pass readily into the stomach so that the line of least resistance for saliva and esophageal content is no longer through the tear in the esophagus. This allows healing of the tear without requiring a major surgical procedure.

Once the Celestin tube has been placed, the patient must be vigorously counseled about the possibility of aspiration. The head of the bed must be elevated at all times and appropriate dietary management should include soft foods. The patient should not go to bed with a full stomach and must be cautioned that if he lies flat he will aspirate and may develop pneumonia. In one case in which a Celestin tube was placed through a tumor for maintenance of nutrition the patient did indeed lie flat, aspirated, developed respiratory arrest, and died.

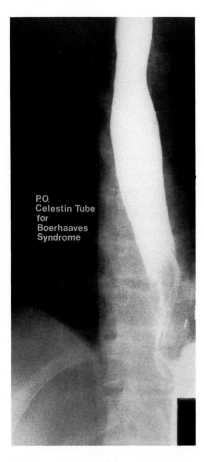

Figure 17–6. Postoperative result in a patient with a perforated esophagus following removal of a Celestin tube.

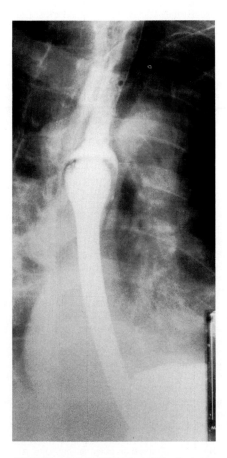

Figure 17–5. Insertion of a Celestin tube in the same patient as Figure 17–4.

■ MALLORY-WEISS SYNDROME

In 1929 Mallory and Weiss reported 15 patients with upper gastrointestinal bleeding following vomiting which was caused by excessive alcohol intake. Autopsy findings on four of these patients showed linear tears of the mucosa in the lower part of the esophagus or the cardia of the stomach.[9] Since this original observation, the syndrome has expanded to include gastrointestinal bleeding caused by mucosal tears elicited by sudden increase in intragastric pressure. The diagnosis was made initially endoscopically in 1956,[32] and since then this has become the diagnostic method of choice.

Most patients have vomiting or retching preceding the onset of painless upper gastrointestinal bleeding. Other preceding events have included coughing, epileptic attacks, and status asthmaticus. The increased intra-abdominal pressure causes a pressure differential across the gastric wall which is accentuated in the presence of a hiatus hernia. This pressure change results in a mucosal tear leading to laceration of the submucosal arteries. The bleeding may be massive and life-threatening because it is arterial or in other instances it will be intermittent and self-limiting. Other patients may present with an ongoing, slow ooze from the gastroesophageal junction. Shock may be present and occurred in 50 per cent of patients in one series.[33] Spontaneous cessation of bleeding is common.[34]

The diagnosis is today routinely made with upper gastrointestinal endoscopy. However, in patients who have massive GI bleeding, the site of bleeding may be obscured by blood clot, or the patient may be unstable enough that the diagnosis is made only at the time of laparotomy. In these instances, following exploration of the abdomen for other sites of gastrointestinal bleeding, a gastrotomy is performed and the stomach blood clot is aspirated. A pack is placed distally in the pylorus and the stomach is inspected to see if blood is coming from above the level of the gastrotomy or if it is coming from the duodenum. If it is coming from the esophagogastric junction the laceration is usually identified with adequate retraction and is treated adequately by oversewing the bleeding tear using a running locking chromic or Vicryl suture. Commonly, other gastrointestinal problems exist such as gastritis, hiatal hernia, and esophagitis. The left side of the chest should be prepared in the event that the tear extends upward above the diaphragm and cannot be entirely closed through the abdomen. Upper gastrointestinal x-rays are not helpful in diagnosing Mallory-Weiss tears.

The treatment of these patients is usually nonoperative. A nasogastric tube is inserted to decompress the stomach because any dilatation of the stomach with blood clot will predispose to ongoing bleeding. As well, it allows for monitoring of the amount of hemorrhage. This does not allow spontaneous cessation of bleeding. Upper gastrointestinal endoscopy with either laser photocoagulation or electrocoagulation of the bleeding site may be of benefit. Infrequently, vasopressin intravenously will help in eliminating GI bleeding. Operative intervention is infrequently necessary. However, in patients with massive bleeding this can be lifesaving if the site is identified through a gastrotomy and oversewn with a running chromic or Vicryl suture. Forty-six per cent of 303 cases of Mallory-Weiss tear treated by Wychulis and Sasso required operation.[35] The mortality rates in this syndrome have ranged from 0[36] to 12 per cent.[34,37]

Present methods of diagnosis and treatment have resulted in decreasing rates of morbidity and mortality from this disease.

■ REFERENCES

1. Samson PC: Injuries and wounds of the esophagus—a classification. Calif Med, 80:363–368, 1954.
2. Jones RJ, Samson PC: Esophageal injury. Ann Thorac Surg, 19:216–230, 1975.
3. Mengoli LR, Klassen KP: Conservative management of esophageal perforation. Arch Surg, 91:238–240, 1965.
4. McInnis WD, Cruz AB, Aust JB: Penetrating injuries to the neck—pitfalls in management. Am J Surg, 130:416–420, 1975.
5. Wychulis AR, Fontana RS, Payne WS: Instrumental perforations of the esophagus. Chest, 55:184–189, 1969.
6. Jones FA, Doll R, Fletcher C, Rodgers HW: The risk of gastroscopy: A survey of 49,000 examinations. Lancet, 1:647, 1951.
7. Smith CCK, Tanner NC: Complications of gastroscopy and oesophagoscopy. Br J Surg, 43:396–403, 1956.
8. Silvis SE, Nebel O, Rogers G, Sugawa C, Mandelstom P: Endoscopic complications. Results of the 1974 American Society of Gastrointestinal Endoscopy Survey. JAMA, 235:926, 1976.
9. Mallory GK, Weiss S: Hemorrhages from lacerations of the cardiac orifice of the stomach due to vomiting. Am J Med Sci, 178:506–515, 1929.
10. Moynihan NH: Pressure perforation and rupture of the esophagus. Lancet, 2:728–732, 1954.
11. Barrett NR: Spontaneous perforation of the oesophagus. Thorax, 1:48–70, 1946.
12. Malt RA, Head JH, Sweet RH: Knife wound of the neck with transection of the esophagus and contralateral hemopneumothorax. N Engl J Med, 268:1353, 1963.
13. Briggs JN, Germann TD: Traumatic perforations of the esophagus. Surg Clin North Am, 48:1297–1302, 1968.
14. Foster JH, Jolly PC, Sawyers JL, Daniel RA: Esophageal perforation: Diagnosis and treatment. Ann Surg, 161:701–709, 1965.
15. Postlethwait RW, Seuk KK, Dillon ML: Esophageal complications of vagotomy. Surg Gynecol Obstet, 128:481–488, 1969.
16. Muller WH Jr, Byron FY, Power HW: Delayed traumatic rupture of the esophagus. J Thorac Surg, 25:371, 1953.
17. Naclerio EA: The "V-sign" in the diagnosis of spontaneous rupture of the esophagus (an early roentgen clue). Am J Surg, 93:291–298, 1957.
18. Bates M: Pressure rupture of the mid-thoracic esophagus. Br J Surg, 56:327–331, 1969.
19. Keighley MR, Girdwood RW, Ionescu MI: Spontaneous rupture of the oesophagus. Br J Surg, 59:649–652, 1972.
20. Loop FD, Groves LK: Esophageal perforations. Ann Thorac Surg, 10:571–586, 1970.
21. Abbott OA: Atraumatic so-called "spontaneous" rupture of the esophagus. J Thorac Cardiovasc Surg, 1:67–83, 1970.
22. Mayer JE: The treatment of esophageal perforation with delayed recognition and continuing sepsis. Ann Thorac Surg, 23:568, 1977.
23. Barrett NR: Report of a case of spontaneous perforation of the esophagus successfully treated by operation. Br J Surg, 35:216–218, 1947.
24. Sawyers JL: Esophageal perforation. Ann Thorac Surg, 19:233–238, 1975.
25. Johnson J, Schwegman CW, MacVaugh H: Early esophagogastrostomy in the treatment of iatrogenic perforation of the distal esophagus. J Thorac Cardiovasc Surg, 55:24–29, 1968.
26. Thal AP, Hatafuku T: Improved operation for esophageal rupture. JAMA, 188:826–828, 1964.
27. Urschel HC, Razzuk MA, Wood RE, Galbraith N, Pockey M, Paulson DL: Improved management of esophageal perforation: Exclusion and diversion in continuity. Ann Surg, 179:587–591, 1974.
28. Grillo HC, Wilkins EW: Esophageal repair following late

diagnosis of intrathoracic perforation. Ann Thoracic Surg, 20:387–399, 1975.

29. Dooling JA, Zick HR: Closure of an esophagopleural fistula using only intercostal pedicle graft. Ann Thorac Surg, 3:553–557, 1967.

30. Hill LD, Billingham RP, Wreggit G: Boerhaave's syndrome. Bull Mason Clin, 32:41–46, 1978.

31. Celestin LR: Permanent intubation in inoperable cancer of the esophagus and cardia. Ann R Coll Surg, 25:165–170, 1959.

32. Hardly JT: Mallory-Weiss syndrome. Report of a case diagnosed by gastroscopy. Gastroenterology, 30:681–685, 1956.

33. Freeark RJ, Norcross WJ, Baker RJ, et al: The Mallory-Weiss syndrome. Arch Surg, 88:882, 1964.

34. Miller AC Jr, Hirschowitz BI: Twenty-three patients with Mallory-Weiss syndrome. South Med J, 63:441, 1970.

35. Wychulis AR, Sasso A: Mallory-Weiss syndrome. Arch Surg, 107:868, 1973.

36. Wells RF: A common cause of upper gastrointestinal bleeding. The Mallory-Weiss syndrome. South Med J, 60:1197–1201, 1967.

37. Weaver DH, Maxwell JG, Castleton KB: Mallory-Weiss syndrome. Am J Surg, 118:887, 1969.

18

Caustic and Medication-Induced Esophagitis

Richard Kozarek

Chemical injury to the esophagus has been estimated to occur in approximately 5000 children under the age of five years annually in this country.[1] Historically, lye has been the most frequently ingested agent, accounting for up to 60 per cent of reported cases.[2,3] Other agents include bleach, various acids, ammonia, potassium permanganate, and iodine. Classically, these substances have been divided into strong and weak alkali and acids and, in turn, subdivided into ingestion of the liquid or crystalline form (Fig. 18–1). More recently, a variety of sclerosing agents have been included as esophageal caustics.[4,5] Moreover, classic caustics are now being packed in unique ways, which can modify the type and extent of esophageal damage. This is particularly true in individuals who ingest alkaline disc batteries.[6–8]

■ Etiology

Alkali ■ Lye, in the form of toilet bowl or drain cleaner, remains the most common caustic agent ingested, accounting for the majority of esophageal burns in series from Finland, the Soviet Union, Denmark, and the United States.[2] Prior to 1967 in this country, lye (sodium hydroxide, NaOH; or potassium hydroxide, KOH) was available primarily in particle or granular form. This form of alkali, while toxic and associated with a chemical burn to exposed tissues, causes significant mucous membrane discomfort and, in turn, expectoration of swallowed particles.[9–11] Toxicity with the granular form is therefore usually localized to the oropharynx. In 1967 liquid forms of lye were introduced by the household cleaning agent industry. From 1967 to 1969, approximately 20 per cent of all caustic ingestions reported occurred with Liquid plumr, a colorless solution of 30.5 per cent NaOH that was associated with a very high rate of esophageal injury and subsequent perforation.[12] Other instances of caustic ingestion occurred with Drano (32 per cent NaOH), Plunge (25 per cent NaOH), Glamorene (25 per cent NaOH), and Down the Drain (36.5 per cent NaOH), as well as additional products.[2] Because of the markedly increased toxicity with these concentrated liquid lye solutions, many have since been reformulated. For instance, Liquid plumr is now 5 per cent KOH intermixed with smaller concentrations of NaOH and sodium hypochlorite.[12,13] Other forms of sodium or potassium hydroxide that have been associated with liquid caustic ingestion include oven cleaners (e.g., Easy-Off) and some liquid cleanser products.

In addition to the above, strong alkali ingestion can occur in two unique settings. The first occurs in the setting of the tablets used to test urine for sugar (Clinitest).[14,15] These tablets contain only small concentrations of NaOH, but may cause both esophageal ulceration and stricture formation related to the intense heat generated during their hydration. The second may occur during disc battery ingestion. These batteries, which may contain manganese dioxide, silver oxide, or mercuric oxide, all contain an alkaline electrolyte that is usually a

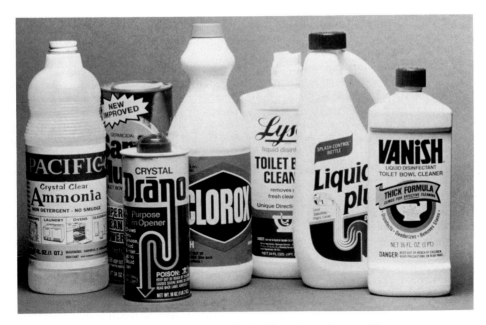

Figure 18-1. Common household items that have been associated with caustic esophagogastritis.

45 per cent solution of KOH.[8] If these batteries become lodged in the esophagus, the combination of local pressure necrosis plus caustic leak has been reported to cause acute esophageal damage including perforation, hemorrhage, and death.

Weak alkali in the form of ammonia has been the third most commonly reported ingested caustic in some series.[2,3,12] Its alkalinity is related to formation of ammonium hydroxide with hydration, but it does not have the deeply penetrating characteristic of either sodium or potassium hydroxide.

Acids ■ In most series, strong acids (pH <5) in the form of hydrochloric, muriatic, or sulfuric acid are the second most common cause of caustic ingestion.[3,5] Such acids are readily available to bring down the pH of swimming pools or Jacuzzi baths and are also commonly available in a number of household products. These include toilet bowl cleaners, such as Mister Plumber, Lysol, and Vanish, and Quaker House steam iron cleaner.[13]

Weak acids may be found in some household cleaners but are more readily available as sodium hypochlorite in bleach. These agents, usually formulated as a 5 to 6 per cent solution, have a pH of approximately 5 and require either a significantly higher amount or a longer contact time to act as significant caustics.[12]

Medications ■ A large number of medications have been reported to act as local caustics. These include various tetracyclines, potassium chloride in tablet form, ascorbic acid, chloral hydrate, and most nonsteroidal anti-inflammatory agents, as well as others.[4,5,16,19] Initially described in patients with enlarged hearts or other relative esophageal

obstructions, it has been shown that up to 60 per cent of barium sulfate tablets, identical in size and shape to aspirin tablets, remain in the esophagus for 5 min or longer.[20] The mechanism of esophageal damage is varied and includes local drug acidity (pH of a 1 per cent solution of doxycycline is 2.5) or venous thrombosis with hemorrhagic infarct (KCl).

Sclerosant ■ In the past several years, endoscopic sclerotherapy has had a resurgence of popularity for the short-term control of esophageal variceal hemorrhage and the subsequent obliteration of these varices. A number of techniques utilizing both para- and intravariceal injections have been described, utilizing a variety of sclerosing agents. Most commonly used in this country, however, are the long-chain fatty acid solutions of sodium morrhuate or sodium tetradecyl to which saline or alcohol has been added. Although neither of these agents has any intrinsic toxicity to the normal esophagus, local injection is associated with acute inflammation, submucosal fibrosis, and possible stricture formation.[21,22] These changes can be similar to the secondary pathology seen with true caustic ingestion and are described in detail in Chapter 24 on esophageal sclerotherapy.

■ *Mechanism of Action and Pathology*

The degree of esophageal and gastric damage following caustic ingestion will depend upon the material swallowed, the amount and form of the caustic agent, its concentration, and the duration of the exposure.

Alkali ■ Ingestion of strong alkali results in the saponification of fats and proteins and the thrombosis of blood vessels.[9,23] These thermal burns are related to the heat of hydration. Microscopically, edema, cell necrosis, and polymorphonuclear leukocyte infiltrations often extend through the submucosa and involve the inner fibers of the muscularis propria. Grossly, the depth of burn has been classified in a fashion similar to cutaneous burns:[24,25] first degree involves mucosal hyperemia, edema, and superficial sloughing; second degree is a transmural burn typified by exudate, mucosal loss, erosions, and deep ulcerations; third degree describes a transmural burn with erosion into the peritoneal or pleural cavities (Fig. 18–2). This is associated with acute clinical perforation or with subacute fistula formation. After the acute inflammatory period that lasts one to two weeks in duration, a latent or postinflammatory period occurs and lasts for two to six weeks.[12] Microscopically, this consists of granulation tissue with chronic inflammatory cells, capillaries, and fibroblast infiltration. The chronic phase is said to occur when sufficient collagen formation has been laid down to result in circumferential stenosis and stricture formation.

The location and degree of esophagogastric damage depend on both the concentration and formulation of ingested alkali. Krey used 3.85, 10.7, and 22.5 per cent NaOH solutions applied for 10 sec to an isolated esophagus.[26] He found that the weakest solution caused necrosis of the mucosa and submucosa, the 10.7 per cent solution caused necrosis which extended to the outer muscle layer, and the 22.5 per cent solution caused necrosis throughout the esophageal wall and into the periesophageal tissues. Ritter, in turn, comments that an 8 per cent solution of KOH for 30 sec results in extensive coagulation necrosis of all walls of the esophagus or stomach.[9]

Ingestion of granular alkali quickly causes punctate mucous membrane burning, limiting the amount of caustic ingested and often causing emesis.[3] Accordingly, burns are often limited to the mouth and pharynx, and the esophagus may be spared entirely or less severely burned than in situations involving liquid alkali[11] (Fig. 18–3). It is unusual to have a normal oropharynx yet have demonstrated esophageal damage following the ingestion of granular alkali. The exception to this is Clinitab ingestion. Liquid alkali, in turn, has a high specific gravity and passes rapidly into the stomach soon after ingestion. Canine studies demonstrate that instillation of 15 ml of concentrated lye into

anesthetized dogs is associated with a violent regurgitation of gastric contents back into the esophagus.[27,28] This regurgitation is followed by cricopharyngeus spasm and subsequent esophageal peristalsis rapidly propelling the alkali back into the stomach. A seesaw action of gastric contents develops and lasts 3 to 5 min. This helps to explain the extensive coagulative and often transmural necrosis that can develop in the esophagus and stomach. The latter has been noted in 10 to 15 per cent of strong alkali ingestions. In addition, mouth, hypopharyngeal, and upper airway damage can be substantial.

In contrast to the above, weak alkali usually causes minor esophageal damage, although significant epiglottis edema and airway obstruction have been reported.[2]

Acids ■ Caustic injury related to strong acids depends upon the amount and type swallowed and upon the postprandial state of the patient. Any acid is diluted and associated with lesser injury in a full stomach. Sulfuric acid, in turn, is the most readily available concentrated acid and has been reported to be both the most common and damaging agent.[29] Clinically, acids have an esophageal sparing effect related to rapid transit and the relative resistance of the squamous mucosa to the acid digestion. Six to 20 per cent of patients ingesting concentrated acid solutions have been reported to develop significant esophageal damage.[29] Tucker and Yarington, on the other hand, reviewed 26 authors reporting 366 ingestions between 1920 and 1971.[12] They found a 33 per cent incidence of stricture and an 18 per cent mortality rate related to such ingestions.

Pathologically, concentrated acids cause a coagulative necrosis covered by a protective eschar, similar to that seen with thermal burns.[12,29,30] The coagulation formation inhibits back diffusion of this acid and is associated with penetration into the deeper muscular coats. The deep penetration is then followed by perforation or sloughing large surface areas of mucosa and subsequent cicatrization. Most of the above-mentioned damage occurs in the stomach and is particularly prominent in the antrum. This is related to pylorospasm and the fact that food and saliva are protectively layered along the greater curvature of the stomach.

In contrast to the above, acids with a pH >5, particularly the hypochloric acid that is present in bleach, are considerably less toxic.[12] In general, a significant amount must be ingested, or prolonged contact time is necessary to produce toxicity. In a review of 837 such patients, only 76 esophageal burns (8.8 per cent) and 13 strictures were found.[12] This low incidence has been confirmed in a more recent review of 214 cases of caustic ingestion.[3]

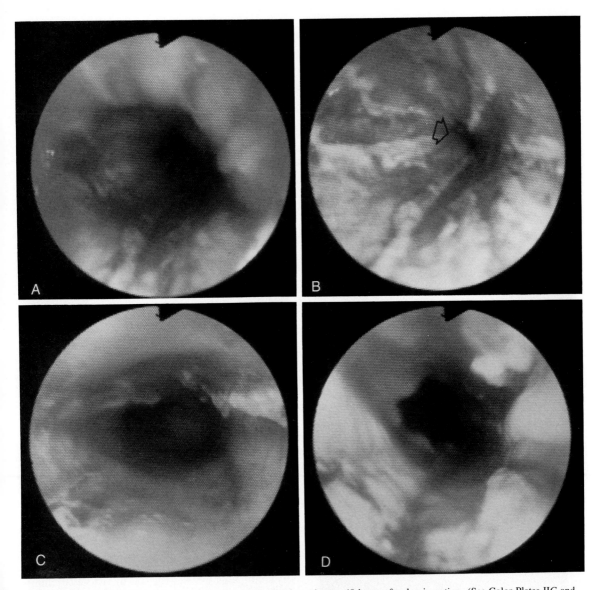

Figure 18–2. *A* and *B,* First degree caustic burns of the distal esophagus; 48 hours after lye ingestion. (See Color Plates II*C* and II*D*.) *C* and *D,* Exudate, esophageal ulcerations one week after liquid lye ingestion. (See Color Plates II*E* and II*F*.)

Medications ■ Patients who develop esophageal sequelae related to medication ingestion seldom develop the diffuse esophageal damage that may be seen after concentrated acid or alkali ingestion. Instead, local punctate ulcerations may be noted, often at sites of extrinsic cardiac enlargement and relative esophageal narrowing. These ulcers and the surrounding esophagus have various degrees of exudate and fibrosis, and there may also be venous thrombosis. Strictures of variable length have been reported in approximately 50 per cent of esophageal ulceration related to slow release KCl tablets[14] as well as with other medications (Fig. 18–4).

■ *Clinical Presentation and Course*

The majority of pediatric caustic ingestions are accidental, whereas most adults swallow caustics with suicidal intent. Presentation acutely depends upon both the ability to communicate as well as the type, form, and amount of ingested agent. Solid alkali usually causes moderate to severe burning of the lips and mouth with a variable degree of dysphagia or odynophagia.[11] Liquid alkali, in turn, may cause the oral symptoms as well as significant respiratory symptoms of wheezing, stridor, cy-

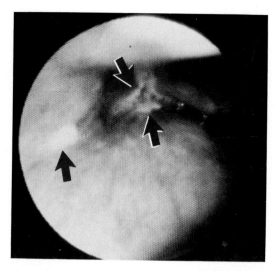

Figure 18–3. Exudate, local hypopharyngeal ulcers 12 hours after granular alkali ingestion. (See Color Plate IIIA.)

anosis, and shortness of breath.[28] The latter are associated with epiglottitis or laryngeal edema or may be related to direct aspiration of the caustic agent deep into the tracheobronchial tree. Salivation related to esophageal edema and severe chest pain are not uncommon. With transmural esophageal involvement, the patient may become acutely and rapidly ill as manifested by fever, tachycardia, and shock.[1] If the patient survives this initial toxic state, bacterial superinfection of the ulcers is common. Mediastinitis, tracheoesophageal fistula with empyema, overwhelming pneumonitis, and sepsis are common causes of death.[31]

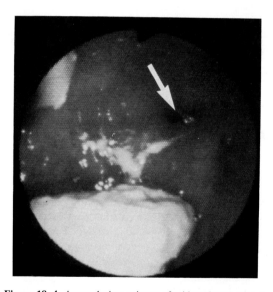

Figure 18–4. Arrow depicts stricture of midesophagus related to KCl tablets. Note partially dissolved pill in lower aspect of photo. (See Color Plate IIIB.)

In addition to the above, concentrated acid ingestion is not infrequently associated with severe and diffuse abdominal pain and retching.[29,30] This pain often localizes to the epigastrium or becomes frankly peritoneal in type. Emesis including hematemesis is not uncommon.

In contrast to the above, acute symptoms related to medication-induced esophageal ulceration are usually those of severe odynophagia.[5] Chest pain, drooling, and dysphagia are also not unusual. Disc battery ingestion, in turn, is usually unassociated with symptoms, and 33 of 56 cases reviewed passed the batteries per rectum without incident.[8] Five of these batteries impacted in the esophagus, and this was a uniform predictor of serious morbidity. Clinical presentation occurred four hours to five days after battery impaction, and symptoms included vomiting, tachypnea, and pneumothorax. Four of the children developed esophageal fistula and three of these died, two from exsanguination and one from a cardiac arrest.

■ *Sequelae*

Patients with first-degree esophageal burns following caustic ingestion usually go on to complete healing over a matter of weeks. Second- and third-degree burns enter a latent period in which collagen laydown is a prominent feature.[12] Such individuals may go on to form esophageal strictures[2,32,33] (Fig. 18–5). These strictures are often long and may totally occlude the esophagus. In a review of 2845 lye ingestions, 812 burns were documented.[12] Of those 812 cases, 126 (14 per cent) developed esophageal strictures. In addition to simple stricturing, third-degree burns involve adjacent organs by contiguous spread (Fig. 18–6). Those strictures include the aorta, trachea, mediastinum, peritoneum, liver, pancreas, and spleen.[34] Tracheoesophageal and aortoesophageal fistulas have been seen at necropsy, as has thrombosis of the hepatic vein. Of 2267 patients with significant caustic burn reviewed by Postlethwait,[2] there was a 13.6 per cent mortality rate. In a more recent study, Hawkins et al. reported a 3.7 per cent mortality rate in 214 patients.[3]

Strong acid ingestion, in turn, may be associated with esophageal stenosis but is more commonly noted to cause antral or pyloric stricturing. Of 25 patients reviewed in one series, 23 required surgical intervention.[30] Eight patients required an emergency operation for peritonitis and perforation, whereas 15 required resection or bypass of an obstructed distal stomach.

The second long-term complication following

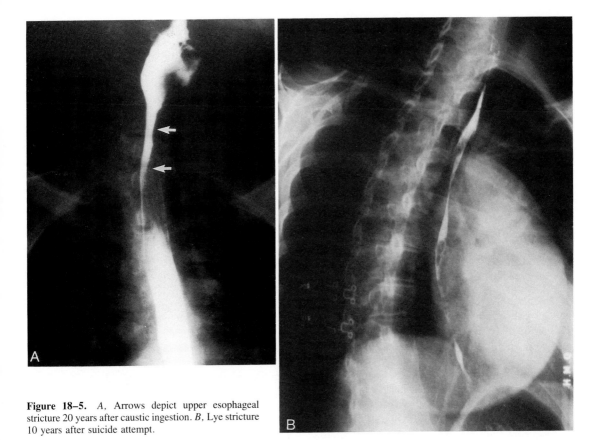

Figure 18–5. *A,* Arrows depict upper esophageal stricture 20 years after caustic ingestion. *B,* Lye stricture 10 years after suicide attempt.

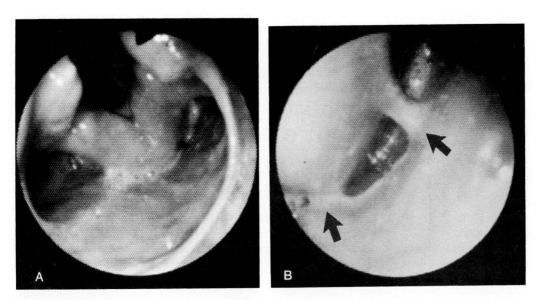

Figure 18–6. *A,* Bifid epiglottis following lye ingestion. (See Color Plate III*C*.) *B,* Adhesive bands (arrows) at esophageal inlet 20 years after liquid alkali ingestion. (See Color Plate III*D*.)

caustic ingestion is development of carcinoma. This incidence is reported to be 0.8 to 4 per cent with a latency period of approximately 40 years.[35,36] A 1000-fold increased risk of developing carcinoma has also been claimed at 24 years after caustic ingestion.[35] In addition, premalignant changes have been reported in the orohypopharynx following such ingestion.[37] Finally, a small number of cases of gastric carcinoma developing in areas of squamous metaplasia have been reported to occur after acid burns of the stomach.[29]

■ *Diagnosis*

Acutely, resuscitation during or prior to diagnostic testing can be of paramount importance. This includes assurance of an adequate airway, vital sign check, and delineation of the type and amount of ingested caustic. Oropharyngeal examination may reveal mucosal damage as necrotic edematous areas or whitish patches, which will later slough and ulcerate (see Fig. 18–3). These changes, however, may not correlate with the degree of esophageal or gastric damage.[11,12,25] In addition to the above, there may be hoarseness, stridor, wheezing, or rales, depending upon the degrees of aspiration or hypopharyngeal injury, and evidence of frank peritonitis or localized abdominal tenderness if the stomach wall has been injured.

Radiographic studies should include a chest x-ray in all patients and flat and upright abdominal films in all individuals with abdominal signs or symptoms. The former may reveal unsuspected pneumonitis, pleural effusion, or mediastinitis, while the latter may reveal free or intramural air. Esophageal contrast studies may reveal irregular or blurred margins caused by diffuse esophageal ulcerations. Alternatively, plaque-like collections and linear streaks may be secondary to deep necrotic ulcerations.[37–39] Intramural collections of air contrast material and gaseous dilatation of the esophagus are ominous radiographic signs.[37] Although similar changes can be seen following concentrated acid ingestion, more commonly antral or pyloric ulceration or stenosis with gastric outlet obstruction occurs.[40] Such stenosis may be seen acutely but more commonly there is a three- to eight-week asymptomatic latent period during which progressive ulceration and fibrosis obstruct the gastric lumen. An additional radiographic sign that is sometimes seen acutely is gastric bullae.[41] In contrast to the above, drug-induced esophagitis is usually typified as focal or multiple closely spaced esophageal ulcers, often present in the mid-

esophagus. Associated stricturing is not uncommon, particularly following oral KCl therapy.

A late sign of caustic ingestion is stricture formation from fibrous replacement and contracture (see Fig. 18–5).[42] This may be complicated not only by malignant degeneration in up to 5 per cent of cases, but by the development of significant superimposed reflux esophagitis.[2] Serial barium swallows have been recommended weekly and then as often as every three months when the depth of caustic injury cannot be accurately gauged.

Prior to the advent of flexible endoscopy, there was considerable debate about the advisability and timing of endoscopy to visualize the location and extent of tissue damage.[12,25,43] This was related to perforations of the necrotic esophagus with the rigid instrument and led to the recommendation that esophagoscopy should be used only to the level of the first detectable area of burn.[2,12] More recent studies suggest that small caliber endoscopes can be safely used in most cases through the entire area of burn and also to evaluate the stomach and proximal duodenum.[44–46]

Because of its safety and superior diagnostic capability, patients should undergo diagnostic flexible endoscopy within the first 24 hours unless obvious perforation necessitating surgical intervention is present. Even in the latter situation, I have undertaken endoscopy in the immediate preoperative setting to assist the surgeon in delineating the length of the intraluminal damage. Such early endoscopy will allow attenuated hospital stay in the patient found to have absent or negligible gastroesophageal damage and will prevent the repeated upper GI radiographs that some other authors recommend. Alternatively, if significant damage is defined, it will allow steps to be taken to minimize further damage and stricture formation.

Finally, some authors use endoscopic findings to initiate immediate operative intervention.[30,32] Endoscopic changes noted initially include linear hyperemic mucositis of the esophagus or stomach (see Fig. 18–2A and B). There may also be extensive exudate formation. Erythematous areas may go on to frank linear or deeply punctated ulcers (Fig. 18–7). Necrosis with black coagulum formation is often seen, particularly after concentrated acid ingestion. The latter has been claimed to represent full-thickness organ injury by some authors.[45] Others suggest that it is related to hematin formation by erythrocytes and therefore does not imply imminent perforation.[46]

In contrast to the above, single, punctate ulcers, often of the midesophagus are usually seen with pill esophagitis.[4,5] I have also seen extensive ulceration, exudate formation, and distal esophageal strictures secondary to both nonsteroidal anti-in-

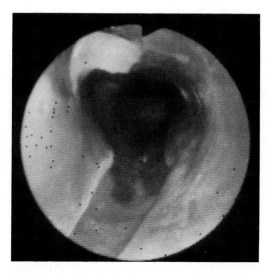

Figure 18–7. Avulsed, ulcerated distal esophagus following sulfuric acid suicide attempt several weeks prior. (See Color Plate III*E*.)

flammatory agents (NSAIAs) and quinidine (see Fig. 18–4).

Both strong acids and alkali can go on to smooth esophageal or gastric stenoses that may be associated with prolonged ulceration. In the stomach, large denuded areas with pseudopolyp formation and evolving cicatrization may be seen.[41,47]

■ *Treatment*

Because strong caustics fix quickly to tissues, efforts at neutralization acutely are unsuccessful. When seen in the hospital or emergency room setting, initial therapy should include instructing the patient to take nothing orally, administration of intravenous fluids, and assessment of the airway. A seriously burned patient may require tracheostomy with or without ventilatory support. If there is no obvious sign of perforation clinically or radiographically on chest and abdominal films, most authors suggest an initial nonoperative approach. This includes early endoscopic as opposed to radiographic evaluation to delineate laryngeal, esophageal, and gastric damage. Because bacterial superinfection is present almost universally in caustic ulcerations, most authors initiate treatment with broad-spectrum antibiotics such as ampicillin, cefazolin, or penicillin-aminoglycoside combination.[3,12]

Historical data suggest that antibiotics used alone have dramatically decreased the incidence of subsequent esophageal stenosis.[12] For this reason some practitioners use only antibiotics and sequential

bougienage in the treatment of caustic ingestion. Most authors, however, advocate the use of a tapered corticosteroid course (adults 60 mg, children 1 mg/kg/day) in addition.[48–51] Steroid use is based upon animal studies that demonstrate decreased stricture formation in dogs, rabbits, and cats as well as documented decrease in fibroplasia, collagen formation, and subsequent scar tissue.[3,10,52] Although there have been a number of small studies in humans, none have conclusively demonstrated corticosteroid efficacy in humans.[3,43] Given this, plus the fact that the doses usually employed increase the risk of perforation, many authors limit steroid use to grade 1 or 2 esophageal burns.[28] Steroid use in grade 3 or concentrated acid burns (almost invariably grade 3) has been claimed to be contraindicated.[3]

Drugs that have been postulated to be useful include the anticollagen drugs β-aminopropionitrile, colchicine, and penicillamine.[2,12,53,54] None have been studied in clinical trials in humans. Total parenteral nutrition, as a means of achieving a positive nitrogen balance and allowing the inflamed GI tract to rest without the trauma of ingested food, has also been espoused as a possible way to decrease subsequent stricture formation.[55]

In addition to antibiotics and steroids, sequential bougienage is the most widely accepted technique for preventing obstructive cicatrization.[12,48] Historically, this technique was accomplished after a small nasogastric tube or string had been passed into the stomach in an attempt to maintain patency of the esophageal lumen. Dilations, usually beginning in the second or third week were accomplished by Maloney dilators in the less severely burned patient and Eder-Peustow olives in the tightly stenotic patient. These dilations, when performed too early or aggressively, however, have been associated with a significant perforation rate in a necrotic esophagus. More recently, hollow polyvinyl, sequentially sized dilators have been marketed (Savary-Gillard, Wilson-Cook, Inc; American, American Endoscopy, Inc.) (Fig. 18–8).[56] Passed fluoroscopically over an endoscopically placed guidewire, they appear to be considerably safer than the previously used metal olives. The timing and need for continued dilation are individualized, although some authors suggest continued dilation for a 6- to 12-month period.[2] In the most severe strictures, gastrostomy and retrograde dilation with Tucker bougies has been undertaken.

Another technique to prevent esophageal stricturing used by some authors is the intraluminal stent.[48,57,58] Placed either surgically or endoscopically, this large-bore Silastic esophageal prosthesis is usually left in place for three weeks or longer. All authors using this technique have also placed

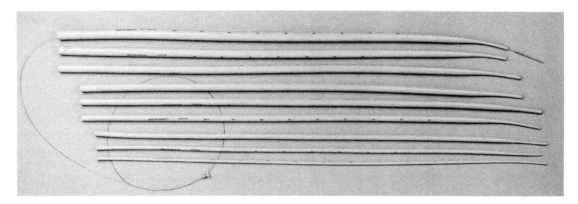

Figure 18–8. Graded, hollow core polyvinyl dilators (American).

their patients on antibiotics and steroids. Because of this and the small number of patients treated, its efficacy remains uncertain. Moreover, given the migration and pressure necrosis potential of esophageal prostheses in general, their use should currently be limited.

Patients with pill-induced esophagitis, on the other hand, require withdrawal of the offending agent and instruction to take all medications with a full glass of water and in the upright position.[4,5] Acutely, narcotics or viscous lidocaine (Xylocaine) analgesia may be required and antacids have often been employed. Chronically, esophageal bougienage may be necessary if stricturing has occurred. Patients with disc battery ingestion also deserve special mention. Impaction in the esophagus requires immediate endoscopic or surgical removal as discussed earlier in this chapter. In a collected series of these patients, only 2 per cent developed a complication (perforated Meckel's diverticulum) when the battery had passed beyond the esophagus.[8] Because of this, surgical removal from the stomach or small bowel does not seem warranted. Instead, radiographs to assure battery passage or careful observation at home appear reasonable. Cathartics and metochlopramide have also been recommended to hasten transit and H_2 blockade to prevent battery corrosion related to gastric acid. Although reasonable theoretically, their value remains to be proved.[8]

In contrast to the medical approach to caustic ingestion outlined above, some clinicians are considerably more aggressive. This includes passing a nasogastric tube into the stomach following liquid alkali ingestion to determine pH. If stomach contents are alkaline, the esophagus and stomach are presumed severely damaged and emergency laparotomy is recommended.[11,28,30] Acute resection then depends upon the extent of demonstrated transmural damage.[59] Because the vast majority of patients ingesting strong acid will require emer-

gency (one third) or semielective resection or bypass operation (two thirds), some authors suggest immediate laparotomy if endoscopy demonstrates gastric damage following concentrated acid ingestion.[30] They reason that earlier operation may prevent sepsis and decrease subsequent complications and fatalities.

For the most part, surgical intervention has been reserved for the acute complications of caustic ingestion: perforation, abscess, fistula formation, and obstruction[2,25,60] (Fig. 18–9). Such surgery includes the aggressive resection of necrotic and questionably viable tissue, appropriate diversion or bypass, and adequate drainage. Of equal importance is the need for surgery in the subacute or chronic setting of esophageal stenosis.[61] Daly and Cardona propose the following indications for esophageal resection following caustic ingestion: (1) complete esophageal stenosis with inability to establish a lumen, (2) chronic fistula formation, (3) dilations that cause a severe periesophageal reaction or mediastinitis, (4) marked irregularity or pocketing of the esophagus, (5) inability to maintain an adequate esophageal lumen, and (6) patients unable or unwilling to undergo repeated esophageal bougienage.[23] A review of postcaustic esophageal resections and reconstructions has been reported by Postlethwait.[2] Best results have been obtained with colon interposition (325 patients, 4.9 per cent mortality rate, 92 per cent good results). Jejunal substitution (104 patients, 8.6 per cent mortality rate, 88 per cent good results) and esophagogastrostomy (161 patients, 14.3 per cent mortality rate, 87 per cent good results) have also been successful. As noted above, surgery is more common following concentrated acid ingestion and was required in 23 of 25 patients reviewed.[30] Eight of the 23 required an emergency procedure for gastric leak, the remaining 15 for pyloric obstruction or suspected cancer. The overall mortality rate in this series was 28 per cent.

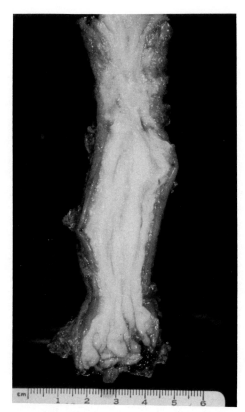

Figure 18–9. De-epithelialized, strictured esophagus resected for undilatable lye stenosis. Radiograph depicts lye stenosis preop. (See Color Plate III*F*.)

■ REFERENCES

1. Leape LL, Ashcraft KW, Scarpelli DG, et al: Hazard to health—liquid lye. N Engl J Med, 287:578–581, 1971.
2. Postlethwait RW: Chemical burns of the esophagus. Surg Clin North Am, 63:915–924, 1983.
3. Hawkins DB, Demeter MJ, Barnett TE: Caustic ingestion: Controversies in management: A review of 214 cases. Laryngoscope, 90:98–109, 1980.
4. Kikendall JW, Friedman AC, Oyewole MA, et al: Pill-induced esophageal injury: Case reports and review of the medical literature. Dig Dis Sci, 28:174–182, 1983.
5. Kikendall JW, Johnson LF: Esophageal injury: Caustics and pills. *In* Castell DO, Johnson LF (Eds): Esophageal Function in Health and Disease. New York, Elsevier, 1983, pp 255–272.
6. Maves MD, Carithers JS, Birck HC: Esophageal burns secondary to disc battery ingestion. Ann Otol Rhinol Laryngol, 93:364–369, 1984.
7. Votteler TP, Nash JC, Rutledge JC: The hazard of ingested alkaline disc batteries in children. JAMA, 249:2504–2506, 1983.
8. Litovitz TL: Button battery ingestions: A review of 56 cases. JAMA, 249:2495–2500, 1983.
9. Ritter FN: Lye burns of the esophagus and their treatments. Adv Oto Rhino Laryngol, 23:104–108, 1978.
10. Oakes DD, Sherck JP, Mark JBD: Lye ingestion: Clinical patterns and therapeutic implications. J Thorac Cardiovasc Surg, 83:194–204, 1982.
11. Kirsh MM, Peterson A, Brown JW, et al: Treatment of caustic injuries of the esophagus: A ten year experience. Ann Surg, 188:675–678, 1978.
12. Tucker JA, Yarington CT Jr: The treatment of caustic ingestion. Otol Clin North Am, 12:343–350, 1979.
13. Lowe JE, Graham DY, Boisaubin EV Jr, Lanza FL: Corrosive injury to the stomach: The natural history and role of fiberoptic endoscopy. Am J Surg, 137:803–806, 1979.
14. Tomsovic EJ, Major MC, Javid H: Cicatricial stenosis of the esophagus following ingestion of single urine sugar reagent tablet. J Pediatr, 53:608–614, 1958.
15. Burrington JD: Clinitest burns of the esophagus. Ann Thorac Surg, 20:400–404, 1975.
16. Bokey L, Hugh TB: Oesophageal ulceration associated with doxycycline therapy. Med J Aust, 1:236–237, 1975.
17. Khera DC, Herschnan BR, Sosa F: Tetracycline-induced esophageal ulcers. Postgrad Med, 68:113–115, 1980.
18. Walta DD, Giddens JD, Johnson LF, et al: Localized proximal esophagitis secondary to ascorbic acid ingestion and esophageal motor disorder. Gastroenterology, 70:766–769, 1976.
19. Lambert JR, Newman A: Ulceration and stricture of the esophagus due to the oral potassium chloride (slow release tablet) therapy. Am J Gastroenterol, 73:508–511, 1980.
20. Evans KT, Roberts GM: Where do all the tablets go? Lancet, 2:1237–1239, 1976.
21. Ayres SJ, Goff JS, Warren GH, Schaefer JW: Esophageal ulceration and bleeding after flexible fiberoptic esophageal vein sclerosis. Gastroenterology, 83:131–136, 1982.
22. Ayres SJ, Goff JS, Warren GH: Endoscopic sclerotherapy for bleeding esophageal varices: Effects and complications. Ann Intern Med, 98:900–903, 1983.
23. Jelenko C III: Chemicals that "burn." J Trauma, 14:65–72, 1974.
24. Hollinger PH: Management of esophageal lesions caused by chemical burn. Ann Otol, 77:819–829, 1968.
25. Cardona JC, Daly JF: Current management of corrosive esophagitis: An evaluation of 239 cases. Ann Otol, 80:521–527, 1971.
26. Krey H: On the treatment of corrosive lesions in the esophagus. Acta Otolaryngol, Suppl, 102:1–49, 1952.
27. Ritter FN, Newman MH, Newman DE: A clinical and experimental study of corrosive burns of the stomach. Ann Otol, 77:830–842, 1968.
28. Ritter FN, Gago O, Kirsh MM, et al: The rationale of emergency esophagogastrectomy in the treatment of liquid caustic burns of the esophagus and stomach. Ann Otol, 80:513–520, 1971.
29. Maull KI: Surgical implications of acid ingestion. Surg Gynecol Obstet, 148:895–898, 1979.
30. Chodak GW, Passaro E Jr: Acid ingestion. Need for gastric resection. JAMA, 239:225–226, 1978.
31. Burington JD: Surgical management of the tracheoesophageal fistula complicating caustic ingestion. Surgery, 84:329–334, 1978.
32. Imre J, Kopp M: Arguments against long-term conservative treatment of esophageal strictures due to corrosive burns. Thorax, 27:594–598, 1972.
33. Stothers HH: Chemical burns and strictures of the esophagus. Arch Otolaryngol, 56:262–276, 1952.
34. Ray JF, Meyers W, Lawton BR, et al: The natural history of liquid lye ingestion. Arch Surg, 109:436–439, 1974.
35. Appleqvist P, Salmo M: Lye corrosion carcinoma of the esophagus: A review of 63 cases. Cancer, 45:2655–2658, 1980.
36. Benirschke K: Time bomb of lye ingestion? Am J Dis Child, 135:17–18, 1981.
37. Kozarek RA, Sanowski RA: Caustic cicatrization of the pharynx associated with dysphagia and premalignant mucosal changes. Am J Gastroenterol, 77:5–8, 1982.

38. Martel WM: Radiologic features of esophagogastritis secondary to extremely caustic agents. Radiology, *103*:31–36, 1972.

39. Laufer I: Radiology of esophagitis. Radiol Clin North Am, *20*:687–699, 1982.

40. Love L, Berkow AE: Trauma to the esophagus. Gastrointest Radiol, *2*:305–321, 1978.

41. Johns TT, Thoeni RF: Severe corrosive gastritis related to Drano: An unusual case. GI Radiol, *8*:25–28, 1983.

42. Edmonson MB: Caustic alkali ingestions by farm children. Pediatrics, *79*:413–416, 1987.

43. Laufer I: Double contrast radiology with endoscopic correlation. Philadelphia, W.B. Saunders Co., 1979.

44. Borga AR, Randell HT Jr, Thomas TV, et al: Lye injuries of the esophagus: Analyses of ninety cases of lye ingestion. J Thorac Cardiovasc Surg, *57*:533–538, 1969.

45. Welsh JJ, Welsh LW: Endoscopic examination of corrosive injuries of the upper gastrointestinal tract. Laryngoscope, *88*:1300–1309, 1978.

46. Chung RSK, Den Besten L: Fiberoptic endoscopy in treatment of corrosive injury of the stomach. Arch Surg, *110*:725–728, 1975.

47. Levitt R, Stanley RJ, Wise L: Gastric bullae: An early roentgen finding in corrosive gastritis following alkali ingestion. Radiology, *115*:597–598, 1975.

48. Goldmann LP, Weigert JM: Corrosive substance ingestion: A review. Am J Gastroenterol, *79*:85–90, 1984.

49. Buttross S, Brouhard BH: Acute management of alkali ingestion in children: A review. Tex Med, *77*:57–60, 1981.

50. Knopp R: Caustic ingestions. *In* Tintinalli JE, Rothstein RJ, Krome RL, eds: Emergency Medicine: A Comprehensive Guide. Dallas, American College of Emergency Physicians, 1985, pp 305–308.

51. Howell JM: Alkaline ingestion. Ann Emerg Med, *15*:820–825, 1986.

52. Webb WR, Koutra S, Ecker RR, et al: An evaluation of steroids and antibiotics in caustic burns of the esophagus. Ann Thorac Surg, *9*:95–102, 1970.

53. Butler C, Madden JW, Davis WM, et al: Morphologic aspects of experimental esophageal stricture, II: Effect of steroid hormones, bougienage, and lathyrisms on acute lye burns. Surgery, *81*:431, 1977.

54. Gehanno P, Guidon C: Prohibition of experimental esophageal lye strictures by penicillamine. Arch Otolaryngol, *107*:145–147, 1981.

55. DiCostanzo J, Nouclere M, Jouglard J, et al: New therapeutic approach to corrosive burns of the upper gastrointestinal tract. Gut, *21*:370–375, 1980.

56. Kozarek RA: Esophageal dilation and prostheses. Endoscopy Rev, *4*:8–20, 1987.

57. Hill JL, Norberg HP, Smith MD, et al: Clinical technique and success of the esophageal stent to prevent corrosive strictures. J Pediatr Surg, *11*:443–449, 1976.

58. Mills LJ, Estrera AS, Platt MR: Avoidance of esophageal stricture following severe caustic burns by the use of an intraluminal stent. Ann Thorac Surg, *28*:60–65, 1979.

59. Ray JF III, Meyers WO, Lawton BR, et al: The natural history of liquid lye ingestion. Rationale for aggressive surgical approach. *109*:436–439, 1979.

60. Moazam F, Talbert JL, Miller D, Mollitt DL: Caustic ingestion and its sequelae in children. South Med J, *80*:187–190, 1987.

61. Stewart JR, Sarr MG, Sharp KW, et al: Transhiatal (blunt) esophagectomy for malignant and benign esophageal disease: Clinical experience and technique. Ann Thorac Surg, *40*:343–348, 1985.

19

Benign Tumors and Cysts of the Esophagus

C. Dale Mercer ▪ *Lucius D. Hill*

Benign tumors and cysts of the esophagus are uncommon problems which are most gratifying for the esophageal surgeon. The operation results in an ultimate cure in a high percentage of cases, with a very low operative mortality rate and a minimal morbidity rate, because most of the tumors and cysts can be removed without opening the mucosa of the esophagus. These lesions occur much less frequently than malignant tumors and are usually single but occasionally may be multiple. Harrington and Moersch[1] found 44 benign esophageal tumors in 7459 postmortem examinations, as compared to 876 cases of esophageal cancer. The highest autopsy incidence reported in the literature is 0.25 per cent by Plachta.[2] The relative incidence of benign versus malignant lesions in the eosphagus is variously reported as 1 to 15 by Johnston et al.[3] and 1 to 150 by Watson et al.[4] Many excellent reviews of these conditions are present in the literature.[2,5–7]

A number of classifications exist. Nemir's classification divides the lesions into epithelial, non-epithelial, and heterotopic tissue,[8] but for simplicity, a division into intramural, extramural, and intraluminal tumors is the best. By far the most frequent of the benign tumors is the intramural leiomyoma. Other less frequent intramural tumors include myomas, fibromas, lipomas, neurofibromas, osteochondromas, and granular cell myoblastomas. Cysts of the esophagus may occur either intramurally or extramurally. Intraluminal tumors include fibrovascular polyps, papillomas, adenomas, and the very rare hemangioma.

▪ *Symptoms and Diagnosis*

The symptomatology for these benign tumors depends on their location within the esophagus and the relationship to the wall of the esophagus. Intraluminal tumors are generally polypoid and freely mobile and therefore cause dysphagia only after they reach a considerable size. A most dramatic type of presentation for these polypoid tumors is regurgitation and rarely asphyxiation and death.[9] Infrequently, they may erode and ulcerate with consequent hemorrhage.

Intramural tumors are usually asymptomatic until they reach a larger size at which time dysphagia is the most prominent symptom. It is extremely uncommon for these tumors to bleed because the mucosa overlying the tumor is intact. This is in contrast to leiomyomas elsewhere in the gastrointestinal tract, particularly in the stomach, which develop umbilication and ulceration.

Extramural tumors cause symptoms of dysphagia but also compress neighboring organs, for instance, the respiratory tract, which may then result in confusing symptoms. Boyd and Hill[5] reported on a patient complaining of pain in the right side of the lower chest, chills, fever, and six months of hemoptysis; this patient had a large leiomyoma weighing 148 g, causing severe atelectasis of the right lower and middle lobes of the lung, necessitating lobectomy in addition to excision of the mass.

The diagnosis of benign esophageal tumors must differentiate these from the more common malignant tumors but also must distinguish between intrinsic esophageal tumors and extrinsic lesions causing distortion of the esophagus. The history and physical examination are generally unremarkable and unhelpful in the diagnosis.

Most of the lesions initially are discovered on routine chest x-ray examination, which commonly identifies the lesion in the mediastinum but does not separate extrinsic from intrinsic esophageal lesions. A barium swallow with cineradiography helps to separate these lesions. The site of the tumor can be identified, and at times these tumors can be differentiated from malignant lesions. As well, they can be radiologically differentiated into mucosal, extramucosal, and extrinsic lesions by certain distinguishing characteristics.[10] Radiologic signs of benignity include mobility of the mass and visualization of a soft tissue mass that fits into the filling defect in the esophagus. The mucosal lesions are irregular, polypoid, and may ulcerate. Although a malignant lesion may produce a soft tissue mass outside the esophagus, its mucosal outline is usually irregular. The intramural tumors produce a sharply defined outline, forming an abrupt angle with the outline of the uninvolved esophagus (Fig. 19–1). The overlying mucosa appears smooth. Extrinsic lesions impinging on the esophagus, on the other hand, produce a gently sloping outline without an abrupt angle with the adjacent uninvolved esophagus. Extrinsic tumors which have become attached to the esophagus over a wide area of their circumference may produce an outline similar to that of an intramural tumor.

Radiologic examination of intraluminal polyps shows that the tumor may be oval or an elongated sausage-like mass, and it may be smooth or lobulated. The attachment of the stalk can be identified easily, and the lesion may be so large that it obstructs the esophagus and may cause proximal dilatation. In these instances the radiologic appearance may be confused with achalasia of the esophagus.

Esophagoscopy is useful in determining the presence or absence of polyps in the esophagus and in identifying the rare hemangioma. When an intramural tumor is suspected, the endoscopy may be helpful to rule out the coexistence of a carcinoma. The findings at the time of examination include a freely movable mass bulging into the lumen but covered by intact normal-appearing mucosa. The endoscope can usually be passed easily beyond the level of the tumor. A biopsy should not be performed because the lesion is within the muscularis and biopsy of the mucosa will not only fail to provide a diagnosis but will hinder the future surgical treatment by violating the mucosa, thereby making the extramucosal excision of the tumor impossible. At times these lesions may be missed entirely at endoscopy because of the mobility of the tumor. If a polypoid lesion is identified, this may be biopsied and, in fact, completely removed with the snare passed through the endoscope.

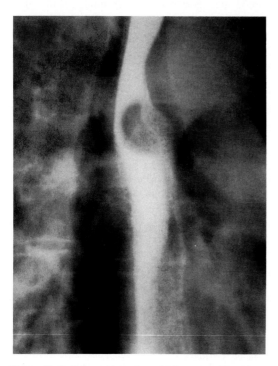

Figure 19–1. Intramural esophageal leiomyoma. Note abrupt angle with the outline of the esophagus. The mucosa is intact.

■ Treatment

All cases of intramural or extramural tumors require operative excision with enucleation of the tumor without incising the esophageal mucosa. The site of the tumor will dictate the type of incison necessary. Lesions in the cervical esophagus can be approached through an incision along the anterior border of the sternomastoid muscle. Lesions in the thoracic esophagus should be approached through a right thoracotomy, which allows adequate visualization of the entire thoracic esophagus. Following exposure of the esophagus, the longitudinal muscles overlying the tumor, which are usually splayed out, are incised down to the level of the lesion. A plane of dissection is then created between the tumor and the esophageal muscularis. With care, most of these tumors can be completely enucleated without opening the mucosa. However, if a previous endoscopic biopsy was obtained or if the lesion has become malignant, this plane of dissection may be difficult to identify. If the mucosa is injured during the dissection, it can be closed with absorbable sutures. Following complete excision, the muscularis of the esophagus is reapproximated with silk sutures.

Frozen section diagnosis should be obtained to rule out any evidence of malignancy. Rarely with leiomyomas that are annular and constricting, the area may need to be excised with an end-to-end anastomosis. The thoracotomy incision is closed with chest tube drainage, and a nasogastric tube is left in place for 24 hours postoperatively.

If the lesion is intraluminal and is a pedunculated polyp, esophagoscopy with snare removal may be all that is required. However, if the lesion is quite large, surgical excision may be necessary. In these cases, identification of the stalk and the site of origin of the polyp is necessary. The esophagus is opened on the wall opposite to the site of origin of the polyp. The polyp is then removed at the base of the stalk, and the integrity of the esophageal wall is reconstituted with sutures following which the esophagotomy incision is closed in two layers.

■ Leiomyoma

The leiomyoma is the most common type of benign tumor of the esophagus[11] but represents less than 10 per cent of the alimentary tract leiomyomas.[12] A recent review by Seremetis et al.,[13] reviewing all foreign literature, found 593 patients requiring surgical treatment for esophageal leiomyoma. Ninety per cent of these lesions are located in the lower two thirds of the esophagus, probably because this area of esophagus is smooth muscle. However, there are reports[5] of a number of leiomyomas occurring in the upper part of the esophagus. Most commonly these lesions are single, but occasionally they may be multiple.[14] Some tumors are quite small and asymptomatic, whereas others can be extremely large, weighing more than 1000 g.[15] Calcification may develop in the leiomyoma.[16] Occasionally cystic changes and malignant transformation may be identified.[17] The typical microscopic appearance is the same as in leiomyomas located elsewhere in the body, with interlacing bundles of spindle-shaped cells containing intracellular myofibrils and nuclei which are narrow, long, and round at the ends.[18] The capsule is usually not well developed; however, interdigitation into the surrounding esophageal tissues is uncommon.

These patients usually present with dysphagia and the typical radiologic findings noted above. Occasionally an x-ray done for other reasons will demonstrate an asymptomatic leiomyoma (see Fig. 19–1). The treatment consists of enucleation of the

mass, in spite of its extremely slow growth.[19] Resection is usually complete with only one documented recurrence.[20] In the 838 cases analyzed by Seremetis, there were no surgical deaths following enucleation of the tumor. However, if resection is necessary, an operative mortality rate of approximately 10.5 per cent is seen.[7] Postoperative complications are extremely rare if enucleation is performed without breaking the esophageal mucosal integrity.

■ Cysts

The complex nomenclature associated with cysts of the esophagus results from the difficulty in determining their origin. These cysts occurring in the thorax lined with gastrointestinal or respiratory epithelium have been described as intrathoracic cysts of foregut origin, periesophageal cysts, diverticula of the esophagus, duplications of the alimentary tract, conglomerate gastroenteric cysts, gastrogenic cysts, accessory esophagus, accessory stomach, enterocystomas, and esophagenic cysts.[5] Some cysts do not have an attachment to the esophagus and have been called mediastinal cysts.

Several theories of causation have been suggested, including the postulate by Lewis and Thyng[21] that they represent pinching off of small diverticula of the gut early in fetal life in which these epithelial nodules become misplaced and subsequently undergo cystic change. A second theory is that of Olenik,[22] more recently supported by Smith,[23] which postulates that all mediastinal enteric cysts are derived from the foregut near the origin of the lung bud. The cells in this area are predestined to become one of the variety of constituents of the different sections of the gastrointestinal and respiratory tracts. They rapidly develop and multiply in close proximity to each other. A few cells may be misplaced from either the tracheal or esophageal anlage into the mesodermal tissue ultimately destined to become the muscular layers of the esophagus.

With esophageal cysts, the separation of cells probably occurs at a later stage, thereby resulting in minimal migration such that the cyst develops close to its source of origin, often within the wall of the esophagus itself. A third hypothesis supported by a number of authors is that there is a failure of coalescence of vacuoles formed in the solid foregut with the lumen of the esophagus bringing about a persistence of the vacuole, ultimately giving rise to an esophagenic cyst. Boyd and Hill[5] point out that the lining of these cysts is variable because the embryologic development of

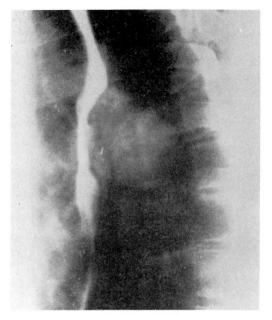

Figure 19–2. Intramural esophagenic cyst excised with recovery.

the mucosa of the esophagus passes through phases of columnar, pseudostratified, ciliated columnar, and ultimately squamous epithelium. Therefore, ciliated epithelial lining in a cyst does not necessarily mean that it is of respiratory origin. Lindquist and Wulff[24] state that the type of mucous membrane lining a cyst need not correspond to the part of the alimentary tract where the cyst originated from or is situated. In Figure 19–2 a large intramural cyst with intact esophageal mucosa is shown. This cyst was excised with recovery. The ciliated columnar lining of the cyst is shown in Figure 19–3.

Symptoms are usually similar to those of other benign esophageal tumors. However, in children, respiratory symptoms may predominate with hemoptysis occurring as an ulceration in the trachea or bronchus owing to the gastric mucosal lining of the cyst.[25] The diagnosis is made, much as with patients with leiomyomas, with plain chest x-ray examination, barium swallow, and esophagoscopy. Surgical excision is the treatment of choice and the intramural cyst can usually be removed from the esophageal wall without opening the mucosa in a similar manner to that of excision of leiomyomas.

■ Polyps of the Esophagus

Polyps of the esophagus are of special interest because they were among the first lesions of the esophagus to be treated surgically. The first treatment was by DuBois in 1818,[26] at which time he ligated the pedicle of an esophageal polyp following which the tumor was regurgitated with asphyxiation of the patient. The first successful therapy was by Annandale in 1878 when a patient regurgitated a polyp and the pedicle was cut with recovery.[26]

Fibrovascular polyps can grow to enormous size and occasionally present catastrophically by prolapsing into the hypopharynx, causing asphyxiation and death. These polyps are composed of varying amounts of fibrous, vascular, and adipose tissue but are covered by normal mucosa. Most of these polyps arise in the cervical esophagus and clinically cause dysphagia and regurgitation which, because of the slow growing polyp, occur late. X-ray shows the lesions as interluminal, oval tumors with a stalk

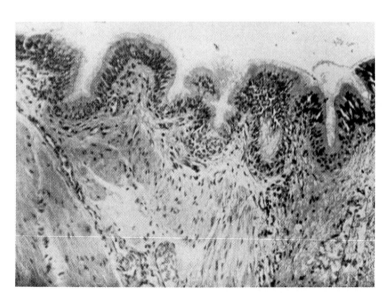

Figure 19–3. Intramural esophagenic cyst lined with ciliated columnar epithelium.

identified by an indentation in the esophageal wall (Fig. 19–4).

Figure 19–4 shows a large polyp of the upper esophagus which was successfully removed with a snare endoscopically. Esophagoscopy is important to rule out malignancy and may be therapeutic if the base of the polyp can be snared with the electrocautery snare. If they cannot be removed in this fashion, an esophagomyotomy on the opposite wall to the base of the polyp is performed, following which the base of the polyp is ligated and transected and the esophagotomy closed. Another pedunculated polyp which has been removed endoscopically is the squamous papilloma, which consists of a papillary structure lined with normal squamous epithelium. These polyps do not increase to the enormous size seen in other benign tumors. They may be multiple.[27]

■ Hemangioma

Hemangioma of the esophagus is extremely rare. Gentry et al.,[28] in a comprehensive review of vascular lesions in the gastrointestinal tract, found 16 benign vascular tumors of the esophagus, one of which may have been esophageal varices. Four of these tumors were recognized clinically, three were treated, and one patient died of hemorrhage without treatment. All three patients treated were dead

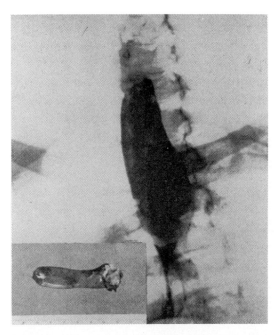

Figure 19–4. Esophageal polyp excised with a snare endoscopically.

within one year of onset in spite of the treatment. Boyd and Hill report a 44-year-old lady followed for 14 years with a large hemangioma of the upper two thirds of the esophagus. No treatment was carried out, and she remained well and free of esophageal bleeding. It is apparent that hemangiomas are exceedingly dangerous lesions and if they are localized they should be treated aggressively.

■ REFERENCES

1. Harrington SW, Moersch HJ: Surgical treatment and clinical manifestations of benign tumors of the esophagus with report of seven cases. J Thorac Surg, *13*:394–414, 1944.
2. Plachta A: Benign tumors of the esophagus. Review of literature and report of 99 cases. Am J Gastroenterol, *38*:639–652, 1962.
3. Johnston JB, Clagett OT, McDonald JR: Smooth muscle tumors of the esophagus. Thorax, *8*:251–265, 1953.
4. Watson RR, O'Connor TM, Weisel W: Solid benign tumors of the esophagus. Ann Thorac Surg, *4*:80–91, 1967.
5. Boyd DP, Hill D: Benign tumors and cysts of the esophagus. Am J Surg, *93*:252–258, 1957.
6. Totten RS, Stout AP, Humphreys GH, Moore RL: Benign tumors and cysts of the esophagus. J Thorac Surg, *25*:606–622, 1953.
7. Postlethwait RW: Benign tumors and cysts of the esophagus. Surg Clin North Am, *63*:925–931, 1983.
8. Nemir P, Wallace HW, Fallahnejad M: Diagnosis and surgical management of benign diseases of the esophagus. Curr Probl Surg, *13*:1, 1976.
9. Allen MS, Talbot WH: Sudden death due to regurgitation of a pedunculated lipoma. J Thorac Cardiovasc Surg, *54*:756, 1967.
10. Schatzki R, Hawes LE: Roentgenological appearance of extramucosal tumors of the esophagus: Analysis of intramural extramucosal lesions of gastrointestinal tract in general. Am J Roentgenol, *48*:1, 1942.
11. Vantrappen G, Pringot J: Benign tumors and cysts of the esophagus. *In* Vantrappen G, Hellemans S (Eds): Diseases of the Esophagus. Berlin, Springer-Verlag, 1974, p 431.
12. Dillow BM, Neis DD, Sellers RD: Leiomyoma of the esophagus. Am J Surg, *120*:615, 1970.
13. Seremetis MG, Lyons WS, deGuzman VC, Peabody JW Jr: Leiomyomata of the esophagus. An analysis of 838 cases. Cancer, *38*:2166–2177, 1976.
14. Godard JE, McCoanie D: Multiple leiomyomas of the esophagus. Am J Roentgenol, *117*:259, 1973.
15. Tsuzuki T, Kakegawa T, Arimori M, Ueda M, Watanabe H, Okamato T, Akakura I: Giant leiomyoma of the esophagus and cardia weighing more than 1000 grams. Dis Chest, *60*:396–399, 1971.
16. Gutman E: Posterior mediastinal calcification due to esophageal leiomyoma. Gastroenterology, *63*:665, 1972.
17. Biasini A: A case of epibronchial fibroleiomyoma of the esophagus with malignant transformation. Pathologica *41*:260, 1949; cited by Lewis and Maxfield, Int Abstr Surg, *99*:105, 1954.
18. Bogedain W, Carpathios J, Najib A: Leiomyoma of the esophagus. Dis Chest, *44*:391–399, 1963.
19. Von Preyss B, Maesen F: Leiomyoma of the oesophagus: Follow-up of 14 years before operation. Br Med J, *285*:1166, 1982.
20. Stranderfer RJ, Paneth M: Recurrent leiomyoma of the oesophagus. Thorax, *37*:478–479, 1982.
21. Lewis FT, Thyng FW: Regular occurrence of intestinal

diverticula in embryos of pig, rabbit, and man. Am J Anat, 7:505, 1907.

22. Olenik JL, Tandotnick JW: Congenital mediastinal cysts of foregut origin. Am J Dis Child, 71:466–476, 1946.

23. Smith EI: The early development of the trachea and esophagus in relation to atresias of the esophagus and tracheoesophageal fistula. Contrib Embryol Carnegie Inst Wash, 36:43, 1975.

24. Lindquist N, Wulff HB: Mediastinal enterocystoma: Report of case in 7 month child with impending suffocation, operation, and recovery. J Thorac Surg, 16:468–476, 1947.

25. Waterston D: Oesophageal diseases in infancy and childhood, excluding esophagotracheal fistula. In Smith PA, Smith RE (Eds): Surgery of the Oesophagus. The Coventry Conference. New York, Appleton Century Crofts, 1972.

26. Postlethwait RW: Surgery of the Esophagus. 2nd ed. New York, Appleton Century Crofts, 1986, p 355.

27. Zeabart LE, Fabian J, Nord HJ: Squamous papilloma of the esophagus. Gastrointest Endosc, 25:18, 1979.

28. Gentry RW, Dockerty MB, Clagett OT: Collective review; vascular malformations and vascular tumors of the gastrointestinal tract. Int Abstr Surg, 88:281–323, 1949.

20

Carcinoma of the Esophagus

Steven D. MacFarlane ▪ Riivo Ilves

▪ *Epidemiology and Etiology*

It is estimated that approximately 9300 cases of esophageal carcinoma were diagnosed in the United States during 1986, accounting for 1 per cent of all new cancers. Approximately 8800 patients died of esophageal carcinoma in 1986—1.8 per cent of all cancer deaths.[1] Five-year survival in white Americans has remained stable at 4 to 7 per cent since 1960. For American blacks the rate is slightly lower at 1 to 4 per cent. Only primary liver and pancreatic malignancies have comparably dismal prognoses. Despite advancements in operative techniques and employment of ever more elaborate treatment modalities, the prognosis has not significantly improved over the past 30 years. Early diagnosis is the only intervention that improves survival, but this is a rarity because clinical manifestations tend to occur late in the disease process.

Incidence rates are fairly constant throughout the world, ranging from 2 to 5 per 100,000 males and 1 to 3 per 100,000 females. However, endemic geographic pockets exist where incidence rates are as high as 263 per 100,000 (females in the Caspian Sea littoral). Other areas include Brittany and Normandy, France (56 per 100,000), northern Iran, Transkei, South Africa, and the Taihag mountain region of Northern China, where the highest death rate from esophageal carcinoma occurs (139 per 100,000 people).[2] Nutrition, soil characteristics, specific carcinogens, tobacco and alcohol habits,

food preparation, and genetic factors have all been implicated as possible etiologic agents.

Nutrition ▪ Nutritional studies in Linxian county, Northern China have revealed deficiencies in vitamins A, B, C, and D and riboflavin in the general population.[3,4] Deficiencies in riboflavin have been shown to alter squamous cell epithelium integrity and lead to precancerous states.[5] Underlying nutritional deficiency may make squamous epithelium more susceptible to environmental carcinogens.

Specific Carcinogens ▪ Nitrites and nitrates are ubiquitous compounds found in plants. They have not been shown to be carcinogenic themselves, but nitroso compounds derived from them are carcinogenic and their concentrations appear to be elevated in grains in the Linxian county region.[6] Molybdenum is a cofactor for the enzyme nitrate reductase in plants and is deficient in the soil in Linxian county and may partially account for the elevated levels of nitrates and nitrites in food.[3]

Fusarin C is a compound metabolized by *Fusarium moniliforme* and is a mutagen.[7] It is predominantly found in millet grains consumed in Linxian county and is also felt to contribute to the pathogenesis of esophageal carcinoma.

Tobacco and Alcohol ▪ Epidemiologic studies have linked tobacco use and alcohol consumption with an increased incidence of esophageal carcinoma, but the causal relationship has not been precisely defined.[8–10] Amount of alcohol consumption appears to be more strongly associated with subsequent esophageal disease than does cigarette smoking, but this is debated[8] as smoking and alcohol consumption are often coexistent. Ethanol may induce or initiate epithelial changes which increase mucosal susceptibility to carcinogenesis.

Genetic ■ A clear-cut inherited basis for esophageal carcinoma has been demonstrated in the autosomal dominant trait keratosis palmaris et plantaris.[11] Also, selected families in Northern China have been found to be predisposed to the disease.[3] No other mendelian patterns have been reported. Sex and race appear to influence susceptibility but vary widely with geography and occurrence of other risk factors. Male-to-female ratio is normally about 3 to 1. However, in Brittany it is 23 to 1, and in Northern Iran the female incidence has been reported to be as high as 263 per 100,000.[2] Racial susceptibility is probably multifactorial, but incidence is 16.9 per 100,000 black U.S. males and only 4.8 per 100,000 white U.S. males.[2]

Esophageal Stasis ■ Incidence of esophageal carcinoma of up to 20 per cent has been documented in patients with achalasia.[12–14] However, a recent review failed to find an association in 91 patients with achalasia followed for a mean period of 6.4 years.[15] In series which showed an association the mean age of tumor occurrence was in the fifth decade. It occurred an average of 17 years after the diagnosis of achalasia. The mechanism appears to be chronic stasis of luminal contents and increased epithelial contact with irritants and potential carcinogens. The most common site is the midesophagus where prolonged contact is maintained. This mechanism may also partially explain why patients with esophageal webs or Plummer-Vinson disease are at higher risk for malignancy.[16]

Caustic Injury ■ History of caustic injury (lye ingestion) is reported in a small minority (1 to 4 per cent) of esophageal carcinoma patients.[17,18] The carcinoma usually appears long (mean period of 40 years) after the injury, but occurs at a younger age than in the general population. Often, lye strictures have required repeated dilatations, and the tumors frequently occur at these sites. Most patients, however, are asymptomatic until the time of tumor manifestation. Whether relative luminal stasis, as in achalasia, plays an etiologic role is unclear and has not been documented. Prognosis may be slightly better in these patients because of younger age and possibly the localizing effects of chronic scarring.

Radiation ■ Radiation-induced esophageal carcinoma is extremely rare, and only 22 cases following therapeutic mediastinal radiation have been reported since 1949.[19] Apparently, neutron irradiation from atomic bomb exposure caused a fourfold increase in the incidence of esophageal carcinoma in Hiroshima.[20]

Barrett's Esophagus ■ Adenocarcinoma has been reported in as many as 15 per cent of patients with known gastric metaplasia of the esophagus.[21–23] This has led to aggressive surveillance of these patients for high-grade dysplasia, a precursor of malignancy. Pathogenesis and treatment of Barrett's esophagus are discussed in detail in Chapter 12. Whether antireflux procedures are effective at reversing this process and reducing the subsequent risk of adenocarcinoma remains controversial.

■ Presentation

The most unfortunate aspect of esophageal cancer is the late stage at which patients present with clinical manifestations. Clinical findings in 155 consecutive patients presenting with esophageal cancer at Virginia Mason Medical Center from 1969 to 1980 are seen in Figure 20–1. Dysphagia, the most common manifestation, does not usually occur until at least two thirds of the circumference of esophageal wall is involved with tumor. Average duration of dysphagia was 3.4 months prior to presentation at Virginia Mason. Dysphagia is usually painless, helping to differentiate it from motor disorders. Odynophagia, or pain with swallowing, is a more grave symptom and implies local tumor extension into mediastinal structures or, in the case of back pain, into the vertebral bodies. Weight loss is also an indication of more extensive disease.

Anemia from occult bleeding of the tumor surface is often seen. Frank bleeding may also occur, and rare cases of erosion into the aorta with exsanguination are seen. Other late signs and symptoms include aspiration pneumonia, vocal cord paralysis from recurrent laryngeal nerve involvement, and cervical or supraclavicular adenopathy.

Physical examination should include thorough upper aerodigestive evaluation to eliminate possible vocal cord involvement or oral-pharyngeal-laryngeal tumors. The neck and supraclavicular areas should be carefully palpated for metastatic lymphadenopathy, confirmation of which would significantly alter subsequent therapy. Abdominal examination should focus on presence of hepatomegaly, ascites, or palpable tumor masses suggesting celiac adenopathy or peritoneal implants. A rectal shelf should be excluded by digital rectal examination and stool examined for occult blood loss.

■ Pathology

Squamous cell carcinoma is the predominant malignancy of the esophagus. The middle and lower

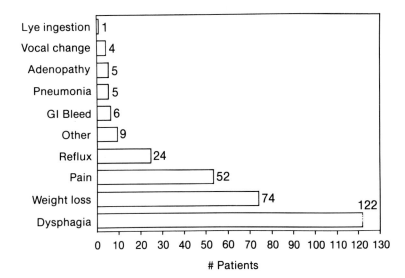

Figure 20–1. Presenting signs and symptoms of esophageal carcinoma in 155 patients at Virginia Mason Medical Center, 1969–1980.

portions of the esophagus are involved more often than the upper. Review of 7000 cases by Postlethwait showed distribution of 17, 47, and 36 per cent in the upper, middle, and lower thirds of the esophagus, respectively.[24]

Morphologically, squamous cell carcinoma may be superficial spreading, ulcerative, papillomatous, or plaque-like. Pleomorphic squamous cells with frequent mitotic features are often connected by intracellular bridges. Tumor grade may range from well to poorly differentiated.[25]

As with most carcinomas, tumor spread is by direct, intraluminal, lymphatic, or hematogenous routes. Unique to the esophagus is its lack of serosal barrier which allows for earlier transmural extension into adjacent structures. Blood-borne metastases most commonly occur in the liver followed by lungs, adrenals, bone, and brain.

Intramural submucosal lymphatic drainage is longitudinal rather than segmental. Tumor cells may travel long distances through these lymphatic channels before they penetrate the esophageal wall to join lymph nodes. Three major lymph node levels have been described: (1) paraesophageal nodes contiguous to the esophagus draining adventitial lymphatics; (2) periesophageal nodes draining structures contiguous to the esophagus (i.e., subcarinal, paratracheal); and (3) regional (or lateral) nodes which secondarily drain the above or drain into periesophageal nodes (i.e., cervical, hilar, suprapyloric, common hepatic, gastric, and celiac).[26]

Primary adenocarcinoma of the esophagus (excluding the gastroesophageal junction) is rare. Three histologic sites of origin have been suggested: (1) esophageal mucosal or submucosal glands; (2) heterotopic gastric mucosa which failed to undergo squamous transformation prior to birth; and (3) metaplastic gastric mucosa (Barrett's

esophagus). Anatomic site of origin is difficult to determine in the lower esophagus as lesions arising from the cardia may extend up into the esophagus proper. The reported incidence of adenocarcinoma of the esophagus ranges from 0.2 to 15 per cent.[27] Incidence increases with more distal location. Analysis of cell type in all patients with middle and upper esophageal tumors (to eliminate confusion with possible gastric origin) at Virginia Mason Medical Center from 1969 to 1985 revealed adenocarcinoma in only 4 of 77 cases (5 per cent).

Gross appearance and malignant behavior of adenocarcinomas are similar to that of squamous cell, though lymphatic penetration may be aggressive. Histologic site of origin determines microscopic characteristics of the tumor. Tumors originating from mucosal or submucosal glands will resemble mucoepidermoid or adenoid cystic tumors. Those from Barrett's esophagus will exhibit features of gastric or intestinal epithelium. Tumors arising from heterotopic gastric mucosa will look like gastric carcinomas.

Miscellaneous esophageal malignancies include adenosquamous carcinomas, carcinosarcomas, oatcell carcinomas, pseudosarcomas, undifferentiated carcinomas, and malignant melanomas, all of which are rare. Treatment and prognosis for these tumors are similar to squamous cell or adenocarcinomas.

Clinical staging is important for prognostic purposes and to aid in proper choice of treatment modality. Methods of clinical staging are described in detail under the diagnostic evaluation section below. Ultimate prognosis following resection is determined by the final histopathologic stage. The American Joint Committee TNM clinical classification system is depicted in Table 20–1. The Japanese have devised a histologic TNM staging sys-

Table 20–1. AMERICAN JOINT COMMITTEE ON CANCER TNM STAGING CLASSIFICATION FOR ESOPHAGEAL CARCINOMA

Primary Tumor (T)

TX	Minimum requirement to assess primary tumor cannot be met
T0	No evidence of primary tumor
Tis	Carcinoma in situ
T1	Tumor involves 5 cm or less of esophageal length, produces no obstruction, and has no circumferential involvement and no extraesophageal spread
T2	Tumor involves more than 5 cm of esophageal length without extraesophageal spread, or any size that produces obstruction, or involves the entire circumference without extraesophageal spread
T3	Tumor with evidence of extraesophageal spread

Nodal Involvement (N)

Cervical nodes:

NX	Minimum requirements to assess regional nodes cannot be met
N0	No clinically palpable nodes
N1	Movable, unilateral, palpable nodes
N2	Movable, bilateral, palpable nodes
N3	Fixed nodes

Thoracic nodes:

NX	Clinical evaluation: regional lymph nodes for the upper, mid-thoracic, and lower thoracic esophagus that are not ordinarily accessible for clinical evaluation

Distant Metastasis (M)

MX	Minimum requirement to assess presence of distant metastasis cannot be met
M0	No evidence of distant metastasis (for thoracic tumor any cervical, supraclavicular, scalene, or abdominal lymph nodes are considered distant metastasis sites)
M1	Distant metastasis present; specify _____

Stage Classification

Stage I	T1, N0, M0
Stage II	T2, N0, M0
Stage III	T3, N0, M0
	Any T, N1–3, M0
Stage IV	Any T, any N, M1

Source: Beahrs O: Manual for Staging of Cancer. American Joint Committee on Cancer, 1986.

tem which places emphasis upon level of tumor penetration rather than size (Table 20–2). Skinner has also recently devised a staging classification based upon wall penetration and lymph node status.[28]

■ *Diagnostic Evaluation*

Screening Cytology ■ High-risk endemic populations have been screened using mesh-covered balloons, encapsulated sponges, and nylon brushes for the early detection of esophageal cancer. In the Henan province of China the accuracy rate is 80 per cent using a fishnet-covered balloon. Three quarters of patients found to have esophageal malignancy had early in situ or stage I cancers.[29] Surgical cure rate in this group as reported by Guojan was 86 per cent at five years.[30] It is estimated that dysplastic changes found in the esophagus may predate frank carcinoma by up to eight years and that periodic screening at intervals of two years will effectively detect early lesions.

The overall incidence of esophageal cancer in the United States would not warrant widespread screening of this type. However, the technique of indirect exfoliative cytologic examination by means of a nylon brush placed inside a nasogastric tube was evaluated in 203 consecutive patients in an esophageal surgery clinic by Dowlatshahi in Chicago.[31] It compared favorably with direct endoscopic biopsy and brushings in the same patients, correctly identifying 78 per cent of patients with esophageal cancer. Application of this technique to high-risk patients with premalignant conditions may be useful, as false positive results were seen in less than 1 per cent of patients with a nonmalignant esophageal condition or normal esophagus.

Contrast Esophagography ■ When history

Table 20–2. JAPANESE TNM STAGING CLASSIFICATION FOR ESOPHAGEAL CARCINOMA

Tumor (T)

m, sm	Confined to mucosa, submucosa
m_p	Confined to muscularis propria
a_1	Invasion reaching adventitia
a_2	Invasion into adventitia
a_3	Invasion into neighboring structures

Lymph Node Metastases (N)

n_0	No metastases
n_1	Metastases to paraesophageal nodes of involved segment
n_2	Metastases to paraesophageal nodes of segments adjacent to tumor and/or to periesophageal nodes of involved or adjacent esophageal segments
n_3	Metastases to paraesophageal or periesophageal nodes of distant esophageal segments and/or metastases to lateral esophageal nodes
n_4	Metastases to nodes beyond group n_3

Organ Metastases (M)

m_0	No organ metastases noted
m_1	Organ metastases positive

Pleural Dissemination (Pl)

pl_0	No pleural dissemination noted
pl_1	Pleural dissemination positive

Histologic Stage

0	m, sm, n_0, m_0, pl_0
I	m_p, n_0, m_0, pl_0
II	a_1, n_1, m_0, pl_0
III	a_2, n_2, m_0, pl_0
IV	a_3, n_{3-4}, m_1, pl_1

Source: Mannell A: Carcinoma of the esophagus. Curr Prob Surg, *19*(10):572, 1982.

and physical examination suggest the possibility of esophageal cancer, further evaluation of the patient should then (1) establish the presence of a lesion, (2) obtain a tissue diagnosis, (3) establish extent of disease (i.e., should treatment be curative or palliative), and (4) determine the medical and nutritional status of the patient (ability to undergo therapy).

Plain chest film may rarely suggest an obstructing lesion by presence of an air-fluid level in the mediastinum or chronic basilar pneumonitis suggestive of chronic aspiration. Double contrast esophagography is the most commonly used initial investigation and can detect small or advanced carcinomas. Small tumors may be identified as only minor irregularities of the mucosa or as diminutive polypoid filling defects (Fig. 20–2). The diagnosis of malignancy becomes more obvious with increase in tumor size. Irregular ulcerations, destruction of surrounding mucosa, abrupt, overhanging margins, and lumen deviation aid in differentiating benign from malignant lesions (Fig. 20–3).

Esophagograms obtained in 141 patients with esophageal cancer at Virginia Mason Medical Center between 1969 and 1980 were highly suggestive of cancer in 135 patients (95.7 per cent). A 5 per cent false negative rate should encourage continued investigation in patients with obvious symptoms and a negative esophagogram.

Although esophagography is used in the United States basically as an initial assessment and not necessarily to stage the disease, it has been used in Japan by Akiyama and Mori to predict resectability based on certain radiologic criteria.[32,33] They found an 85 per cent correlation between tortuosity of the proximal tumor along with excess angulation or deviation of the esophageal axis, and tumor invasion of adjacent structures at exploration which precluded curative resection. However, other modalities such as computed tomography appear to be more effective means to assess extent of extra-esophageal disease.

Esophagoscopy ■ Endoscopic evaluation of the esophagus is mandatory in any patient with dysphagia and signs or symptoms suggesting possible esophageal cancer. Approximately 5 per cent of upper GI contrast studies will miss lesions identified otherwise, and it is likely that these may be early, potentially more curable lesions (Fig. 20–4). A positive tissue diagnosis implements further pretreatment staging and patient evaluation. Fiberoptic endoscopy is initially employed by most endoscopists. However, rigid esophagoscopy is very helpful in screening high-risk patients for early lesions. Four morphologic types of preinvasive cancers have been identified by Monnier using rigid esophagoscopy: type I—elevated, white (leukoplastic) dysplastic lesions which are usually single;

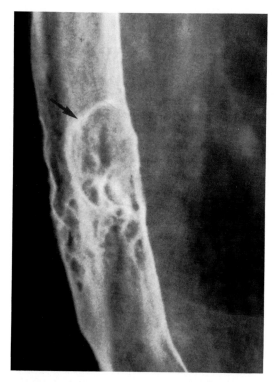

Figure 20–2. Early esophageal carcinoma. Double contrast barium examination of the esophagus shows a focal area of mucosal irregularity (arrow) due to a superficial squamous cell carcinoma of the esophagus.

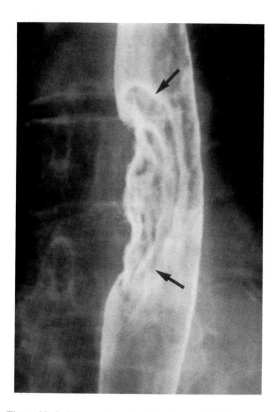

Figure 20–3. Advanced esophageal carcinoma. Double contrast barium examination of the esophagus shows a large, eccentric intraluminal mass involving the right lateral wall of the esophagus (arrows) due to squamous cell carcinoma of the esophagus.

type II—depressed, reddish (erythroplastic) lesions which are usually multicentric; type III—mixed lesions; and type IV—occult lesions identified only after a vital stain such as toluidine blue has been applied.[34]

Dilatation is sometimes necessary to allow passage of the endoscope for biopsy and cytologic evaluation in the presence of nearly obstructing lesions. Examination of the esophagus and stomach distal to the lesion is important to exclude multiple tumors or intraluminal implants. If the patient is totally or near totally obstructed, laser excavation of the tumor may be necessary. This does not necessarily preclude subsequent resection and has been useful at Virginia Mason in some gastroesophageal junction tumors. Brush cytologic examination as well as tissue biopsies should be performed, as sensitivity was improved 8 per cent over biopsy alone in a series of 155 patients at Virginia Mason. If local inflammatory changes preclude positive tissue diagnosis at flexible endoscopy, rigid esophagoscopy may be a more effective means of obtaining sufficient tissue for diagnosis. Rigid endoscopy also allows for more thorough evaluation of postcricoid tumors.

There were 183 endoscopic biopsies performed in 155 patients at Virginia Mason Medical Center

between 1969 and 1980. Rigid endoscopy was used more often early in this series, and was used later only if fiberoptic endoscopy was negative. Overall sensitivity using brush cytology and biopsy was 76 per cent, which meant that tissue diagnosis was obtained either at exploration or by biopsy of met-

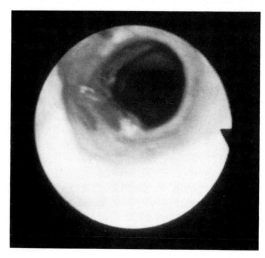

Figure 20–4. Early intramural squamous cell cancer not seen on initial esophagography. (See Color Plate IV*A*.)

astatic lymph nodes in one fourth of patients.

The presence of an esophageal stricture may mask an underlying cancer. Malignancy associated with stricture is one of the most difficult esophageal lesions to detect. In our experience as many as seven different biopsies have been necessary to find the malignancy. In these difficult cases, the rigid esophagoscope and larger biopsy forceps are needed to obtain deep biopsies. Otherwise, stricture-associated cancers will be missed.

Computed Tomography ■ Computed tomographic (CT) scanning is generally regarded as the most useful single pretreatment staging modality, as it evaluates both local and metastatic extent of disease. Thoracic and upper abdominal scans will generally include all likely sites of disease. Cervical scanning is warranted as well for upper esophageal tumors. Intravenous contrast medium helps to enhance vascular structures and improve resolution. Normal esophageal wall thickness should be no greater than 3 to 5 mm, depending upon degree of luminal distention. Presence of tumor is manifested by asymmetric wall thickening and often loss of esophageal lumen (Fig. 20–5). If obstruction has been present long enough, the proximal esophagus may be excessively dilated. Tumor invasion outside the muscularis propria (Fig. 20–6) is characterized by loss of normal periesophageal fat planes, which should be present above or below the level of the tumor to lend validity to this sign. However, patients with esophageal cancer are often cachectic, and normal periesophageal fat planes may not be present for comparison.

Invasion of contiguous mediastinal structures can also be appreciated on CT scan. Normally, the membranous trachea and left mainstem bronchus bow outward or are flat. Concavity of the posterior membranous airway correlates highly with tumor invasion of these structures (Fig. 20–7).[35,36] Invasion of the left atrium or aorta distally is more difficult to detect as there is less of a natural fat plane between these structures and the esophagus. Picus et al. quantified the "angle of abutment" between the esophagus and aorta.[37] If over 90 per cent of the circumference of the aorta was abutted by esophagus, this correlated with an 80 per cent chance of tumor invasion at exploration. However, other studies have not found this sign to be helpful.[36]

CT is an excellent modality for staging of gastroesophageal junction tumors. Freeny and Marks accurately staged 18 of 21 (86 per cent) patients, with two false negative scans (both missed lymph node metastases).[38] The most reliable signs of unresectability of gastroesophageal junction tumors are detection of distant metastases (liver, adrenal) and local tumor extension (Fig. 20–8).

Assessment of lymph node status is the "Achilles heel" of CT scan evaluation.[35,36,39] Increased lymph node size may often correlate with the presence of metastatic tumor (τ 0.6 cm in the retrocrural space, τ 1.5 cm elsewhere) but, alternatively, may be due to inflammatory changes (Fig. 20–9). Periesophageal metastases are often overlooked as they become incorporated into the primary tumor mass. Halverson's analysis of three major series showed that accuracy for periesophageal nodes was 57 per cent but for abdominal nodes it was 87 per cent.[35] Lea et al., on the other hand, found a predictive accuracy of 72 per cent for mediastinal lymph nodes and only 39 per cent for abdominal nodes in 18 patients.[39]

Extranodal metastatic disease usually involves the liver, adrenals, lungs, or bone. The incidence

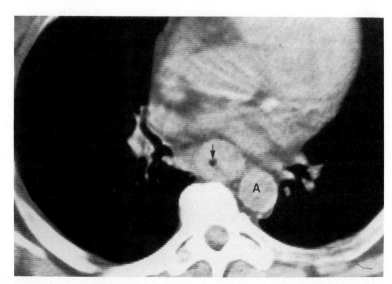

Figure 20–5. Computed tomography: Esophageal carcinoma. CT scan of the chest at the level of the distal third of the esophagus shows marked thickening of the esophageal wall. The esophageal lumen (arrow) is slightly eccentric. A = aorta.

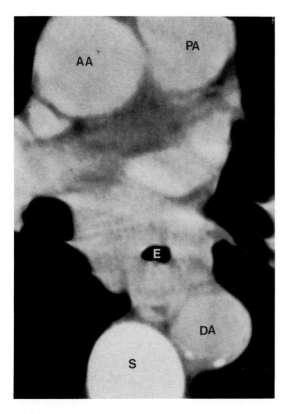

Figure 20–6. Computed tomography: Invasive esophageal carcinoma. CT scan of the thorax at the level of the middle third of the esophagus (E) shows obliteration of the normal periesophageal soft tissue planes anteriorly between the esophagus and pericardium and posteriorly between the esophagus and the descending thoracic aorta (DA). AA = ascending aorta; PA = pulmonary artery; S = spine.

of bone metastases is low enough so that routine bone scan is not usually recommended.[36] CT scan does evaluate the remaining sites. Liver metastases characteristically appear as low attenuation lesions (Fig. 20–10). If necessary, CT-guided fine-needle aspiration may be performed for cytologic diagnosis. Adrenal metastases may appear as solitary masses, but CT-guided needle aspiration may, again, be necessary to differentiate nodular adrenal enlargement from metastatic disease.

Ultimately, for the surgeon, the information derived from CT scan evaluation is used to determine if the tumor is resectable and the patient potentially curable. CT staging criteria vary from institution to institution and, unlike the TNM staging system, do not take into account lymph node involvement. The CT staging system developed by Moss is commonly used: stage I—intraluminal mass without wall thickening; stage II—esophageal wall thickening (τ 5 mm); stage III—esophageal wall thickening and contiguous spread of tumor into adjacent mediastinal structures; and stage IV—any stage with evidence of distant metastatic disease.[40] The underlying philosophy of the surgeon (whether resection is done for potential cure or for palliative purposes) dictates the importance of CT staging. The more selective the indications for surgery, the more important will be the CT scan findings, and also the need for further preliminary staging.

Bronchoscopy ■ Bronchoscopy is usually recommended for evaluation of possible tracheal or bronchial involvement from upper esophageal tumors. However, lower esophageal cancers may often spread via transmural lymphatics to the proximal esophageal wall and periesophageal nodes and if CT scan or patient symptoms suggest possible airway involvement bronchoscopy should be performed. Choi, using rigid bronchoscopy, found that approximately one third of 86 patients with cervical or upper third esophageal tumors had tracheal impingement and another fourth had actual tracheal invasion.[41,42] He also found that 12 per cent of patients with lower third and gastroesophageal junction tumors had airway impingement and 5 per cent had frank invasion of the airways.

Bronchoscopic findings suggesting tumor involvement range from frank tumor invasion and fistula formation to inward bulging or widening of the membranous portion of the tracheobronchial tree. Since the esophagus is slightly to the left of the carina in the mediastinum, usually the left mainstem bronchus will be involved at this level by primary tumor. However, right mainstem bronchus involvement is often seen if nodal spread occurs from lower esophageal tumors. Simple bulging does not necessarily imply invasion (as it apparently seems to on CT scan) and approximately one half of these tumors may be totally resectable.[43] Loss of normal mucosal rippling means probable invasion and resection for cure is unlikely. Rarely, a synchronous lung primary may be detected by bronchoscopy, which would alter the treatment course.

Other Diagnostic Tests ■ Uncommonly used methods of evaluating esophageal cancer for resectability and staging are described in the literature. Azygography has been employed in Japan looking for shift, narrowing, or obstruction of the azygos vein after injection of 20 ml of methylglucamine iodamide into the marrow of the tenth spinous process of the thoracic vertebrae.[33] Gallium scanning may also detect metastatic disease but has high false positive and false negative rates. Liver-spleen scan has not been shown to add significantly to CT evaluation.[36] Mediastinoscopy is rarely used to stage esophageal cancer. Unlike lung cancer, patterns of nodal involvement are not predictable. Usually, lymph node involvement which would preclude exploration is identified in the abdomen

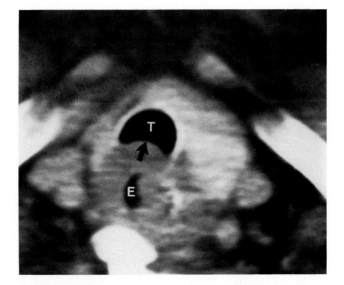

Figure 20–7. Computed tomography. Invasive esophageal carcinoma. CT scan of the upper esophagus (E) at the level of the thoracic inlet shows a thick esophageal wall due to squamous cell carcinoma. The tumor bulges anteriorly (arrow), indenting the trachea (T).

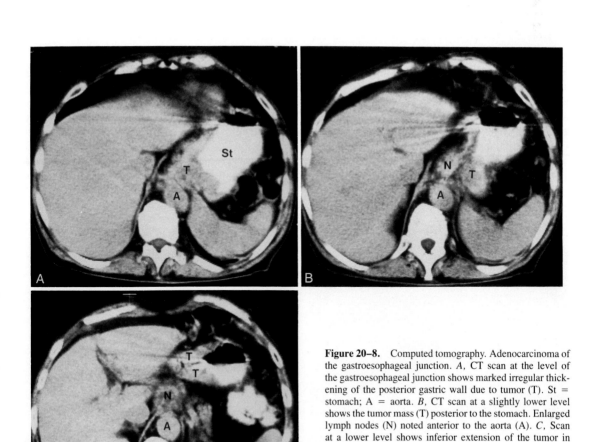

Figure 20–8. Computed tomography. Adenocarcinoma of the gastroesophageal junction. *A,* CT scan at the level of the gastroesophageal junction shows marked irregular thickening of the posterior gastric wall due to tumor (T). St = stomach; A = aorta. *B,* CT scan at a slightly lower level shows the tumor mass (T) posterior to the stomach. Enlarged lymph nodes (N) noted anterior to the aorta (A). *C,* Scan at a lower level shows inferior extension of the tumor in the gastric wall (T) and a persistent large nodal mass (N) anterior to the aorta (A).

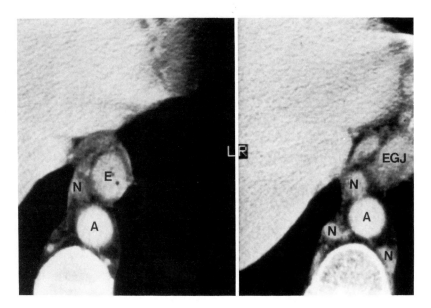

Figure 20–9. Computed tomography. Adenocarcinoma of the gastroesophageal junction. Contiguous CT scans at the level of the distal esophagus (E) and esophagogastric junction (EGJ) show marked thickening of the esophagus and esophagogastric junction owing to adenocarcinoma. Multiple enlarged lymph nodes (N) are demonstrated adjacent to the esophagus and in the retrocrural space adjacent to the aorta (A).

or is often evident on physical examination. Periesophageal node metastases are usually identified pathologically only at the time of resection. The role for cervical mediastinoscopy may be in patients with upper third esophageal cancers, or when CT scan shows paratracheal lymph node enlargement which, if metastatic, would preclude resection for cure. The suprasternal incision may then form the proposed neck incision for proximal

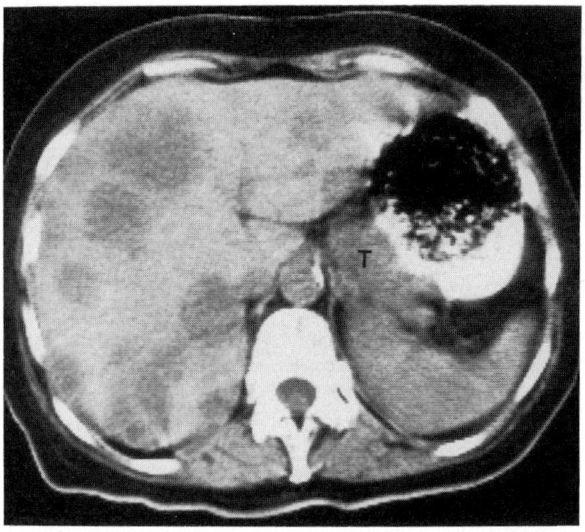

Figure 20–10. Computed tomography. Esophagogastric junction adenocarcinoma and liver metastases. CT scan at the level of the esophagogastric junction shows a large tumor mass (T). There are multiple low attenuation lesions within the liver owing to metastases.

esophageal mobilization and anastomosis if resection is carried out.

Application of magnetic resonance imaging (MRI) to esophageal disease is in its infancy. Normal features of the esophagus have been described by Quint.[43] In his series of 10 patients with esophageal cancer, MRI and CT scan were similarly poor predictors of local tumor invasion and node status. MRI correctly staged only four of 10 tumors. It was suggested that further technologic advances, including respiratory gating, are needed to improve accuracy of MRI in staging mediastinal disease.

■ Chemotherapy and Radiation Treatment

Primary chemotherapy has traditionally been reserved for palliative purposes in advanced disease. Partial and complete response rates as measured by clinical parameters such as degree of dysphagia, palpable change in metastatic disease, chest x-ray, CT scan, or endoscopy have been poor.[44–46] Single agent and combination chemotherapy also cause undesirable side effects including renal dysfunction, alopecia, nausea and vomiting, bone marrow suppression, and susceptibility to infection. Survival has not been improved by chemotherapy alone and the likely role for this modality is in combination with radiation or surgery.

Other than surgery, radiotherapy has been the only treatment modality shown to improve survival. Radiation therapy offers an alternative primary treatment modality when surgical resection is contraindicated. Approximately two thirds of patients achieve satisfactory short-term palliation from dysphagia. Adjunctive use of laser treatment or intraluminal stent placement may improve these results. Survival has been best following treatment of proximal third tumors. Pearson reported a 25 per cent five-year survival in 76 patients with proximal third squamous cell tumors following 4800 to 5300 rads tumor dose over four weeks.[47] Five-year survival rate in 288 patients with tumors at all levels was 17 per cent. No other series has reported similarly good results, and the overall five-year survival rate usually ranges from 0 to 9 per cent.[48] Results following radiotherapy may be poor because treatment is so often reserved for patients who are not deemed surgical candidates. However, van Andel reported only one five-year survivor in 115 patients who were operable candidates, but chose radiation as a primary treatment modality.[49]

At Virginia Mason Medical Center 145 esophageal cancer patients were treated nonoperatively from 1969 to 1985. Eighty-one (56 per cent) completed at least 4000 rads tumor dose and 64 (44 per cent) either failed to complete full treatment or did not undergo radiation therapy. Mean survival time was 9.9 ± 1 month in those able to receive 4000 rads of radiation and 4.2 ± 0.5 months in the remaining patients ($p <0.01$ Mantel-Cox statistical test). Only one patient survived beyond two years, ultimately dying of a stroke with no evidence of disease at four years.

■ Surgical Treatment

Most patients present with advanced disease with little chance for cure. They are typically malnourished and physically debilitated secondary to their inability to swallow. Owing to their generally poor overall prognosis, the objective of surgical treatment of these patients should be prompt restoration of the ability to swallow and improvement in quality of life. A philosophy of rapid palliation using a ''least cost'' strategy (in terms of patient morbidity) is usually appropriate in most patients.

Esophageal intubation has been a useful approach with the understanding that, although it may minimize invasiveness and achieve luminal patency, it does not minimize morbidity.[50,51] The ideal situation for esophageal intubation is bypass of tracheoesophageal fistulas. Laser therapy has even been used in this situation to open up the lumen

prior to placement of the stent.[52] The method of placement varies from endoscopic ''pulsion'' techniques using specialized loading devices placed over a guidewire through an endoscope to ''traction'' techniques via gastrotomy. Tube-related deaths and complications occur from perforation, bleeding, erosion, aspiration, or obstruction. Between 1969 and 1980 45 patients at Virginia Mason Medical Center had intraluminal stents placed across esophageal tumors, nine via pulsion and 36 via traction techniques. Four were placed for tracheoesophageal fistulas. Tube-related morbidity occurred in 20 patients (44 per cent).

Nonresectional operative bypass was first introduced by Kirschner of Germany in 1920,[53] but because of high mortality and morbidity rates it has been largely abandoned. Kirschner's operation consisted of bringing the stomach subcutaneously up to the divided cervical esophagus. The distal esophagus was then drained into a roux-en-Y loop of jejunum. Roehrer has subsequently described a modified double bypass version of the Kirschner operation in 1981 for palliation of esophagobronchial fistulas in six patients which resulted in two operative mortalities.[54] He suggested it as an alternative to intubation. Wong described using the Kirschner bypass in 142 patients with a 42 per cent hospital mortality rate.[55] Other routes of bypass and choices of conduit have been used for palliative bypass and vary, depending upon location of the primary tumor, extent of disease, and nature of previous treatment.

Intraluminal laser tumor excavation has come to the forefront of palliative therapy because of its immediate effectiveness, low morbidity, and suitability for outpatient treatment (see Chapter 25 for a discussion of laser therapy). With the introduction of laser treatment, other alternative treatments designed to minimize tumor morbidity, such as intraluminal stent placement or operative bypass, have been used less frequently.

Tumor resection is probably the most commonly performed treatment for esophageal cancer in patients who are operative candidates. Aside from intent, it is extremely difficult to determine whether resection is actually ''palliative'' or ''curative'' at the time of operation. As a result, the separation of resective treatment into ''palliative'' or ''curative'' categories may be at times arbitrary. Table 20–3 depicts results following major operative series and suggests that survival statistics may be better following intended ''curative'' resections. However, even in series where apparently palliative resections were carried out five-year survival has been 5 to 8 per cent, an improvement over most nonresection therapies.

Survival has been shown to correlate well with

Table 20–3. OPERATIVE RESULTS FOLLOWING RESECTION OF ESOPHAGEAL CARCINOMA

Author/Date	Intent of Resection	Number of Patients	Operative Mortality Rate	Operative Morbidity Rate	Survival Rate	Technique
Fisher, 1972[56]	Palliative	31	13%	NA	7 of 31 alive at 6–24 months	Lewis; esophagogastrostomy
Belsey, 1974[57]	Palliative	119	NA	NA	25% 1 year/19% >2 years	Right thoracotomy—all mid third tumors Esophagogastrostomy
	Curative	21	28%		43% 1 year/24% >2 years	
Skinner, 1976[58]	Palliative	58	NA	NA	8% 5 years	Left thoracotomy lower third Right thoracotomy upper third Majority esophagogastrostomy
Griffen, 1976[59]	Palliative	10	20%	60%	NA	Substernal Gastric tube
Ellis, 1979[60]	Palliative	72	2.8%	15.3%	Mean 20.8 months	Lewis or left thoracotomy Colon or esophagogastrostomy
Dark, 1981[61]	?	449	7.6%	22%	21% alive 9 months–2 years 18% 5 year predicted	Left thoracotomy Esophagogastrostomy
McKeown, 1981[61]	Palliative	154	15.7%	20%	NA	Lewis ± cervical incision Esophagogastrostomy
Hoffman, 1981[68]	Palliative	44	16%	NA	Mean 11.5 months	Lewis or left thoracotomy Esophagogastrostomy
Akiyama, 1981[64]	Curative	210	1.4%	35%	35% 5 years	Regional mediastinectomy Colon or esophagogastrostomy
Maillet, 1982[65]	Palliative	197	21% > 5.4%	26%	2.3% 5 years	Lewis; esophagogastrostomy
	Curative	74			28% 5 years	
Le-Tian, 1982[66]	Curative	664	10%	NA	22% 5 year	Lewis or left thoracotomy Colon or esophagogastrostomy
Keagy, 1984[67]	Palliative	60	6.7%	43%	27% 2 years 5% 5 years	Lewis; esophagogastrostomy
Fein, 1985[68]	Curative	73	8.2%	NA	14/73 alive, median 11 months	Lewis or thoracoabdominal Esophagogastrostomy
Gatzinsky, 1985[69]	Curative	84	18%	NA	5 yr { 12% penetration of esophagus—67 patients / 94% no penetration of esophagus—17 patients }	Colon or esophagogastrostomy
Galandiuk, 1986[70]	Palliative	21	7.1%	72%	5.8% 5 years	Lewis or left thoracotomy Esophagogastrostomy
	Curative	63			15.4% 5 year	
Skinner, 1986[28]	Palliative	21	5%	50%	14% 18 months	Enbloc mediastinectomy
	Curative	31	9.7%	43%	55% 18 months	Lewis or left thoracotomy Esophagogastrostomy
Virginia Mason (see text)	Curative	91	6.6%	27%	12.7% 5 year	See text

tumor stage at resection. Gatzinsky reported 94 per cent two-year survival in 17 patients who had no penetration of the muscular wall compared to 12 per cent two-year survival in 67 patients who had microscopic or macroscopic penetration.[69]

It is not as clear to what degree the extent of regional resection contributes to recurrence or survival statistics. Akiyama reported a 15.3 per cent five-year survival in patients with extensive regional resections who had positive lymph nodes which improved to 55 per cent if nodes were negative.[64] In his series he also demonstrated that the site of lymph node involvement may be far removed from the site of primary tumor. Skinner advocates careful pre- and intraoperative staging to determine extent of esophageal wall penetration and lymph node status. En bloc regional mediastinal resection including pleura and pericardium is then carried out for disease confined to the limits of the proposed en bloc resection and lymph nodes within 10 cm of the primary tumor. Otherwise, a standard esophagectomy is performed for palliation.[28] Giuli on the other hand did not demonstrate any benefit from extended lymph node resection in 703 patients evaluated in a survey conducted by the International Organization for Statistical Studies of Esophageal Diseases (OESO) in Europe.[71]

Strategy for resection must take into account several factors including choice of incision and exposure, extent of resection, choice of conduit, and technical factors involving reconstruction. For gastroesophageal junction tumors, there are three main choices of exposure, left thoracotomy alone, left thoracoabdominal, or combined midline abdominal incision and right thoracotomy as originally described by Lewis.[72] The advantages of a right thoracotomy in combination with an abdominal incision are increased exposure of possible intra-abdominal metastatic sites, improved ease of mobilizing the stomach into the chest, and improved exposure of the proximal esophagus in the chest. The Lewis approach is excellent for middle esophageal tumor resection and the addition of a cervical incision as described by McKeown[62] allows for more proximal resection and anastomosis of the stomach to the cervical esophagus. A right thoracotomy alone as described by Belsey[57] may also be adequate for midesophageal tumors but does not allow thorough exploration of the gastric or celiac lymph nodes. The left thoracotomy approach lends itself to excellent exposure of the gastroesophageal junction through a single incision but may be inadequate if it is found that more proximal resection is necessary.

Choice of conduit includes the stomach, colon, and less commonly the small bowel. The stomach is the most often used organ for substitution in the chest as it has an excellent blood supply and is easily mobilized for this purpose. Mobilization can also be accomplished all the way into the neck, basing the blood supply on the right gastric and right gastroepiploic arteries after performing an adequate Kocher maneuver. The greater curve of the stomach may have a tendency to rotate in the chest resulting in problems with gastric emptying. Tacking sutures secured to the pleural surface will prevent this as well as reduce tension on the anastomosis. A cervical anastomosis offers a potential advantage as leaks are more likely to be limited and not involve the mediastinum. However, potential for mediastinitis still exists.[71]

A modified gastric tube (reversed or nonreversed) using the greater curvature of the stomach has been described by Griffen and Heimlich.[59,73] Advantages are that only a laparotomy and cervical incision are necessary for palliative bypass if resection is deemed unwarranted at abdominal exploration. However, reports using this technique describe high leakage rates along the staple lines and at the anastomosis.

Colon interposition has been in use for many years as a replacement conduit, both for malignant and nonmalignant esophageal disorders. The colon may be placed either in a peristaltic or antiperistaltic configuration, based on the left, right, or middle colic arteries. Care must be taken to ensure an adequate vascular supply to the colon transplant, which may entail use of preoperative angiogram. Preoperative contrast study is necessary to exclude other colon disease including colon carcinoma. It is important that the colon vascular pedicle be configured behind rather than in front of the stomach. Gastric outlet obstruction will result from the latter, and dilation of the stomach may also compromise the vascular supply to the colon leading to necrosis. Disadvantages of colon interposition include the possible need for multiple staging of the operation in patients with short-term life expectancy, the need for additional anastomoses, and reports of higher operative morbidity.[74,75] Advantages would seem to be associated with the more extensive esophageal resection with which colon interposition is associated and the acid resistance of the colon mucosa.

Jejunal interposition has been described for replacement of the cervical esophagus using both pedicled or free grafts.[76] However, these procedures should be performed by surgeons who have developed special expertise in these techniques. Others have successfully replaced the cervical esophagus using the stomach.[77]

Total esophagectomy without thoracotomy has been advocated by Orringer.[78,79] A blind one-stage esophagectomy is performed via abdominal and cervical incisions. Mobilization of the esophagus is carried as high as possible through the diaphragmatic hiatus after confirming that the tumor is not adherent. The upper esophageal blood supply is ligated as far caudally as possible via the cervical incision. Usually a few midesophageal vessels are not accessible and are avulsed when the esophagus is pulled out through the hiatus after dividing the cervical portion. Stomach is then brought up through the posterior mediastinum and a cervical esophagogastrostomy constructed. Use of colon or small bowel retrosternally has also been described.[80,81] Orringer claims lower operative mortality and morbidity rates (particularly with respect to pulmonary complications) compared to standard transthoracic techniques. Surprisingly, bleeding was not a significant problem. However, recurrent laryngeal nerve injury occurred to some degree in 21 per cent of his patients.

Nonthoracotomy transhiatal esophagectomy appears to be an acceptable alternative for lower esophageal, gastroesophageal, or cervical tumors where wide tumor dissection can be carried out under direct vision. Total removal of the esophagus with cervical anastomosis may theoretically reduce anastomotic recurrence because of intramural lymphatic spread. Adequacy of resection for middle esophageal tumors remains in doubt, and this technique is contraindicated if invasion of contiguous structures is suspected. Orringer's mortality rate was higher than that of Mitchell, who performed 40 esophageal resections with no mortality.[101]

At Virginia Mason Medical Center surgical resection has been the cornerstone of treatment for patients with esophageal carcinoma who are operative candidates. The intent at the time of resection usually has been "curative." Between 1969 and July of 1985, 134 of a total of 235 patients seen for esophageal cancer (57 per cent) were explored with intent of tumor resection. Ninety-one of the 134 (68 per cent) had resectable tumor.

Table 20–4 depicts the types of operations performed, and Table 20–5 lists the cell types and locations of the tumors in the 91 patients who had resection. The majority of single-stage resections were performed through a right thoracotomy and midline laparotomy. All periesophageal lymphatics were resected en bloc with the tumor. Proximal and distal margins of at least 5 cm were obtained and confirmation of tumor-free margins was obtained by frozen section microscopic analysis at operation. End-to-side configuration and invagination or inkwelling of the anastomosis along with pyloroplasty or pyloromyotomy for gastric drainage were performed in the majority of esophagogastrostomies. Six of 16 planned multiple-stage resections and colon interpositions were not completed because of recurrent esophageal tumor in four patients, pneumonia in one patient, and colon cancer in one patient.

The operative mortality rate was 6.6 per cent (6 of 91) and included 2 of 16 multiple-stage patients and 4 of 75 single-stage patients. Operative morbidity in operative survivors most commonly occurred secondary to pulmonary, cardiac, and anastomotic problems (Table 20–6). Palliation from dysphagia was accomplished in 83 operative survivors (97 per cent), 19 of whom required postoperative dilation.

Anastomotic problems included benign strictures in 21 patients (25 per cent of survivors) and anastomotic leak in 10 patients (12 per cent). No deaths resulted directly from anastomotic leaks. Mean hospital stay was 27 ± 19 days following single-stage resection and 63 ± 42 days following staged resections. This represented 3.7 and 7.0 per cent of these respective patients' mean remaining life span.

Improvements in operative techniques such that reconstruction-related morbidity is minimized include use of "inkwelling" and end-to-side techniques at the esophagogastric anastomosis, thereby reducing anastomotic leak rates and gastroesophageal reflux.[58,82] Gastric drainage procedures did not significantly reduce gastric stasis or outlet obstruction following surgery at Virginia Mason and others have also questioned their effectiveness.[83,84] The continued high incidence of pulmonary complications requires careful patient selection and perioperative vigilance.

Use of preoperative hyperalimentation has been suggested to reduce operative morbidity and mor-

Table 20–4. RESECTIONS FOR ESOPHAGEAL CARCINOMA: 91 OPERATIONS, VIRGINIA MASON MEDICAL CENTER, 1969–1985

Number of Patients		Type of Resection
75		Single-stage resections
	70	Esophagogastrostomies (66 chest, 4 cervical)
	3	Esophagojejunostomies
	2	Colon interpositions
16		Multiple-stage resections
	11	Two-stage colon interposition
	5	Three-stage colon interposition

Table 20–5. RESECTION OF ESOPHAGEAL CARCINOMA: 91 PATIENTS,
VIRGINIA MASON MEDICAL CENTER, 1969–1985

Location	Adenocarcinoma	Squamous Cell Carcinoma	Other	All
Proximal third	0	2	1	3
Middle third	1	13	0	14
Distal third	13	11	1	15
GE junction	45	3	1	49
Total	59	29	3	81

tality rates. Biochemical reversal of gluconeogenesis and protein turnover have been demonstrated following hyperalimentation in esophageal cancer patients. However, clinical trials have not shown particularly encouraging improvements in complication or mortality rates.[85]

Virginia Mason five-year survival statistics following resection alone were analyzed in 65 consecutive patients who received no preoperative adjuvant therapy. Five-year survival was 12.7 per cent (mean of 29.5 ± 5.1 months). Age, sex, and tumor cell type were not predictors of survival. The most important predictor of survival was status of regional lymph nodes. Lymph nodes were not involved with tumor in 29 patients and five-year survival was 21.5 per cent (mean of 44.6 ± 8.7 months). Regional lymph nodes were involved with tumor in 36 patients and five-year survival was 6 per cent (mean of 15.9 ± 3.9 months); p <0.01.

Tumor recurrence was the major cause of death following resection of esophageal cancer. In 33 patients in whom the site of recurrence was known, the liver was involved in 14 patients. Anastomotic recurrence occurred in 10 patients. Less common sites of recurrence included lungs, stomach, bone, brain, and peritoneum. Further evaluation showed that tumor recurrence following resection remained proportionately high throughout the follow-up period, even after five years. Isono demonstrated cancer recurrence in 79 per cent of 151 patients who

survived less than five years and in 28 per cent of 21 patients who survived more than five years.[86] Careful follow-up is necessary even in long-term survivors.

■ *Preoperative Chemotherapy*

Chemotherapy alone has provided little clinical satisfaction in terms of survival. Poorly quantitated, often subjective, clinical end points have made the interpretation of tumor response confusing. Adjuvant preoperative chemotherapy has recently provided the opportunity to histologically evaluate the tumor effects of chemotherapy. Shields reports confinement of the tumor to the esophageal wall in six patients who underwent resection following cisplatin and fluorouracil.[87] Bains reported 7 of 34 patients with only microscopic disease at resection following cisplatin, vindesine, and bleomycin.[88] Follow-up is not sufficient to determine the effects on survival.

■ *Preoperative Radiation*

The rationale for preoperative radiation is reduction of local tumor mass and sterilization of regional lymphatics with the hope of improved re-

Table 20–6. OPERATIVE MORBIDITY RATE OF ESOPHAGEAL RESECTION: 85 OPERATIVE
SURVIVORS, VIRGINIA MASON MEDICAL CENTER, 1969–1985

	Single-Stage (N = 71)	Multiple-Stage (N = 14)	Total (N = 85)
Pulmonary	16	7	23 (27%)
Benign stricture	16	5	21 (25%)
Cardiac	11	2	13 (15%)
Abscess/fistula	6	5	11 (13%)
Anastomotic leak	7	3	10 (12%)
Diarrhea/dumping	8	1	9 (11%)
Gastric emptying	7	0	7 (8%)
Wound infection	4	1	5 (6%)
Bowel obstruction	4	0	4 (5%)
Reflux esophagitis	2	0	2 (3%)
Vocal cord paralysis	0	2	2 (3%)

sectability, reduced recurrence rates, and prolonged survival. Initial fears that radiation fibrosis would make resection more difficult have not been substantiated, especially if resection is carried out at a reasonably short time interval from treatment. In fact, tumor shrinkage and reduced blood loss from fibrosis appear to aid in the dissection.[89]

Survival statistics have been marginally improved in some series. Nakayama showed a five-year 22 per cent survival rate in 304 patients following four doses of 500 rads of cobalt therapy.[90] Sugimachi reported 16.7 per cent five-year survival rate in 104 patients following 2500 to 3000 rads in 18 to 22 fractions. Five-year survival rate was 45 per cent in 15 patients with histologically no viable tumor found at resection.[91] Van Andel reported resectability in 61 per cent of 133 patients following 4000 rads of tumor dose in 20 fractions over four weeks. Five-year survival rate was 21 per cent.[92] Launois noted no difference in resectability, operative mortality, morbidity, or pathologic stage at resection between two groups of irradiated and nonirradiated patients. Tumor dose was 4000 rads over 8 to 12 days. Five-year survival rate was about 10 per cent in each group.[93] Wilson found improved one-year, but not two-year, survival, comparing 26 patients who received a mean tumor dose of 4229 rads over four weeks preoperatively to 25 patients with no preoperative therapy.[89]

Treatment techniques, tumor doses, and fractionation vary greatly with the institution, making comparisons and interpretation of results difficult. It appears that lower doses are associated with less perioperative morbidity and still result in significant tumor response.

■ *Preoperative Combined Chemotherapy and Radiation*

The most recent promising therapeutic results described in the literature have followed combined preoperative chemotherapy, radiation, and tumor resection. For the first time, total eradication of local disease has been seen at resection in a significant percentage of patients. Initial reports using various chemoradiation protocols are summarized in Table 20–7. Theoretically, these protocols combine the local control of radiation and resection with the systemic effects of chemotherapy.

At Virginia Mason, 22 patients (13 with adenocarcinoma, 9 with squamous cell carcinoma) have had explorations following preoperative chemotherapy and radiation since January 1983.

Two months prior to operation, radiation (3000 cGY tumor dose) was given in 15 treatments over 19 days. Two cycles of cisplatin, 75 to 100 mg/ m^2 on days 1 and 29, and 5-FU, 750–1000 mg/m^2 continuous infusion days 1 through 4 and 29 through 32, were given to patients with squamous cell cancer. Mitomycin, 7.5 mg/m^2 on days 1 and 29, was added for patients with adenocarcinoma. Follow-up ranged from 2 to 44 months.

Nineteen of the 22 patients had resectable tumor (86 per cent). Three adenocarcinomas were unresectable. Operative death occurred in three patients (13.6 per cent). Eight patients (36 per cent) (three adenocarcinoma, five squamous cell carcinoma) had no evidence of disease on histopathologic examination of the resected specimen. Six of the eight patients are alive, five with no recurrence and one with lung recurrence. The two deaths in patients with no evidence of disease at resection were from operative mortality in one patient and lung and liver metastases in the other.

Four of 19 resected patients (21 per cent) have had recurrences, all at distant sites (three adenocarcinomas, one squamous cell carcinoma). One patient died of lung and liver metastases at one year, and three patients remain alive. Mean time to recurrence was 27.2 ± 6.5 months. Two of the recurrences followed resections with no evidence of disease at histologic examination.

Overall, 14 of 22 patients (64 per cent) are alive at 2 to 44 months follow-up with a mean survival of 29.6 ± 5.5 months. Comparison with 65 patients who had received no preoperative therapy revealed mean survival improvement approaching statistical significance ($p = 0.13$ Mantel-Cox statistical test).

Disappointment in combined preoperative chemotherapy and radiation protocols is based on two observations. First, many patients who begin the treatments are unable to complete the full protocol owing to overall poor health, treatment toxicity, disease progression, poor operative risk, or operative death. Second, the majority of recurrences are distant, sometimes occurring in unusual locations such as the lungs, and the subsequent clinical course is often fulminant.

Based on these observations, some have advocated eliminating the surgical arm of treatment, suggesting that resection will not prevent distant recurrence and the elimination of surgery may decrease treatment morbidity and mortality rates.[96] However, clinical restaging using CT scan, esophagography and endoscopic biopsy following preoperative treatment are not accurate compared to surgical-pathologic evaluation of the resected specimen.[98] Commonly, preoperative restaging will find no evidence for disease, but histologic ex-

Table 20–7. PREOPERATIVE COMBINED CHEMOTHERAPY AND RADIATION TREATMENT FOR ESOPHAGEAL CANCER

Group	Preoperative Therapy	Number of Patients	Clinically Downstaged	Resected	No Evidence of Disease at Resection	Treatment Mortality Rate	Survival Rate
Werner, 1979[94]	Methotrexate 2000 cGy	93 (squamous cell carcinoma)	NA	55 (59%)	15 (16%)	8 (14.5%)	Mean 26 months resected
Andersen, 1984[95]	Bleomycin 3000 cGy	65 (squamous cell carcinoma)	NA	35 (52%)	NA	8 (23%)	24.6% 2 year survival
Leichman, 1984[96]	5-FU* and mitomycin 3000 cGy	30 (squamous cell carcinoma)	NA	23 (77%)	6 (20%)	8 (27%)	Median 12 months
Leichman, 1984[96]	5-FU* and cisplatin 3000 cGy	21 (squamous cell carcinoma)	NA	15 (71%)	5 (24%)	5 (24%)	Median 24 months
Poplin, 1986[97]	5-FU* and cisplatin 3000 cGy	113 (squamous cell carcinoma)	NA	75 (66%)	18 (16%)	NA	Median 32 months, NED; Median 24 months, residual resected; Median 6 months, residual left
Campbell, 1985[98]	5-FU and cisplatin 300 cGy	21 (squamous cell carcinoma)	11 (52%)	15 (71%)	NA	3 (14%)	52% 2 year if curative resection performed
Popp, 1986[99]	5-FU, cisplatin or mitomycin, and vincristine 3000 cGy	27 (squamous cell carcinoma)	18 (66%)	10 (37%)	2 (7.4%)	6 (22%)	35% 30 months if resected
Parker, 1986[100]	5-FU and mitomycin 3000 rads	NA	NA	31 (squamous cell carcinoma)	11 (36%)	NA	33% 2 year in 21 patients followed >2 years
Virginia Mason Medical Center, 1986	See text	22 (13 adenocarcinoma and 9 squamous cell carcinoma)	NA	19 (86%)	8 (36%)	3 (13.6%)	See text

*Postoperative radiation given for residual disease at resection.
NA = not available; NED = No evidence of disease.

amination of the specimen after resection will find residual microscopic tumor. By omitting the surgical arm, many of the patients who would not go on to develop distant recurrence may theoretically be deprived of cure from local disease. Campbell found a 20 per cent two-year nonresected survival rate versus 50 per cent two-year resected survival rate following combined therapy.[98] Popp found that swallowing difficulties were present in 56 per cent of patients not resected following combined therapy while only 17 per cent of resected patients had dysphagia.[99]

Balancing the risks and benefits of combined modality treatment in these debilitated patients is difficult at best. Results of the various combined treatment series are difficult to interpret because the role of patient selection is not well defined. The effects of preoperative chemotherapy and radiation on operative morbidity and death may prove to be prohibitive in many patients. As statistics on morbidity and survival accrue, the ultimate effects of this promising new therapy will become clearer.

■ REFERENCES

1. Silverberg E, Lubera J: Cancer Statistics, 1986. CA-A Cancer J Clinicians, 36(1):9–25, 1986.
2. Schottenfeld D: Epidemiology of cancer of the esophagus. Sem Oncol, 11:92–100, 1984.
3. Yang CS: Research on esophageal cancer in China: A review. Cancer Res, 40:2633–2644, 1980.
4. Yang CS, Sun Y, Yang Q, Miller KW, Li G, Zheng SF, Ershow AG, Blot WJ, Li J: Vitamin A and other deficiencies in Linxian, a high esophageal cancer incidence area in northern China. J NCI, 73:1449–1453, 1984.
5. Foy H, Kondi A: The vulnerable esophagus: Riboflavin deficiency and squamous cell dysplasia of the skin and the esophagus. J NCI, 72:941–943, 1984.
6. Fraser P: Nitrates: Epidemiological evidence. IARC Sci Pub, 65:183–194, 1985.
7. Cheng SJ, Jiang YZ, Lo HZ: A mutagenic metabolite produced by Fusarium moniliforme isolated from Linxian county, China. Carcinogenesis, 6:903–905, 1985.
8. Burch PRJ: Variance and dissent: Esophageal cancer in relation to cigarette and alcohol consumption. J Chron Dis, 11:793–808, 1984.
9. Schoenberg BS, Bailor JC, Fraumeri JF: Certain mortality patterns of esophageal cancer in the United States. J NCI, 6:63–73, 1971.
10. Tuyns AJ, Pequignot G, Gignoux M, Valla A: Cancers of the digestive tract, alcohol and tobacco. Int J Cancer, 30:9–11, 1982.
11. Harper PS, Harper RMJ, Howel-Evans AW: Carcinoma of the oesophagus with tylosis. Q J Med, New Series XXXIX, 155:317–333, 1970.
12. Carter R, Brewer LA: Achalasia and esophageal carcinoma: Studies in early diagnosis for improved surgical management. Am J Surg, 130:114–120, 1975.
13. Just-Viera JO, Haight C: Achalasia and carcinoma of the esophagus. Surg Gynecol Obstet, 128:1081, 1967.
14. Joske RA, Benedict EB: The role of benign esophageal obstruction in the development of carcinoma of the esophagus. Gastroenterology, 36:749–755, 1959.
15. Chuong JJH, Dubovik S, McCallum RW: Achalasia as a risk factor for esophageal carcinoma: A reappraisal. Dig Dis Sci, 29:1105–1108, 1984.
16. Larsson LG, Sandstrom A, Westling P: Relationship of Plummer-Vinson disease to cancer of the upper alimentary tract in Sweden. Cancer Res, 35:3308–3316, 1975.
17. Appelqvist P, Salmo M: Lye corrosion carcinoma of the esophagus: A review of 63 cases. Cancer, 45:2655–2658, 1980.
18. Hopkins JRA, Postlethwait RW: Caustic burns and carcinoma of the esophagus. Ann Surg, 194:146–148, 1981.
19. Marchese MJ, Liskow A, Chang CH: Radiation therapy associated cancer of the esophagus. NY State J Med, 152–153, 1986.
20. Beebe GW, Kato H, Land CE: Studies of the mortality of A-bomb survivors. Radiat Res, 75:138–201, 1978.
21. Rosenberg JC, Budev H, Edwards RC, Singal S, Steiger ZWI, Sundareson AS: Analysis of adenocarcinoma in Barrett's esophagus utilizing a staging system. Cancer, 55:353–360, 1985.
22. Sarr MG, Hamilton SR, Marrone GC, Cameron JL: Barrett's esophagus: Its prevalence and association with adenocarcinoma in patients with symptoms of gastroesophageal reflux. Am J Surg, 149:187–193, 1985.
23. Saubier EC, Gouillat C, Samaniego C, Guillaud M, Moulinier B: Adenocarcinoma in columnar-lined Barrett's esophagus. Am J Surg, 150:365–369, 1985.
24. Postlethwait RW: Surgery of the Esophagus. New York, Appleton Century Crofts, 1979.
25. Ming S: Tumors of the esophagus and stomach. In Hartmanan WH (Ed): Atlas of Tumor Pathology. Washington, D.C., Armed Forces Institute of Pathology, 1985, pp 52–58.
26. Mannell A: Carcinoma of the esophagus. Curr Probl Surg, 19:569–570, 1982.
27. Faintuch J, Shepard KV, Levin B: Adenocarcinoma and other unusual variants of esophageal cancer. Sem Oncol, 11:196–202, 1984.
28. Skinner DB, Ferguson MK, Soriano A, Little AG, Staszak VM: Selection of operation for esophageal cancer based on staging. Ann Surg, 204:391–401, 1986.
29. Lightdale CJ, Winawer SJ: Screening diagnosis and staging of esophageal cancer. Sem Oncol, 11:101–112, 1984.
30. Guojun H, Linfang S, Dawei Z, Zhangcai L, Guoqing W, Shuxian L, Fubao C: Diagnosis and surgical treatment of early esophageal carcinoma. Chin Med J, 94:229–232, 1981.
31. Dowlatshahi K, Skinner DB, DeMeester TR, Zachary L, Bibbo M, Wied GL: Evaluation of brush cytology as an independent technique for detection of esophageal carcinoma. J Thorac Cardiovasc Surg, 89:848–851, 1985.
32. Akiyama H, Kogure T, Itai Y: The esophageal axis and its relationship to the resectability of carcinoma of the esophagus. Ann Surg, 176:30–36, 1972.
33. Mori S, Kasai M, Watanabe T, Shibuya I: Preoperative assessment of resectability for carcinoma of the thoracic esophagus. Part 1. Esophagogram and azygogram. Ann Surg, 190:100–105, 1979.
34. Monnier P, Savary M, Pasche R, Anani P: Intraepithelial carcinoma of the oesophagus: Endoscopic morphology. Endoscopy, 13:185–191, 1981.
35. Halvorsen RA, Thompson WM: Computed tomographic evaluation of esophageal carcinoma. Sem Oncol, 11:113–126, 1984.
36. Inculet RI, Keller SM, Dwyer A, Roth JA: Evaluation of noninvasive test for the preoperative staging of carcinoma of the esophagus: A prospective study. Ann Thorac Surg, 40:561–565, 1985.
37. Picus D, Balfe DM, Koehler RE, Roper CL, Owen JW:

Computed tomography in the staging of esophageal carcinoma. Radiology, *146*:433–438, 1983.

38. Freeny PC, Marks WM: Adenocarcinoma of the gastroesophageal junction: Barium and CT examination. AJR, *138*:1077–1084, 1982.

39. Lea JW, Prager RL, Bender HW: The questionable role of computed tomography in preoperative staging of esophageal cancer. Ann Thorac Surg, *38*:479–481, 1984.

40. Moss AA, Schnyder P, Thoeni RF, Margulis AR: Esophageal carcinoma: Pretherapy staging by computed tomography. AJR, *136*:1051–1056, 1981.

41. Choi TK, Siu KF, Lam KH, Wong J: Bronchoscopy and carcinoma of the esophagus. I. Findings of bronchoscopy in carcinoma of the esophagus. Am J Surg, *147*:757–759, 1984.

42. Choi Tk, Siu KF, Lam KH, Wong J: Bronchoscopy and carcinoma of the esophagus. II. Carcinoma of the esophagus with tracheobronchial involvement. Am J Surg, *147*:760–762, 1984.

43. Quint LE, Glazer GM, Orringer MB: Esophageal imaging by MR and CT: Study of normal anatomy and neoplasms. Radiology, *156*:727–731, 1985.

44. Kelson D: Chemotherapy of esophageal cancer. Semin Oncol, *11*(2):159–168, 1984.

45. Dinwoodie WR, Bartolucci AA, Lyman GH, Velez-Garcia E, Martelo OJ, Sarma PR: Phase II evaluation of Cisplatin, bleomycin, and vindesine in advanced squamous cell carcinoma of the esophagus: A southeastern cancer study group trial. Ca Treat Rep, *70*(2):267–270, 1986.

46. Resbeut M, Prise-Fleury EL, Ben-Hassel M, et al: Squamous cell carcinoma of the esophagus: Treatment by combined vincristine-methotrexate plus folinic acid rescue and cisplatin before radiation. Cancer, *56*:1246–1250, 1985.

47. Pearson JG: Radiotherapy for esophageal carcinoma. World J Surg, *5*:489–497, 1981.

48. Hancock S, Glatstein E: Radiation therapy of esophageal cancer. Semin Oncol, *11*(2):144–158, 1984.

49. van Andel JG, Dees J, Eijkenboom WM, van Howten H, Jobsen JJ, Mud HJ, et al: Therapy of esophageal carcinoma. Results from the Joint Group on Esophageal Carcinoma in Rotterdam. Acta Radiol [Oncol], *25*(2):115–120, 1986.

50. Angorn IB: Intubation in the treatment of carcinoma of the esophagus. World J Surg, *5*:535–541, 1981.

51. Ogilvie AL, Dronfield MW, Ferguson R, Atkinson M: Palliative intubation of esophagogastric neoplasms at fiberoptic endoscopy. Gut, *23*:1060–1067, 1982.

52. Ghazi A, Nussbaum M: A new approach to the management of malignant esophageal obstruction and esophagorespiratory fistula. Ann Thorac Surg, *41*:531–534, 1986.

53. Kirschner M: Ein neues verfahrender Oesophagus plastik. Arch Klin Chir, *114*:604, 1920.

54. Roeher HD, Horeyseck G: The Kirschner bypass operation—a palliation for complicated esophageal carcinoma. World J Surg, *5*:543–546, 1981.

55. Wong J, Lam KH, Wei WI, Ong GB: Results of the Kirschner operation. World J Surg, *5*:547–552, 1981.

56. Fisher RD, Brawley RK, Kieffer RF: Esophagogastrostomy in the treatment of carcinoma of the distal two-thirds of the esophagus. Ann Thorac Surg, *14*:658–669, 1972.

57. Belsey R, Hiebert CA: An exclusive right thoracic approach for cancer of the middle third of the esophagus. Ann Thorac Surg, *18*:1–15, 1974.

58. Skinner DB: Esophageal malignancies: Experience with 110 cases. Surg Clin North Am, *56*:137–147, 1976.

59. Griffen WO, Daugherty ME, McGee EM, Utley JR: Unified approach to carcinoma of the esophagus. Ann Surg, *183*:511–516, 1976.

60. Ellis FH, Gibb SP: Esophagogastrectomy for carcinoma: Current hospital mortality and morbidity rates. Ann Surg, *190*:699–705, 1979.

61. Dark JF, Mousalli H, Vaughan R: Surgical treatment of carcinoma of the oesophagus. Thorax, *36*:891–895, 1981.

62. McKeown KC: Resection of midesophageal carcinoma with esophagogastric anastomosis. World J Surg, *5*:517–525, 1981.

63. Hoffman TH, Kelley JR, Grover FL, Trinkle JK: Carcinoma of the esophagus: An aggressive one-stage palliative approach. J Thorac Cardiovasc Surg, *81*:44–49, 1981.

64. Akiyama H, Tsurumaru M, Kawamura T, Ono Y: Principles of surgical treatment for carcinoma of the esophagus: Analysis of lymph node involvement. Ann Surg, *194*:438–446, 1981.

65. Maillet P, Baulieux J, Boulez J, Benhaim R: Carcinoma of the thoracic esophagus: results of one-stage surgery (271 cases). Am J Surg, *143*:629–634, 1982.

66. Le-Tian X, Zhen-Fu S, Ze-Jian L, Lian-Hun W: Surgical treatment of carcinoma of the esophagus and cardiac portion of the stomach in 850 patients. Ann Thorac Surg, *35*:542–547, 1983.

67. Keagy BA, Murray GF, Starek PJ, Battaglini JW, Lores ME, Wilcox BR: Esophagogastrectomy as palliative treatment for thoracic esophageal carcinoma: Results obtained in the setting of a thoracic surgery residency program. Ann Thorac Surg, *38*:611–616, 1984.

68. Fein R, Kelsen DP, Geller N, Bains M, McCormack P, Brennan MF: Adenocarcinoma of the esophagus and gastroesophageal junction: Prognostic factors and results of therapy. Cancer, *56*:2512–2518, 1985.

69. Gatzinsky P, Berglin E, Dernevik L, Larsson I, William-Olsson G: Resectional operations and long-term results in carcinoma of the esophagus. J Thorac Cardiovasc Surg, *89*:71–76, 1985.

70. Galandiuk S, Hermann RE, Gassman JJ, Cosgrove DM: Cancer of the esophagus: The Cleveland Clinic experience. Ann Surg, *3*:101–108, 1986.

71. Giuli R, Sancho-Garnier H: Diagnostic, therapeutic, and prognostic features of cancers of the esophagus: Results of the international prospective study conducted by the OESO group (790 patients). Surgery, *99*:614–622, 1986.

72. Lewis I: The surgical treatment of carcinoma of the esophagus with special reference to a new operation for growths of the middle third. Br J Surg, *34*:18, 1946.

73. Heimlich HJ: Esophagoplasty with reversed gastric tube. Am J Surg, *123*:80, 1972.

74. Bernstein JM, Juler GL: Colon interposition versus esophagogastrostomy for esophageal carcinoma. Am Surg, *46*(4):216–222, 1980.

75. Wilkins EW: Long-segment colon substitutions for the esophagus. Ann Surg, *192*:722–725, 1980.

76. Kasai M, Nishihira T: Reconstruction using pedicled jejunal segments after resection for carcinoma of the cervical esophagus. Surg Gynecol Obstet, *163*::145–152, 1986.

77. Kakegawa T, Yamana H, Ando N: Analysis of surgical treatment for carcinoma situated in the cervical esophagus. Surgery, *97*:150–156, 1985.

78. Goldfaden D, Orringer MB, Appleman HD, Kalish R: Adenocarcinoma of the distal esophagus and gastric cardia: Comparison of results of transhiatal esophagectomy and thoracoabdominal esophagogastrectomy. J Thorac Cardiovasc Surg, *91*:242–247, 1986.

79. Orringer MB: Transhiatal esophagectomy without thoracotomy for carcinoma of the esophagus. *In* Mannick JA, ed: Advances in Surgery. Chicago, Year Book Medical Publishers, Inc., 1986, pp 47–49.

80. Finley RJ, Grace M, Duff JH: Esophagogastrectomy without thoracotomy for carcinoma of the cardia and lower part of the esophagus. Surg Gynecol Obstet, *160*:49–56, 1985.

81. Kirk RM: A trial of total gastrectomy, combined with total thoracic oesophagectomy without formal thoracotomy, for carcinoma at or near the cardia of the stomach. Br J Surg, *68*:577–579, 1981.

82. Chassin JL: Esophagogastrectomy: Data favoring end-to-side anastomosis. Ann Surg, *188*:22–27, 1978.

83. Shapiro S, Hamlin D, Morgenstern L: The fate of the pylorus in esophagoantrostomy. Surg Gynecol Obstet, *135*:216–218, 1972.

84. Angorn IB: Oesophagogastrostomy without a drainage procedure in oesophageal carcinoma. Br J Surg, *62*:601–604, 1975.

85. Burt ME, Brennan MF: Nutritional support of the patient with esophageal cancer. Semin Oncol, *11*:127–135, 1984.

86. Isono K, Onoda S, Ishikawa T, Sato H, Nakayama K: Studies on the causes of deaths from esophageal carcinoma. Cancer, *49*:2173–2179, 1982.

87. Shields TW, Rosen ST, Hellerstein SM, Tsang T, Ujiki GT, Kies MS: Multimodality approach to treatment of carcinoma of the esophagus. Arch Surg, *119*:558–562, 1984.

88. Bains MS, Kelsen DP, Beattie EJ, Martini N: Treatment of esophageal carcinoma by combined preoperative chemotherapy. Ann Thorac Surg, *34*:521–528, 1982.

89. Wilson SE, Hiatt JR, Stabile BE, Williams RA: Cancer of the distal esophagus and cardia: Preoperative irradiation prolongs survival. Am J Surg, *50*:114–121, 1985.

90. Nakayama K: My experience in the management of esophageal cancer. Internat Surg, *64*:7–11, 1979.

91. Sugimachi K, Matsufuji H, Kai H, Masuda H, Ueo H, Inokuchi K, Jingu K: Preoperative irradiation for carcinoma of the esophagus. Surg Gynecol Obstet, *162*:174–176, 1986.

92. van Andel JG, Dees J, Dijkhuis CM, Fokkens W, vanHouten H, deJong PC, van Woerkom-Eykenboom WM: Carcinoma of the esophagus: Results of treatment. Ann Surg, *190*:684–689, 1979.

93. Launois B, Delarue D, Campion JP, Kerbaol M: Preoperative radiotherapy for carcinoma of the esophagus. Surg Gynecol Obstet, *153*:690–692, 1981.

94. Werner ID: The multidisciplinary approach in the management of squamous carcinoma of the oesophagus. Gastrointest Res, *5*:130–135, 1979.

95. Andersen AP, Berdal P, Edsmyr F, Hagen S, Hatlevoll R, Nygaard K, Ottosen P, Peterffy P, Kongsholm H, Elgen K: Irradiation, chemotherapy and surgery in esophageal cancer: A randomized clinical study. Radiotherapy Oncol, *2*:179–188, 1984.

96. Leichman L, Steiger Z, Seydel HG, Vaitkevicius VK: Combined preoperative chemotherapy and radation therapy for cancer of the esophagus: The Wayne State University, Southwest Oncology Group and Radiation Therapy Oncology Group experience. Sem Oncol, *11*:178–185, 1984.

97. Poplin E, Leichman L, Seydel G, Steiger L, Fleming C: SWOG 8037: Combined therapy for squamous cell carcinoma of the esophagus (SCCE). Proc Am Soc Clin Oncol, *5*:80, 1986.

98. Campbell WR, Taylor SA, Pierce GE, Hermreck AS, Thomas JH: Therapeutic alternatives in patients with esophageal cancer. Am J Surg, *150*:665–668, 1985.

99. Popp MB, Hawley D, Reising J, Bongiovanni G, Weesner R, Moomaw CJ, Martelo O, Aron B: Improved survival in squamous esophageal cancer. Arch Surg, *121*:1330–1335, 1986.

100. Parker EF, Marks RD, Kratz JM, Chaikhouni A, Warren T, Bartles DM: Chemoradiation therapy and resection for carcinoma of the esophagus: Short-term results. Ann Thorac Surg, *40*:121–125, 1985.

101. Mitchell RL: Abdominal and right thoracotomy approach as standard procedure for esophagogastrectomy with low morbidity. Thorac Cardiovasc Surg *93*:202–211, 1987.

21

Esophageal Replacement, Bypass, and Intubation

G. Alec Patterson

In the surgical management of benign and malignant disease of the esophagus, replacement, bypass, or intubation of the esophagus is often necessary. Although carcinoma of the esophagus has necessitated performance of these procedures for years, they have been increasingly employed for benign disease as thoracic surgeons embark on ever more complex attempts at reconstruction. This chapter will not be a comprehensive review of all available methods for replacement, bypass, or intubation, but rather will serve to indicate the preferences and techniques employed by the Thoracic Surgical Group in Toronto. Our group performs 35 to 40 esophagectomies annually.

■ *Esophageal Replacement*

This discussion is restricted, for the most part, to the replacement of the entire thoracic esophagus as well as the replacement of the esophagus and pharynx following pharyngolaryngectomy. Several organs are readily available, including stomach, either as a whole pedicled graft or as a gastric tube leaving the remaining gastric remnant intact. The colon is advocated by many authors as the replacement of choice, particularly for benign disease.[1] The left colon is most favored as a substitute, but the right colon can also be employed. Jejunum is also available for use as a pedicle or a free graft using a microvascular anastomosis to the mesenteric vessels.

■ STOMACH

Stomach is our first choice for esophageal replacement following resection for malignant esophageal disease, as well as most benign esophageal conditions. The advantages of the stomach are many. The conduit is readily constructed, establishing natural continuity in the GI tract. Only a single anastomosis is required between the stomach and the esophageal or pharyngeal remnant. Adequate length of stomach is available in virtually all patients to reach as high as the nasopharynx following esophageal resection. The vascular supply is excellent, as long as care is taken to preserve the arterial and, in particular, venous supply to the stomach.

The preferred route of reconstruction is transthoracic, placing the gastric pedicle in the posterior mediastinum and in the natural bed of the esophagus. This is the shortest route between the abdomen and the neck. In addition, it is not necessary to excise a portion of manubrium to enlarge the thoracic inlet, as is often required following substernal transposition. The incidence of anastomotic leak is lessened when the anastomosis is placed in the posterior neck, surrounded by healthy local tissue.[2] Certainly the stomach can be placed substernally in situations in which the posterior mediastinum has been obliterated, such as following major sepsis, after attempted previous reconstruction, or in certain cases of lye ingestion. Substernal gastric positioning is a valuable option in bypass procedures, as will be discussed later.

It is our usual practice to establish an esophago-gastric anastomosis in the neck for a variety of reasons. First, the procedure is readily performed without great technical difficulty. If meticulous anastomotic technique is employed, anastomotic disruption will occur in about 5 to 10 per cent of cervical esophagogastric anastomoses. This usually presents no significant problem.[3,4] These patients are usually able to maintain their nutrition orally by application of local pressure over the site of leak until healing occurs, usually in a period of a week to 10 days. Injury to the recurrent laryngeal nerve can occur during dissection necessary for esophagogastric anastomoses in the neck. However, with careful dissection and avoidance of the use of retractors in the neck, particularly over the tracheal esophageal groove, the incidence of vocal cord paralysis is less than 5 per cent.[5,6]

Another advantage of neck anastomosis is the avoidance of the inevitable esophagogastric reflux, which occurs following intrathoracic esophagogastric anastomoses. However, Wong[7] prefers to use a high intrathoracic esophagogastric anastomosis following a total thoracic esophagectomy. This anastomosis can be readily performed at the apex of the chest through the thoracotomy incision, usually employing an EEA stapling instrument. A hand-sewn anastomosis high in the chest provides a technical challenge. In addition, although the incidence of anastomotic leak in the thorax is less than that observed following a neck anastomosis,[3] the consequences of a major anastomotic disruption in the chest are catastrophic.

It was our past practice to establish a gastro-esophageal anastomosis high in the right side of the chest, as is preferred by Wong. However, for reasons stated above, we have in the past decade converted to cervical gastroesophageal anastomoses in almost every case. We would choose to transpose the stomach to the neck regardless of the level of esophageal lesion. Adenocarcinoma or squamous cell cancer of the lower third are treated by total esophagectomy with cervical gastric anastomosis if adequate length of stomach is available.

In selected patients we would choose limited esophagogastrectomy with the anastomosis below the aortic arch in the left side of the chest. This thoracoabdominal operation is well tolerated and should be employed in those patients whose lower third tumors are so extensive as to require excision of a portion of gastric fundus. Other patients suitable for this procedure are those with lower third lesions and extensive nodal metastatic disease along the lesser curve or celiac axis. These patients tolerate limited resection well and enjoy good swallowing for their short period of survival. In these patients there is minimal risk of long-term reflux problems and associated anastomotic stricture.

The stomach is a suitable conduit for esophageal replacement in the vast majority of patients undergoing esophageal replacement. An existing feeding gastrostomy is not a contraindication to use of the stomach. Often the gastrostomy site can be incorporated into the lesser curve suture line. In such cases in which the gastrostomy is placed remote from the lesser curve, the gastrostomy can be easily closed longitudinally without compromising length or vascularity of the stomach.

Technical Details ■ The stomach is prepared in a standard fashion, dividing between ligatures the short gastric vessels as well as the vessels along the greater curve outside the gastroepiploic arcade (Fig. 21–1). We have avoided the use of clips particularly on the gastric side since they often fall off during the passage of the stomach through the mediastinum to the neck. This greater curve dissection should be carried to the level of the pylorus, taking extreme care to preserve the arterial supply and venous drainage of the right gastroepiploic arcade. Rough handling or excessive traction at this point can result in injury to the gastroepiploic vein at its union with the middle colic vein, producing annoying hemorrhage as well as compromise to the venous drainage of the pedicle. Following mobilization of the greater curve, by lifting the stomach upward and to the right, the left gastric vessels can easily be exposed and ligated. The gastrohepatic omentum is divided. A generous Kocher maneuver is performed, allowing the pylorus to be elevated to the level of esophageal hiatus.

If the pyloric canal appears narrowed and does not admit a thumb easily, then a pyloromyotomy is performed. It is certainly not our usual practice to perform a pyloroplasty because transverse closure of the pyloroplasty does sacrifice gastric length necessary for passage of the stomach to the neck.

A generous length of gastric conduit can be obtained by increasing the length of the lesser curve suture line. Cutting well down along the lesser curve increases the length of the gastric conduit as well as reducing its bulk for passage through the mediastinum. We employ the GIA stapling instrument to create the suture line, reinforcing the staple line with a continuous absorbable suture.

Passing the stomach up through the mediastinum is particularly easy when a three-incision approach (laparotomy, right anterolateral thoracotomy, and right-sided neck incision) is employed (see Fig. 21–1). Another advantage of this approach is that the greater curvature of the stomach can be sewn to the mediastinal tissue preventing rotation and subsequent gastric dilatation during the postoperative period (Fig. 21–2). If a nonthoracotomy ap-

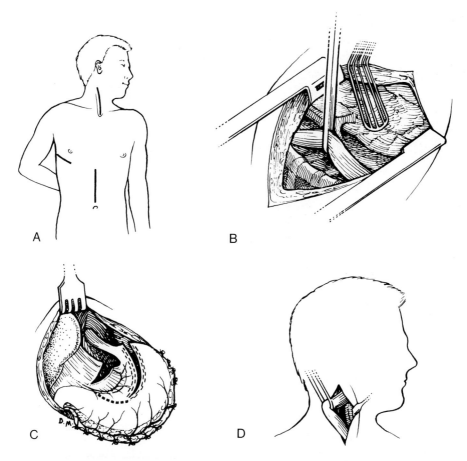

Figure 21–1. *A,* Positioning of the patient and location of incisions for a ''three hole'' esophagectomy. *B,* With the upper hand retractor in place, exposure of the upper abdomen is excellent, enabling complete mobilization of the stomach, preserving the gastroepiploic arcade and dividing the lesser curve using multiple applications of the stapling instrument. Excision of a generous portion of lesser curve allows suitable gastric length for transposition to the neck. *C,* Single lung ventilation allows retraction of the atelectatic right lung anteriorly. This exposes the posterior mediastinum and enables easy mobilization of the esophagus posteriorly. *D,* The esophagus is mobilized in the neck, thereby minimizing risk of recurrent laryngeal nerve injury.

proach is selected for resection, particular care must be taken to avoid traumatizing or twisting the stomach during passage to the neck. Passage of the stomach through the mediastinum is facilitated by use of a clear plastic arthroscopy bag. The stomach is placed in the bag. A long instrument is passed down from the neck through the mediastinum and esophageal hiatus into the abdomen. The bag is grasped and drawn up into the neck (Fig. 21–3). The stomach passes easily along the bag up into the neck without placing any traction whatsoever on the fundus of the stomach. The bag is then easily pulled away and discarded.

The early and late results of whole stomach transpositions are excellent and support its use as the conduit of choice in the majority of patients. We have recently reviewed 25 patients who have survived one to four years following esophagectomy for squamous carcinoma. Each patient had a reconstruction using stomach with a cervical esoph-

agogastric anastomosis. All patients were able to take a regular diet within two weeks of surgery. Six patients had some degree of dysphagia at follow-up. In three patients it was effectively treated by several dilatations. Three others developed recurrent carcinoma at the anastomosis and periodic dilatations were required. Two patients experienced mild regurgitation and one patient has nocturnal aspiration and cough. Three patients had anorexia and all of them were found to have systemic recurrent carcinoma. Two patients had vomiting in association with chemotherapy. Only one patient had symptoms of delayed gastric emptying requiring pyloroplasty.

Our group has reported results of gastric reconstruction in 22 patients undergoing pharyngolaryngectomy.[8] Most had undergone previous high-dose cervical irradiation. There was one operative death. Three of four anastomotic leaks closed within 10 days. Only one leak required surgical

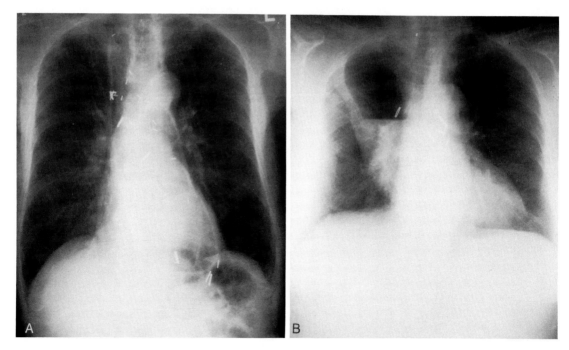

Figure 21–2. *A,* Proper positioning of the gastric transposition in the mediastinum by securing the greater curve aspect to the posterior mediastinum, preventing rotation of the stomach on its lesser curve axis and subsequent dilatation. *B,* Rotation and the gastric transposition on its lesser curve aspect have placed the greater curve aspect of the stomach adjacent to the right superolateral chest wall. The transposition is dilated. The large air-fluid level is indicative of chronic stasis within the gastric conduit.

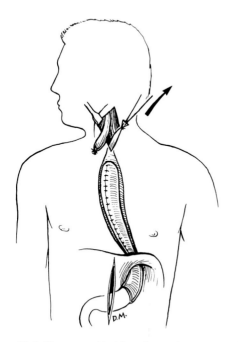

Figure 21–3. Placement of incisions for esophagectomy without thoracotomy. The gastric conduit is placed within the clear plastic arthroscopy bag. Traction on the bag is exerted superiorly pulling the conduit up through the posterior mediastinum and into the neck without any direct traction being placed on the gastric conduit itself. When the stomach has reached suitable position in the neck the bag is pulled directly up through the mediastinum out through the neck incision and discarded.

closure. Mean hospital stay was 31 days. All patients leaving hospital could take a regular diet. Palliation was excellent in all 21 operative survivors. Lam and his colleagues have had similar good results in a large number of patients who survived pharyngoesophagectomy and reconstruction by gastric transposition.[9]

Reversed and nonreversed gastric tubes can be employed as esophageal replacement. However, we have generally employed this therapeutic option in esophageal bypass situations. The added problems of the long suture line and tenuous vascular supply are added risks, and there are no additional advantages over the use of the entire stomach as a conduit.

■ COLON

Colon provides a useful and effective substitute for the esophagus in many situations. It has been used for both total esophageal replacement as well as short segments of distal esophagus. It is the preferred conduit of several authors, particularly for benign disease.[10] The right or transverse colon can be employed as an isoperistaltic graft on the middle colic artery. The left colon is then readily employed as an isoperistaltic segment based on the left colic artery or as an antiperistaltic conduit on the middle colic artery. It has been stated that it makes little difference whether colic grafts are placed iso- or antiperistaltic with respect to long-term function. However, the colon retains some motor function in its transposed position. Troublesome discomfort and regurgitation can occur in patients with antiperistaltic segments. Pearson and Belsey have personal experience with a small number of such patients. The clinical results are better with isoperistaltic colon interposition.[11] Our preference is to employ isoperistaltic left colon as the colonic conduit of choice.

The vascularity of the colon in general is excellent. It is useful to obtain mesenteric angiograms preoperatively, particularly in elderly patients. By extensive mobilization of the colonic mesentery the vessels can be well visualized with a bright light source directed on the opposite side of the mesentery. A sterile fiberoptic light source is particularly useful in this regard. Multiple fine vascular occlusion clamps can be used to temporarily occlude feeding vessels to determine viability on the main pedicle. There are several disadvantages with the use of colon as a substitute. Two additional anastomoses are required: cologastric and colocolonic. The colon tends to dilate and become redundant over time. Patients often develop increasing dysphagia, bloating, and pain when this occurs. Placement of the colon in the posterior mediastinum, substernal, or subcutaneous position does not prevent subsequent dilatation and redundancy. It is a very difficult problem to prevent. Placement of the colon without redundancy tends to lessen the subsequent problems but does not eliminate them altogether.

Nonetheless, colon has been used extensively for esophageal replacement. It is an excellent esophageal substitute in children.[12] Kelly et al.[13] reported long-term follow-up in 23 children undergoing long segment esophageal replacement using right or left colon. There was one operative death. Early complications, primarily colonic ischemia, anastomotic leak, or stricture, were seen in 14 patients. However, long-term function was excellent in 19 of 22 patients.

■ JEJUNUM

We have little experience with small bowel for long segment esophageal substitution. However, in patients in whom the stomach and colon are unsuitable for use, the jejunum can be employed. Varco's group reported long-term results into adulthood in 16 staged jejunal grafts placed during childhood.[14] The jejunum was brought to the neck as a pedicled graft in every case. By division of the mesentery overlying arcade vessels, as well as dividing an occasional secondary arcade, adequate length can be achieved.[15] There were no deaths in this series of patients. Long-term function was excellent.

Similar techniques can be employed in adults, achieving long lengths of jejunum as a pedicled graft for esophageal replacement. Free jejunal grafts can be used as short segment replacements. This has been recently advocated for reconstruction of the hypopharynx and cervical esophagus. Excellent results have been obtained using microvascular techniques to provide adequate viability to these free grafts. Multiple free grafts have also been employed in sequence to reconstruct the entire thoracic esophagus. We have experience in one such patient whose esophagus was reconstructed with three separate free jejunal grafts.

■ *Esophageal Bypass*

Locally advanced carcinoma of the esophagus is the usual indication for esophageal bypass. When life expectancy is short, palliation is the only important consideration. Patients with locally unresectable carcinoma, malignant tracheoesophageal fistulas, or extensive metastatic disease require immediate and effective short-term relief of their local esophageal symptoms. Unfortunately, esophageal bypass is associated with significant operative mortality rates. Postlethwaite[16] reported mortality rates of 41 per cent employing a variety of bypass conduits.

Our preference is to use stomach as a conduit. Whole stomach can be brought up readily in the substernal position for anastomosis to the cervical esophagus, thereby excluding the remaining thoracic esophagus. Mobilization of the stomach is identical to that described above. The substernal tunnel must be spacious. A generous opening in the thoracic inlet is required. It is often necessary to resect a portion of the manubrium and medial head of the clavicle to achieve a satisfactory opening for the fundus of the stomach. With a sizable opening, the vascularity to the stomach will not be compromised. Despite these precautions, the incidence of anastomotic disruption is high. Wong reported an esophagogastric leak rate of 47 per cent in patients undergoing bypass.[7]

Management of the remaining esophagus is somewhat controversial. Attempts at oversewing both the proximal and distal excluded ends have usually met with failure.[2] If both ends of the esophagus heal, an esophageal mucocele can occur over the long term. Certainly, this is not a concern in the vast majority of patients requiring esophageal bypass, for most patients die of local or distant metastatic disease in a very short time. We have experience with only one such patient who developed a symptomatic mucocele six years following esophageal bypass for carcinoma. This patient's symptoms of airway compression were relieved by excision of the esophageal remnant.

The Kirschner bypass operation has been used effectively by Wong and his colleagues.[17] The distal esophagus is anastomosed to a roux-en-Y loop of jejunum to establish drainage of the distal esophagus following substernal or subcutaneous gastric transposition. This adds a moderate amount of operating time to a palliative procedure. However, Wong reports only one complication attributable to esophagojejunostomy in 142 patients undergoing Kirschner bypass procedures.[17]

To avoid problems of distal esophageal drainage, a reversed gastric tube (Gavriliu) constructed from the greater curvature can be employed to achieve satisfactory esophageal bypass. This procedure is readily performed, constructing an adequate tube of stomach using multiple applications of the GIA stapling instrument. The tube can then be passed substernally to the neck. These tubes are associated with a very high incidence of anastomotic leak. Postlethwaite[16] reported cervical bypass using an isoperistaltic greater curvature tube. In his series only seven of 34 colonic bypasses and one of seven substernal gastric bypasses were complicated by anastomotic leak.

Because of the tenuous blood supply and very high incidence of anastomotic disruption following anastomosis to the esophagus and the gastric tube, we have advocated carrying out this procedure as a staged procedure, placing the gastric tube in its bed and exteriorizing the upper end of the tube for subsequent anastomosis seven to ten days following creation of the tube. This allows adequate protection against widespread contamination should a leak occur in the neck.

Other organ substitutes are available for bypass procedures, with colon being the most readily available and widely employed.

■ *Esophageal Intubation*

Morbidity and mortality rates of bypass procedures are high. Survival time is usually short, and it is unreasonable to subject many of these patients to procedures associated with such increased mortality rate. Esophageal intubation offers a valuable option in patients with locally advanced unresectable tumors who are either not candidates for rad-

ical resection or develop local recurrence following radiation. Patients with malignant tracheo-esophageal fistulas benefit from intubation, particularly when there is a major degree of esophageal obstruction in association with the fistula. A wide variety of prosthetic tubes have been designed for esophageal intubation.

Tubes can be placed by "pulsion" or "traction" techniques. With the availability of small caliber flexible gastroscopes and improved dilating equipment, tubes usually can be placed by the pulsion technique. This is particularly true of upper and middle thoracic esophageal lesions. Lesions of the lower third are usually best intubated using a traction technique.

The standard tube used in our institution is a Celestin tube. This tube is designed for use by traction technique, pulling the tube through the tumor via a laparotomy and gastrotomy. Payne[18] reported a 10 per cent mortality rate and a 90 per cent acceptable swallowing among 150 patients having this tube placed by traction technique. However, recent improvements in instrumentation have allowed placement of Celestin tubes from above without the need for laparotomy in the majority of patients.

The malignant stricture is dilated to a size 36 or 38 French bougie under fluoroscopic control. The tube is cut to size, allowing its inferior end to be well below the inferior border of the tumor. The tube is placed over a well-lubricated small gauge fiberoptic gastroscope. The gastroscope is then placed under direct vision into the stomach, and the Celestin tube is advanced over the gastroscope into an appropriate position. Its position can then be checked as the gastroscope is withdrawn. A firm seating of the tube is possible using a rigid esophagoscope.

Angorn of Durban has reported results of esophageal intubation in a very large series of patients with squamous cell carcinoma of the esophagus treated in a recent five-year period.[19] This group has a depth of experience which would be impossible to accumulate in other parts of the world where esophageal carcinoma is not nearly so common. Most of these patients present very late and are, as a result, technically inoperable. Their management of such patients should serve as a guide for other centers with much less experience.

Upper thoracic lesions in 1045 patients were intubated with a Procter-Livingstone tube (Latex Products, Johannesburg). This soft latex tube is easily placed by pulsion technique. During the same period 90 patients with lower thoracic lesions had Celestin tubes inserted by traction. The mean age of both patient groups was similar, as was duration of dysphagia prior to presentation. Mortality rates were similar: 16 per cent for pulsion and 20 per cent for traction. However, complications were seen in 39 per cent of traction tubes and only 26 per cent of pulsion tubes. Bronchopneumonia was the commonest complication in both groups. Local problems, such as wound infection, subphrenic abscess, and gastric fistula, accounted for the increased morbidity in the laparotomy group.

Pulsion intubation was successful in 80 per cent of patients. Tube migration (usually proximal) occurred in 6 per cent but was corrected by reintubation in each case. Average duration of hospital stay was 3.4 days and mean survival was 6.8 months. Traction intubation was successful in 73 per cent of patients. Average hospital stay was 15.4 days and mean survival period was 5.9 months. In a much smaller series of patients using a variety of tubes, Hankins et al.[20] reported a mortality rate greater than 40 per cent. Very poor results were obtained in upper third esophageal carcinomas.

Angorn[19] also described his experience with pulsion intubation in 184 patients with malignant esophagorespiratory fistulas. The communication was to the trachea in 57 per cent, bronchus in 40 per cent, and a pulmonary abscess cavity in 3 per cent. Mortality rate was 25 per cent. Effective palliation was achieved in all survivors.

Other tubes are available but we have little experience with their use. We have employed soft Silastic salivary tubes in a number of circumstances. Patients with high cervical lesions pose a difficult management problem, particularly following radiation. They usually have significant pain, as well as severe dysphagia. While there is an adequate "shelf" on which to seat a Celestin tube, there is not adequate length superiorly to place the large funnel within the esophagus. The funnel would sit well up in the pharynx in an unacceptable position. The short, wide flange of the salivary tubes sits nicely in the superior esophagus or indeed at the cricopharyngeus. We have also employed this same tube successfully to stent a large cervical esophagogastric anastomotic leak.

Improved laser technology and equipment will enable endoscopers to palliate many of these patients without intubation (see Chapter 25). Nd-YAG contact laser probes are now available, which can be easily employed to core out lengthy esophageal lesions without transmural injury or perforation. We are just beginning our experience with the use of such contact probes, but anticipate that this technology will avoid the necessity for palliative esophageal intubation in many patients with unresectable carcinoma.

■ Summary

Our preference is to employ whole stomach as a conduit to replace the thoracic esophagus. We prefer to perform esophagogastric anastomosis in the neck. If properly mobilized, a normal stomach will always reach the neck following generous removal of lesser curvature. Left colon is our preference if stomach is unavailable. If the stomach and colon cannot be employed, then a free jejunal graft would be selected.

Whole stomach is the bypass conduit of choice for malignant or benign disease. The majority of patients requiring esophageal intubation for palliation can be intubated from above using the pulsion technique. A variety of tubes can be inserted in this manner, providing acceptable results with less morbidity and mortality than that associated with a traction technique.

■ REFERENCES

1. Belsey R: Reconstruction of the esophagus with left colon. J Thorac Cardiovasc Surg, 49:33, 1965.
2. Orringer MB: Substernal gastric bypass of the excluded thoracic esophagus. Results of an ill-advised operation. Surgery, 96:467, 1984.
3. Orringer MB: Trans-hiatal esophagectomy for benign disease. J Thorac Cardiovasc Surg, 90:649, 1985.
4. Skinner DB: En-bloc resection for neoplasms of the esophagus and cardia. J Thorac Cardiovasc Surg, 85:59, 1983.
5. Shahian DM, Neptune WB, Ellis FH, et al: Trans-thoracic vs. extra-thoracic esophagectomy: Mortality, morbidity and long term survival. Ann Thorac Surg, 41:237, 1986.
6. Kirk RM: Palliative resection of esophageal carcinoma without formal thoracotomy. Br J Surg, 61:689, 1974.
7. Wong J: Personal communication, 1986.
8. Moores DWO, Ilves R, Cooper JD, et al: One stage reconstruction for pharyngolaryngectomy: Esophagectomy and pharyngogastrostomy without thoracotomy. J Thorac Cardiovasc Surg, 85:330, 1983.
9. Lam KH, Wong J, Lim STK: Pharyngogastric anastomosis following pharyngolaryngoesophagectomy: Analysis of 151 cases. World J Surg, 5:509, 1981.
10. Skinner DB: Surgical treatment for esophageal carcinoma. Semin Oncol, 11:136, 1984.
11. Clark J, Modri A, Moosa AR, et al: Functional evaluation of the interposed colon as an esophageal substitute. Ann Surg, 183:93, 1976.
12. Campbell JR, Webber BR, Harrison MW, et al: Esophageal replacement in infants and children by colon interposition. Am J Surg, 144:29, 1982.
13. Kelly JP, Shackelford GD, Roper CL: Esophageal replacement with colon in children: Functional results in long-term growth. Ann Thorac Surg, 36:634, 1983.
14. Ring WS, Varco RL, R'Heureux PR, et al: Esophageal replacement with jejunum in children. J Thorac Cardiovasc Surg, 918, 1982.
15. Folker JE, Ring S, Varco RL: Technique of jejunal interposition for esophageal replacement. J Thorac Cardiovasc Surg, 83:928, 1982.
16. Postlethwaite RW: Complications and deaths after opera-

tions for esophageal carcinoma. J Thorac Cardiovasc Surg, 85:827, 1983.

17. Wong J, Lam KH, Wei WI, et al: Results of the Kirschner operation. World J Surg, 5:547, 1981.

18. Payne SW: Palliation of esophageal carcinoma. Editorial. Ann Thorac Surg, 208, 1979.

19. Angorn IB: Intubation and treatment of carcinoma of the esophagus. World J Surg, 5:535, 1981.

20. Hankins JR, Cole FN, Attar S, et al: Palliation of esophageal carcinoma with intraluminal tubes: Experience with thirty patients. Ann Thorac Surg, 28:224, 1978

22

Gastroesophageal Reflux in the Pediatric Patient

Dennis L. Christie

Gastroesophageal reflux (GER) is a common disease in the pediatric population and it probably occurs once in every 500 patients. Fortunately, about 65 per cent of all infants with GER will be symptom-free by two years of age. Thirty per cent will have prolonged clinical symptoms that last beyond four years of age, and approximately 5 per cent may develop esophageal stricture (Fig. 22–1).[1]

Reflux symptoms in infants and children are different from those in adults. Vomiting is the most frequent symptom and is seen in 72 to 90 per cent of patients. In infancy, the vomiting can be projectile and generally begins in the first month of life.[2,3] For this reason, it is important to remember other causes of projectile vomiting that can occur in early infancy such as pyloric stenosis, antral web, duodenal band, or malrotation with volvulus. Since any of these conditions can present with projectile vomiting, the diagnosis of GER is based upon the concept that the other anatomic causes of vomiting have been excluded. Often the material will be regurgitated. The regurgitation can occur immediately after feeding, several hours after, or just before the next feeding (Table 22–1).

If the amount of vomited formula is significant, the infant can fail to thrive on the basis of inadequate calorie intake (Fig. 22–2). These infants usually have vomiting and regurgitation from birth and demonstrate a falloff in weight in the first two to four months of life. Historically, these patients will vomit at least 50 per cent of oral intake.

Pulmonary complications are present in approximately 12 per cent of pediatric patients with GER. There are at least three reasons why these patients develop pulmonary complications: (1) aspiration of excessive quantities of gastric contents into the lungs, causing chemical pneumonitis, (2) aspiration of very small quantities into the upper airway, causing vagal stimulation and airway obstruction, and (3) stimulation of mucosal receptors in the esophagus, causing secondary bronchospasm.[4–6]

The major symptoms associated with pediatric GER and pulmonary disease are chronic bronchitis, recurrent pneumonia, intractable asthma, and awake apnea (Table 22–2).

More than 20 years ago Carré recognized the association between pediatric GER and recurrent acute pulmonary disease. He noted in a large number of patients with reflux and nocturnal vomiting that there was a significantly higher incidence of pulmonary infections compared with those patients who did not have nocturnal vomiting. He believed that nocturnal aspiration might contribute to the recurrent pulmonary disease.[7]

Danus et al. evaluated recurrent obstructive bronchitis in young children and concluded that reflux was an important cause of their symptoms. Forty-three patients with recurrent episodes of bronchial infections were evaluated by upper gastrointestinal radiograph and esophageal manometry. Radiographic evidence of GER was found in 26 patients, all of whom had an abnormally low lower esophageal sphincter pressure (LESP). Fifteen of 20 patients treated medically for reflux showed significant improvement in their pulmonary disease.[8]

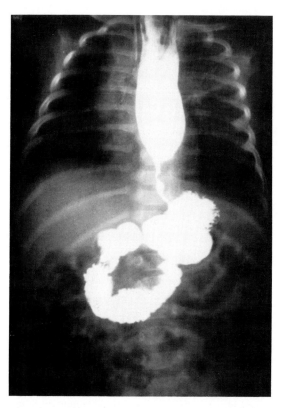

Figure 22–1. Tight esophageal stricture in two-year-old with chronic vomiting.

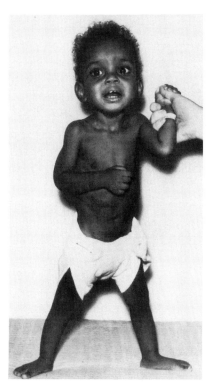

Figure 22–2. A 15-month-old child with failure to thrive who had a history of projectile emesis since early infancy. Evaluation showed severe reflux esophagitis.

Christie et al. studied 15 infants and young children with recurrent acute respiratory symptoms. Ten had GER on the basis of acid reflux testing and five by barium esophagogram. There was a high prevalence of infiltrates on chest radiographs and histories characterized by excessive regurgitation and episodic nocturnal cough (Fig. 22–3). No other cause for their chronic recurrent respiratory disease could be ascertained by thorough evaluation.[9]

Establishing a definite relationship between GER and recurrent respiratory symptoms can be difficult. Radiographic evaluation of the oropharynx, esophageal body, stomach, and duodenum is usually the first screening test when reflux is thought to be present. Because so many children with neurologic disease have aspiration during swallowing,

it is important to look at cricopharyngeal function and oropharyngeal disease as causes of aspiration before deciding that GER is the only cause of the patient's recurrent respiratory symptoms. Several criteria should be fulfilled before one can assume that aspiration or reflux bronchospasm is present (Table 22–3).[5] Prolonged esophageal pH monitoring should be performed. The per cent of time that the pH is less than 4 should be greater in patients with aspiration pneumonia than in control subjects. Also, the mean duration of reflux during sleep usually will be greater in aspirating patients than in asymptomatic control subjects. If there is a delay in clearance following a single reflux episode, this also supports aspiration as a cause of the recurrent respiratory symptoms.

Another clinical problem commonly attributed

Table 22–1. COMMON MANIFESTATIONS OF PEDIATRIC GASTROESOPHAGEAL REFLUX

Vomiting
Failure to thrive
Recurrent respiratory symptoms
Apnea
Heartburn
Hematemesis
Dysphagia

Table 22–2. COMPATIBLE HISTORY FOR GASTROESOPHAGEAL REFLUX AND RESPIRATORY DISEASE

Apnea
Choking episodes
Recurrent pneumonia
Recurrent wheezing
Chronic nocturnal cough
Nocturnal emesis

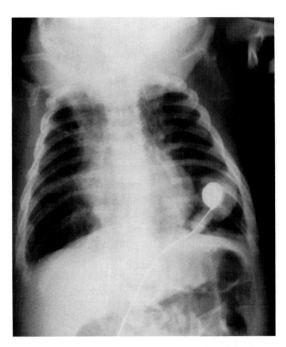

Figure 22–3. Chest radiograph of an infant with recurrent pneumonia caused by gastroesophageal reflux.

to GER is intractable asthma.[10–12] Asthma is thought to occur because of a neurally mediated reflex bronchoconstriction or because small quantities of acid reach the trachea. Mansfield et al. demonstrated *increased pulmonary flow resistance in asthmatic patients following intraesophageal acid provocation.*[13] Boyle et al. used the cat model to evaluate airway responses to acid reflux. Infusion of as little as 0.05 ml of 0.2 normal hydrochloric acid through a tracheostomy caused dramatic increases in total lung resistance, whereas similar esophageal infusion produced no such effects. Much larger volumes of 10 ml of 0.2 normal hydrochloric acid in the esophagus of the cat also evoked an increase in total resistance. Boyle believes that microaspiration in the trachea is a more likely mechanism for bronchospasm than reflux of

Table 22–3. CRITERIA FOR ASSOCIATING GASTROESOPHAGEAL REFLUX AND RESPIRATORY DISEASE

Compatible history
Percentage of time pH <4.0 greater than in control group
Duration of reflux during sleep greater than in control subjects
Acid clearance time in esophagus abnormal
Observed respiratory symptoms following drop in pH
Increased airway resistance after intraesophageal acid infusion
Pulmonary aspiration of ^{99m}Tc sulfur colloid

acid into the esophagus.[4] Not all investigators evaluating pediatric patients with bronchospasm believe that reflux is an important cause of intractable asthma. Hughes et al. could find no evidence of increased incidence of GER in patients with chronic asthma and concluded that reflux played no role in production of their nighttime respiratory symptoms.[14] Shapiro and Christie studied 19 children with chronic allergic steroid-dependent asthma. All were atopic based upon family history, skin testing, serum IgE concentrations, and a history of chronic wheezing exacerbated by allergens. Forty-seven per cent of these patients had positive acid reflux tests, and 42 per cent had LESP less than 12 mm Hg. All were treated for three weeks with medical antireflux therapy. There was no significant improvement in their asthma symptoms or pulmonary function tests.[15] This study could not define whether reflux was the result of medical therapy for asthma or whether reflux played a significant role in their chronic asthma symptoms. Since theophylline lowers LESP, it may be that medications used in treating asthma contribute to reflux.[16] However, Berquist et al. could not demonstrate that chronic asthmatic children on standard bronchodilator therapy had adverse effects of reflux on pulmonary function.[17]

Infants under six months of age may present with apnea and cyanosis secondary to reflux.[18,19] Spitzer described awake apnea as occurring within one hour after feeding and characterized by a sudden startle or staring expression with rigid posturing and subsequent hypotonia.[20] Eighty-seven per cent of the 15 infants studied by Spitzer demonstrated significant GER by pH monitoring with airway obstruction occurring during the reflux event. Leape et al. reported 10 cases of children under six months of age with apnea thought to be secondary to GER.[21] These patients suffered from recurrent cyanotic spells, vomiting, aspiration pneumonia, and respiratory arrest. Herbst also described a similar group of infants and demonstrated that reflux episodes preceded apnea. In some of these infants he was able to induce apnea by placing acid in the esophagus.[22]

Anemia, hematemesis, esophagitis, and esophageal stricture are more likely to occur in the older pediatric patient. However, in patients with disordered motility such as tracheoesophageal fistula or trisomy 21, esophageal stricture is more common and can be a significant cause of chronic morbidity. The infant with significant esophagitis will commonly be extremely irritable and a poor feeder. The older child will complain of heartburn and have regurgitation of acid into the back of the oropharynx. Chronic inflammation may lead to the development of Barrett's esophagus.

Table 22–4. COMMON ASSOCIATED
CONDITIONS IN PEDIATRIC
GASTROESOPHAGEAL REFLUX

Mental retardation
Trisomy 21
Spastic cerebral palsy
Tracheoesophageal fistula
Bronchopulmonary dysplasia
Scoliosis
Congenital heart disease
Hypotonia syndromes

Certain conditions appear to predispose to the development of significant reflux. Patients with mental retardation, spastic cerebral palsy, and scoliosis are particularly prone to develop incapacitating GER (Table 22–4, Fig. 22–4).

■ Diagnostic Tests

Radiographic examination of the oropharynx, the esophageal body, stomach, and duodenum is the first screening test that should be done in infants and children when GER is considered. Barium esophagogram can evaluate stomach, pylorus, and duodenal bulb to exclude other causes of chronic vomiting. If there is concern about aspiration, a cine study of the oropharynx should be performed to look for abnormal movements in the soft palate

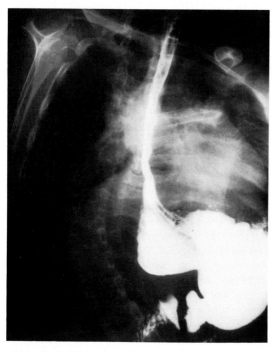

Figure 22–4. Adolescent with severe scoliosis and esophageal stricture.

and tongue or nonpropulsive pharyngeal contractions, inadequate upper esophageal sphincter relaxation, or evidence of aspiration. Reflux will be present by radiograph in approximately 40 per cent of pediatric patients with suggestive symptoms. There is good correlation between spontaneous reflux of barium and positive pH probe testing. While barium esophagography with the water siphon test has been used to evaluate GER, its false-positive rate of 29 per cent makes it an obsolete test.[23] If there is a strong history of GER and the barium esophagogram shows spontaneous reflux, further tests usually are not indicated.

Intraluminal pH monitoring has been used to evaluate the significance of GER. The one-hour esophageal pH probe study or the acid reflux test has been the most widely employed. This test is performed by placing the pH probe at a point equal to 87 per cent of the distance from the nares to the lower esophageal sphincter. The esophageal pH is then monitored for a short time, after which either acid or glucose is introduced into the stomach by a nasogastric tube. The volume of liquid placed in the stomach is equal to 300 mm per 1.73 m^2 of body surface area. The test is continued for 60 min while the patient is in the supine position. Valsalva maneuvers can be done to elicit GER. Two episodes of a drop in the esophageal pH to less than 4 identifies the presence of significant reflux in children. The acid reflux test will define the majority of patients with symptomatic GER but still has a false positive rate of approximately 15 per cent.[24,25]

Recently, one-hour esophageal pH monitoring has been extended for 24 hours as a way to evaluate the temporal relationship of reflux to clinical symptomatology in patients with such problems as recurrent pneumonia, apnea, cyanotic spells, chronic asthma, and atypical chest pain. The 24-hour esophageal pH tracing can be evaluated for the number of reflux episodes, total esophageal exposure to an acid pH of less than 4, and acid clearance time. This test is valuable if a significant symptom such as apnea, cyanosis, or coughing can be correlated with a drop in esophageal pH.[25] Normal children have reflux less than 5 per cent of the time during a 24-hour period. Euler and Byrne found that symptomatic infants had approximately 281 min of reflux compared to 33 min in an asymptomatic group ($p < 0.001$).[25] Jolley et al. evaluated the relationship of esophageal pH during sleep correlated with respiratory symptoms in children with GER and found greater reflux during sleep in these children. Prolonged clearance of refluxed material and the clustering of reflux events may precipitate respiratory symptoms in pediatric patients.[26]

There are still problems with 24-hour pH monitoring. First, the pH electrode does not measure the volume of material refluxed but only its presence in the esophagus. Second, alkaline reflux goes undetected by pH monitoring. Third, there is no physiologic way that 24-hour pH monitoring can be done in a young infant, because the procedure is uncomfortable and the patient is often restrained or daily activity is restricted.

■ **ESOPHAGOSCOPY AND ESOPHAGEAL BIOPSY**

Fiberoptic endoscopy provides a method to directly visualize the effects of acid reflux on the esophageal mucosa. If esophagitis is seen endoscopically and confirmed by biopsy, one has a diagnosis that significant GER is occurring. Barium esophagogram is insensitive to diagnose esophagitis, so in a patient with extreme irritability or hematemesis, fiberoptic endoscopy is the method of choice for evaluation of acute or chronic esophagitis. Fiberoptic endoscopy can be performed easily and requires little sedation. Younger infants are usually sedated with chloral hydrate while older pediatric patients generally require intravenous Valium and Demerol. General anesthesia is no longer required routinely for fiberoptic endoscopy in the pediatric patient.

Esophageal biopsy confirms the presence of inflammation in the esophagus and can exclude other causes of inflammation such as monilial or herpetic esophagitis.[27] A few pediatric patients will demonstrate columnar esophageal epithelium. The risk of malignancy in the pediatric patient from Barrett's esophagus is not defined.

The isotopic methods available for evaluating GER and esophageal function include radionuclide gastroesophagography and radionuclide transit. Radionuclide transit is valuable for patients with dysphagia because it is more sensitive in detecting esophageal motor abnormalities than esophageal manometry or radiographic studies. The transit test is performed by using a bolus of water and 250 millicuries of technetium sulfur colloid. The bolus is ingested with a single swallow and further dry swallows follow 30 s later. The passage of the bolus to the proximal third, middle third, and distal third of the esophagus is monitored, and abnormalities in transit are then detected.

Radionuclide gastroesophagography is used in children to demonstrate reflux of gastric contents into the esophagus.[28] It is superior to a barium esophagogram but less sensitive than pH monitoring. The stomach is loaded with ^{99m}Tc sulfur colloid and a gamma camera detects reflux into the esophagus. This method is useful for quantitating the number of reflux events that occur during one hour of monitoring and also evaluates esophageal clearance as well as pulmonary aspiration of ^{99m}Tc sulfur colloid (Fig. 22–5). Because some patients with GER have delayed gastric emptying of liquids and solids, the ^{99m}Tc test is also useful in evaluating gastric emptying. Hillemeier recently suggested that infants with severe GER have significant delays in gastric emptying.[29] Gastric retention may contribute to pulmonary symptoms and failure to thrive.

Esophageal manometry is used to determine basal LESP and esophageal peristalsis in the body of the esophagus following swallowing. Most patients with reflux esophagitis have basal LESPs of less than 10 mm Hg to 12 mm Hg. Pediatric patients with esophageal strictures generally have sphincter pressures of less than 12 mm Hg, whereas normal children without reflux have pressures from 15 to 30 mm Hg.[30] The measurement of LESP by itself, however, is not specific or sensitive enough to separate pediatric patients with or without GER. The test can be done easily without sedation and should be performed on patients with complications from GER (Fig. 22–6).

■ *Treatment*

Previously, medical treatment for GER sought only to increase LESP and thereby sphincter competence. However, it is now evident that increased intra-abdominal pressure and inappropriate relaxation of the lower esophageal sphincter following eating or during sleep can lead to reflux.[31] Factors that may contribute to complications of reflux are the volume and acidity of gastric fluid and the rate of clearance of refluxed material from the esophagus. Patients with GER and delayed gastric emptying have a larger volume of gastric contents available to be refluxed. Patients with abnormal esophageal clearance have an increased incidence of esophagitis and esophageal stricture because exposure to reflux acid or bile is prolonged. Medical treatment is thus designed to increase the pressure in the lower esophageal sphincter and to alter the nature of gastric contents and to reduce intragastric pressure.

Methods for improving lower esophageal sphincter competence remain the first mode of medical therapy. Antacids neutralize gastric contents and alter the amount of acid coming into contact with esophageal mucosa. Although antacids are effective in helping to relieve heartburn, they are not successful in the prevention of reflux over a long period of time.

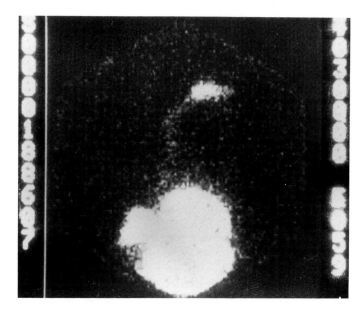

Figure 22–5. Radionuclide study demonstrating activity in oropharynx following gastroesophageal reflux.

Bethanechol, a cholinergic agent, has been demonstrated by several authors to be useful in increasing LESP and alleviating symptoms of reflux in young infants with GER.[32,33] Esophageal pH probe studies demonstrate a significant decrease in the frequency and duration of reflux episodes with bethanechol treatment. Thanik et al. demonstrated the effectiveness of oral bethanechol in adult patients when the medication was taken four times daily combined with antacid use.[34] Bethanechol resulted in complete endoscopic healing of reflux esophagitis in 10 of 22 patients compared with only 3 of 22 controls. Bethanechol improves lower esophageal sphincter competence and increases the force of esophageal contractions in the body of the esophagus. The drug, however, has certain adverse effects. It can cause abdominal cramps and diarrhea and may produce irritability in the young infant. Also, it may significantly increase gastric acid secretion and thus could increase the risk of aspiration.

Metoclopramide has been studied in adult patients with GER. The medication is usually given four times each day—before meals and at bedtime. It increases the resting LESP through mechanisms that are not defined. The drug also increases the amplitude of contractions in the esophagus, gastric antrum, and proximal small intestine. There appears to be increased coordination of mechanical activities so that relaxation of the pylorus and duodenum are coordinated with stomach contractions. Because metoclopramide increases antral contractions and antroduodenal coordination, the rate of gastric emptying is accelerated.[35] Side effects of metoclopramide are nervousness, dystonia, drowsiness, agitation, and anxiety. It should not be used in patients using phenothiazines.

A rational treatment plan for esophageal reflux based on experience and evaluations to date should combine methods to improve sphincter competence and esophageal and gastric emptying and to alter gastric secretions. In pediatric patients, especially infants, frequent low volume feedings thickened with cereal are given every two to three hours and the infant is kept upright 24 hours a day using an infant seat or placed on a prone wedge.[36] These

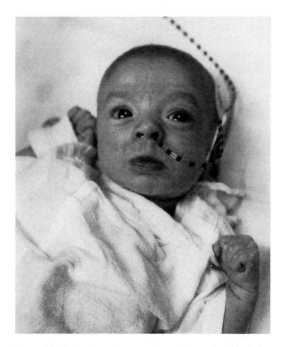

Figure 22–6. Esophageal manometry catheter placed in infant without sedation.

maneuvers are useful ways to avoid gastric distention and decrease episodes of reflux. Antacids can be given one and three hours postprandially and at bedtime at a dose of 5 to 20 ml per dose, depending upon the patient's weight. Because cimetidine has not been well studied in children and is not free of adverse effects, its use should be carefully monitored. It is indicated for patients with severe reflux esophagitis and may be applicable in patients with recurrent respiratory disease. The daily dose of cimetidine is 20 mg to 40 mg per kilogram of body weight, given in four divided doses. Bethanechol is given usually four times daily at a total dose of 8.7 mg/m². This medication should be used in pediatric patients with intractable vomiting, failure to thrive, or delayed gastric emptying. Metoclopramide may also be useful particularly in patients with delayed gastric emptying. The pediatric dose is 0.4 mg/kg/day.

In the adolescent patient, frequent feedings may also be useful. The patient should sleep in the upright position at night with the head of the bed elevated on 8-inch blocks. We recommend avoidance of coffee or chocolate. The patient should not consume excessive amounts of carbohydrate, which may also slow gastric emptying. Patients with heartburn may benefit from decreasing their intake of orange juice and tomato juice which sometimes aggravates their discomfort. Cimetidine may be used in the adolescent at a dose of 300 mg four times each day. Bethanechol is used at a dose of 25 mg four times daily. If metoclopramide is indicated, the dose is approximately 10 mg four times a day. These drugs are usually used individually rather than in combination and should not be prescribed without close follow-up.

■ SURGERY

Surgery is reserved for pediatric patients with significant sequelae of GER when medical management is not adequate.[37–42] Infants who fail to thrive in spite of aggressive medical therapy, which may include continuous drip feedings, will require an antireflux surgery. Patients with stricture formation or recurrent respiratory disease are also candidates for antireflux surgery. In the pediatric patient, the Nissen fundoplication has been widely used with varied results. Hicks et al. demonstrated complete resolution of esophageal stricture in 10 of 13 patients following Nissen fundoplication.[30] Stricture resolution occurred in nine patients without the need for postoperative dilatations. Recent evidence has demonstrated that severely retarded patients with GER respond poorly to medical therapy. These unfortunate children appear to have a high incidence of recurrent aspiration pneumonia and significant reflux esophagitis and stricture formation. An antireflux procedure may be useful in these patients but there is significant morbidity with the operation.[43] Postoperative bowel obstruction, a "slipped Nissen," and severe gas bloat syndrome are more common in the severely retarded patient with GER than in otherwise normal children who have significant sequelae from GER (Figs. 22–7 and 22–8).

There is little information about the effects of surgery on respiratory disease in adults, and there is controversy regarding antireflux surgery in pediatric patients with recurrent respiratory symptoms. A major problem in evaluating and comparing results is precise definition of the population studied. At present there are no clearly established methods to determine who aspirates and who has reflex bronchospasm. Several criteria should be fulfilled before one can assume that aspiration or reflex bronchospasm is occurring in patients with recurrent acute respiratory disease. In the older patient, the classical symptoms of an acid taste in the back of the mouth followed by bronchospasm is convincing evidence that aspiration has occurred. Prolonged esophageal pH monitoring should be performed, and the percentage of time that the pH is less than 4 should be abnormal. The mean duration of reflux during sleep should also be greater in these patients. The pH monitor should be observed to document a delay in clearance of a single reflux

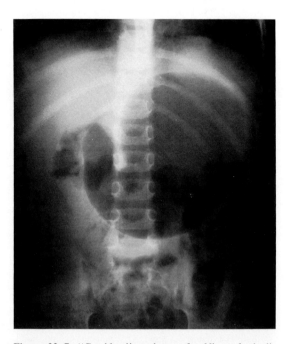

Figure 22–7. "Gas bloat" syndrome after Nissen fundoplication.

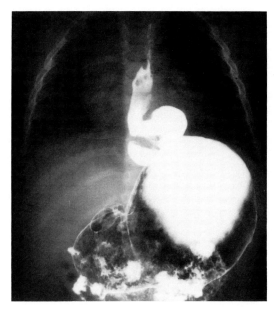

Figure 22–8. "Slipped" Nissen in an infant one year after Nissen fundoplication.

episode and clustering of reflux episodes as well as possible correlation with respiratory symptoms. Esophageal transit studies should be considered to demonstrate whether abnormal esophageal motility is present and to demonstrate aspiration into the oropharynx after swallowing. Increased airway resistance following intraesophageal acid infusion supports the reflex bronchospasm concept. The patient with respiratory disease who satisfies these criteria and fails to respond to medical intervention may respond to an antireflux procedure. This patient may be an infant with apnea or an older child with aspiration pneumonia and spasmodic nocturnal cough. As mentioned previously, the patient with asthma who is free of pneumonia and nocturnal choking and vomiting fails to satisfy the criteria for surgery.

■ REFERENCES

1. Carré IJ: Management of gastro-oesophageal reflux. Arch Dis Child, 60:71, 1985.
2. Herbst JJ: Gastroesophageal reflux. J Pediatr, 98:859, 1981.
3. Weissbluth M: Gastroesophageal reflux: A review. Clin Pediatr, 20:7, 1981.
4. Boyle JT, Tuchman DN, Altschuler SM, et al: Mechanisms for the association of gastroesophageal reflux and bronchospasm. Am Rev Respir Dis, 131:S16, 1985.
5. Christie DL: Pulmonary complications of esophageal disease. Pediatr Clin North Am, 31:835, 1984.
6. Barish CF, Wu WC, Castell DO: Respiratory complications of gastroesophageal reflux. Arch Intern Med, 145:1882, 1985.
7. Carré IJ: Pulmonary infections in children with a partial thoracic stomach (hiatus hernia). Arch Dis Child, 36:481, 1961.
8. Danus O, Casar C, Larrain A, et al: Esophageal reflux: An unrecognized cause of recurrent obstructive bronchitis in children. J Pediatr, 89:220, 1976.
9. Christie DL, O'Grady LR, Mack DV: Incompetent LES and GER in recurrent acute pulmonary disease of infancy and childhood. J Pediatr, 93:23, 1978.
10. Nelson HS: Gastroesophageal reflux and pulmonary disease. J Allergy Clin Immunol, 73:547, 1984.
11. Wilson NM, Charette L, Thomson AH, et al: Gastro-esophageal reflux and childhood asthma: The acid test. Thorax, 40:592, 1985.
12. Mitsuhashi M, Tomomasa T, Tokuyama K, et al: The evaluation of gastroesophageal reflux symptoms in patients with bronchial asthma. Ann Allergy, 54:317, 1985.
13. Mansfield LE, Stein MR: Gastroesophageal reflux and asthma: A possible reflex mechanism. Ann Allergy, 41:224, 1978.
14. Hughes DM, Spier S, Rivlin J, et al: Gastroesophageal reflux during sleep in asthmatic patients. J Pediatr, 102:666, 1983.
15. Shapiro GG, Christie DL: Gastroesophageal reflux in steroid-dependent asthmatic youths. Pediatrics, 63:207, 1979.
16. Goyal RK, Rattan S: Mechanism of the lower esophageal sphincter relaxation: Action of prostaglandin E and theophylline. J Clin Invest, 52:337, 1973.
17. Berquist WE, Rachelefsky GS, Rowshan N, et al: Quantitative gastroesophageal reflux and pulmonary function in asthmatic children and normal adults receiving placebo, theophylline, and metaproterenol sulfate therapy. J Allergy Clin Immunol, 73:253, 1984.
18. Ariagno RL, Guilleminault C, Baldwin R, et al: Movement and gastroesophageal reflux in awake term infants with "near miss" SIDS, unrelated to apnea. J Pediatr, 100:894, 1982.
19. Walsh JK, Farrell MK, Keenan WJ, et al: Gastroesophageal reflux in infants: Relation to apnea. J Pediatr, 99:197, 1981.
20. Spitzer AR, Boyle JT, Tuchman DN, et al: Awake apnea associated with gastroesophageal reflux: A specific clinical syndrome. J Pediatr, 104:200, 1984.
21. Leape LL, Holder RM, Franklin JD, et al: Respiratory arrest in infants secondary to GER. Pediatrics, 60:924, 1977.
22. Herbst JJ, Minton SD, Book LS: Gastroesophageal reflux causing respiratory distress and apnea in newborn infants. J Pediatr, 95:763, 1979.
23. Blumhagen JD, Christie DL: GE reflux in children: Evaluation of the water siphon test. Radiology, 131:345, 1979.
24. Christie DL: The acid reflux test for gastroesophageal reflux. J Pediatr, 94:78, 1979.
25. Euler AR, Byrne WJ: Twenty-four-hour esophageal intraluminal pH probe testing: A comparative analysis. Gastroenterology, 80:957, 1981.
26. Jolley SG, Herbst JJ, Johnson DG, et al: Esophageal pH monitoring during sleep identifies children with respiratory symptoms from gastroesophageal reflux. Gastroenterology, 80:1501, 1981.
27. Shub MD, Ulshen MH, Hargrove CB, et al: Esophagitis: A frequent consequence of gastroesophageal reflux in infancy. J Pediatr, 107:881, 1985.
28. Rudd TG, Christie DL: Demonstration of GE reflux in children by radionuclide gastroesophagography. Radiology, 131:483, 1979.
29. Hillemeier AC, Grill BB, McCallum R, et al: Esophageal and gastric motor abnormalities in gastroesophageal reflux during infancy. Gastroenterology, 84:741, 1983.
30. Hicks LM, Christie DL, Hall DG, et al: Surgical treatment

of esophageal stricture secondary to GER. J Pediatr Surg, *15*:863, 1980.

31. Werlin SL, Dodds WJ, Hogan WJ, et al: Mechanisms of gastroesophageal reflux in children. J Pediatr, *97*:244, 1980.

32. Euler AR: Use of bethanechol for the treatment of GER. J Pediatr, *96*:321, 1980.

33. Sondheimer JM, Mintz HL, Michaels M: Bethanechol treatment of gastroesophageal reflux in infants: Effect on continuous esophageal pH records. J Pediatr, *104*:128, 1984.

34. Thanik KD, Chey WY, Shah AN, et al: Reflux esophagitis: Effect of oral bethanechol on symptoms and endoscopic findings. Ann Intern Med, *93*: 805, 1980.

35. Hyman PE, Abrams C, Dubois A: Effect of metoclopramide and bethanechol on gastric emptying in infants. Pediatr Res, *19*:1029, 1985.

36. Orenstein SR, Whitington PF, Orenstein DM: The infant seat as treatment for gastroesophageal reflux. N Engl J Med, *309*:760, 1983.

37. Harnsberger JK, Corey JJ, Johnson DG, et al: Long-term follow-up of surgery for gastroesophageal reflux in infants and children. J Pediatr, *102*:505, 1983.

38. Tunell WP, Smith EI, Carson JA: Gastroesophageal reflux in childhood: The dilemma of surgical success. Ann Surg, *197*:560, 1983.

39. Berquist WE, Fonkalsrud EW, Ament ME: Effectiveness of Nissen fundoplication for gastroesophageal reflux in children as measured by 24-hour intraesophageal pH monitoring. J Pediatr Surg, *16*:872, 1981.

40. Jolley SG, Herbst JJ, Johnson DG, et al: Surgery in children with gastroesophageal reflux and respiratory symptoms. J Pediatr, *96*:194, 1980.

41. Wesley JR, Coran AG, Sarahan TM, et al: The need for evaluation of gastroesophageal reflux in brain-damaged children referred for feeding gastrostomy. J Pediatr Surg, *16*:866, 1981.

42. Johnson DG: Current thinking on the role of surgery in gastroesophageal reflux. Pediatr Clin North Am, *32*:1165, 1985.

43. Wilkinson JD, Dudgeon DL, Sondheimer JM: A comparison of medical and surgical treatment of gastroesophageal reflux in severely retarded children. J Pediatr, *99*:202, 1981.

23 Surgical Aspects of Congenital Anomalies of the Esophagus

R. W. Postlethwaite ■ *Howard C. Filston*

No discussion of surgery for congenital anomalies should begin without acknowledgment of the major contribution of Haight, when he performed the first successful anastomosis for esophageal atresia over 40 years ago.

Esophageal atresia and tracheoesophageal fistula, singly or together, have justifiably received emphasis, although other disorders such as gastroesophageal reflux are common in infants. The latter, however, does not invariably require operative treatment. As diagnosis has been considered in another chapter, this discussion will first outline preoperative care for infants with esophageal atresia.

■ Esophageal Atresia

Preoperative Care ■ The greatly improved measures for the care of seriously ill neonates have included better transport facilities, the intensive care nursery, sensitive hardware for monitoring of vital signs, infant ventilators, readily available blood gas determinations, and provision of nutritional support. This has allowed deferral of operation until appropriate evaluation and treatment can be carried out. Urgent operation may be required for associated anomalies but seldom for the esophageal anomaly. The appropriate care and the timing of operation depend on a number of factors which include (1) the type of the esophageal lesion, (2) the presence and severity of associated anomalies, (3) the birth weight and vigor of the infant, (4) the

severity of pulmonary involvement and the respiratory functional status, and (5) the presence of infection. The implications regarding prognosis are evident.

An open palette with overhead warmer and a hood for oxygen and mist or an incubator with temperature and humidity controls and equipped to provide oxygen is utilized. A temperature of approximately 32°C in the incubator should keep the temperature of the infant normal, but "servocontrol" of heating devices is essential to allow adjustment to the needs of the individual infant. Humidity is adjusted to 90 to 100 per cent. Oxygen in the incubator is maintained to keep the PaO_2 above 60 but less than 100 mm Hg because of the possible relationship of an elevated PaO_2 to retrolental fibroplasia in the premature infant. The infant is placed in prone, head-up position at a 30- to 45-degree angle, which will decrease the regurgitation of acid from the stomach and will pool gastric content anteriorly away from the esophagus. Frequent turning from side to side aids in the prevention of atelectasis and pneumonitis.

Mucus should not be allowed to accumulate in the proximal pouch. Continuous aspiration is better than intermittent, and a sump catheter such as that described by Replogle[38] has been found to function effectively. Replogle maintained satisfactory suction of 25 to 30 mm Hg in some infants for several weeks. Mucolytic agents may be helpful in liquefying tracheobronchial secretions. Tracheobronchial aspiration may be necessary and is best accomplished using an infant laryngoscope to avoid trauma to the vocal cords. Gentle suction of short duration, controlled through a Y-side arm, may be required several times a day. With a tracheoesophageal fistula, productive coughing is impaired; endotracheal intubation may be required to allow adequate clearing of secretions. Rarely is tracheostomy necessary to clear secretions.

The details of the fluid and electrolyte requirements in these infants are beyond the scope of this discussion. Error should be on the side of mild dehydration rather than overhydration. One suggested schedule of fluid maintenance for neonates one or two days old is 65 ml per kg of body weight per 24 hours; over seven days of age the maintenance dosage is 100 ml per kg per 24 hours. Using 5 per cent dextrose and 0.25 per cent normal saline provides about 3.8 mEq of sodium. Potassium may be added in the amount of 2.0 mEq per kg of body weight per 24 hours. A multivitamin preparation should be given. Urinary output should be monitored, and unusual losses, as from a gastrostomy, provided for appropriately.

If operation must be postponed more than a few days, total parenteral feeding should be considered to maintain nutrition, as suggested by Holder et al.[21] This may be crucial in the case of the small premature infant. After appropriate cultures are obtained, particularly from the respiratory tract, most surgeons favor the administration of antibiotics.

Selection of the most favorable time for operation may or may not be a problem. When the infant is vigorous, the lungs clear, hydration adequate, and fever and tachycardia are absent, then the best time for operation has been reached. These objectives can nearly always be achieved with proper preoperative care. A minimum room-air arterial Pao_2 of 60 mm Hg is an excellent gauge of readiness. If this status cannot be attained, then a compromise will have to be made if any hope of survival is to be held.

Gastrostomy ■ A consensus has not been reached on the performance of gastrostomy routinely. Tyson[43] believes that progress in the management of these neonates obviates the need for routine gastrostomy in the most frequent anomaly: atresia and fistula to the distal segment. He performs gastrostomy only if anastomotic leak develops. Others[19,20,30] have strongly recommended gastrostomy in the past. We do not favor routine gastrostomy when primary repair is indicated.

The immediate advantage of gastrostomy is decompression of the distended stomach and removal of gastric secretions, which should decrease pulmonary aspiration and possibly improve respiratory function. Later, the gastrostomy provides a route for aspiration or feeding, depending on the stage of treatment; should a stricture develop, it permits retrograde dilatation.

Logically, the decision should be made for each infant, based on the type of anomaly and the severity of complications. Gastrostomy should be performed if primary repair must be delayed. Even in the pure atresia type, when regurgitation is not a problem, gastrostomy facilitates nutritional support of the infant and provides access to the intestinal tract for further evaluation; the significant incidence of associated intestinal atresia makes gastrostomy necessary in order to identify the accompanying lesions and to prevent a closed-loop obstruction.

Gastrostomy in the neonate, in whom primary esophageal repair must be delayed because of poor lung compliance and severe respiratory distress syndrome, may become a formidable procedure because of the inability to secure adequate ventilation with the stomach open. Filston et al.[11] describe telescopic bronchoscopy and occlusion of the fistula with a Fogarty balloon catheter in this situation.

Premature and Critically Ill Infants ■ These patients present a challenge to the neonatologist and surgeon. Staged operations may be required. A gastrostomy must be done gently but rapidly, occasionally under local anesthesia; often these infants require intubation for respiratory support so that general anesthesia is appropriate. Despite the presence of the gastrostomy, some reflux and aspiration may continue when the fistula from the distal segment remains. The possibility of blocking the fistula with a Fogarty balloon catheter should be kept in mind. This can be achieved transtracheally or transgastrostomy in a retrograde fashion.

The safest course for the very critically ill neonate would be careful nursing care with particular attention to the prone head-up position, continuous aspiration of the proximal pouch, and frequent tracheal and gastric aspiration until improvement occurs. The use of total parenteral nutrition enhances the possibility of success. With it, the premature infant will gain weight, and time can be gained for resolution of the respiratory insufficiency. Atelectasis and pneumonitis may be resolved, but of equal importance, as the lungs mature the pulmonary reserve increases. Expert nursing care is vitally important, and modern neonatal care can protect infants from most complications so the necessity for multistage operations (other than initial gastrostomy) has decreased considerably. For example, Rickham[39] reported six infants weighing between 2 and 3 lb with five surviving primary or delayed primary operation. Obviously, some infants with severe respiratory distress syndrome will not respond to treatment and some may have associated anomalies that cannot be corrected and are incompatible with life.

Atresia without Fistula ■ The critical factor in this type of anomaly is the length of the atresia, i.e., the gap between the two segments of esophagus (ignoring prematurity, pneumonitis, and associated anomalies). The gap may be short, making anastomosis easy, but more likely will be of appreciable length. With no attachment to the trachea, the distal segment will retract toward the stomach making the gap appear very wide; when later stretched out, it may be longer than anticipated.

Absence of air in the stomach and intestines suggests this variety of esophageal atresia, and gastrostomy will be necessary to evaluate the rest of the intestinal tract. Telescopic esophagoscopy and bronchoscopy are indicated to rule out the very rare esophageal stenosis and confirm the absence of a distal fistula; unusual fistulas from the blind proximal pouch are also best identified endoscopically. The length of the distal esophageal segment may be determined later through the gastrostomy by a probe, by refluxing barium, or by catheterization through an endoscope. Should the lower segment be too short (and the gap too long) for anastomosis, some method of pouch elongation may be considered. In the same month Howard and Myers[22] and Johnston[23] reported successful anastomosis after proximal pouch lengthening by repeated bougienage; a number of confirmatory reports have subsequently appeared. As will be noted below, forceful elongation may be unnecessary because over time, the natural sequence of swallowing will elongate the proximal segment and by reflux, the distal segment.

Filston et al.[9] described the management of these patients at Duke Medical Center as follows: (1) gastrostomy and sump tube decompression of the proximal pouch; (2) gastrostomy feeding after demonstration of adequate gastric emptying; (3) contrast material injection of the stomach under fluoroscopy to fill the distal segment; (4) if the distal pouch is clearly rudimentary or absent, cervical esophagostomy to clear secretions and sham feedings while waiting for adequate growth for an interposition operation; (5) with a distal segment of reasonable length, gastrostomy feeding and proximal pouch decompression until the stomach is sufficiently adherent to the abdominal wall to allow safe manipulation, usually in three to four weeks; (6) under fluoroscopy, the passage of small Bakes dilators into the proximal segment and through the gastrostomy into the distal segment to determine their extensibility and the length of the gap; (7) when the initial gap can be reduced to less than three vertebral bodies, allowance of three to six weeks to stretch the proximal and distal segments by swallowing and by reflux, and to permit weight gain (the gap can be checked weekly as noted above); (8) the gap having been decreased to one vertebral body, anastomosis with a circular myotomy in the proximal segment if needed; (9) if anastomosis is impossible, cervical esophagostomy and later interposition operation.

■ Operation

Anesthesia in these infants presents unusual problems. The necessities of a clear airway and adequate oxygenation are made difficult by the excessive secretions, the parenchymal involvement of lung tissue, and the fistula from the trachea. Preoperative bronchoscopy will identify the site of any unusual fistula and help the anesthesiologist in positioning the endotracheal tube to obtain satisfactory ventilation. A secure flexible cannula is established, preferably percutaneously rather than by cut-down, which will permit administration of fluid and blood needed. Preservation of normal body temperatures is required, as a decrease to an abnormally low level may result in cardiac irregularities or even cardiac arrest. Constant temperature and arterial pressure monitoring is necessary, and blood gases should be determined as indicated. With controlled respiration, frequent aspiration, light plane of anesthesia, full muscle paralysis, good oxygenation, and a dependable route for blood administration to aid the anesthesiologist, the surgeon needs only to plan the operation to secure closure of the fistula at the earliest possible time to eliminate this complicating factor.

The infant is turned on the left side in a semiprone position for the surgical approach through the right side, and a 30- to 45-degree elevated position of the infant is maintained. A straight lateral thoracotomy incision begins just below the nipple and allows entry through the fourth or fifth intercostal space.

The approach to the posterior mediastinum may be transpleural or retropleural, and the question of which is best has not been definitely answered. The retropleural route has at least two advantages: (1) should a leak at the anastomosis develop, an empyema is unlikely to occur, and (2) the disturbances in pulmonary function are less severe. The transpleural approach gives excellent exposure more rapidly so the fistula can be occluded earlier, thus obtaining better control of respiratory exchange. The major disadvantage of the transpleural route is the probable development of empyema should anastomotic deficiency occur. Holder and

Ashcraft[20] collected a series totaling 747 infants who had primary anastomosis. They found in 603 transpleural approaches, anastomotic leak occurred in 104 with a 60 per cent mortality rate; a retropleural approach in 144 resulted in 20 anastomotic leaks and a 40 per cent mortality rate. The differences are significant. Saron et al.[41] reported all leaks closed spontaneously after a retropleural approach, whereas anastomotic leak after the transpleural route required multiple operations for reconstruction. Louhimo and Lindahl,[29] however, after their very extensive experience, prefer the transpleural route. Current neonatal intensive care should result in a much lower mortality rate for this complication, regardless of the route; furthermore, in experienced surgical hands, the incidence of significant anastomotic leakage should be minimal.

For the retropleural approach, the plane outside the pleura is developed and extended gradually above, below, and toward the mediastinum. As the azygos vein is approached, the pleura becomes more difficult to dissect, and care must be taken not to tear into the pleural space. The azygos vein is ligated and divided (Fig. 23–1). Through a transpleural approach, the pleura is opened longitudinally over the mediastinum, and the azygos vein is ligated and divided. The posterior aspect of the trachea and the right vagus nerve are identified without extensive dissection. The distal segment of the esophagus is identified by following the right vagus nerve inferiorly. The upper portion of the distal segment of the esophagus is exposed to the point of entry into the trachea or, infrequently, into one of the main bronchi. This point is usually just above the bifurcation of the trachea. Further dissection of the distal esophageal segment is as limited as possible.

Division of the fistula and closure of the tracheal component is now performed. The fistulous structure should be divided near the trachea in order to preserve all possible length of the lower segment of esophagus, but an adequate cuff must be left on the trachea to permit secure closure. The latter is an important step in the operation, for a breakdown may result in recurrence of the fistula. Interrupted 5–0 or 6–0 silk sutures on a small atraumatic needle are traditionally used to obtain closure (Fig. 23–2). The use of one of the synthetic absorbable sutures may be considered, however, as use of silk may cause a suture granuloma in the trachea. A reinforcing pleural flap is then sutured over the closure if this can be secured. If not, mediastinal soft tissues or even a free muscle graft may be used. Haight,[17] and subsequently many others, emphasized the necessity for this buttress over the tracheal closure, interposed between it and the anastomosis. Equally important is atraumatic handling of the

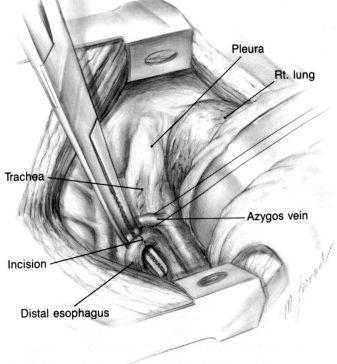

Figure 23–1. The azygos vein should be ligated prior to exposure of the fistula. The distal segment is shown with the site of division.

Pleura

Rt. lung

Trachea

Azygos vein

Incision

Distal esophagus

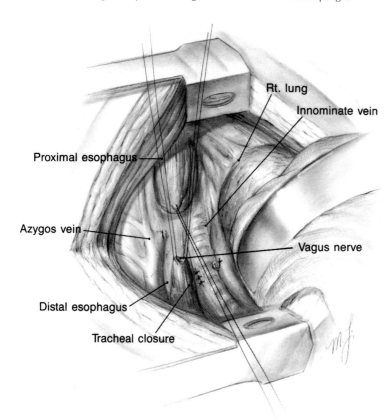

Figure 23–2. The closure of the trachea has been accomplished. The proximal and distal segments are controlled by traction sutures.

tissue and air-tight closure. The latter can be tested by filling the chest with saline as the anesthesiologist increases the intratracheal pressure.

The proximal segment of the esophagus can usually be easily identified in its retrotracheal position, but at times it is short and found only with difficulty. A soft tube passed into the upper pouch by the anesthesiologist facilitates its identification by palpation and can extend it further into the mediastinum. A suture is placed in the lower tip of the proximal segment to make dissection easier and to avoid the use of forceps on the wall of the esophagus. The proximal segment has a good blood supply coming from above, as well as a thicker wall than the lower segment, so that dissection can be extended well into the thoracic inlet (Fig. 23–3). As noted above, the upper end of the lower segment is mobilized only enough to permit anastomosis, as it is thin-walled and the blood supply less robust. It is segmental in character and loss of each vessel results in loss of about 1 cm of esophagus. The gap between the segments should, therefore, be overcome by mobilization of the proximal pouch.

Livaditis et al.[28] described circular myotomy in the esophagus of piglets to increase length and decrease anastomotic tension; they found no dysfunction in bolus passage. Subsequent experimental studies and then clinical utilization have

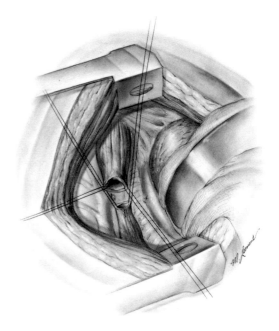

Figure 23–3. The proximal segment is opened and the anastomosis can be started.

demonstrated the accomplishment of increased length of the proximal pouch to overcome the gap and relieve tension on the anastomosis. The circular myotomy extends to a plane between the muscularis propria and the submucosa. Accidental opening through the mucosa may be closed and has resulted in no leaks in reported cases. Later studies show only moderate dilatation at the myotomy site, although Otte et al.[36] reported two infants who developed huge diverticula. Esophageal exclusion and colon interposition were eventually necessary. The myotomy, however, remains a valuable adjunctive maneuver.

As with any alimentary tract anastomosis, well-vascularized segments that can be accurately apposed without tension are required for a successful result. Most surgeons prefer to avoid the use of forceps by placing traction sutures, which are gently handled to manipulate the ends of the two segments of the esophagus. A small button of the muscle layers is excised from the upper pouch through this, the mucosa is pulled out and opened. The limited opening in the distal segment may be enlarged by making a 1-mm longitudinal cut, which will increase the circumference by 2 mm and make the anastomosis easier (Fig. 23–4).

Several types of anastomosis have been employed. Haight[16] recommended suturing all layers of the lower segment to the mucosa of the proximal pouch (Fig. 23–5). The cut edge of the muscle layers of the upper pouch is then brought down over the first suture line and attached to the outer wall of the lower segment. This telescopes the lower segment into the upper slightly and buttresses the inner layer. Most surgeons prefer a simple one-layer anastomosis with sutures passing through all layers of both segments. Others utilize two layers with mucosa to mucosa and muscularis to muscularis. A most important factor in avoiding anastomotic leak and stricture is precise mucosal apposition, a technical consideration that deserves special emphasis. Another type of anastomosis that has not attained wide acceptance was described by Sulamaa et al.[42] The fistula from the lower segment is ligated, but not divided, after minimal dissection. The open end of the proximal pouch is sutured into an opening in the side of the distal segment with a one-layer technique. Using this method Cumming[8] found anastomotic leak, recurrent fistula, and stricture to be more frequent than after end-to-end anastomosis.

In the survey by Holder and Ashcraft[20] describing 747 anastomoses, the one-layer anastomosis leaked in 21.4 per cent, the two-layer procedure leaked in 14.6 per cent, and the Haight type leaked in 10.5 per cent. Of those who had anastomotic leak, survival was highest with the Haight anastomosis (62 per cent) and the lowest with the one-layer technique (31 per cent). These series predate modern neonatal supportive care and more effective modern antibiotics. Although stricture is more frequent after the Haight anastomosis, Holder and Ashcraft prefer it because of the greater safety. Nason and Gillis[34] state that the decisions should be made on the basis of the amount of tension on the anastomosis: the Haight technique is preferable when tension is present, and a one-layer anastomosis is recommended when tension is absent or minimal.

Silk has usually been the recommended suture for anastomosis. Cowley,[7] however, believed the capillarity of silk increased the possibility of a small localized abscess and that led to fistula reformation. He indicated that fine wire would avoid this. In animal experiments, Belin et al.[4] found chromic catgut most satisfactory and used this for end-to-end anastomosis in 50 neonates with only three leaks. Santos et al.[40] took generous full-thickness bites with 6–0 polypropylene sutures and reported no leaks in a series of 24 infants.

After anastomosis, a catheter traversing the two segments is usually unnecessary, although a small plastic (Silastic) tube does have certain advantages. Leaving such a tube in place is routine with some surgeons and opposed by others. Certainly a large tube will stimulate nasopharyngeal secretions, and increase aspiration, and possibly interfere with normal healing at the anastomosis. A very small Silastic tube will not irritate or block and should not affect healing but will provide a route for aspiration

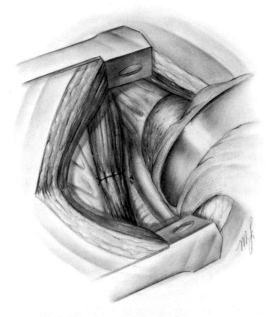

Figure 23–4. The anastomosis is complete.

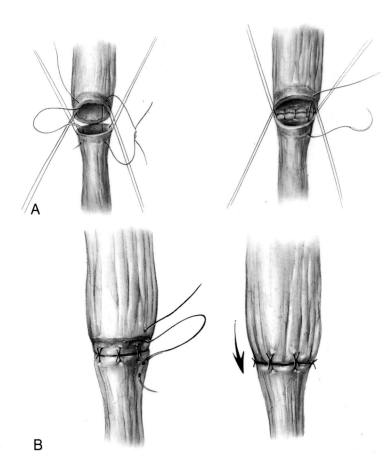

Figure 23–5. The Haight anastomosis. Mucosa of proximal segment is sutured to full thickness of lower segment (*A*), then the muscular layer of upper to lower is sutured to overlap the inner suture lines (*B*).

of air and gastric secretions if necessary and will permit administration of enteral fluids earlier than oral feeding might be advisable, assuming a gastrostomy has not been done. However, before the anastomosis is complete, a tube should be passed routinely into the stomach to exclude the presence of a distal web or stenosis.

The anastomosis having been completed, a 12 French plastic chest tube is brought in through a small stab wound with the tip of the tube placed near but not on the line of anastomosis. This may be anchored with a fine catgut suture. The tube is led to underwater seal but preferably is not placed on suction because of the danger of a small eversion of mucosa through the anastomosis. In a transpleural approach, the pleura may be loosely and incompletely reapproximated over the mediastinum with interrupted sutures. The chest is closed in the usual manner.

Rarely, the proximal pouch is so high as to leave a hopelessly long gap. A cervical esophagostomy will be necessary with later esophageal substitution. In others, while a primary anastomosis cannot be performed, the gap may be such that a subsequent operation will allow anastomosis. After ligation and division of the fistula, the distal esophageal segment is closed and sutured to mediastinal tissue; the proximal pouch is not further disturbed. Attempts may be made to elongate the segments or, after continuing close nursing care for several weeks, a second operation may be performed. Following this plan, Koop et al.[25] were "happily surprised" in staged operations after division of the fistula to find esophageal segments to have elongated so that what had seemed an impossible gap to overcome now permitted direct anastomosis (Fig. 23–6).

Extensive procedures such as mobilization of the stomach to decrease the gap are not justified.

Esophageal Substitution ■ Every effort should be made to restore continuity of the esophagus, as no replacement will function as well. Even an anastomosis under tension with the increased danger of leak and stricture is an acceptable risk, as long as adequate drainage is provided and maintained.

The timing of the reconstruction will depend on the progress of each infant; intervals of 6 to 24 months have been recommended, so one year of age seems a reasonable time. The weight should have increased to at least 20 lb. The choices for the substitute are jejunum, colon, stomach, or greater curvature gastric tube, but the majority of

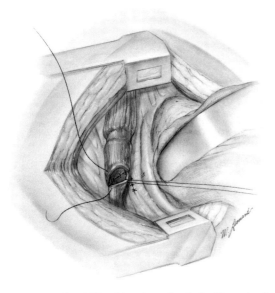

Figure 23–6. Additional length can be obtained by a circular myotomy in the proximal segment.

surgeons prefer a segment of the transverse colon. The routes for placement of the substitute are intrathoracic, substernal, or subcutaneous.

The transverse colon based on a left colic artery vascular pedicle provides adequate length, the lumen is of appropriate size, and most important, the blood supply is good. The constant left colic artery gives off a long ascending branch which is seldom deficient; venous return is also good. The details of substernal colon interposition do not require description here, but the intrathoracic technique described by Waterston[45] should be noted. A left thoracotomy or abdominothoracic incision is used. The mobilized segment of colon is brought posterior to the stomach and pancreas. The vascular pedicle goes through a small incision in the diaphragm near the hiatus. The proximal anastomosis is made at the appropriate level, usually in the neck. Distally, the esophageal stump is dissected, opened, and the distal end of interposed colon anastomosed to the esophagus (later studies have shown a functional sphincter remains). Many surgeons recommend delaying the cervical anastomosis to avoid leakage into the mediastinum and chest.

The gastric tube has been utilized less frequently than colon. The blood supply to the reversed tube is from the left gastroepiploic vessels; for an isoperistaltic tube, the blood supply is from the right gastroepiploic vessels. Cohen et al.[6] have utilized both techniques: 23 infants had the reversed tube, and 12 had the isoperistaltic. They are convinced the greater curvature gastric tube is a safer operation and gives a better functional result than colon.

Lindahl et al.[27] after 34 reconstructions with either colon or gastric tube conclude that either substitute is satisfactory and functions equally well. The gastric tube operation, however, was for them easier to perform and had a lower mortality rate and fewer complications.

Postoperative Care ■ After closure of the fistula and esophageal anastomosis for the usual esophageal atresia with distal fistula, the postoperative care continues the same principles followed before operation. The major threat to life remains the pulmonary complications. Appropriate temperature, humidity, and oxygen atmosphere control must be assured. Nebulized mist will maintain liquidity of secretions and result in more effective cough. Without it, frequent suctioning becomes essential; endotracheal intubation appears to be superior to repeated laryngoscopy and tracheal aspiration for this purpose. The infants are not extubated until they can maintain on room air a PaO_2 of 60 mm Hg and not retain CO_2. Respiratory failure requires continued mechanical ventilation. The infant's head must be supported at all times to prevent inadvertent extension, as this "levers" the esophageal anastomosis across the bony spine and may disrupt it.

Cultures are repeated after operation, and antibiotic therapy is given as indicated. With good progress, feeding through the gastrostomy or nasogastric tube may begin on the third postoperative day. About the fifth day, a barium swallow is obtained to ensure that the anastomosis is intact. If this is satisfactory, the chest tube is removed and feedings of formula are started. Care is exercised in giving oral feedings because there is continued danger of aspiration.

■ POSTOPERATIVE MORBIDITY AND MORTALITY

Factors affecting morbidity and mortality rates include the type of the esophageal anomaly, birth weight, presence and severity of associated malformations, degree of pulmonary involvement, experience of the surgeon and the anesthetist, and the skill of nursing care before and after operation. A useful classification indicating prognosis was suggested by Waterston et al.:[44]

Type A: Birth weight over 5.5 lb (2500 g) and well.

Type B: (1) Birth weight 4 to 5.5 lb (1800 to 2500 g) and well. (2) Higher birth weight; moderate pneumonia or anomaly.

Type C: (1) Birth weight under 4 lb (1800 g). (2) Higher birth weight; severe pneumonia or severe associated anomaly.

Although persistent or recurrent pulmonary complications are most common, four causes of morbidity and, at times, death, which are more or less specific for these infants, are anastomotic leak, recurrent fistula, stricture, and gastroesophageal reflux.

Anastomotic leak has been noted to occur in about 23 per cent of anastomoses, although this has decreased to 13 per cent in recently reported series. The causes include a small friable lower segment, impaired blood supply, infection, inaccurate mucosal apposition, technically poor suturing, the location in the mediastinum, and the movement of the joined segments during respiration and swallowing. In addition, chest tube suction may evert mucosa and cause a leak. Diagnosis is usually not difficult. Treatment depends on the extent of the anastomotic disruption which can only be estimated by the amount of drainage and the radiographic findings. A small opening adequately drained will usually close spontaneously if oropharyngeal and gastrostomy suction is continued, antibiotics are administered, and nutrition is maintained. A large or total disruption of the anastomosis requires immediate reoperation. The choice of attempted reanastomosis or exteriorization of the proximal segment with closure of the distal segment depends on the operative findings, especially the condition of the two ends of the esophagus and the severity of infection.

Recurrent fistula may be an early or late complication and occurs in about 6 per cent of the patients. The causes include leak of the anastomosis either directly through the tracheal closure or by way of abscess. The mechanical trauma of dilatations may be a factor. Diagnosis is frequently a problem and is best accomplished by cine-esophagograph and telescopic bronchoscopy as described by Filston et al.[10] Operative closure of the fistula is necessary, and most important is interposition of tissue such as pleura or intercostal muscle between the trachea and esophagus.

Narrowing at the anastomosis is almost inevitable because the upper pouch has a relatively large lumen, which is now in continuity with the narrow lumen of the lower segment; a true stricture, however, is rare. A survey of recent reports shows that stricture occurs in about 30 per cent, but with meticulous apposition it can occur far less frequently. Gastroesophageal reflux may contribute to its persistence. Diagnosis is usually on the basis of barium swallow. A number of surgeons routinely perform dilatation two to three weeks after successful anastomosis, but many find this unnecessary. A major advantage of gastrostomy at this point is to allow retrograde dilatation, which is safer than antegrade in infants. Response to dilatation is usually good, but a small number will require resection of the stricture and reanastomosis.

Gastroesophageal reflux has been implicated both in causing the stricture at the anastomosis as well as in initiating a new stricture in the lower esophagus. Ashcraft et al.[1] suggested that reflux is more prevalent in infants who have had atresia and a distal fistula compared with normal infants. Eight of their patients in this group required an antireflux operation.

Mortality Rate ■ The remarkable decrease in the mortality rate has been evident in all reported series. Two large series[29,32] report zero mortality in recent years for Waterston type A infants and nearly zero for type B. The type C group mortality rate decreased from nearly 100 per cent to about 40 per cent. We have had occasion to note mortality rates in reported series, based on the year of publication as follows: for all admissions to 1959, 577 infants and a mortality rate of 58.2 per cent; from 1960 to 1976, 1295 infants and 42.2 per cent; from 1977 to 1984, 1046 infants and 30 per cent. For those who had anastomosis, the percentages for the same intervals were 53.3 per cent, 24.6 per cent, and 18.7 per cent, respectively.

Currently, chromosomal abnormalities and cardiovascular anomalies are the major cause of death. A representative series is that of Louhimo and Lindahl[29] of operations beginning in 1947. In their 500 patients, the causes of death were pulmonary (65), intracranial hemorrhage (16), anastomotic leak or refistula (55), associated anomalies (57), and others (10). An irreducible minimal mortality rate is being approached as the surgeon has little chance to influence the major contributing causes of death. In the most recent decade almost all deaths are due to severe associated anomalies or unrelenting pulmonary complications, rather than technical failures.

Late Results ■ Most studies relate to esophageal function. Haight[18] early noted problems with swallowing after primary anastomosis and described the absence of peristalsis in the segment below the anastomosis. This has been confirmed by numerous studies, including manometric. The sphincters have been found to be normal, but the body of the esophagus, usually below the anastomosis, shows abnormal motility. This may be no peristalsis, feeble contractions, or spasm but infrequently a coordinated peristaltic contraction. Some problem in swallowing may be apparent clinically, usually not to a major degree. The alteration, however, may be responsible for recurrent tracheobronchitis or pneumonitis due to poor clearing or refluxed stomach content after gastroesophageal reflux. For example, Myers[31] followed 58 patients at least 13 years and reported resection of a stricture was necessary in ten and closure of a recurrent fistula in one. Only one patient currently had dysphagia, but many had to be careful when eating. He concluded that esophageal function is not normal, dysphagia is an early problem, recurrent respiratory infections occur in the early years, and demonstrable radiologic and manometric abnormalities are present; nevertheless, the end results are very satisfactory.

■ OTHER TYPES OF FISTULA

The preceding discussion has mainly considered the two most common types of abnormality: atresia with fistula into the distal segment (86 per cent) and atresia without fistula (7.5 per cent). The less frequent configurations are atresia with fistula into the upper pouch, atresia with fistula into both segments, and tracheoesophageal fistula without atresia. In each, the problem may be more one of diagnosis rather than of surgical correction. The first two are compounded by the fact that the proximal fistula usually does not enter at the tip of the upper pouch but may be found at any point, especially as high as the neck, and may be missed during operation. Radiologic demonstration is difficult so that telescopic endoscopy is important for diagnosis and localization.

In the infant with atresia, the proximal fistula can be easily identified if preoperative bronchoscopy is routinely utilized; if not, the fistula may be identified and corrected during mobilization of the upper pouch. If missed, the postoperative course of continued pulmonary problems will suggest either a proximal or recurrent fistula. The importance of accurate diagnosis is obvious, especially since the second operation may be possible through a neck incision.

Fistula without atresia is of interest for several reasons. Although usually recognized during infancy, approximately 25 per cent are not found until after the age of 15 years and the majority in adults over 30 years of age. In the adult, the fistula is more likely to be into a bronchus rather than the trachea and an appreciable number are into a pulmonary sequestration.

The fistulas vary in length and diameter: 0.5 to 2.0 cm long with a diameter about 0.5 cm. Most are buried in a common tracheoesophageal wall. At operation, simple ligation is not advisable because of the danger of recanalization. Division or excision are followed by careful closure of the esophagus and trachea and interposition of tissue such as a pleural flap or muscle. Preoperative placement of a catheter through the fistula greatly facilitates identification at operation.

Numerous unusual variants of esophageal atresia and tracheoesophageal fistula occur. Kluth[24] has illustrated over 100 configurations that have been reported.

■ *Other Congenital Anomalies*

Stenosis and Web ■ These lesions are seen so infrequently in infants that very limited experience has been reported. Stenosis may respond to dilatation. Webs are usually thin and may be disrupted by an endoscope or bougie. Infrequently, esophagotomy and excision or incision of the web may be needed.

Duplications, Rests, and Cysts ■ Duplications may be small and localized or extensive. If the duplication opens into the esophageal lumen at both ends, a double esophagus is present; if it is open proximally, a diverticulum; if closed, an elongated cyst. Surgical treatment depends on the size and configuration. Local excision may be possible. A long double esophagus may have a common wall, which can be divided.

Embryonic rests, where cells from the tracheal or esophageal anlage are displaced into the mesodermal tissues which are to become esophageal muscle, usually take the form of a cyst. The lining is most frequently ciliated columnar epithelium, resembling the bronchial lining. Predominantly gastric epithelium is next in occurrence; pure squamous epithelium is least frequent. A mixture of more than one type may be found.

In infants, cysts may be large enough to cause severe respiratory distress and require urgent operation. Waterston[46] has found that some duplications and cysts in infants are vascular and adherent to vital mediastinal structures, making excision hazardous; others are readily excised with clearly demarcated tissue planes. He advises making a small incision in the cyst and removing the mucosal lining, a submucosal plane being readily established. In the adult, a cyst can nearly always be removed without opening into the esophageal lumen or damaging the esophageal muscle.

One form of embryonic rest merits special mention. This is the solid intramural tracheobronchial rest termed choristoma. Nearly always in the lower third of the esophagus, the choristoma partly or completely encircles the esophagus and, because of the cartilaginous content, does not respond to dilatation. Operation is necessary; in five of the 40 reported cases, the choristoma was removed by intramural dissection without opening the mucosa. Most of the others had a limited resection. These may first become symptomatic when solid foods are begun in late infancy.

Muscle Hypertrophy ■ The muscle hypertrophy occasionally found with achalasia and usually with diffuse spasm is well known. A third form appears to be congenital and is most often reported as an unexpected autopsy finding. The majority had been asymptomatic with relation to swallowing, so the anomaly is compatible with normal esophageal function. The few symptomatic patients reported had excellent results after a long myotomy.

A possibly related but very rare condition shows marked muscle hypertrophy and massive dilatation of the esophagus (not achalasia). Resection and esophageal replacement will be necessary.

Columnar Epithelium–Lined Lower Esophagus ■ We have previously suggested that the term Barrett's esophagus, as currently used, represents two different diseases: one congenital and the other acquired. The embryology of the esophagus is consistent with a congenital basis. If our interpretation of Barrett's original description is correct, a congenital origin seems most likely for his cases and the eponym is correct. The many patients described with reflux esophagitis and progressively more proximal replacement of epithelium leaves no doubt as to the acquired type, for which Naef and Savary[33] have suggested the term "extensive columnar metaplasia." An extensive discussion of the differentiation would not be appropriate here; from the surgical standpoint, the complications of either type may require surgical treatment.

In the congenital form, gastroesophageal reflux does occur, but less frequently than in the acquired type. Depending on the severity of the symptoms, an antireflux operation may be needed. Probably the most frequent complication is a stricture at the squamocolumnar junction, usually in the vicinity of the aortic arch. In our limited experience, these strictures dilate easily and no resection has been necessary.

Another complication, Barrett's ulcer, is to be differentiated from the longitudinal esophagitis and ulceration seen in the acquired type. This is a solitary ulcer, above the esophagogastric junction, which simulates the usual gastric ulcer, i.e., it may penetrate, perforate, or bleed. Bleeding is most frequent and may respond to medication and an antireflux operation. In two of our patients, continued bleeding required resection.

Cardial Incompetence and Hiatal Hernia ■ Although an occasional article appeared in the American literature, most early reports of gastroesophageal reflux came from other countries, especially England. In 1947, Neuhauser and Berenberg[35] reported 12 infants and suggested the term chalasia to describe the incompetence of the lower esophageal sphincter. Subsequently, an increasing number of patients have been reported, particularly in the past 10 years. For example, Leape and Ramenofsky[26] state they now see over 400 cases annually. Two groups merit special mention: the severely mentally retarded and those who have had repair of esophageal atresia. Byrne et al.,[5] for example, reported 42 mentally retarded children with reflux and just over half required operation. Gauthier et al.[14] reported that 53 of 113 infants with atresia developed gastroesophageal reflux and 15 had to have operation.

The cause of incompetence of the lower esophageal sphincter, with or without hiatal hernia, is usually described as an autonomic or a neuromuscular dysfunction. The diagnosis is based on the symptoms, the radiologic examination, and more definitively, the manometric and pH studies. Radionuclide scans have also been reported to be useful. Diagnosis is obviously important for several reasons, not the least being the avoidance of severe stricture formation by early treatment of esophagitis.

In the absence of complications, postural treatment is initiated; the recommended trial period varies from six weeks to six months. The various reports state the response rate has been from 75 to 90 per cent. Generally, the indications for operation are failure of postural treatment, large hiatus hernia, esophagitis, bleeding, anemia, recurrent aspiration, failure to thrive, and any suggestion of stricture development. More specifically, we summarized the indications for operation in reports of 935 infants and children with gastroesophageal reflux (Table 23–1): recurrent pneumonia, 26.3 per cent; croup and choking, 5.2 per cent; apnea, 14.7 per cent; vomiting, 21.8 per cent; failure to thrive, 26.1 per cent; bleeding or anemia, 1.6 per cent; esophagitis, 4.1 per cent; stricture, 6.5 per cent; CNS disorder, 12.4 per cent; and prior atresia, 3.2 per cent. (The percentages total greater than 100

Table 23–1. INDICATIONS FOR OPERATION IN REPORTS OF 935 INFANTS AND CHILDREN WITH GASTROESOPHAGEAL REFLUX

Indication	Percentage*
Recurrent pneumonia	26.3
Failure to thrive	26.1
Vomiting	21.8
Apnea	14.7
CNS disorder	12.4
Stricture	6.5
Croup and choking	5.2
Esophagitis	4.1
Prior atresia	3.2
Bleeding or anemia	1.6

*The percentage total is greater than 100 because some patients had more than one major indication

because some patients had more than one major indication.)

Surgeons are remarkably in agreement as to the operation; currently some form of the Nissen fundoplication is almost universally performed. Injury to the spleen is carefully avoided, and the vagus nerves are protected. A loose complete wrap is usually employed. A number of minor modifications such as a partial wrap have been described but the basic principle remains the same. In a few infants, the stomach will be small and not adequate for fundoplication. A gastropexy, usually posterior, may then be performed, but this procedure has given inconsistent results.

Several authors have described disturbances in gastric emptying termed antral dysmotility in these infants. Fonkalsrud[13] reported that ten of his patients responded to medical treatment, including bethanechol or metoclopramide, but eight had to have pyloroplasty.

The treatment after stricture development depends on the severity of the stricture and the amount of acquired shortening of the esophagus. A soft stricture, with major components of spasm and edema, should respond promptly to dilatations and postural treatment, to be followed shortly by the antireflux operation. A more resistant stricture may be dilated intraoperatively with the fundoplication. Dilatations postoperatively will usually be necessary until stabilization occurs. No information is available on the role of gastroplasty when the esophagus is short. A rigid, undilatable stricture will usually eventually require resection with reconstruction by a short colon interposition (esophagogastrostomy is less satisfactory because of continued reflux and recurrent stricture).

We have summarized the results of antireflux operations as reported in 12 articles published during the past 10 years. Four postoperative deaths occurred in the 1053 infants and children. Follow-up for variable periods was recorded for 994 patients: results were good in 896 (90 per cent) and poor in 98. The latter include 33 with recurrent reflux, 9 with paraesophageal hernia, and 5 with wrap malalignment who had a second operation with a satisfactory outcome.

Dysphagia Lusoria ■ For completeness, the vessel anomalies causing dysphagia will be noted, as properly they should be discussed by a cardiovascular surgeon. Of the several variations described, the anomaly is usually one of three types: double aortic arch, right aortic arch with left ligamentum arteriosum, and right aberrant subclavian artery.

■ REFERENCES

1. Ashcraft KW, Goodwin C, Amoury RA, Holder TM: Early recognition and aggressive treatment of gastroesophageal reflux following repair of esophageal atresia. J Pediatr Surg, 12:317, 1977.
2. Barrett NR: The oesophagus lined by columnar epithelium. Gastroenterologia, 86:183, 1956.
3. Barrett NR: The lower oesophgaus lined by columnar epithelium. Surgery, 41:881, 1957.
4. Belin RP, Lieber A, Segnitz RH: A comparison of technics of esophageal anastomosis. Am Surg, 38:533, 1972.
5. Byrne WJ, Euler AR, Ashcraft E, et al: Gastroesophageal reflux in the severely retarded who vomit; criteria for and result of surgical intervention in 22 patients. Surgery, 91:95, 1982.
6. Cohen DH, Middleton AW, Fletcher J: Gastric tube esophagoplasty. J Pediatr Surg, 9:451, 1974.
7. Cowley LL: Congenital tracheo-esophageal fistula: Recurrence after repair. Am Surg, 33:409, 1967.
8. Cumming WA: Esophageal atresia and tracheoesophageal fistula. Radiol Clin North Am, 13:277, 1975.
9. Filston HC, Merten DF, Kirks DR: Initial care of esophageal atresia to facilitate potential primary anastomosis. South Med J, 74:1530, 1981.
10. Filston HC, Rankin JS, Kirks DR: The diagnosis of primary and recurrent tracheoesophageal fistulas: Value of selective catheterization. J Pediatr Surg, 17:144, 1982.
11. Filston HC, Chitwood WR Jr, Schkolne B, Blackmon LR: The Fogarty balloon catheter as an aid to management of the infant with esophageal atresia and tracheoesophageal fistula complicated by severe RDS or pneumonia. J Pediatr Surg, 17:149, 1982.
12. Filston HC, Rankin JS, Grimm JK: Esophageal atresia. Prognostic factors and contribution of preoperative telescopic endoscopy. Ann Surg, 199:532, 1984.
13. Fonkalsrud EW, in discussion of Velasco N, Hill LD, Ganna RM, Pope CE II: Gastric emptying and gastroesophageal reflux. Effects of surgery and correlation with esophageal motor function. Am J Surg, 144:58, 1982.
14. Gauthier F, Gaudiche O, Baux D, Valayer J: Esophageal atresia and gastro-esophageal reflux. Chir Pediatr, 21:253, 1980.
15. Haight C, Towsley HA: Congenital atresia of the esophagus with tracheo-esophageal fistula; extrapleural ligation of fistula and end-to-end anastomosis of esophageal segments. Surg Gynecol Obstet, 76:672, 1943.
16. Haight C: Congenital atresia of the esophagus with tracheoesophageal fistula. Reconstruction of esophageal continuity by primary anastomosis. Ann Surg, 120:623, 1944.
17. Haight C: Congenital tracheo-esophageal fistula without esophageal atresia. J Thorac Surg, 17:600, 1948.
18. Haight C: Some observations on esophageal atresia and tracheoesophageal fistulas of congenital origin. J Thorac Surg, 34:141, 1957.
19. Hendren WH: Esophageal atresia and tracheoesophageal fistula. Principles of management. Clin Pediatr, 3:30, 1964.
20. Holder TM, Ashcraft KW: Esophageal atresia and tracheoesophageal fistula. Ann Thorac Surg, 9:445, 1970.
21. Holder TM, Leape LL, Mann CM Jr: Esophageal atresia, tracheoesophageal fistula, and associated anomalies—hyperalimentation as an aid in treatment. J Thorac Cardiovasc Surg, 63:838, 1972.
22. Howard R, Myers NA: Esophageal atresia: A technique for elongating the upper pouch. Surgery, 58:725, 1965.
23. Johnston PW: Elongation of the upper segment in esophageal atresia: Report of a case. Surgery, 58:741, 1965.
24. Kluth D: Atlas of esophageal atresia. J Pediatr Surg, 11:901, 1976.
25. Koop CE, Schnaufer L, Broennie AM: Esophageal atresia

and tracheoesophageal fistula: Supportive measures that affect survival. Pediatrics, *54*:558, 1974.

26. Leape LL, Ramenofsky ML: Surgical treatment of gastro-esophageal reflux in children. Am J Dis Child, *134*:935, 1980.
27. Lindahl H, Louhimo I, Virkola K: Colon interposition or gastric tube? Follow-up study of colon-esophagus and gastric tube-esophagus patients. J Pediatr Surg, *18*:58, 1983.
28. Livaditis A, Bjorck G, Kangstrom LE: Esophageal myomectomy. An experimental study in piglets. Scand J Thorac Cardiovasc Surg, *3*:181, 1969.
29. Louhimo I, Lindahl H: Esophageal atresia: Primary results of 500 consecutively treated patients. J Pediatr Surg, *18*:217, 1983.
30. Martin LW: Management of esophageal anomalies. Pediatrics, *36*:342, 1965.
31. Myers NA: Oesophageal atresia with distal tracheo-oesophageal fistula—a long-term follow-up. Prog Pediatr Surg, *10*:5, 1977.
32. Myers NA: Oesophageal atresia and/or tracheo-oesophageal fistula—a study of mortality. Prog Pediatr Surg, *131*:141, 1979.
33. Naef AP, Savary M: Conservative operations for peptic esophagitis with stenosis in columnar-lined lower esophagus. Ann Thorac Surg, *13*:543, 1972.
34. Nason HO, Gillis DA: Transpleural end-to-end repair of esophageal atresia and tracheoesophageal fistula. Can J Surg, *22*:168, 1979.
35. Neuhauser EBO, Berenberg W: Cardioesophageal relaxation as a cause of vomiting in infants. Radiology, *48*:480, 1947.
36. Otte JB, Gianello P, Wese FX, et al: Diverticulum formation after circular myotomy for esophageal atresia. J Pediatr Surg, *19*:68, 1984.
37. Postlethwaite RW: Surgery of the Esophagus. Norwalk, Conn, Appleton Century Crofts, 1986, pp 1–82.
38. Replogle RL: Esophageal atresia: Plastic sump catheter for drainage of the proximal pouch. Surgery, *54*:296, 1963.
39. Rickham PP: Infants with esophageal atresia weighing under 3 pounds. J Pediatr Surg, *16*:595, 1981.
40. Santos AD, Thompson TR, Johnson DE, Foker JE: Correction of esophageal atresia with distal tracheoesophageal fistula. J Thorac Cardiovasc Surg, *85*:229, 1983.
41. Saron IJ, Spitz L, Isdale J: The influence of respiratory complications on the outcome of oesophageal atresia. S Afr J Surg, *13*:251, 1975.
42. Sulamaa M, Gripenberg L, Ahvenainen EK: Prognosis and treatment of congenital atresia of the esophagus. Acta Chir Scand, *102*:141, 1951.
43. Tyson KRT: Primary repair of esophageal atresia without staging or preliminary gastrostomy. Ann Thorac Surg, *21*:378, 1976.
44. Waterston DJ, Bonham-Carter RE, Aberdeen: Oesophageal atresia: Tracheo-oesophageal fistula. A study of survival in 218 infants. Lancet, *1*:819, 1962.
45. Waterston DJ: Colonic replacement of the esophagus (intrathoracic). Surg Clin North Am, *44*:1441, 1964.
46. Waterston DJ: Oesophageal disease in infancy and childhood, excluding oesophagotracheal fistula. *In* Smith RA, Smith RE (Eds): Surgery of the Oesophagus. The Coventry Conference. New York, Appleton Century Crofts, 1972, pp 81–92.

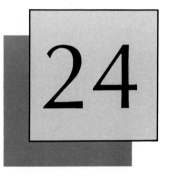

24

Endoscopic Variceal Sclerotherapy

Richard A. Kozarek

As an isolated phenomenon, gastroesophageal varices as a consequence of portal hypertension would have little clinical importance. The fact that once they are present, approximately one-third of individuals will bleed massively from such varices[1] and that death at six weeks in patients who have bled approaches 40 to 50 per cent[2] adds considerable significance to the diagnosis. Add to this the enormous costs associated with variceal hemorrhage and lack of a satisfactory medical or surgical approach to the condition and varices assume even more importance.

■ Current Therapy of Bleeding Varices

Because the vast majority of patients with bleeding varices have cirrhosis, standard medical therapy is directed to both conditions and includes volume replacement, correction of underlying coagulopathy, and prevention of encephalopathy with cathartics, lactulose, or neomycin. Beyond that, measures to control bleeding include infusion of pitressin or glypressin and balloon tamponade. The former reduces blood flow in the mesenteric vascular system and decreases portal pressure by approximately 25 per cent.[3] Bolus or drip infusion has been reported to control bleeding initially in 50 to 75 per cent of patients.[4] The mortality rate from rebleeding, liver or renal failure, or infection, however, may be unchanged. Pitressin infusion in-

duces falling cardiac output and coronary blood flow with bradycardia and ischemia often the rate-limiting factors in its use. Glypressin (triglycl lysine vasopressin), a synthetic pitressin analog without the cardiovascular side effects, has been released recently in Europe and currently is undergoing testing in this country.[5] Balloon tamponade with the Sengstaken-Blakemore or Linton tubes is associated with control of acute bleeding in the majority of patients. Significant side effects include pressure necrosis, esophageal or gastric perforation, and aspiration pneumonitis.[6]

Procedures that have been tried and largely abandoned in the treatment of bleeding esophageal varices include endoscopic laser photocoagulation and percutaneous transhepatic obliteration of varices. Beta blockade with propranolol as a method of decreasing cardiac output and portal pressure was initially reported as promising in the prevention of rebleeding.[7] This has not been substantiated, and as of this writing, no medication has been shown to conclusively prevent the rebleeding that occurs in 50 to 100 per cent of patients once an initial hemorrhage has occurred.

■ Surgery

Three large surgical trials have shown decreased survival compared to a medically managed group in patients who underwent prophylactic portacaval shunting to prevent a bleeding episode.[8–10] Surgical therapy to control acute bleeding includes emergency portacaval shunting, esophageal devascularization with or without transection, and esophageal stapling or vein ligation.[11] With the exception of Orloff's series in which there was a 58 per cent operative survival with emergent portocaval shunting, most series report surgical mortality rates in excess of 50 per cent when these procedures are performed in the acute setting.[11]

Surgical treatment to prevent rebleeding basically has been limited to decompressive portosystemic shunts in this country. Of the four large controlled trials that have been reported, bleeding was decreased in all, but there was no statistically significant improvement in survival when compared to a group of matched patients treated medically.[13-16] Add to this the additional expense of surgery and the significant (one-third) development of portosystemic encephalopathy following the shunting procedures, and results are less than satisfactory.

With the current management of esophageal varices as described above, it has been obvious to physicians caring for such patients that additional treatment modalities are desirable both in the treatment of acute hemorrhage and in the prevention of rebleeding once hemorrhage has occurred.

■ *Acute Bleeding*

Injection of sclerosant material into esophageal varices, despite recent enthusiasm for its use, was initially described by Crafoord and Frenchner in 1939.[17] Their sclerosant was quinine injected through a rigid endoscope. Despite numerous reports in the 1940s and 1950s demonstrating its efficacy,[18] the procedure was never widely used, in part because of the need for rigid esophagoscopy and general anesthesia. With the emergence of fiberoptic endoscopy, and with the limitations of current medical and surgical therapy that have been outlined above, sclerotherapy has been used with increasing frequency over the past several years.

■ TECHNIQUE

Less is known about sclerotherapy than has been defined with certainty, and the plethora of sclerosing agents and injection techniques attests to this lack of knowledge. Most sclerosing agents currently used are derivatives of long-chain fatty acids and include sodium morrhuate, sodium tetradecyl, and ethanolamine oleate (the last is not currently available in this country). Other caustic or thrombotic agents often added include variable concentrations of ethyl alcohol, paraffin, cefazolin, hypertonic dextrose, and thrombin. Using a canine model of portal hypertension, Jensen et al. recently demonstrated that 1.5 per cent tetradecyl and 5 per cent ethanolamine were the most efficacious single agents for sclerotherapy, and that a mixture of 1 per cent tetradecyl, 33 per cent alcohol, and 33 per cent saline was ultimately the least damaging but most effective sclerosant combination.[19] These agents, whether injected intra- or paravariceally, induce acute phlebitis with thrombosis.[20-21] Perivenular as well as esophageal wall fibrosis occurs later.[22,23] This fibrosis is related both to submucosal sclerosant injection and deep ulceration of the esophageal wall in up to 50 per cent of patients undergoing sclerotherapy.[24] Wall fibrosis, in turn, is associated with shunting of venous blood into vessels within and deep to the esophagus and its muscular layers.[25] It is this shunting phenomenon as well as the perivenular fibrosis that is thought to be associated with the reduction of bleeding episodes in patients who have undergone chronic sclerotherapy.

Although there are a variety of sclerotherapy techniques utilizing rigid endoscopes, paravariceal injections, and balloon tamponade either during or immediately after injection,[26-30] most endoscopists in this country attempt intravariceal injections "free-hand" using a flexible endoscope and use balloon tamponade sparingly (Fig. 24–1).[18,31-33] I currently use a large channel endoscope (Olympus 1-T, New Hyde Park, NY) which has capabilities for both aspirating blood and washing the injection

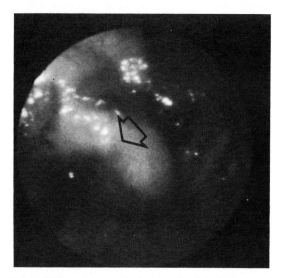

Figure 24–1. Bulging varix (arrow) after injection of 1 ml sodium tetradecyl. Note injection needle within varix (7 o'clock). (See Color Plate IV*B*.)

site. A commercially available polyethylene catheter with a 23-gauge, 4-mm retractable needle is used (Microvasive, Belmont, MA), and the patient is sedated with either a topical throat spray alone or with 50 to 100 mg of meperidine intravenously. Neither proximal balloon tamponade, which has been claimed to facilitate sclerotherapy by increasing the size of the distal vessels, nor an overtube with a rotatable window through which varices project to facilitate ease of injection[34,35] has been found to be necessary. I currently use 1.5 per cent sodium tetradecyl as the sclerosant and attempt to inject intravariceally. Studies incorporating simultaneous venography and sclerotherapy have shown that "intravariceal" injections result in local sclerosant accumulation 40 per cent of the time, presumably related to either vein rupture or due to an unintentional paravariceal injection (Fig. 24–2).[36,37] In another 40 per cent of injections, sclerosant is cleared rapidly in a cephalad direction, whereas 14 per cent of injections were cleared in a caudal fashion (Fig. 24–3).

The esophageal venous plexus has been noted to have three components[38]: (1) intrinsic veins consisting of subepithelial plexus in the lamina propria plus a second layer deep to the muscularis mucosa, the submucous plexus; (2) associated veins which

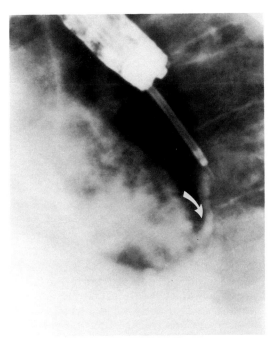

Figure 24–3. Note retrograde contrast flow into gastric varices (arrow). Needle injector is in distal esophageal varix.

are longitudinal veins on the external aspect of the esophagus; and (3) extrinsic veins which anastomose distally with the left gastric vein and proximally with the azygous system. This interconnecting venous plexus explains the bidirectional flow of injected sclerosant material noted at fluoroscopy. It may also offer a clue as to why sclerotherapy is efficacious in the long run (shunting of blood into a deeper and less likely to bleed venous network).

Originally limited to Childs' class C patients or in better operative risk patients who developed rebleeding after initially stopping, I currently use sclerotherapy in all massive variceal bleeders in lieu of pitressin or balloon tamponade or after initial control with these agents. I inject 0.5 to 2.0 ml per injection site, starting below the bleeding varix. If bleeding persists, I inject an additional 1.0 to 2.0 ml above as well as into the bleeding site on the varix. If bleeding has stopped prior to endoscopy, I begin at or just below the gastroesophageal junction, using 0.5 to 2.0 ml in each varix at that level. Similar amounts of sclerosant are circumferentially injected every 2 to 3 cm up to the mid or proximal third of the esophagus, using a total of 15 to 30 ml of sclerosant per session. If bleeding persists after this, I will employ a balloon for tamponade.

The condition of the patient, as well as subsequent plans to undertake portosystemic shunt or other surgical decompressive procedures, deter-

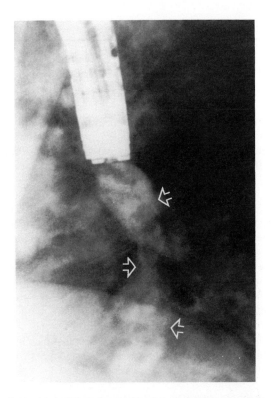

Figure 24–2. Arrows outline local accumulation of contrast sclerosing mixture injected at time of simultaneous sclerotherapy venography.

mines the timing of follow-up sclerotherapy sessions. At our institution, shunt surgery is undertaken only in patients in whom sclerotherapy cannot control the acute or recurrent bleeding episodes. This is currently approximately 10 per cent of patients with variceal hemorrhage. For patients in whom chronic sclerotherapy is planned, I repeat sclerotherapy three to four days after the initial injection session and then every two to four weeks until variceal obliteration has been effected. As obliteration proceeds, progressively smaller sclerosing volumes are required for subsequent sessions.

■ RESULTS

The goals of endoscopic sclerotherapy can be defined as control of acute hemorrhage, reduction in transfusion requirements, and the prevention of rebleeding. Its use acutely has been shown to control bleeding in 75 to 100 per cent of cases.[26–28,30,31,33,39,40] In one of the largest series to date, Paquet utilized a rigid endoscope and paravariceal injections to stop bleeding in 93 per cent of 359 patients with active variceal hemorrhage.[41] Overall short-term mortality rate was 22 per cent, two-thirds of patients expiring from liver failure and portosystemic encephalopathy, whereas 7 per cent died from exsanguination. Using intravariceal injections through a flexible endoscope, the Cleveland Clinic's experience in 105 patients demonstrated cessation of hemorrhage in 84 per cent with a consequent reduction in transfusion requirements but uncertain effect on mortality.[31] Denck, in turn, demonstrated an acute survival rate of 87.5 per cent of 277 patients undergoing sclerotherapy for massive hemorrhage.[42] This compares to a 50 per cent mortality rate in patients treated with balloon tamponade, 16 per cent mortality rate in patients undergoing elective portacaval shunt, and an 80 per cent mortality rate in patients undergoing emergency shunting procedure. Terblanche, in turn, was able to stop acute or recurrent variceal hemorrhage in 95 per cent of patients admitted to the hospital during a prospective five-year study period,[43] compared to a 40 per cent definitive control rate with balloon tamponade in a previous study at his institution. Acute mortality rate was 28 per cent in sclerotherapy patients and 60 per cent in the patients treated with balloon tamponade.

In one of the few randomized prospective studies to be reported, Cello et al. studied 52 patients with severe cirrhosis (Childs' class C) who required at least 6 units of blood for acute variceal hemorrhage.[44] These patients were randomized to treatment with sclerotherapy versus portacaval shunt.

During the index hospitalization, short-term survival rates were equivalent and the shunt group required approximately twice as much blood replacement. After a mean follow-up time of 263 days, there was no difference in survival, although the sclerotherapy group required significantly more hospitalization days for subsequent rebleeding. Total health care costs for the sclerotherapy group were approximately one half those of the shunted group. The author concluded that sclerotherapy was less costly and as effective as shunt surgery. In a second study that addressed cost, Chung and Lewis compared four groups of patients admitted to the University of Iowa with bleeding varices.[45] Group I was treated with portosystemic shunts; group II, standard medical therapy; group III underwent emergency variceal ligation; and group IV, sclerotherapy. The authors found that the cost per patient and cost per survivor at two years was lowest for the sclerotherapy group. These costs were approximately one half those for patients treated medically and one fourth those for the patients treated surgically.

In summary, acute sclerotherapy can stop bleeding, is cost-effective when compared to conventional medical or surgical regimens, and appears to be associated with improved short-term survival when compared to current therapies.

■ *Chronic Sclerotherapy*

Because of the problems of subsequent rebleeding in patients who have bled from gastroesophageal varices, most endoscopists institute a course of chronic sclerosis in an attempt to obtain variceal obliteration or fibrosis. In the largest series reported to date Paquet used monthly injection sessions in 1123 patients at the time of acute bleeding or during bleed-free intervals.[41] Variceal obliteration was usual, but subsequent recurrence was common (35 per cent at four months). Death usually was related to liver failure or infection, occurring in 16 per cent acutely with a 19 per cent secondary mortality rate. Six per cent of patients were lost to follow-up, and 60 per cent were still alive, 50 per cent after five years or longer. Terblanche et al. prospectively randomized patients who bled into follow-up sclerotherapy or standard medical management.[43] Recurrent hemorrhage occurred in 60 per cent of the medically treated group and in 36 per cent of the chronic sclerotherapy group. Once variceal obliteration was effected, there was no further bleeding in patients who had been sclerosed. There was no difference in the two-year mortality rate, with patients in the sclerotherapy group expiring from liver failure or infection.

Clark and his associates studied 64 patients randomized to medical or injection treatment after an initial variceal bleed.[46] Thirty-three per cent of sclerotherapy and 68 per cent of medically treated patients rebled. The eventual risk of bleeding in medically treated patients was threefold at 2, 6, and 12 months when compared to patients treated with sclerosis. One-year survival was 46 per cent in the sclerotherapy group and 6 per cent in the medically treated group ($p < 0.02$). In contrast, results of a retrospective study of patients treated at the Mayo Clinic found no improvement in sclerotherapy patients when compared to historical control subjects.[47] Some of the discrepancies between the various series may be related to the underlying etiology of the cirrhosis, Childs' classification of the patient, injection technique and timing, sclerosant used, cessation of alcohol by the patient with alcoholic liver disease, and the skill and perseverance of the endoscopist. Despite the above, chronic sclerotherapy appears to obliterate varices and decrease but not eliminate recurrent hemorrhage. Its effect upon survival is uncertain and results might be expected to parallel those of surgically treated patients, i.e., rebleeding episodes are fewer but survival does not necessarily improve. Rather, it is defined by the hepatic reserve of the patient.

■ Prophylactic Sclerotherapy

In contrast to use in acute variceal hemorrhage and in patients in whom variceal obliteration is attempted, variceal sclerotherapy has been used prophylactically in a single controlled trial to date.[48] Paquet randomized 71 patients with large (grade III or IV) varices plus reduced coagulation factors to serial endoscopies every four months, or weekly sclerotherapy sessions until variceal obliteration was accomplished. Over a two-year period, 67 per cent of medically treated patients bled and 42 per of these died at the time of first hemorrhage. In contrast, 6 per cent of the sclerotherapy patients bled, and hemorrhage was controlled in each case with further sclerosis. By the third year, 90 per cent of conservatively treated patients had died of bleeding or hepatic coma compared with 12.5 per cent of the sclerosant group.[49] Although this study suggests that prophylactic sclerotherapy may have benefit in a subset of patients with large varices and coagulopathy, the lack of additional controlled trials plus previous data on prophylactic shunting

should make one cautious in accepting these data.[50,51]

■ Complications

Reported complications in variceal sclerotherapy have ranged between 2 per cent and 25 per cent.[26,29,31,35,46] In two surveys of American Society for Gastrointestinal Endoscopy (ASGE) members, complications were 9 per cent per procedure and 19 per cent per patient prior to 1981.[24] These complications fell to 16.7 per cent per patient and 6.4 per cent per procedure by 1982. Such complications are for the most part self-limiting and often the direct result of the sclerosant itself.

Chest discomfort, often described as burning or crushing and substernal in location, can occur in a quarter of patients and may be the result of esophageal spasm or a direct chemical esophagitis related to the sclerosant. Low-grade fever, occurring in 10 to 15 per cent of patients, may be related to bacteremia at the time of injections, but is more commonly self-limited and probably also related to a chemically induced esophagitis.[52] This fever usually lasts 24 to 48 hours.[53]

Ulceration, occurring in well over one half of the patients treated with sclerotherapy in my series, was the most common complication in the ASGE survey (42 per cent of total complications) (Fig. 24–4).[24] This ulceration may, in part, be related to the type, volume, and concentration of sclerosant used.[19] More commonly, finding these ulcers may

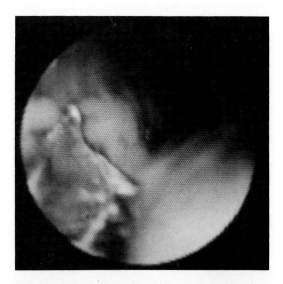

Figure 24–4. Extensive esophageal ulceration, 7 to 9 o'clock, after sclerotherapy. Ulcers are commonly colonized by yeast (see text). (See Color Plate IVC.)

simply be related to the timing of follow-up endoscopy after initial sclerotherapy. The presence of shallow ulcerations may actually be beneficial, as they are associated with intramural fibrosis and prevention of rebleeding.

Deep ulceration, on the other hand, may be associated with rebleeding or perforation which may present as local mediastinitis or empyema (Fig. 24–5).[22,54,55] Reported perforation rates vary widely but averaged 1.8 per cent in the ASGE survey.[31] Most, but not all, of these perforations can be managed conservatively. Deep ulceration may also be associated with stricture formation,[56] and such strictures occurred in 20 per cent of patients in my series and 9.1 per cent in the ASGE survey.[50] These strictures are usually readily dilated and are partly related to the aggressiveness and frequency of follow-up sclerotherapy sessions. They may be related to reflux with decreased acid clearance secondary to wall fibrosis or chronic monilial infection of the ulceration. More frequent than stricture formation, however, is the development of esophageal dysmotility plus a variable effect upon lower esophageal sphincter pressure.[57,58] The long-term significance of these changes remains to be defined.

After ulceration, precipitation of bleeding appears to be the most common complication of sclerotherapy.[24] Occurring in 5 to 10 per cent of patients, this bleeding can ususally be controlled by additional injections above and below the bleeding site. Occasionally, pitressin or balloon tamponade may be necessary. As mentioned above, bleeding may also be delayed and the result of sclerotherapy-induced ulcers. Paradoxically, such bleeding can usually be controlled with further sclerosant injected around the ulcer base.

In addition to the above, there have been several cases of portal vein thromboses related to sclerotherapy, probably as a result of retrograde sclero-

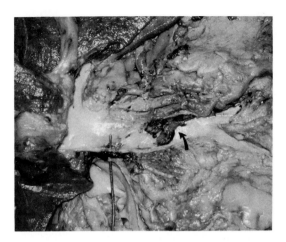

Figure 24–6. Autopsy specimen demonstrates probe through patent portacaval anastomosis in a patient who died from bleeding gastric varices. Arrow shows portal vein clot propagated from left gastric veins after sclerotherapy. (See Color Plate IV*E*.)

sant (Fig. 24–6).[34] Intramural hematomas and abscess formation have also been reported, as has aspiration pneumonitis and a variety of other cardiopulmonary reactions.[55,59,60]

■ Conclusions

Sclerotherapy can stop acute variceal hemorrhage in the majority of instances and appears to offer short-term survival advantages over conventional medical management. Long-term sclerotherapy can obliterate varices and appears to protect from rebleeding. Data regarding long-term survival rates are too sparse to make any definite conclusions. It appears to be as effective as shunt therapy in Childs' class C patients and consistently more cost-effective. What its place should be in Childs' class A and B patients remains to be defined. Because of initial operative mortality rates, cost, and the encephalopathy associated with shunting procedures, many centers use sclerotherapy as the definitive treatment modality in patients with bleeding varices. Complications, most often self-limiting but occasionally life-threatening, can occur with sclerotherapy, and once obliterated, varices may eventually return and require resclerosis. Only prospectively controlled clinical trials will define the ultimate place sclerotherapy will finally play in the treatment of portal hypertension.[61–63]

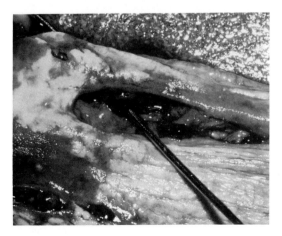

Figure 24–5. Probe demonstrates deep esophageal ulceration with free mediastinal perforation. (See Color Plate IV*D*.)

■ REFERENCES

1. Fleischer D: Review of the results of shunt surgery. *In* Sivak

MV (ed): Endoscopic Sclerotherapy of Esophageal Varices. New York, Praeger Publishing, 1984, pp 17–21.

2. Graham DY, Smith JL: The course of patients after variceal hemorrhage. Gastroenterology, 80:800–809, 1981.

3. Barr JW, Lakin RC, Rosch J: Similarity of arterial and intravenous vasopressin on portal and systemic hemodynamics. Gastroenterology. 69:13–19, 1975.

4. Carey WD: The medical therapy for variceal hemorrhage. In Sivak MV (ed): Endoscopic Sclerotherapy of Esophageal Varices. New York, Praeger Publishing, 1984, pp 11–15.

5. Freeman JG, Lishman AH, Corden I, et al: Controlled trial of terlipressin (glypressin) versus vasopressin in the early treatment of esophageal varices. Lancet, 1:66–68, 1982.

6. Pitcher JL: Safety and effectiveness of the modified Sengstaken-Blakemore tube: A prospective study. Gastroenterology, 61:291–298, 1971.

7. Lebrec D, Poynard T, Hillon P, et al: Propranolol for prevention of recurrent gastrointestinal bleeding in patients with cirrhosis. N Engl J Med, 305:1371–1374, 1981.

8. Resnick RH, Chalmers TC, Ishihara AM, et al: The Boston interhospital liver group: A controlled study of the prophylactic portacaval shunt. A final report. Ann Intern Med, 70:675–688, 1969.

9. Jackson FC, Perrin EB, Smith AG, et al: A clinical investigation of the portacaval shunt. II: Survival analysis of the prophylactic operation. Am J Surg, 115:22–42, 1968.

10. Conn HO, Lindermuth WW: Prophylactic portacaval anastomosis in cirrhotic patients with esophageal varices: A progress report of a continuing study. N Engl J Med, 272:1255–1263, 1965.

11. Wexler MJ: Esophageal procedures to control bleeding from varices. Surg Clin North Am, 63:905–914, 1983.

12. Orloff MJ, Bell RH, Hyde PJ: Long-term results of emergency portacaval shunt for esophageal varices in unselected patients with alcoholic cirrhosis. Ann Surg, 192:325–340, 1980.

13. Jackson FC, Perrin EB, Felix WR, et al: A clinical investigation of the portacaval shunt. V: Survival analysis of the therapeutic operation. Ann Surg, 174:672–701, 1971.

14. Resnick RH, Iber FL, Ishihara AM, et al: A controlled study of the therapeutic portacaval shunt. Gastroenterology, 74:843–857, 1974.

15. Rueff B, Degos F, Degos JD, et al: A controlled study of therapeutic portacaval shunt in alcoholic liver cirrhosis. Lancet, 1:655–659, 1976.

16. Reynolds TB, Donovan AJ, Mikkelsen WP, et al: Results of a twelve-year randomized trial of portacaval anastomosis: To shunt or not to shunt. Gastroenterology, 80:1005–1011, 1981.

17. Crafoord C, Frenchner P: New surgical treatment of varicose veins of the oesophagus. Acta Otolaryngol, 27:422–429, 1939.

18. Williams R, Westaby D: History and development of sclerotherapy. In Sivak MV (ed): Endoscopic Sclerotherapy of Esophageal Varices. New York, Praeger Publishing, 1984, pp 29–33.

19. Jensen DM: Evaluation of sclerosing agents in animal models. In Sivak MV (ed): Endoscopic Sclerotherapy of Esophageal Varices. New York, Praeger Publishing, 1984, pp 51–53.

20. Halpap B, Bollweg L: Morphologic changes in the terminal oesophagus with varices, following sclerosis of the wall. Endoscopy, 13:229–233, 1981.

21. Ayres SJ, Goff JS, Warren GH, Schaefer JW: Esophageal ulceration and bleeding after flexible fiberoptic esophageal vein sclerosis. Gastroenterology, 83:131–136, 1982.

22. Matsumoto S: Clinicopathological study of sclerotherapy of esophageal varices. I. A review of 26 autopsy cases. Gastroenterol Jpn, 21:99–105, 1986.

23. Evans DMD, Jones DB, Cleary BK, Smith PK: Oesophageal varices treated by sclerotherapy: A histopathological study. Gut, 23:615–620, 1982.

24. Sivak MV Jr: Endoscopic injection sclerosis of esophageal varices: ASGE survey (Letter). Gastrointest Endosc, 28:41, 1982.

25. Lewis JW: Histologic changes in the eosphagus after sclerotherapy. In Sivak MV (ed): Endoscopic Sclerotherapy of Esophageal Varices. New York, Praeger Publishing, 1984, pp 55–58.

26. Paquet KJ, Oberhammer E: Sclerotherapy of bleeding oesophageal varices by means of endoscopy. Endoscopy, 10:7–12, 1978.

27. Hennessy TPJ, Stephens RB, Keane FB: Acute and chronic management of esophageal varices by injection sclerotherapy. Surg Gynecol Obstet, 154:375–377, 1982.

28. Johnston GU, Rodgers HW: A review of 15 years experience in the use of sclerotherapy in the control of acute hemorrhage for oesophageal varices. Br J Surg, 60:797–800, 1982.

29. Hughes RW Jr, Larson DE, Viggiano TR, et al: Endoscopic variceal sclerosis: A one-year experience. Gastrointest Endosc, 28:62–66, 1982.

30. Johnson AG: Injection sclerotherapy in the emergency and elective treatment of oesophageal varices. Ann Royal Coll Surg (Engl), 59:497–501, 1977.

31. Sivak MV, Stout DJ, Skipper G: Endoscopic injection sclerosis (EIS) of esophageal varices. Gastrointest Endosc, 27:52–57, 1981.

32. Yassin YM, Sherif SM: Randomized controlled trial of injection sclerotherapy for bleeding oesophageal varices: An interim report. Br J Surg, 70:20–22, 1983.

33. Jensen DM, Silpa M, Sue M, et al: Emergency sclerotherapy for active variceal bleeding in poor risk cirrhotics (abstract). Gastrointest Endosc, 31:130, 1985.

34. Goodale RL, Silors SE, O'Leary JF, et al: Early survival after sclerotherapy for bleeding esophageal varices. Surg Gynecol Obst, 155:523–528, 1982.

35. Lewis J, Chung RS, Allison J: Sclerotherapy of esophageal varices. Arch Surg, 115:476–480, 1980.

36. Grobe JL, Kozarek RA, Sanowski RA, et al: Venography during endoscopic injection sclerotherapy of esophageal varices. Gastrointest Endosc, 30:6–8, 1984.

37. Barsoum MS, Khattar NY, Riak-Allah MA: Technical aspects of injection sclerotherapy of acute oesophageal variceal hemorrhage as seen by radiography. Br J Surg, 65:588–589, 1978.

38. Butler H: The veins of the eosphagus. Thorax, 6:276–296, 1951.

39. Terblanche J, Northover JMA, Bornman P, et al: A prospective evaluation of injection sclerotherapy in the treatment of acute bleeding from esophageal varices. Surgery, 85:239–245, 1979.

40. Terblanche J, Northover JMA, Bornman P, et al: A prospective controlled trial of sclerotherapy in the long-term management of patients after esophageal variceal bleeding. Surg Gynecol Obstet, 148:323–333, 1979.

41. Paquet KJ: Endoscopic paravariceal injection sclerotherapy of the esophagus: Indications, technique, complications, results of a period nearly fourteen years. In Sivak MV (ed): Endoscopic Sclerotherapy of Esophageal Varices. New York, Praeger Publishing, 1984, pp 99–114.

42. Denck H: Endoesophageal sclerotherapy of bleeding esophageal varices. J Cardiovasc Surg, 12:146, 1977.

43. Terblanche J, Yakoob HI, Bornman PC, et al: A five-year prospective evaluation of tamponade and sclerotherapy. Ann Surg, 194:521–530, 1981.

44. Cello JP, Grendell JH, Cross RA, et al: Endoscopic sclerotherapy versus portacaval shunt in patients with severe

cirrhosis and variceal hemorrhage. N Engl J Med, *311*:1589–1600, 1984.

45. Chung R, Lewis JW: Cost of treatment of bleeding esophageal varices. Arch Surg, *118*:482–485, 1983.

46. Clark AW, Westaby D, Silk DBA, et al: Prospective controlled trial of injection sclerotherapy in patients with cirrhosis and recent variceal hemorrhage. Lancet, *1*:552–554, 1980.

47. DiMagno EP, Zinsmeister AR, Larson DE, et al: Influence of hepatic reserve and cause of esophageal varices on survival and rebleeding before and after introduction of sclerotherapy: A retrospective analysis. Mayo Clin Proc, *60*:149–157, 1985.

48. Paquet KJ: Prophylactic endoscopic sclerosing treatment of the esophageal wall in varices: A prospective controlled randomized trial. Endoscopy, *14*:4–5, 1982.

49. Paquet KJ: A controlled trial of prophylactic endoscopic sclerotherapy of esophageal varices. *In* Sivak MV (ed): Endoscopic Sclerotherapy of Esophageal Varices. New York, Praeger Publishing, 1984, pp 59–68.

50. Lieberman DA: Sclerotherapy for bleeding esophageal varices after randomized trials. West J Med, *145*:481–484, 1986.

51. Paquet KS, Koussouris P: Is there an indication for prophylactic endoscopic paravariceal injection sclerotherapy in patients with liver cirrhosis and portal hypertension? Endoscopy, *18*:32–35, 1986.

52. Brayko CM, Kozarek RA, Sanowski RA, Testa AW: Bacteremia during esophageal variceal sclerotherapy: Its cause and prevention. Gastrointest Endosc, *31*:10–12, 1985.

53. Roark GD, Patterson M: Endoscopic sclerotherapy for the management of variceal bleeding. South Med J, *76*:494–496, 1983.

54. Soederlund C, Wiechel K-L: Oesophageal perforation after sclerotherapy for variceal hemorrhage. Acta Chir Scand, *149*:491–495, 1983.

55. Sarin SK, Nanda R, Sachdev G, et al: Intravariceal versus paravariceal sclerotherapy: a prospective, controlled, randomized trial. Gut, *28*:657–662, 1987.

56. Sørenson TIA, Burcharth F, Pedersen ML, Lindahl F: Oesophophageal stricture and dysphagia after endoscopic sclerotherapy for bleeding varices. Gut, *25*:473–477, 1984.

57. Cohen LB, Simon C, Korsten MA, et al: Esophageal motility and symptoms after endoscopic injection sclerotherapy. Dig Dis Sci, *30*:29–32, 1985.

58. Fleig WE, Butters M, Dehmel M: Effects of endoscopic paravariceal sclerotherapy on LES function and esophageal motility (abstract). Gastrointest Endosc, *31*:128–129, 1985.

59. Palani CK, Abuabara S, Draff AR, Jonasson O: Endoscopic sclerotherapy in acute variceal hemorrhage. Am J Surg, *141*:164–168, 1981.

60. Schuman BM: The systemic complications of sclerotherapy of esophageal varices. Gastrointest Endosc, *31*:348–349, 1985.

61. Smith PM: Variceal sclerotherapy: Further progress. Gut, *28*:645–649, 1987.

62. Sarin SK, Sachdev G, Nanda R: Follow-up of patients after variceal eradication. A comparison of patients with cirrhosis, noncirrhotic portal fibrosis and extrahepatic obstruction. Ann Surg, *204*:78–82, 1986.

63. Warren WD, Henderson JM, Millikan WJ, et al: Distal splenorenal shunt versus endoscopic sclerotherapy for long-term management of variceal bleeding. Preliminary report of a prospective, randomized trial. Ann Surg, *203*:454–462, 1986.

25

Neodymium-YAG Laser Applications in the Esophagus

Richard A. Kozarek

Laser is an acronym for light amplification by stimulated emission of radiation.[1] It is a phenomenon which occurs when an electron from a light-stimulated atom is excited to a higher energy state and subsequently emits a photon of light upon return to its original resting orbit. This photon stimulates other atoms, producing a chain reaction and subsequent burst of light energy. With the use of a mirror system, this light energy is passed back and forth through a substance that emits additional photons. This, in turn, results in light amplification. Amplified light can then be directed through a lens system which concentrates it to an extremely small point. In the case of the neodymium-YAG (Nd-YAG) laser, it can be further transmitted through a quartz fiber which is passed through the biopsy channel of a conventional endoscope.

Laser energy is intense and nondivergent (parallel) and can be easily focused. Unlike white light, which consists of a variety of wavelengths, laser light consists of a single wavelength. The tissue absorption characteristics of this wavelength determine its clinical application. Tissue effect is dependent upon light absorption, which is subsequently converted to heat energy.

The three lasers that are currently in medical use in this country include the carbon dioxide, argon, and Nd-YAG lasers.[2] The argon laser has a wavelength of 476.5 and 514.5 nm and emits a blue-green color. It is highly absorbed by melanin and hemoglobin and therefore useful in coagulating surface vessels. Its primary use has been coagulation of blood vessels in diabetic retinopathy, but it also has been used in the skin to remove local tumors, tattoos, and hemangiomas.[3]

The carbon dioxide (CO_2) laser has an infrared wavelength of 10,600 nm. This wavelength is strongly absorbed by water in living cells. It causes intracellular water to boil and superficial cells to vaporize. Its major clinical application is as a surgery scalpel, and it has been used particularly in gynecologic procedures (tubal ligation, cervical cone).[3]

The Nd-YAG laser has an intermediate wavelength of 1060 nm and penetrates tissue 5 to 18 times more deeply than the respective argon and CO_2 lasers. Because of this deeper penetration and a maximum power output greater than 10 times that delivered by the argon laser, it is ideally suited for the heating and coagulation of underlying vessels. It has been applied by a variety of subspecialties. Uses include endometrial ablation in dysfunctional uterine bleeding, resection of bladder neoplasms, palliative vaporization of obstructing endobronchial neoplasms, and subcapsular cataract extractions, among others.[4]

■ Technique

There are now a number of commerically available Nd-YAG laser units in this country. Each consists of an operating console which contains a power supply, control unit, and cooling coils. The laser is transmitted through a small quartz fiber

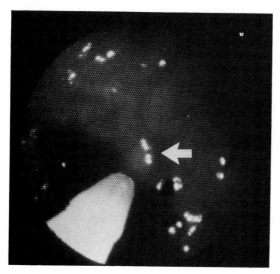

Figure 25–1. Sheath containing quartz fiber through which Nd-YAG laser is transmitted. Aiming beam (arrow) is a low power argon laser. (See Color Plate IV*F*.)

which can be passed through the biopsy channel of a standard fiber endoscope. This fiber is encased in a sheath through which air or CO_2 flows, thereby clearing blood or debris from the treatment site (Fig. 25–1). There is also a special gas evacuation valve which is attached to the endoscope that helps to prevent gastric or intestinal overinflation.

Most laser units incorporate a computer system that allows the operator to set the power between 10 and 100 watts (W) and the pulse time between 0.1 and 9.9 s (Fig. 25–2). Cumulative energy in

joules (W·s) is automatically tabulated. Low powers (50 to 70 W) and short pulse times (0.1 to 0.5 s) cause tissue charring and coagulation of blood vessels.[5] They are particularly useful for achieving hemostasis. Powers in excess of 80 W, particularly when delivered for longer time periods, cause intense local heat (greater than 100°C) and tissue vaporization. These effects are useful for tumor photoablation. After the desired power and pulse times have been registered, the quartz fiber delivery system is passed into the endoscope biopsy channel until the fiber protrudes 0.5 to 1.5 cm from the endoscope tip. Light pulses can be delivered using a foot-operated switch. Tissue effect depends not only on power and pulse settings, but also on distance from the treatment site, angle of laser beam delivery, and amount of blood or debris on the lesion being treated.[5]

Because the laser beam can also be reflected back through the instrument to the operator or assistants, and because such light can cause permanent retinal damage, all individuals in the laser suite are required to wear special glasses which filter out the laser light wavelength. The patient's eyes are covered with a towel. Light sedation with intravenous meperidine or diazepam is used for the treatment sessions which average 30 to 90 min.

■ *Applications*

■ GENERAL

Nd-YAG lasers have had three major applications in the gastrointestinal tract.[6] First, they have

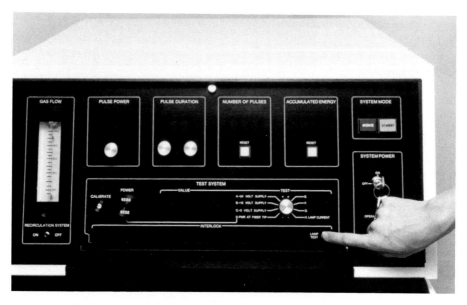

Figure 25–2. Cooper Nd-YAG laser. Note console allowing control of pulse power and duration. Accumulated energy in joules is calculated and recorded by a minicomputer.

been demonstrated to stop acutely bleeding mucosal lesions in over 90 per cent of patients treated.[7,8] Such lesions include duodenal and gastric ulcers, hemorrhagic gastritis, Mallory-Weiss tears, and a variety of vascular anomalies. Studies have confirmed that bleeding, operative, and rebleeding rates all can be decreased by laser therapy.[9,10] The data is uncertain, however, whether laser treatment improves survival in patients with upper GI bleeding. This is probably related to the fact that only one third to one half of patients with gastrointestinal hemorrhage who end up dying actually die of the hemorrhage itself.[11]

The second indication for laser therapy is treatment of chronically bleeding gastrointestinal lesions in an attempt to minimize transfusions and recurrent hospitalizations.[6] Lesions treated most commonly have been vascular anomalies, including telangectasia and angiodysplasia, and bleeding, unresectable neoplasms of the esophagus, stomach, and colon. In the largest series reported to date, Jensen et al. showed that both transfusion requirements and hospitalization were dramatically decreased in patients with hereditary hemorrhagic telangiectasia who were prophylactically treated with the laser.[13] However, treatment of incidentally found nonbleeding vascular lesions in patients being evaluated for chronic or recurrent hemorrhage is not necessarily associated with prevention or reduction in subsequent bleeding episodes.[13,14] Because all such lesions can re-form over time, periodic retreatments are often necessary.

The third gastrointestinal application of the Nd-YAG laser is treatment of unresectable, obstructing neoplasms. Originally used for recurrent or unresectable esophageal cancers,[15–18] use has been extended to gastroesophageal junction adenocarcinomas and gastric and rectal cancer.[19–25] Because high laser power settings are associated with tissue vaporization, new lumina can be formed in such a setting, offering palliative bowel continuity.

■ ESOPHAGEAL APPLICATIONS

The major uses of laser therapy in the esophagus have been control of acute hemorrhage and palliative tumor ablation.

Hemorrhage ■ There have been a variety of bleeding esophageal lesions successfully treated with laser therapy.[6] Using short pulses (0.5 to 1.0 s) and coagulative power settings (50 to 70 W), it is highly effective against Mallory-Weiss tears (Fig. 25–3). These tears are circumferentially treated, allowing tissue edema and temperature-dependent coagulation to effect hemostasis. Bleeding esophageal ulcerations and Osler-Weber-Rendu

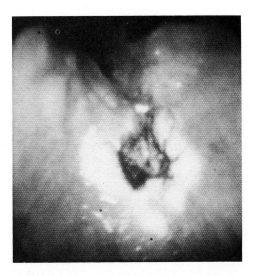

Figure 25–3. Laser-treated Mallory-Weiss tear of the gastroesophageal junction. Note edema and tissue blanching related to circumferential treatment of the laceration. (See Color Plate VA.)

telangiectasias are also easily amenable to treatment. More diffuse esophageal lesions that have been treated include severe esophagitis with multiple oozing points and bleeding esophageal varices.[8,9] Both situations require a modification of conventional laser technique and are most readily treated by using long pulse times (1 to 5 s) and slighly higher power. Coagulation is undertaken using a Z technique in which the endoscope and laser beam are broadly moved to trace the letter Z.[5] This allows large areas of mucosa to be treated sequentially. Laser treatment allows control of 90 to 95 per cent of localized mucosal hemorrhage from the esophagus, and its use can obviate the need for emergency surgery in a substantial number of patients. In contrast, the efficacy rates for control of variceal hemorrhage are significantly lower.[8] Because treatment can be associated with the development of deep ulceration and does not obliterate varices by itself, most endoscopists have abandoned its use in variceal hemorrhage, using sclerotherapy instead.

Neoplasm ■ Because high powers (greater than 80 W) and longer pulse time (1 to 5 s) are associated with vaporization and tissue cavitation, the Nd-YAG laser is an ideal palliative tool for obstructing esophageal or GE junction tumors.

More than 75 per cent of patients with esophageal or GE junction malignancies have local tumor invasion or distant metastases at the time of diagnosis, precluding curative surgical resction.[26] Of the 83,383 cases reviewed by Earlam and Cunha-Melo, there was a 29 per cent mortality rate in patients undergoing resection and a 17 per cent mortality rate for exploration without resection.[27] These authors state: "Out of any 100 patients, including all in the community who actually visit a doctor, 58 will be explored, 39 resected, 26 leave the hospital with the tumor excised, 18 survive for one year, 9 for two years, and 4 for five years. If there is a surgeon, accepting all the patients in the population he serves, who can improve upon these figures, he has not yet written an article with his results. . . ." Because radiation therapy is no more effective than surgical treatment, and the benefit of chemotherapy is even more uncertain,[28] palliative maneuvers become of prime concern in the treatment of esophageal and GE junction cancers. Such palliation may be directed to nutritional supplementation and control of local pain but is most often directed to the progressive dysphagia that is almost universal. In the past and currently, this dysphagia has been treated with rigid and flexible dilators, passage of peroral esophageal prostheses (particularly if tracheoesophageal fistula is present), and various palliative surgical maneuvers.[26,29-34]

More recently, the Nd-YAG laser has been used as an additional palliative maneuver. Based on the finding that long application with higher power is associated with tissue vaporization, Fleischer and Kessler initially described its use in obstructing esophageal malignancy[15] and later expanded its application to advanced adenocarcinoma of the gastric cardia.[19] Mean luminal size increased in the latter series from 3.3 to 12.1 mm with treatment. This was associated with decreased dysphagia, increased food intake, and significant palliation. Mean survival time approximated five months in the 15 patients reported. More recently Mellow and Pinkas compared laser-treated patients who had disease recurrence after radiation or surgical therapy with historical control subjects treated with irradiation.[16] They found that not only were dysphagia and performance status improved with laser, but so was survival. An additional report by Cello et al. confirmed the ability to debulk tumor with laser and that this debulking was associated with substantial and immediate palliation.[19]

Finally, Nd-YAG laser therapy is frequently used in our institution in obstructed patients undergoing preoperative chemotherapy (cisplatin) and irradiation prior to surgical resection. Such treatment allows the patient to mobilize his saliva and eat a general diet, and usually precludes the need for prolonged home hyperalimentation or feeding gastrostomy placement prior to definitive resection.

Patients are sedated with meperidine or diazepam, and large channel endoscopes (e.g., Olympus IT, Olympus Corporation, New Hyde Park, NY) are used. Unless previous bougienage has been successful in transiently increasing luminal size to allow scope passage through the tumor, treatment is directed at the uppermost margin of the neoplasm. Using power settings between 80 and 100 W and pulse time of 1 to 2 s, the beam is transmitted onto the tissue circumferentially with a vaporizing or cavitating effect. Necrotic debris can be removed with an electrocautery snare or biopsy forceps, after which more distal esophageal tumor can be treated in a similar fashion.

Using the Nd-YAG laser in this manner, I usually deliver 5 to 10,000 joules of energy per treatment session. These sessions take 30 to 90 min and are repeated every other day until adequate luminal enlargement has occurred (Fig. 25-4). The mean number of treatment sessions required in our institution has been 3.4, and total energy delivered per patient approximates 20,000 joules. The subsequent luminal enlargement allows the patient to mobilze secretions, eat a soft diet, and maintain weight. Tumor regrowth, which can occur from weeks to months later, may require simply bougienage or a second course of laser treatments.

Two recent developments have the potential to modify current treatment delivery. The first entails intravenous injection of a photosensitizing porphyrin.[35] This allows deeper tissue penetration of laser light delivered to tumor and accelerated destruction of neoplasm. The second is the development of contact laser probes. These probes consist of a synthetic sapphire tip which can be attached to the end of the quartz fiber delivery system, allowing tissue contact without damage to the fiber.[26] They have several advantages which include high-power density at the tip, minimal backscatter, and depending upon the tip used, variable patterns of tissue penetration. Using these tips, lesser power outputs (10 to 20 W) can be used for photoablation, and unseen tissue burn is greatly reduced. Using this system, I have been able to effect a reasonable esophageal lumen in obstructed patients in one to two treatment sessions, using considerably less energy than with conventional fibers (Fig. 25-5). When commercially available, these contact probes may dramatically alter current laser techniques.

■ Methodology

In our institution palliative tumor photoablation is done in either an inpatient or outpatient setting.

■ Complications

Complications of laser use for bleeding include those of diagnostic endoscopy (drug reaction, as-

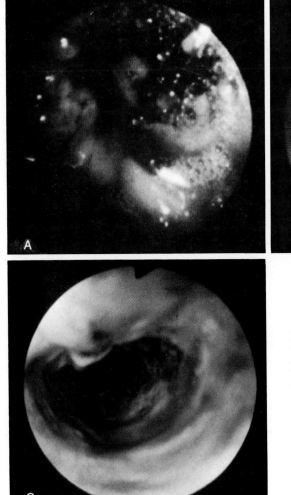

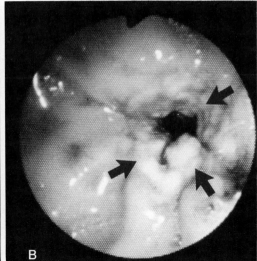

Figure 25–4. *A*, Gastroesophageal junction neoplasm with 2 mm opening into stomach. (See Color Plate V*B*.) *B*, Arrows delineate necrotic tissue after initial laser treatment of 4800 J. (See Color Plate V*C*.) *C*, Gastroesophageal junction of patient depicted in *A* and *B* after second laser treatment. Note progressive increase in luminal size. Patient required two additional treatments to increase lumen to 15 mm. (See Color Plate V*D*.)

piration, vasovagal reaction, arrhythmia, bleeding, instrument perforation) as well as those unique to laser therapy. The incidence of laser therapy complications ranges between 0 and 10 per cent and is highly dependent upon the skill and experience of the user.[1,10,38–41] Paradoxically, the most common complication appears to be acceleration of arterial bleeding and can occur when the laser beam is aimed directly at a visible vessel causing clot lysis. For this reason it is preferable to treat a bleeding site circumferentially to effect tissue edema prior to direct laser application to a vessel. Because of the high power used and the degree of tissue penetration associated with conventional application of the Nd-YAG laser, a 40 to 80 per cent incidence of transmural injury to the bowel wall has been reported.[37–39] This has translated into a clinical perforation rate of 1 per cent in some studies.[10] In addition, air embolism and gas bloat, related to gas infusion to clear the bleeding site, are potential problems, as is an intraluminal fire.

In addition to the complications noted above, use of the Nd-YAG laser for palliation of esophageal or GE junction neoplasm carries special risks. These are related primarily to the amount of tissue being treated, the depth of tissue penetration required, and the multiple treatment sessions that are often needed. Minor complications that occur in 25 to 50 per cent of patients include variable degrees of chest discomfort and fever, usually less than 38.5°C, which can last for several days.[15] Free and contained perforations, with or without development of tracheoesophageal fistula, also have been reported.[15–18] Finally, significant amount of tissue vaporization can be associated with inhalation of potentially toxic hydrocarbon and smoke by both the patient and laser personnel. For this reason, most laser suites are equipped with a vacuum system which minimizes inhalation risk.

What improvement in complication rates will be achieved with the use of the contact laser tips remains to be seen. However, the increased focusing

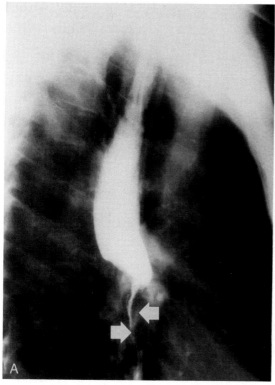

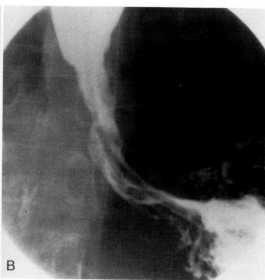

Figure 24–5. *A,* Arrows demonstrate extensive gastroesophageal junction carcinoma extending into distal esophagus. Note proximal esophageal dilation. *B,* Same patient after two laser sessions. Luminal enlargement is noted but residual tumor shouldering in the esophagus is still evident.

ability, improved control of depth of laser penetration, and the lesser amount of smoke generated during the procedure are all potential advantages and may improve both efficacy and safety.

▪ Summary

Despite gastrointestinal applications spanning less than a decade, medical lasers are now firmly entrenched as treatment modalities in esophageal disease. In particular, the Nd-YAG laser has received widespread use to treat both acute and chronically bleeding lesions and to palliatively enlarge GE junction or esophageal lumens obstructed by recurrent or unresectable malignancy. The latter treatments appear to improve patient quality of life, although survival benefits remain to be clearly defined. New technologies, including pretreatment of tumor patients with porphyrins and the development of contact laser tips, appear promising. The future use of medical lasers appears to depend upon development of instruments which can be set to deliver variable wavelengths. Each of these laser beams will react in a slightly different fashion (tissue cutting, deep or superficial vaporization) in the tissue to which it is being applied.

▪ REFERENCES

1. Kozarek RA: Laser: gastrointestinal applications. Am Fam Phys, *29*:187–190, 1984.
2. Dwyer RM, Bass M: Lasers in medicine. *In* Ross M (ed): Laser Applications. Vol 3. New York, Academic Press, 1977, pp 107–134.
3. Bernstein LH: Horizons of laser light therapy. Endosc Rev, *1*:51–55, 1984.
4. Kozarek RA, Ball TJ: Use of the neodymium-YAG laser in gastroenterology. Bull Mason Clin, *38*:25–35, 1984.
5. Dwyer RM: The technique of gastrointestinal laser endoscopy. *In* Goldman L (ed): The Biomedical Laser. Technology and Clinical Applications. New York, Springer-Verlag, 1981, pp 255–269.
6. Fleischer D: The current status of gastrointestinal laser activity in the United States. Gastrointest Endosc, *28*:157–161, 1982.
7. Laurence B, Vallon A, Cotton P, et al: Endoscopic laser photocoagulation for bleeding peptic ulcers. Lancet, *1*:124–125, 1980.
8. Kiefhaber P, Nath G, Moritz K: Endoscopic control of massive gastrointestinal hemorrhage by irradiation with a high power neodymium-YAG laser. Progr Surg, *15*:140–155, 1977.
9. Rutgeerts P, Vantrappen G, Broeckaert L, et al: Controlled trial of YAG laser treatment of upper digestive hemorrhage. Gastroenterology, *83*:410–416, 1982.
10. Silverstein FE, Gilbert DA, Auth DC: Endoscopic hemostasis using laser photocoagulation and electrocoagulation. Dig Dis Sci, *26*:31S–40S, 1981.
11. Allan R, Dykes P: A study of the factors influencing mortality rates from gastrointestinal hemorrhage. Q J Med, *180*:533–550, 1976.
12. Bonheim NA: Endoscopic therapy of bleeding gastrointes-

tinal hemangiomas and angiodysplasia. Am J Gastroenterol, *80*:727–729, 1985.

13. Jensen DM, Machicado GA, Tapia JF, et al: Endoscopic argon laser photocoagulation of patients with severe gastrointestinal bleeding. Gastroenterology, *84*:572, 1983.

14. Jensen DM, Machicado GA: Endoscopic treatment of incidental angioma in patients with severe gastrointestinal bleeding (abstract). Gastrointest Endosc, *31*:147, 1985.

15. Fleischer D, Kessler F: Endoscopic Nd-YAG laser therapy for carcinoma of the esophagus: A form of palliative treatment. Gastroenterology, *85*:600–606, 1983.

16. Mellow MH, Pinkas H: Endoscopic therapy for esophageal carcinoma with Nd-YAG laser: Prospective evaluation of efficacy, complications, and survival. Gastrointest Endosc, *30*:334–339, 1984.

17. Cello JP, Gerstenberger PD, Wright T, et al: Endoscopic neodymium-YAG laser palliation of nonresectable esophageal malignancy. Ann Intern Med, *102*:610–612, 1985.

18. Fleischer D: Endoscopic laser therapy for carcinoma of the esophagus. Endosc Rev, *1*:37–49, 1984.

19. Fleischer D, Sivak M: Endoscopic Nd-YAG laser therapy as palliative treatment for advanced adenocarcinoma of the gastric cardia. Gastroenterology, *87*:815–820, 1984.

20. Sakita T, Kogama S, Ishii M, et al: Early cancer of the stomach treated successfully with an endoscopic neodymium-YAG laser. Am J Gastroenterol, *76*:441–445, 1981.

21. Cello JP, Melnick S, Meiselman MS: Endoscopic neodymium-YAG laser treatment of nonresectable gastrointestinal tract cancer. West J Med, *142*:42, 1985.

22. Groisser VW: YAG laser therapy of gastrointestinal tumors. Gastrointest Endosc, *30*:311–312, 1984.

23. Kiefhaber P, Kiefhaber K: Present endoscopic laser therapy in the gastrointestinal tract. Gastroenterology, *85*:439–446, 1983.

24. Brunetaad JM, Mosquet L, Bourez J, et al: Laser applications in nonhemorrhagic digestive lesions. *In* Atsumi K (Ed): New Frontiers in Laser Medicine and Surgery. Amsterdam, Excerpta Medica, 1983, pp 455–461.

25. Jensen DM: Lasers in the GI cancer war and on other fronts. Gastroenterology, *87*:974–976, 1984.

26. Orringer MB: Palliative procedures for esophageal cancer. Surg Clin North Am, *63*:941–950, 1983.

27. Earlam R, Cunha-Melo JR: Oesophageal squamous cell carcinoma: I. A critical review of surgery. Br J Surg, *67*:381–390, 1980.

28. Boyce HW Jr: Palliation of advanced esophageal cancer. Semin Oncol, *11*:186–195, 1984.

29. Heit AH, Johnson LF, Siegel SR, et al: Palliative dilation for dysphagia in esophageal carcinoma. Ann Intern Med, *89*:629–631, 1978.

30. Cassidy DE, Nord HJ, Boyce HW Jr: Management of malignant esophageal strictures: Role of esophageal dilation and peroral prosthesis. Am J Gastroenterol, *76*:173, 1981.

31. Olgilvie AL, Bomfield MW, Ferguson R, et al: Palliative intubation of oesophagogastric neoplasms. Gut, *23*:1060–1067, 1982.

32. Boyce HW, Jr: Medical management of esophageal obstruction and esophageal-pulmonary fistula. Cancer, *50*:2597–2600, 1982.

33. Balmes JL, Baghdad H, Michel H: Palliative endoscopic treatment of malignant esophageal stenosis using a Häring prosthesis. Digestion, *23*:31–38, 1982.

34. Valbeuna J: Palliation of gastroesophageal carcinoma with endoscopic insertion of new antireflux prosthesis. Gastrointest Endosc, *30*:241–243, 1984.

35. Lambert R, Sabben G: Photoradiation therapy (PRT) for cancer in the esophagus (abstract). Gastrointest Endosc, *30*:134, 1984.

36. Joffe HLJ, Sanker MY, Brackett KM, et al: Comparison of ''touch'' and ''nontouch'' techniques of Nd-YAG laser in experimental hepatic resections (abstract). Gastrointest Endosc, *31*:155. 1985.

37. Dixon JA, Berenson MM, McCloskey DW: Neodymium-YAG laser treatment of experimental canine gastric bleeding: Acute and chronic studies of photocoagulation, penetration, and perforation. Gastroenterology,*77*:647–651, 1979.

38. Overholt B: Laser treatment of esophageal cancer. Am J Gastroenterol, *80*:719–720, 1985.

39. Jensen DM, Silpa ML, Tapia JI, et al: Comparison of different methods for endoscopic hemostasis of bleeding canine esophageal varices. Gastroenterology, *84*:1455–1461, 1983.

40. Mellow MH, Pinkas H: Endoscopic laser therapy for malignancies affecting the esophagus and gastroesophageal junction. Analysis of technical and functional efficacy. Arch Intern Med, *145*:1443–1446, 1985.

41. Pietrafitta JJ, Dwyer RM: Endoscopic laser therapy of malignant esophageal obstruction. Arch Surg, *121*:395–400, 1986.

26

Esophageal Foreign Bodies and Food Impaction

Richard A. Kozarek

Foreign body impaction in the esophagus is not an uncommon occurrence. It can occur in any age group and in any part of the esophagus and can be associated with discomfort alone or potentially fatal perforation into the mediastinum. Clinically, the problem can be divided into the adult and pediatric age groups, the presence or absence of underlying esophageal disease, and the type of material impacted. All impactions, however, are associated with the unique symptom complex of chest or neck discomfort, odynophagia, increased salivation, and persistent feeling of esophageal obstruction on swallowing. Retching, vomiting, expectoration of bloody saliva, previous history of gagging or choking during meals, and refusal to eat in children are also commonly seen.

■ *Children*

During the learning and exploration associated with childhood, it is the norm to suck, place in the mouth, and in some cases swallow a variety of nondigestible objects. Fortunately, less than 10 per cent of these objects are retained in the gastrointestinal tract, and a smaller portion still in the esophagus.[1] In both the adult and pediatric age groups, the majority of nonfood bolus foreign bodies impact in the cervical esophagus.[2-4] These objects usually hang up at one of the normal areas of anatomic narrowing, the cricopharyngeus muscle, or the aortic arch.[5] Less frequently, they can be

302

held up where the left mainstem bronchus crosses the esophagus (Fig. 26–1*A*) or at the cardioesophageal junction. Usually, there is intrinsic esophageal disease in these children, and the impaction is related to the size and shape of the object swallowed.[6] For instance, in 343 children seen with esophageal foreign bodies, Nandi and Ong found the offending object to be a fishbone (146) or coin (134) in 82 per cent.[4] Seventy-six per cent of 2394 cases reviewed in this series had impactions in the cervical esophagus, 12 per cent in the hypopharyngeal area, and 7.7 per cent in the thoracic esophagus. Other objects included fruit, stones, glass, toothpicks, wire, pieces of plastic toy, and buttons. A less common cause of esophageal foreign body in children occurs in the setting of congenital anomalies.[3] These include congenital stenoses, webs, tracheoesophageal fistulas, and anomalous or enlarged vascular channels, among others.

As mentioned above, symptoms may be those of classical dysphagia with pain and increased salivation or may be simply recurrent emeses or failure to eat. Complications of foreign body ingestion in the pediatric group are much less common than in the adult population.[4] Nevertheless, such complications may include aspiration with subsequent chemical or bacterial pneumonitis, Mallory-Weiss or Boerhaave's laceration of the esophagus associated with recurrent retching, and esophageal perforation with possible mediastinitis, pneumothorax, and lung abcess.[4,7-11] Eighty-four cases of esophagoaortic fistulas have also been reported in relation to impacted foreign body and pressure ne-

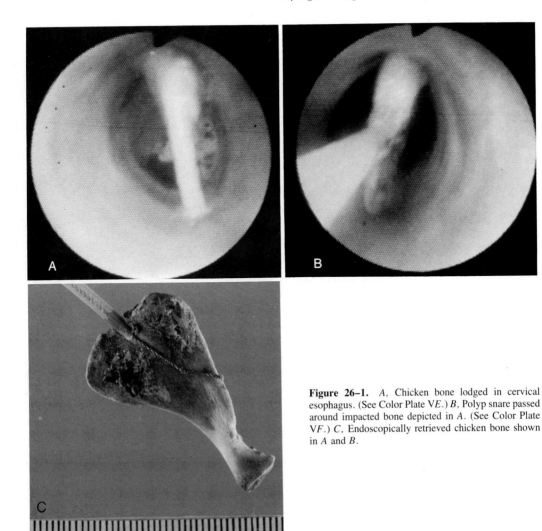

Figure 26–1. *A*, Chicken bone lodged in cervical esophagus. (See Color Plate V*E*.) *B*, Polyp snare passed around impacted bone depicted in *A*. (See Color Plate V*F*.) *C*, Endoscopically retrieved chicken bone shown in *A* and *B*.

crosis or local infection.[4,12–14] Finally, it should be noted that certain ingested objects have intrinsic local and systemic toxicity that goes beyond simple impaction with the attendant edema and local inflammatory response. This is especially true in children who ingest and obstruct alkali disc batteries.[15,17] These batteries may not only cause tissue saponification with local ulceration, perforation or stricture formation, but may also cause systemic toxicity related to blood levels of absorbed metals. This topic is covered in more detail in the chapter on caustic ingestion.

■ *Adults*

Foreign body impaction in the adult can be subdivided into food impactions and the inadvertent or deliberate ingestion of nondigestible materials. In the latter category are individuals who swallow fruit pits, pieces of denture material, or bits of meat with attached bone. Such impactions are more common in inebriated patients or in individuals wearing dentures who have lost the tactile sensation of the palate. The majority of these materials lodge above the thoracic inlet, similar to the pediatric age group.[4–6,18,19] As many as one third, however, can lodge more distally. In contrast to the pediatric population, local complications are more common and perforation rates up to 1 per cent are reported.[4,20]

In addition to inadvertent foreign body ingestion, some impactions occur when foreign objects are deliberately swallowed. These include narcotic-filled balloons swallowed by ''body packers'' as a method of smuggling.[21,22] A more lethal consequence of this ingestion is balloon disruption in the stomach or leakage in the more distal gastrointestinal tract, leading to systemic absorption, respiratory depression, and death. Mentally disturbed or psychotic patients may also ingest foreign bodies, many repeatedly so.[23–27] These objects may spontaneously pass per rectum or may remain in the stomach and cause remarkably few symptoms. Alternatively, they may require surgical removal because of local bleeding, perforation (Fig. 26–2), or obstruction of the intestinal tract, or they may impact in the esophagus. Objects that have been documented to obstruct the esophagus in these individuals include cigarette lighters, coins, and checkers, among others.[27] Finally, I have seen prisoners who have repeatedly ingested objects—spoons, salt shakers, metal bed springs—in order to escape incarceration. Some of these individuals who preferred hospitalization and repeated endoscopic or surgical retrieval to jail settled into foreign body ingestion as a career, and would virtually devour large chunks of their jail cells.

In contrast to the ingestion of foreign bodies in which impaction can occur even in the normal esophagus, patients who impact food usually have underlying esophageal disease and most commonly obstruct their esophagus distally (Fig. 26–3).[18,28–30] Food impactions can be seen in patients with chronic dysphagia secondary to reflux or lye stricture, achalasia, or carcinoma of the esophagus or gastric cardia. More commonly, however, these patients learn their swallowing limitations quickly and either limit their diet accordingly or chew their food well while washing it down with copious liq-

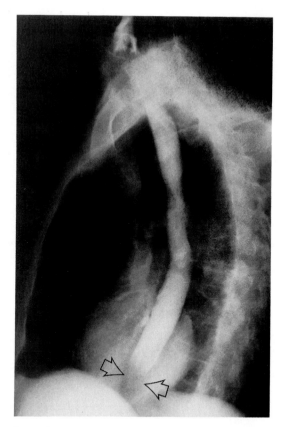

Figure 26–3. Arrows delineate impacted food bolus, distal esophagus.

uids. The majority of patients who develop food impaction have intermittent dysphagia with normal periods of swallowing interspersed. Such individuals usually have a lower esophageal ring in conjunction with a hiatal hernia (Fig. 26–4). Esophageal dysmotility, frequently present before the obstruction, becomes almost invariable at time of impaction.[28] Associated factors include faulty mastication in individuals who are either edentulous or have ill-fitting dentures.[31] Alcoholism and intoxication also predispose to impaction, as normally chewed pieces of food may be swallowed whole.[32] Although I have seen bread, olives, and garbanzo beans impacted in a lower esophageal ring, the majority of instances occur with meat ingestion, particularly steak. This has led some authors to coin the phrase "backyard barbeque"[32] or "steakhouse" syndrome[33] when describing this phenomenon.

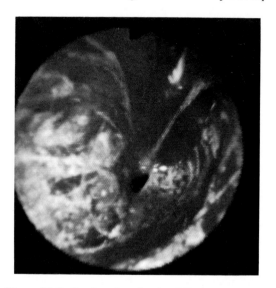

Figure 26–2. Esophageal perforation following emergency room attempt to dislodge impacted food bolus with mercury bougie. Photograph is per os view of mediastinum. (See Color Plate VI*A*.)

■ *Diagnosis*

The diagnosis of foreign body or food impaction is usually not difficult in the adult population. In

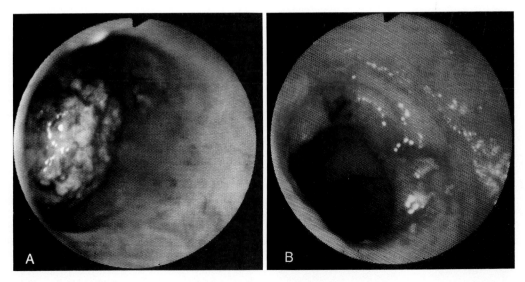

Figure 26–4. *A*, Food bolus impacted at gastroesophageal junction. Esophageal fluid has been endoscopically aspirated. (See Color Plate VI*B*.) *B*, Tight Schatzki's ring noted after endoscopic retrieval of food impaction depicted in *A*. Hiatal hernia can be seen distally. (See Color Plate VI*C*.)

addition to the previously defined symptoms of dysphagia, odynophagia, chest or neck pain, retching, and excess salivation, patients will often bring a cup to the physician's office or emergency room to expectorate saliva. Children, in contrast, may simply complain of pain or cough related to the aspiration of saliva, or they may refuse feedings. Physical signs other than excess salivation and the tachycardia associated with patient discomfort are usually minor unless a complication has supervened. In such cases, pulmonary rhonchi or wheezing, fever, neck abscess, or signs of mediastinal air (mediastinal crunch, subcutaneous emphysema) may be noted.[4,9,34]

In almost all instances, diagnostic workups should include plain film radiographs of the neck and chest.[35–37] These films will detect both radiopaque objects such as metal or glass as well as evidence of local perforation such as abscess or free or contained air. They will also confirm suspected aspiration and may even show unsuspected foreign body aspiration into the tracheobronchial tree.[38] Neck films usually are not required with suspected food impaction in the distal esophagus. Chest films, however, may detect unsuspected bone fragments and evidence of local leak. Diagnosis of esophageal foreign body can be confirmed either radiographically or endoscopically. The method of confirmation depends both upon endoscopic availability and the type of foreign body ingested. In general, Gastrografin is irritating to the lungs and should be avoided if there is a risk of aspiration. In cases of food obstruction in which initial definition is radiographic, a nasogastric tube

may need to be passed to the level of obstruction, so that fluid can be aspirated from the esophagus. Such patients often continue to eat or drink after impaction, hoping to dislodge the offending food piece. Alternatively, some patients salivate prolifically after impaction, filling the esophagus in this manner. After aspiration, barium is inserted through the nasogastric tube to delineate the obstruction and configuration of the adjacent esophagus (Fig. 26–5). It is both unnecessary and uncomfortable to the patient to completely fill the esophagus.

In the setting of bone fragments and most other foreign bodies, endoscopy is the preferred method of diagnosis and, in addition, can be used for retrieval.[5,18,20,29,30] Caution must be exercised in the systemically toxic patient or in the individual in whom local perforation is suspected clinically or radiographically. In addition, aspiration associated with endoscopic intubation must be guarded against if esophagoscopy is used for either diagnosis or treatment.

■ *Treatment*

■ FOOD IMPACTION

Treatment of distal esophageal food impaction as well as some distally impacted foreign bodies which are relatively small, smooth, and likely to pass through the remaining GI tract without incident should begin with initial pharmacologic mea-

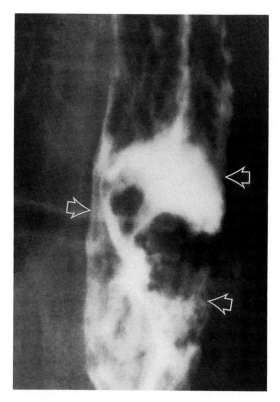

Figure 26–5. Arrows depict partially obstructing food bolus in fluid-filled esophagus.

sures. A number of smooth muscle relaxants have been used. The rationale is the elimination of associated spasm or dysmotility and dilation of an obstructing lower esophageal ring. The most commonly used agent has been glucagon, administered as a 0.5-mg to 1-mg intravenous bolus. This hormone causes a transient reduction in lower esophageal sphincter pressure without demonstrable change in esophageal wave speed, amplitude, or duration.[39] Originally reported in 1977 as effective in three of six cases of esophageal food impactions,[40] a number of subsequent reports have documented its efficacy in up to 50 per cent of such cases.[41-43] This medication can be repeated in 5 to 10 min if bolus passage is not immediate. Postingestion nausea is common, and vomiting, ileus, and dizziness are occasionally seen. Transient hyperglycemia is an invariable consequence of glucagon, and it should not be used in patients with hypersensitivity, insulinoma, or pheochromocytoma. Other medications that have been tried for similar reasons include atropine, diazepam, and nitroglycerin.[18]

If pharmacologic maneuvers are unsuccessful, enzymatic digestion of an impacting meat bolus is considered the treatment of choice by some authors.[28] Originally described in 1945 by Richard-

son,[31] a variety of proteolytic agents have since been used to treat meat impactions.[44,45] Papain, a trypsin-like enzyme derived from the pawpaw or melon tree *(Carica papaya)*, is currently the enzyme which is most commonly used. Available commercially as Adolf's Meat Tenderizer, it has been purported to digest up to 45 times its weight in lean meat.[46] The technique includes ingesting a teaspoon of papain in 4 oz of water and repeating this amount every 15 to 30 min until bolus passage. This method usually allows passage of a meat bolus within two to four hours, but can require up to eight hours. Initial aspiration of a fluid-filled esophagus with a nasogastric tube may be required. Papain digestion is generally safe, is often effective, and can be used in the emergency room setting without requiring endoscopic expertise. However, symptomatic relief can be delayed. Moreover, both hemorrhagic pulmonary edema related to aspiration (dog model)[47] and esophageal perforation secondary to transmural enzymatic digestion have been reported.[47,48] For the foregoing reasons, its use should be limited to settings in which other therapies have failed or are unavailable.

Other treatments for food impaction have included meat extraction by a balloon catheter[49] and, in the veterinary literature, esophageal lavage.[50] Both of these methods carry a significant risk of aspiration and are, therefore, not recommended. Blind or fluoroscopically guided passage of a mercury dilator in an attempt to push the offending bolus into the stomach is another procedure used not infrequently in the emergency room setting. The risk of Mallory-Weiss laceration and esophageal perforation make this a dangerous technique, even in experienced hands (see Fig. 26–2). Similar reservations are registered for the use of gas-forming agents (tartaric acid plus sodium bicarbonate ingested in an attempt to push the obstruction into the stomach).[51] A technique that has been used successfully in communities in which endoscopic capabilities are limited, however, involves a modified 34 French gastric lavage tube, the end of which has been trimmed off and filed smooth.[52] After initial barium swallow delineates the level of obstruction, the tube is placed per os and passed to the obstructing bolus. Suction is applied using a 120 ml syringe and the tube and foreign body are subsequently retrieved (Fig. 26–6). Although the technique was originally described without using fluoroscopy, in my opinion fluoroscopy is helpful and improves the procedure's safety. It has proved effective in approximately two thirds of cases of impacted meat bolus in which it has been employed in my practice.

Despite the variety of treatment modalities outlined above, most practitioners still prefer endoscopic retrieval of impacted food bo-

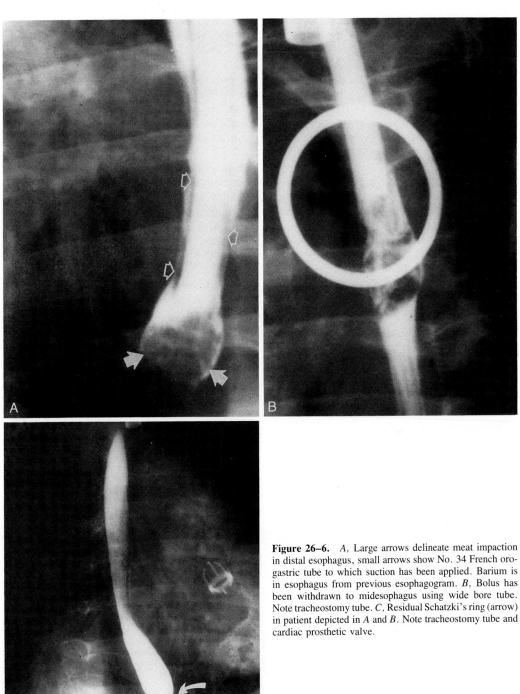

Figure 26–6. *A*, Large arrows delineate meat impaction in distal esophagus, small arrows show No. 34 French orogastric tube to which suction has been applied. Barium is in esophagus from previous esophagogram. *B*, Bolus has been withdrawn to midesophagus using wide bore tube. Note tracheostomy tube. *C*, Residual Schatzki's ring (arrow) in patient depicted in *A* and *B*. Note tracheostomy tube and cardiac prosthetic valve.

luses.[4,5,18,20,29,30] This allows both directed removal as well as precise delineation of the underlying disease, ring stricture, or neoplasm. Historically, most disimpactions were accomplished with the rigid endoscope. Because of the necessity of general anesthesia, the need for hospitalization, and a 0.3 to 1 per cent perforation rate,[4,5,18] the majority of practitioners now use flexible endoscopes to remove food impactions. A large variety of endoscopic tools have been adapted by resourceful endoscopists for such tasks. They include standard rat's tooth and alligator biopsy forceps, stone baskets, polyp snares, and a variety of blunt foreign body grabbers (Fig. 26–7). Despite the variety of available implements, however, removal of impacted food can be tedious and time-consuming. Such impacted food is often removed piecemeal, resulting in numerous endoscopic passages through the cricopharyngeus. This increases the risk of aspiration unless an overtube is also used (Fig. 26–8).[53] This is discussed in the next section.

■ FOREIGN BODY

Small, smooth objects which are impacted in the distal esophagus may respond to glucagon given as outlined above. Blunt esophageal foreign bodies can also be removed using Foley catheter extraction. With this technique, the patient is placed in the head-down position in the fluoroscopic suite to prevent subsequent aspiration. Using a 14 or 16 French Foley catheter passed beyond the object and subsequently inflated, Campbell and Foley were able to safely remove foreign bodies from over 100 children.[54] All objects were radiographically ascertained to be blunt, and 92 per cent were located in the mid or proximal esophagus.

For the most part, however, esophageal foreign bodies traditionally have been removed with the rigid endoscope.[4,18] Since Lerche's initial report in 1911,[2] over 7000 cases of foreign body extraction have been reported with the rigid esophagoscope.[18] In the 2650 cases in which morbidity and mortality were reported in these series, the perforation rate was 0.34 per cent, and the mortality rate of the procedure was 0.05 per cent.[18] Because of the necessity for hospitalization and general anesthesia, rigid endoscopy today is reserved in most centers for situations in which foreign body removal by flexible endoscopy is not successful.[5,20,29,30,55,56] I currently employ a small caliber endoscope (see Fig. 26–1A, B, C) inserted through a 60-cm long, 34 French overtube for removal of most food impactions or foreign bodies. After inserting both the overtube and endoscope through the cricopharyngeus, the airway is protected upon subsequent endoscope removal. Moreover, multiple insertions are possible without additional patient discomfort. Finally, sharp objects such as pins, bones, or toothpicks can be pulled into the overtube without fear of lacerating either the esophagus or hypopharynx upon scope removal.

■ *Complications*

Complications of esophageal foreign body or food impaction include bleeding from Mallory-Weiss laceration, local perforation (see Fig. 26–2) with neck abscess or mediastinitis, aspiration pneu-

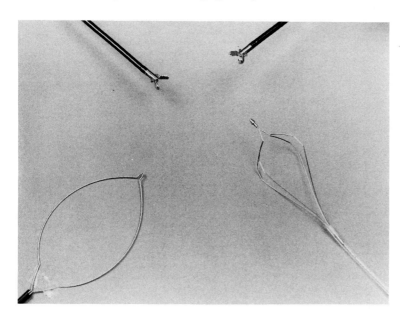

Figure 26–7. Flexible endoscopic accessories that can be used for foreign body extraction.

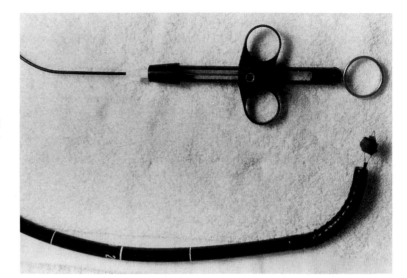

Figure 26–8. Meat bolus removed with flexible endoscope in patient depicted Figure 26–4A and B.

monitis, and esophagoaortic fistula formation. These topics and the surgery required to correct some of them will receive additional coverage in other chapters.

■ REFERENCES

1. Davidoff E, Towne JB: Ingested foreign bodies. NY State J Med, 75:1003, 1975.
2. Lerche W: The esophagoscope in removing sharp foreign bodies from the esophagus. JAMA, 56:634–637, 1911.
3. Hollinger PH, Johnston KC, Greenland J: Congenital anomalies of the oesophagus related to oesophageal foreign bodies. Am J Dis Child, 78:467–476, 1949.
4. Nandi P, Ong GB: Foreign body in the esophagus: A review of 2394 cases. Br J Surg, 65:5–9, 1978.
5. Sanowski RA: Foreign body removal from the upper gastrointestinal tract. Arizona Med, 41:161–163, 1984.
6. Spitz L: Management of ingested foreign bodies in childhood. Br Med J, 4:469, 1971.
7. Michel L, Grillo HC, Malt RA: Esophageal perforation. Ann Thorac Surg, 33:203–210, 1982.
8. Jones RJ, Sampson PC: Esophageal injury. Ann Thorac Surg, 19:216–218, 1975.
9. Barber GB, Peppercorn MA, Ehrlich C, Thurer R: Esophageal foreign body perforation: Report of an unusual case and review of the literature. Am J Gastroenterol, 79:509–511, 1984.
10. Brewster ES: Traumatic perforation of the esophagus caused by self-catheterization with heavy electric wire. Am J Surg, 93:1021, 1957.
11. Keszler P, Buzna E: Surgical and conservative management of esophageal perforation. Chest, 80:158–162, 1981.
12. Vella EE, Booth PJ: Foreign body in the oesophagus. Br Med J, 2:1042, 1965.
13. Marcello FB Jr: Aorto-esophageal fistula: An unusual case of massive hematemesis and melena. Acta Med Philippines, 2:27–34, 1966.
14. Sloop RD, Thompson JC: Aorto-esophageal fistula: Report of a case and review of the literature. Gastroenterology, 53:768–777, 1967.
15. Litovitz TL: Button battery ingestions: A review of 56 cases. JAMA, 249:2495–2500, 1983.
16. Votteler TP, Nash JC, Rutledge JC: The hazard of ingested alkaline disk batteries in children. JAMA, 249:2504–2506, 1983.
17. Maves MD, Carithers JS, Birck HC: Esophageal burns secondary to disc battery ingestions. Ann Otol Rhinol Laryngol, 93:364–369, 1984.
18. Giordano A, Adams G, Boies L Jr, Meyerhoff W: Current management of esophageal foreign bodies. Arch Otolaryngol, 107:249–251, 1981.
19. Savary M, Miller G: The esophagus. In Grassman AG (Ed): Handbook and Atlas of Endoscopy. Solothurn, Switzerland, Schweiz, 1978, p 45.
20. Vizcarrondo FJ, Brady PG, Nord HJ: Foreign bodies of the upper gastrointestinal tract. Gastrointest Endosc, 29:208–210, 1983.
21. Suaraz CA, Arango A, Lester JL: Cocaine-condom ingestion: Surgical treatment. JAMA, 238:1391–1392, 1977.
22. Weber F, Williams G, Swartz MA: Effect of ipecac in "body packers." Ann Emerg Med, 11:699, 1982.
23. Ghani A, Masud S, Hashmi S: Large foreign bodies of the gastrointestinal tract. Int Surg, 66:271–272, 1981.
24. Eldredge WW: Foreign bodies in the gastrointestinal tract. JAMA, 178:665–668, 1961.
25. Cigtay DS, Quesada R: Foreign bodies in the gastrointestinal tract. AFR, 3:104–110, 1971.
26. Teimourian B, Gigtay AS, Smyth NPO: Management of ingested foreign bodies in the psychotic patient. Arch Surg, 88:915–920, 1964.
27. Roark GD, Subramanyam K, Patterson M: Ingested foreign material in mentally disturbed patients. South Med J, 76:1125–1127, 1983.
28. Hargrove MD Jr, Boyce HW Jr: Meat impaction of the esophagus. Arch Intern Med, 12:277–281, 1970.
29. Ricote GL, Tome LR, De Ayala VP, et al: Fiberendoscopic removal of foreign bodies of the upper part of the gastrointestinal tract. Surg Gynecol Obstet, 160:499–504, 1985.
30. Selivanov V, Sheldon GF, Cello J, Crass RA: Management of foreign body ingestion. Ann Surg, 199:187–191, 1984.
31. Richardson JR: A treatment for esophageal obstruction due to meat impaction. Ann Otol Rhinol Laryngol, 54:328–348, 1945.

32. Palmer E: Backyard barbeque syndrome. JAMA, 235:2637–2638, 1976.
33. Norton RA, King GD: "Steakhouse syndrome": The symptomatic lower esophageal ring. Lahey Clin Found Bull, 13:55–59, 1963.
34. Sullivan PK, Jafek BW: Esophageal injury. ENT J 63:34–39, 1984.
35. DeLuca SA, Rhea JT: Foreign bodies in the hypopharynx and esophagus. Am Fam Phys, 28:142–143, 1983.
36. McArthur DR, Taylor DF: A determination of the minimum radiopacification necessary for radiograph detection of a aspirated swallowed object. Oral Surg, 39:329–338, 1975.
37. Fodor J III, Malott JC: The radiographic detection of foreign bodies. Radiol Technol, 54:361–370, 1983.
38. DaSilva AMM: Foreign body aspiration. S Afr Med J, 61:130–134, 1982.
39. Hogan WJ, Dodds WJ, Hoke SE, et al: Effect of glucagon on esophageal motor function. Gastroenterology, 69:160–165, 1975.
40. Ferrucci JT Jr, Long JA Jr: Radiologic treatment of esophageal food impaction using intravenous glucagon. Radiology, 125:25–28, 1977.
41. Fredlund GW: The treatment of acute esophageal food impaction. Radiology, 149:601–602, 1983.
42. Glauser J, Lilja GP, Greenfield B, et al: Intravenous glucagon in the management of esophageal food obstruction. JACEP, 8:228–231, 1979.
43. Marks HW, Lousteau RJ: Glucagon and esophageal meat impaction. Arch Otolaryngol, 105:367–368, 1979.
44. Nighbert E, Dorton H, Griffen WO Jr: Enzymatic relief of the "steakhouse syndrome." Am J Surg, 116:467–469, 1968.
45. Miller JM, Godfrey GC: Treatment of impaction of cooked meat in the esophagus with trypsin. Arch Otololaryngol, 62:202–203, 1958.
46. Robinson AS: Meat impaction in the esophagus treated by enzymatic digestion. JAMA, 181:1142–1143, 1962.
47. Anderson HA, Bernatz PE, Grindlay JG: Perforation of the esophagus after use of a digestive agent: Report of a case and experimental study. Ann Otol Rhinol Laryngol, 68:890–896, 1959.
48. Holsinger JR Jr, Fuson RL, Sealy WC: Esophageal perforation following meat impaction and papain ingestion. JAMA, 204:734–735, 1968.
49. Dieter RA Jr, Norbeck DE, Acuna A, et al: Fogarty catheter removal of cervical esophageal meat bolus. Arch Surg, 105:790–791, 1972.
50. Kerz PD: A technique for relieving esophageal obstruction in the horse. Vet Med Small Anim Clin, 71:216, 1976.
51. Rice BT, Spiegel PK, Dombrowski PJ: Acute esophageal food impaction treated by gas-forming agents. Radiology, 146:299–301, 1983.
52. Kozarek RA, Sanowski RA: Esophageal food impaction: Description of a new method for bolus removal. Dig Dis Sci, 25:100–103, 1980.
53. Rogers BH, Kot C, Meiri S, et al: An overtube for the flexible fiberoptic esophagogastroduodenoscope. Gastrointest Endosc, 28:256–257, 1982.
54. Campbell JB, Foley LC: A safe alternative to endoscopic removal of blunt esophageal foreign bodies. Arch Otolaryngol, 109:323–325, 1983.
55. Kleinman MS: Management of foreign bodies in the esophagus. JAMA, 236:2054, 1976.
56. Brady PG, Johnson WF: Removal of foreign bodies: The flexible fiberoptic endoscope. South Med J, 70:702–704, 1977.

Index

Note: Numbers in *italics* refer to illustrations; numbers followed by *(t)* refer to tables.